140.00

This book should be returned by the last date stamped
above. You may renew the loan for a further period
if the book is not required by another reader.

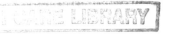

Early Breast Cancer
From screening to multidisciplinary management

Edited by

Guidubaldo Querci della Rovere MD(Padua) FRCS(Eng) FRCS(Ed) Comm OMRI
The Royal Marsden NHS Foundation Trust London/Surrey, United Kingdom

Ruth Warren MD FRCP FRCR
Cambridge Breast Unit, Addenbrooke's Hospital, Cambridge, United Kingdom

John R Benson MA(Oxon) DM FRCS(Eng) FRCS(Ed)
Cambridge Breast Unit, Addenbrooke's Hospital, Cambridge
and Hinchingbrooke Hospital, Huntingdon, United Kingdom

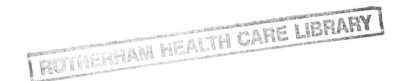

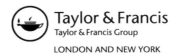
Taylor & Francis
Taylor & Francis Group
LONDON AND NEW YORK

© 2006 Taylor & Francis, an imprint of the Taylor & Francis Group

First published in the United Kingdom in 2006 by Taylor & Francis, an imprint of the
Taylor & Francis Group, 2 Park Square, Milton Park, Abingdon, Oxon OX14 4RN

Tel.:   +44 (0)20 7017 6000
Fax.:   +44 (0)20 7017 6699
E-mail: info.medicine@tandf.co.uk
Website: www.tandf.co.uk/medicine

Although every effort has been made to ensure that all owners of copyright material
have been acknowledged in this publication, we would be glad to acknowledge in
subsequent reprints or editions any omissions brought to our attention.

The Author has asserted his right under the Copyright, Designs and Patents Act 1988 to
be identified as the Author of this Work.

Although every effort has been made to ensure that drug doses and other information are
presented accurately in this publication, the ultimate responsibility rests with the
prescribing physician. Neither the publishers nor the authors can be held responsible for
errors or for any consequences arising from the use of information contained herein. For
detailed prescribing information or instructions on the use of any product or procedure
discussed herein, please consult the prescribing information or instructional material
issued by the manufacturer.

A CIP record for this book is available from the British Library.

Library of Congress Cataloging-in-Publication Data

Data available on application

ISBN 1 84184 384 9
ISBN 978-1-84184-384-1

Distributed in North and South America by

Taylor & Francis
2000 NW Corporate Blvd
Boca Raton, FL 33431, USA

Within Continental USA
Tel: 800 272 7737; Fax: 800 374 3401
Outside Continental USA
Tel: 561 994 0555; Fax: 561 361 6018
E-mail: orders@crcpress.com

Distributed in the rest of the world by
Thomson Publishing Services
Cheriton House
North Way
Andover, Hampshire SP10 5BE, UK
Tel.: +44 (0)1264 332424
E-mail: salesorder.tandf@thomsonpublishingservices.co.uk

Composition by Scribe Design, Ashford, Kent, UK
Printed and bound in Great Britain by CPI Bath

Contents

Multidisciplinary management of breast cancer

Consent and litigation

Contributors

Jean Abraham
University of Cambridge and Addenbrooke's
Hospital, Cambridge, UK

Kusum Agarwal
Formerly at St Margaret's Hospital, Epping
and Princess Alexandra Hospital, Harlow
Essex, UK

Salam Z. Al-Sam
Broomfield Hospital
Chelmsford, Essex
UK

Daniela Ambrogietti
Centre for the Study and Prevention of Cancer
Florence, Italy

Lia Bartella
St Bartholomew's Hospital
London, UK

Bristi Basu
University of Cambridge and Addenbrooke's
Hospital, Cambridge, UK

Michael Baum
University College London
and The Portland Hospital
London, UK

John Benson
Addenbrooke's Hospital, Cambridge
and Hinchingbrooke Hospital, Huntingdon
UK

Simonetta Bianchi
University of Florence
Florence, Italy

Lynda Bobrow
University of Cambridge and Addenbrooke's
Hospital, Cambridge, UK

Peter Britton
Cambridge Breast Unit, Addenbrooke's Hospital
Cambridge, UK

Gina Brown
The Royal Marsden NHS Foundation Trust
Sutton, UK

Luigi Cataliotti
University of Florence
Florence, Italy

Angelo Cerofolini
City Hospital,
Schio, Vicenza, Italy

Jenny Chang
Baylor College of Medicine Breast Center
Houston, Texas, United States of America

Catherine Chinyama
Princess Elizabeth Hospital
Guernsey, UK

Stefano Ciatto
Centro per la prevenzioine Oncologica
Firenze, Italy

Mario Ciocca
European Institute of Oncology
Milan, Italy

Charlotte Coles
Addenbrooke's Hospital,
Cambridge, UK

Jean Darymple
Formerly at St Margaret's Hospital, Epping
and Princess Alexandra Hospital, Harlow
Essex, UK

Nicholas Day
Strangeways Research Laboratory
University of Cambridge
Cambridge, UK

Erika Denton
Norfolk and Norwich University Hospital
Norwich, UK

Vito Distante
University of Florence
Florence, Italy

Helena Earl
University of Cambridge and Addenbrooke's
Hospital, Cambridge, UK

Ian Ellis
City Hospital NHS Trust,
Nottingham, UK

Gareth Evans
St Mary's and Christie Hospitals
Manchester, UK

Gianantonio Farello
City Hospital,
Schio, Vicenza, Italy

Charlotte Fowler
Department of Radiotherapy
Addenbrooke's Hospital
Cambridge, UK

Giovanna Gatti
European Institute of Oncology
Milan, Italy

Massimiliano Gennaro
Istituto Nazionale tumori
Milano, Italy

Rosalind Given-Wilson
St George's Hospital
London, UK

Marco Greco
Istituto Nazionale Tumori
Milan, Italy

Delilah Hassanally
The Royal Marsden NHS Foundation Trust
Sutton, UK

Mattia Intra
European Institute of Oncology
Milan, Italy

Samar N Jader
St Margaret's Hospital, Epping
and Princess Alexandra Hospital, Harlow
Essex, UK

Ismail Jatoi
National Naval Medical Center and Uniformed
Services University of the Health Sciences,
Bethesda, Maryland, United States of America

Chris Jones
The Breakthrough Toby Robins Breast Cancer
Research Centre
The Royal Marsden NHS Foundation Trust
London, UK

Caroline M Kissin
Jarvis Breast Screening Centre
Guildford, Surrey, UK

Mark Kissin
Royal Surrey County Hospital and Jarvis Breast
Screening Centre,
Guildford, Surrey, UK

Sunil Lakhani
The University of Queensland
Herston, Australia

Gillian Lawrence
West Midlands Cancer Intelligence Unit
University of Birmingham, UK

Simon Levene
Chambers,
199 Strand,
London, UK

Alberto Luini
European Institute of Oncology
Milan, Italy

Tarik Massoud
Department of Radiology
University of Cambridge
Cambridge, UK

Jolanta McKenzie
St Margaret's Hospital, Epping
and Princess Alexandra Hospital, Harlow
Essex, UK

Michael Michell
King's College Hospital,
London, UK

Michael Morgan
Formerly at St Margaret's Hospital, Epping
and Princess Alexandra Hospital, Harlow
Essex, UK

Iain Morrison
St Bartholomew's Hospital
London, UK

Eleanor Moskovic
The Royal Marsden NHS Foundation Trust,
London, UK

Susan Moss
Cancer Screening Evaluation Unit, ICR
Sutton, Surrey, UK

Susan O'Mahony
Department of Surgery
Addenbrooke's Hospital
Cambridge, UK

Roberto Orecchia
European Institute of Oncology
Milan, Italy

Lorenzo Orzalesi
University of Florence
Florence, Italy

Michael Osborne
Weill Medical College of Cornell University
New York Presbyterian Hospital
New York, United States of America

Cheryl Palmer
University of Cambridge and Addenbrooke's
Hospital, Cambridge, UK

Ashraf Patel
St Margaret's Hospital
Epping, Essex, UK

Julietta Patnick
NHS Cancer Screening Programmes
Sheffield, UK

Nicholas Perry
St Bartholomew's Hospital,
London, UK

Sarah Pinder
University of Cambridge and Addenbrooke's
Hospital, Cambridge, UK

Linda Pointon
The Royal Marsden NHS Foundation Trust
London, UK

Trevor J Powles
Parkside Oncology Clinic
London, UK

Anand Purushotham
Cambridge Breast Unit
Addenbrooke's Hospital
Cambridge, UK

Guidubaldo Querci della Rovere
The Royal Marsden NHS Foundation Trust
Sutton, UK

Nicola Roche
Royal Marsden NHS Foundation Trust
Sutton, UK

Assem Rostom
The Royal Marsden NHS Foundation Trust
Sutton, UK

Simon Russell
Department of Radiotherapy
Addenbrooke's Hospital
Cambridge, UK

Melvin Silverstein
Keck School of Medicine
University of Southern California,
Los Angeles, California

Rache Simmons
Weill Medical College of Cornell University
New York Presbyterian Hospital
New York, United States of America

Kristin Skinner
Keck School of Medicine
University of Southern California
Los Angeles, California

Judith Spencer-Knott
Formerly at St Margaret's Hospital, Epping
Essex, UK

Will Teh
Department of Radiology
Northwick Park Hospital
Harrow, Middlesex, UK

Hazel Thornton
University of Leicester
Leicester, UK

Peter Trott
The London Clinic
London, UK

Umberto Veronesi
European Institute of Oncology
Milan, Italy

Vincent Wallace
Teraview Ltd
Cambridge, UK

Ruth Warren
Cambridge Breast Unit
Addenbrooke's Hospital
Cambridge, UK

Clive Wells
St Bartholomew's Hospital
London, UK

Robin Wilson
Breast Screening Unit
City Hospital NHS Trust
Nottingham, UK

Carol Woo
Keck School of Medicine
University of Southern California
Los Angeles, California

Foreword

Medicine is in the midst of a revolution which will greatly modify our attitudes towards the patients of tomorrow. The three major areas of new development are: (i) the biomolecular approach; (ii) the achievements of imaging technology; and (iii) stem cell research. The first and second will have a substantial influence on oncology in general and on breast cancer in particular. Breast cancer, the most common cancer in women worldwide, is in fact undergoing a considerable upheaval in terms of its biological concepts, such as the predictive value of gene profiling and the cancer stem cell hypothesis and, even more importantly, the revolution in imaging, which has totally changed the possibilities for the detection of early breast lesions.

On the other hand we also have to consider that the greatest change in breast cancer treatment can be summarized in the transition from the 'maximum tolerable treatment' paradigm of the 1960s to the 'minimal effective treatment' paradigm of today. In other words the old concept that treatment should be as aggressive as possible (extended mastectomies, very extensive radiotherapy fields, hypophysectomy, adrenalectomy and high dose chemotherapy) was the result of our limited knowledge on the biology of breast cancer.

When, 30 years ago, we showed that a small resection of the breast had long term results equal to those of mastectomy, we ushered in a new era, not only in terms of new techniques but also in terms of conceptual breakthroughs which led to new ideas, such as sentinel node biopsy and partial breast irradiation.

This evolution has been made possible by two important factors. The first being the consciousness-raising of women towards early detection programmes: the idea that the discovery of an early tumour leads to a minimal change in their breast has played an important role in motivating women towards detection. The second is the availability of diagnostic tools, which are able to identify very tiny carcinomas. These changes are reflected in the fact that, while in the 1970s the majority of breast cancers were classified as T2, today the majority lie in the category T1. Even more important is the fact that 15–30% of the cases are non-palpable. These cases, which can only be discovered by imaging, now enjoy a curability rate greater than 95%. The same applies to in situ tumours, a type of lesion which was occasionally seen in the 1970s, and today represents a considerable portion of the tumours of the breast, with a curability close to 100%.

The trend is therefore towards smaller and smaller proliferative lesions, borderline with precancerous lesions so that the problem that we will have to face in the next two decades will not be one of 'breast cancer' but of 'early breast cancer', which is exactly the title of this book. This volume, whose contributors are all competent experts in the field, is devoted to the innumerable problems of early breast carcinomas, problems which are much more complex compared to the ones of more advanced cases. In the 1970s all cases were unhesitatingly treated with mastectomy followed by radiotherapy, whereas today an early case can undergo a wide range of treatment options.

The main problem which remains, however, is this: how can we detect this disease in asymptomatic women, which is so frequent and so highly curable at the early stages? For this reason large sections of the book are devoted to breast cancer screening, breast imaging and the histological diagnosis of very small lesions.

We must congratulate the editors for focussing their attention on breast cancer 'at its debut'. We are all convinced that if great strides are to be made in mortality reduction for this disease, they will be linked to the progress we make in its very early discovery.

Umberto Veronesi

Acknowledgements

The Editors are very grateful to the following individuals for their assistance in preparing this book:

Ms Yvonne Glendenning, Hinchingbrooke Hospital, Huntingdon

June New, The Royal Marsden Hospital, Sutton, UK

Preface

Despite a modest decrease in mortality rates over the past two decades, the incidence of breast cancer continues to rise inexorably in Western society where it remains the commonest malignancy amongst women with a lifetime risk of approximately 10%. Almost half a million women die of the disease annually worldwide with 15,000 and 45,000 deaths per annum in the United Kingdom and United States, respectively. Though breast cancer is predominantly a disease of post-menopausal women, almost one-third of cases occur in women under 50 years of age and it represents a major cause of death in the age group 40-50 years. Breast cancer diagnosis has an emotional dimension which is manifest disproportionately in younger women for whom the psychosocial impact of the disease can reverberate collectively amongst family members, friends and colleagues. Many of these patients are not only a wife and mother, but nowadays often have demanding careers and may be the primary breadwinner for the family.

The fall in mortality from breast cancer in the face of rising incidence rates is testimony to the success of interventional strategies in the form of screening and adjuvant systemic therapies, which reduce the burden of micrometastatic foci and perturb the natural history of this enigmatic disease. Though the radical mastectomy has been abandoned in favour of less invasive surgical procedures (skin-sparing modified radical mastectomy and breast conservation), the Halstedian paradigm is now acknowledged as pertinent to the behaviour of some breast cancers. There is an emerging 'spectrum' paradigm which incorporates elements of Halsted's centrifugal theory of cancer spread and Fisher's hypothesis of biological predeterminism. Modern methods of molecular profiling may permit tumours to be assigned to a particular group with appropriate intensities of loco-regional and systemic treatments. An increasing proportion of patients are presenting with node negative disease and in situ forms of cancer. This 'stage migration' is due to better public awareness of the disease combined with screening programmes. The technique of sentinel node biopsy has found relevance in this era of earlier stage disease but there are persistent and unresolved issues relating to standardization of methodology and the significance of micrometastatic deposits in sentinel nodes. More intense scrutiny of nodal tissue with immunohisto-chemistry/PCR potentially upstages 20-30% of patients with risk of overtreatment. Conversely, the consequences in terms of local relapse and overall survival from failure to remove non-sentinel nodes remain unknown. Ironically, in recent years there has been a trend towards lesser forms of surgical extirpation, but more aggressive adjuvant therapies (radiotherapy/chemotherapy). The sophisticated methods of genetic profiling with DNA microarrays and their integration with proteomics may ultimately allow treatments to be better tailored. However, these newer technologies must be rigorously validated against conventional indices and independent data sets prior to any meaningful conclusions and assimilation into routine clinical practice.

Translational research from laboratory to clinic is a slow and unpredictable process which somewhat infrequently yields advances in treatment of proven and sustained clinical utility. The tremendous progress in cellular biology at the molecular level is likely to accelerate translational work through improved understanding of carcinogenesis and therapeutic approaches based on sound biological rationale and robust pre-clinical models. Furthermore, a small number of well-designed clinical trials, which are adequately powered, may in the future provide definitive answers to key clinical questions with less reliance on meta-analysis of many imperfect and/or flawed trials.

It is essential to ensure that current patients have access to consistently high standards of care which accord with accepted guidelines and consensus statements based on collective expert opinion. Management of breast cancer is centred around the multidisciplinary team (MDT). This multidisciplinary approach facilitates optimum patient management decisions with input from various specialities including surgery, radiology, pathology, radiation/medical oncology, genetics and plastic surgery. This pan-integration of diagnostic and therapeutic modalities is epitomized by breast cancer and has contributed to improvements in treatment outcomes and quality of life for this group of patients.

This book discusses the principles and practice of breast cancer management within the context of multidisciplinary team working and places emphasis on pragmatism. The text provides a comprehensive and contemporary account of the subject and should permit the reader to develop a firm understanding of the disease from epidemiology, genetics and screening, to pathology, diagnosis, treatment and prevention. This in turn will enable healthcare personnel to deliver a high quality and up-to-date service to breast cancer sufferers.

The initial enthusiasm which followed identification and cloning of the breast cancer specific genes, BRCA-1 and BRCA-2, has been tempered by the realization that the phenotypic heterogeneity of breast cancer cannot be attributed to simple changes in one or two autosomally dominant genes, but more likely results from an accumulation of mutations in a larger number of less highly penetrant genes. This hasn't stemmed the tide of public interest and demand for genetic testing whose meaning and relevance are limited and the risk:benefit unclear for many individuals seeking information on familial predisposition to breast cancer. These important issues are discussed alongside surveillance protocols in the first section of the book. The text includes a separate chapter on the biological basis for breast cancer screening and its relevance to current screening strategies both within the NHS screening programme and elsewhere. Chapters 7 and 8, respectively, offer critical appraisal of breast screening in women over and, more controversially, under 50 years of age where transatlantic differences in practice exist. The section on breast imaging includes a chapter on radiology of benign breast lesions and the emerging role of newer techniques such as MRI and PET scanning. There is comprehensive coverage of breast pathology from normal and benign breast lesions, through pre-malignant, in situ and finally invasive carcinoma. The future of breast pathology is considered in Chapter 28 and the role of cytopathology discussed at a time when image-guided core biopsy is the preferred method for obtaining definitive preoperative diagnosis.

In accordance with the general ethos of the book, the therapeutic aspects of breast cancer have been grouped together into a section entitled 'Multidisciplinary management of breast cancer.' This incorporates a chapter dedicated to the multidisciplinary team. Controversial areas such as management of the axilla and intra-operative radiotherapy are included in this section, together with a succinct and authoritative account of systemic adjuvant therapies. The latter is a useful distillation of evidence from many clinical trials/meta-analyses and encompasses newer developments such as aromatase inhibitors, taxanes and targeted therapies with biological response modifiers (e.g. herceptin).

Clinical practice takes place within an increasingly litigious and regulated working environment. Furthermore, there are shifting social and ethical mores coupled with increased patient rights and expectations. The advent of the internet has allowed ease of access to unprecedented volumes of 'literature' on breast cancer with creation of 'webwise' patients who come along to the clinic forearmed with information. It is particularly important that less highly specialized clinicians who work in the field of breast disease maintain a critical and up-to-date knowledge base and can make sensible judgements and appropriate clinical decisions. It is therefore contemporaneous to include some comment on informed consent and litigation, with the former constituting a very important and substantial portion of this final section of the book.

This is an intermediate sized text which should be of value not only to established practitioners but also trainees working in the sub-speciality of breast diseases. It may also be of assistance to some clinical scientists researching at the laboratory-clinical interface and other healthcare professionals involved in the treatment and support of patients with breast cancer.

John Benson
G Querci della Rovere
Ruth Warren

1 An introduction to screening for breast cancer

Linda J Pointon, Nicholas E Day

Introduction

Although mortality from breast cancer has fallen over the last decade, it is still the leading cause of death from cancer among women in the UK. In 2000, over 40 000 cases were diagnosed and there were nearly 13 000 deaths.[1–4] The aetiology of the disease is not fully understood, although the risk is known to be associated with reproductive and family history. Screening for breast cancer has been shown to advance the diagnosis of the disease, which can lead to more successful treatment and therefore reduced mortality. This chapter details the evidence upon which breast screening has been introduced on a national scale, with particular reference to the UK.

The natural history of breast cancer is well documented.[5] The disease is believed to usually have a pre-invasive stage where the carcinoma cells are confined to the duct system within the breast. This may then become invasive and begin to invade the surrounding tissue, and thereafter possibly spread to the lymph nodes or other secondary sites within the body. Breast tumours may disseminate at different stages in their natural history. In some women, and for some types of tumour, this could take years, while in others metastatic spread may take only weeks, depending on the aggressiveness of the cancer. Ideally, screening should detect tumours while they are still small and before any metastases have developed.[6] In order for screening to be effective, the disease must have a recognisable early stage. In the case of breast cancer, this is the preclinical detectable phase where a tumour can be seen on a mammogram but before it becomes palpable (about 1 cm in diameter). Tumours in this phase are more likely to be non-invasive or, if already invasive, less likely to have local regional or distant spread.

For screening to be beneficial, treating breast cancer at this earlier stage must also improve the prognosis compared with more advanced cancers. It is not, however, sufficient to compare the survival of women with screen-detected cancers with the survival of those who present symptomatically without removing the effect of various biases. Figure 1.1 illustrates the stages through which the disease passes as it progresses. Lead-time bias occurs because survival is measured from time of diagnosis. As screening will advance the date of diagnosis, the survival time will automatically be longer even if there is no effect on the actual date of death. Also, less aggressive, slowly growing cancers will spend more time in the preclinical detectable phase than will rapidly growing cancers, which are more likely to present symptomatically. Screening will therefore detect proportionally more of the slow growing, or non-invasive, cancers, which in turn have a better

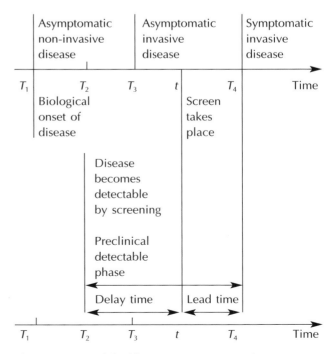

Figure 1.1 Model of breast cancer progression.

prognosis. This is known as length bias. There is also the problem of selection bias in which those who attend for screening are more likely to be health-conscious individuals than those who refuse, and would probably have a better prognosis anyway. These biases can be removed by comparing mortality in a population that was offered screening with that in a population that was not offered screening, in the context of a randomised controlled trial.

The suitability of any screening test depends on its accuracy. It must be able both to detect the majority of women who have breast cancer (high sensitivity) and therefore give few false-negative results, and to eliminate the majority of women who do not have the disease (high specificity), thereby minimising the number of false-positive results. Sensitivity is defined as the proportion of all those with breast cancer present who test positive; specificity is defined as the proportion of all those without the disease who test negative. Ideally, both sensitivity and specificity would be 100%, but there is an inevitable compromise as no test is perfect and the two are inversely related to one another. Different screening modalities will be discussed in more detail later.

For public health, the acceptability of a screening test by the general population is of paramount importance. The acceptability will be reflected by the rate of compliance with invitation to screening. Levels of between 80% and 90% have been seen in Sweden.[7] A level of 70% compliance has been shown to be effective in reducing breast cancer mortality in the target population.[8] Latest figures show that an acceptance rate of 75.3% has been achieved in the UK as a whole,[9] although there are regional differences and specific groups where more work is needed. Women from minority ethnic groups and women with learning disabilities have particular needs. A major research project is now underway to look at the information needs of women from a diverse range of social and cultural backgrounds.[10]

Another important consideration in a screening test is that it should do no harm, either physical or psychological. The potential physical hazards from screening by mammography are the risk from ionising radiation (X-rays) and unnecessary surgical procedures resulting from overdiagnosis of tumours that may never have become invasive in the lifetime of the patient. The radiation risk from mammography has been very much reduced in recent years. Due to technical advances, the maximum dose is now about 2.2 mGy (compared with 2–3 cGy in the past).[11,12] There is no evidence that this level of radiation induces breast cancer, but from the excess breast cancer incidence seen in women exposed to higher doses, it has been inferred that modern mammography may induce one breast cancer in a population of two million women above the age of 50, after a latent period of 10 years. When compared with the expected natural breast cancer incidence of 1400 cases per million women per year at age 50 and 2000 cases per million women per year at age 65, the risk is considered to be insignificant compared with the potential benefits.

High-quality screening techniques and highly trained technical and radiological staff should minimise the risk of overdiagnosis. Ideally, the recall rate should be as low as possible. It is also important that adequate assessment and treatment facilities exist to ensure that women are seen as quickly as possible. In addition, there is a range of non-invasive investigative techniques stopping short of open biopsy that should be employed to reduce the risk of unnecessary surgery. These include ultrasound, spot views, micromagnification, fine needle aspiration and needle core biopsy. These techniques have greatly reduced the benign biopsy rate.

Screening for breast cancer was introduced in the UK following the recommendations of the Forrest Report published in 1986.[12] The NHS Breast Screening Programme (NHSBSP) initially offered single mediolateral oblique-view mammography to women aged 50–64 with an interval of 3 years. Following further research, the programme has been expanded to invite women up to the age of 69 and to offer two-view mammography at all screens.

Screening must be repeated at regular intervals to ensure its effectiveness, as the risk of developing breast cancer increases with age and the growth rate of the disease is variable. There has to be a compromise taking into account the cost and practicality of screening too frequently while aiming to let as few cancers as possible escape detection by screening. In the UK, the interval was initially set to 3 years, which reflected the 33-month interval in the Swedish Two-County Trial, with a recommendation for more research into the screening interval. In the UKCCCR Breast Screening Frequency Trial, 76 000 women were randomised to either 3-yearly or annual screening.[13] The Nottingham Prognostic Index (NPI) was used to compare predicted mortality in the two groups. No significant improvement in predicted mortality was seen in the annual screening group. The screening interval in the NHSBSP therefore remains unchanged at 3 years.

Screening modalities

There are three basic potential mass screening tools: mammography, physical examination by trained staff and breast self-examination (BSE). Mammography has been shown to be effective in reducing breast cancer mortality. The Swedish Two-County Trial[14] used single mediolateral oblique-view mammography alone and achieved a mortality reduction of 32% in women aged 40–74. The sensitivity was 91–100% for women aged over 50 and 83% for women in the 40–49 age group. This may be due to denser breast tissue in younger women, and sensitivity could possibly be improved by using two-view mammography. The main reason for using a single view in this case was the perceived need in the 1970s to minimise radiation dose. As has already been discussed, with modern mammography techniques this risk is now insignificant. A study of one- versus two-view mammography[15] has shown that by adding a second (craniocaudal) view, the sensitivity of screening during the prevalence round of a population screening programme was increased from 83% to 89% and 14 additional cancers were detected out of a total of 217. The recall rate was also reduced by the addition of a second view, from 8.8% to 6.6%. In conclusion, mammography, particularly with two views, is effective, acceptable and sensitive as a primary screening method.

The effectiveness of clinical examination alone has not been tested, although some trials have used it in conjunction with mammography. In Edinburgh between 1979 and 1981, 45 130 women were entered into a randomised controlled trial in which approximately half were invited to screening.[16] At the prevalence round, the study group were offered two-view mammography and clinical examination. Subsequent screens involved clinical examination alone in years 2, 4 and 6, and one-view mammography plus clinical examination in years 3, 5 and 7. Although the compliance at the initial screen was poor (61%), and fell at subsequent screens, there did not appear to be any difference in the acceptance of clinical examination and mammography. An analysis has shown the sensitivity of mammography to be 63% and that of clinical examination to be 40%.[17] The Edinburgh data lack statistical power, however, and there is no conclusive evidence to show that clinical examination is effective in reducing mortality. Similar analyses on the HIP data result in sensitivities of 39% and 47% respectively for mammography and clinical examination.

BSE is very difficult to assess, as the only intervention possible is education, and failure to practise seems to be a major disadvantage to the use of BSE as a sole screening method. The sensitivity of BSE is very difficult to measure, but it is assumed that frequent BSE will enable a woman to detect a cancer earlier than less frequent visits for a professional clinical examination. There is some evidence that BSE may lead to a reduction in tumour size at diagnosis.[12] There is no evidence that BSE contributes to a reduction in mortality, but women should not be discouraged from practising it, as it may contribute to an earlier diagnosis.

Magnetic resonance imaging (MRI) is a relatively new technology that has been shown to have high sensitivity for detecting abnormalities in the breast.[18–23] In general, the population at greatest risk of breast cancer is that of women over the age of 50. In this group, X-ray mammography has been shown to be a relatively cheap, quick and effective modality for breast screening. It is therefore not appropriate to consider MRI as a mass screening tool in the same way. It is more expensive, resources in terms of machines and expertise are scarce at present, and scans and their analyses can be time-consuming. However, MRI may have a particular application in screening younger women (aged less than 50) who are at high risk of developing breast cancer. In these younger, premenopausal women, the breast can be mammographically dense and mammograms are often difficult to interpret. There is a recognised need to screen women at high familial risk of breast cancer, since the disease may develop at an earlier age than in the general population, but there are concerns about repeated radiation exposure. With the advent of genetic testing, groups of women at high risk will be identified, for whom X-ray mammography does not provide a satisfactory method of screening for breast cancer. MRI avoids radiation exposure while providing high sensitivity in detecting breast cancer, even in the mammographically dense breast. Its role in screening is currently under evaluation. Two studies to assess the effectiveness of annual MRI scans compared with annual mammography in the high-genetic-risk group have recently reported from Canada and the Netherlands.[24,25] The sensitivity of MRI versus mammography in the Canadian and Dutch studies are 79% versus 32%, and 79.5% versus 33.3% respectively. A similar MRC-funded study (MARIBS) was recently published in the UK.[26,27]

Another group who are considered at high risk of breast cancer are women who have been previously exposed to supradiaphragmatic radiotherapy for Hodgkin's disease at a young age.[28] MRI is currently recommended for breast screening in this group for young women (aged 25–29) and those aged 30–50 who have dense breasts. No screening is recommended for women aged 25 or under; women aged 30–50 with predominantly fatty breasts should have annual two-view mammography; women over the age of 50 will have 3-yearly mammography as normal in the NHSBSP.

Evidence for mortality reduction from randomised controlled trials

The Health Insurance Plan Study of Greater New York (HIP) was the first trial of breast cancer screening.[8] The population consisted of approximately 62 000 women aged 40–64 who were selected from 23 of the 31 HIP medical centres. From each group, two systematic random samples of women with membership in HIP for at least a year were selected and entered into the programme from December 1963 to June 1966. These two groups then formed the study and control populations. The study group were offered screening by clinical examination and two-view mammography first at entry to the trial and then yearly for the next 3 years. The control group were not invited to screening. The compliance at the first screen was 67%, and 80% of these women attended the first annual repeat examination, 75% the second and 69% the third. Overall, 40% attended all four screens. Ten years after the start of the trial, the breast cancer mortality reduction in the study group was 30%. After 18 years, the reduction was around 25%.

The Swedish Two-County Trial took place in Östergotland and Kopparberg counties.[14] Women aged 40–74 were entered into the programme from 1977 to 1981. The trial population was randomised by population cluster rather than by individual. Later analyses have shown the loss of power to be minimal. In Östergotland, one cluster in each block of two was randomised to invitation to screening, while in Kopparberg, it was two clusters in each block of three. This resulted in a study group of 77 080 and a control group of 55 985. Women aged 40–49 were invited to screening by one-view mammography alone every 24 months, and those in the age range 50–74 were invited every 33 months on average. The control group were not invited to screening in the initial study. In 1985, after four rounds of screening in the younger age range, three in the 50–69 range and two in the 70–74 range, the control group were invited to screening. All breast cancers in both arms of the trial diagnosed between randomisation and the end of the first screen of the controls were included in the final analysis of the trial results. Compliance was good. In women aged under 70, participation was consistent at approximately 90% at all screens. For women aged between 70 and 74, the participation rate was 79% at the first screening round and 67% at the second. Consequently, no further invitations were issued to this age group. The first results of the study, before the controls were invited to screening, were published in 1985 and showed a mortality reduction in the study group of 31%. After 20 years, the main result of the trial remained the same: the mortality reduction in the study group was 32%.

The Malmö mammographic screening trial started in October 1976 to determine whether breast cancer mortality in women over 45 could be reduced by mammographic screening.[29] All women born in 1908–32 were identified from the population registry of Malmö, Sweden. Half the women in each birth-year cohort were randomly selected as the study group and invited to mammographic screening at intervals of 18–24 months. The remaining women were allocated to the control group and were not offered screening. In the first two rounds, two views were taken. In subsequent rounds, either both views or just the oblique view were taken, depending on the density of the breasts. The attendance rate was higher in the first round (74%) than in subsequent rounds (70%) and higher among younger than among older women. The predetermined end of the trial was 31 December 1986, and by this stage no significant reduction in mortality was seen in the study group. In fact, during the first 7 calendar years of the screening programme, the cumulative number of deaths from breast cancer was higher in the study group than in the controls, although by the end of the trial this situation had been reversed. The Malmö study suffered from loss of power due in part to the attendance rate but also to dilution of the control group. A random sample of 500 of the control group showed that 24% had undergone mammography during the study period.

The randomised controlled trial in Edinburgh, Scotland has been described previously.[30] Like the Two-County Trial, population clusters (general practices) rather than individuals were randomised. Initially, there was evidence that the cluster randomisation did not achieve comparability between the two groups in, for example, cardiovascular mortality, although when this was adjusted for socio-economic status using logistic regression, these differences disappeared. After 14 years, there was a significant mortality reduction of 29% in those invited to screening (relative risk (RR) 0.71, 95% confidence interval (CI) 0.53–0.95).

In Stockholm, Sweden, a randomised controlled trial was begun in March 1981 to compare single-view mammography with no intervention in women aged 40–64.[31] Selection was individually by birth date, and 40 000 women were randomised to the study population and 20 000 to the controls. The study group were invited twice to attend for mammography, with a screening interval of about 30 months. The compliance was over 80% in the first and second screening rounds, with little difference between the age groups. After the second round was completed in 1985, the control group were invited for one screen by mammography, where the compliance was approximately 77%. After 11 years of follow-up, there was a non-significant mortality reduction of 26% (RR 0.74, 95% CI 0.5–1.1). However, in the 50–64 age group, a significant 38% mortality reduction was observed (95% CI 0.38–1.0). In the 40–49 age group, no effect on mortality was seen (RR 1.08, 95% CI 0.54–2.17).

The Canadian National Breast Screening Study (NBSS) was planned in the late 1970s and started screening women in January 1980. The study was in two parts: women aged 40–49[32] and women aged 50–59[33] followed different screening regimes. In the younger age group, 50 430 women with no history of breast cancer who had not undergone mammography in the previous 12 months were invited to an initial physical examination. At this initial visit, half were then randomly assigned to the MP (study) group, who would be offered annual mammography and physical examination, and the other half to the UC (control) group, who would be returned to usual community care with annual follow-up by mailed questionnaire. The first 62% of the study women were eligible for a 4-year programme; the remainder were offered a 3-year programme. All women were taught BSE. The mean follow-up time was 8.5 years. Over 90% of the women in each group attended the screening sessions or returned the annual questionnaires or both over years 2–5. The ratio of the proportions of death from breast cancer in the MP group compared with the UC group was 1.36 (95% CI 0.84–2.21), which was not significant. The study concluded that screening with mammography and physical examination had no impact on the rate of death from breast cancer after 7 years.

The entry criteria and randomisation techniques were the same in the older age group. In this part of the study, 39 405 women attended the initial physical examination and were randomly assigned to undergo either annual mammography and physical examination (MP group) or annual physical examination only (PO group). The first 62% of the women who entered the study were offered five annual screens and the remainder were offered four. Again, all women were taught BSE at the initial examination. These women were followed up for an average of 8.3 years. Over 85% of the women in each group attended the screening sessions after the initial screen. The survival rates were similar in the two groups. Women whose cancer had been detected by mammography alone had the highest survival rate. The ratio of the proportions of death from breast cancer in the MP group compared with the PO group was 0.97 (95% CI 0.62–1.52). which again was not significant. The conclusions were similar to those in the younger age group. Unfortunately, conclusions from the Canadian study must be tentative because the quality of the mammography, as assessed by independent review, was unacceptably poor.[34] There were also concerns about the randomisation in this trial, although these have been discounted after an investigation.[35]

Recruitment of women aged 40–59 in the screening trial in Gothenburg, Sweden, started in December 1982. Approximately 21 000 women were randomly allocated to the study group and 29 000 to the controls. The randomisation was largely by individual in the age range 40–49 and by cluster from 50–59, according to day of birth. The study group were invited to two-view mammography at intervals of 18 months. The control group was not invited to screening. The compliance at the first round was 84% and the mortality reduction was found to be 14%, although this result was not significant. The controls were invited to screening from November 1987 onwards.[36] Results have been published for the younger age group (40–49 years) only, and show a 45% reduction in mortality in this group (RR 0.55, 95% CI 0.31–0.96).[37]

Table 1.1 Randomised controlled trials of breast cancer screening with mammography

Study	Year started	Age group	Approximate no. of subjects (total)	Mortality reduction (%)[a]
HIP, New York[8]	1963	40–64	62 000	25 (not stated)
Two-County Trial, Sweden[14]	1977	40–74	133 000	30 (15 to 42)
Malmö, Sweden[29]	1976	45–69	42 000	4 (–35 to 32)
Edinburgh, Scotland[30]	1979	45–64	45 000	17 (–18 to 42)
Stockholm, Sweden[31]	1981	40–64	60 000	29 (–20 to 60)
NBSS(1), Canada[32]	1980	40–49	50 000	–36 (–121 to 16)
NBSS(2), Canada[33]	1980	50–59	39 000	3 (–52 to 38)
Gothenburg, Sweden[36]	1982	40–59	50 000	14 (–37 to 46)

[a]95% confidence interval in parentheses.

The results of all these randomised controlled trials are summarised in Table 1.1.

Age effects

The most important risk factor for breast cancer is age. In addition to screening those most likely to develop breast cancer, one should also consider whose prognosis will be improved by early detection. The Swedish Two-County Trial is the only randomised trial to have analysed the mortality benefit in the older age group (aged 65–74). This analysis shows a mortality reduction of 32% (RR 0.68, 95% CI 0.51–0.89).[38] These findings are supported by other studies showing that the sensitivity of mammography is high in this age group.[39–41] The UK NHSBSP has now been extended to routinely invite women up to the age of 69.

No trial has yet been published, except for the controversial Canadian NBSS study, which was specifically designed to look at the issue of screening women in the younger age range, i.e. the 40–49 age group. Although the results showed no benefit from screening, the trial has been criticised with regard to technical screening quality, staff training and statistical power. In general, concerns over widespread population screening of women in this age range relate to the efficacy, increased radiation exposure and the likelihood of false positives leading to psychological distress.[42]

Some of the trials already described have included women in this age range, and subgroup analyses have generally shown that with high-quality mammography and a 12- to 18-month screening interval, there may be some benefit to screening younger women. The HIP study shows an overall mortality reduction across all ages, but questions the utility of screening the under-50s at randomisation, as most of the benefit in this group was seen in cancers actually diagnosed after the age of 50.[8] An overview of the Swedish trials demonstrated a 23% mortality reduction in women aged 40–49 at randomisation, with a median follow-up time of 12.8 years and a screening interval of 18–24 months.[43] The Gothenburg trial found a 45% mortality benefit in this age group for the screened population compared with the controls, where two-view mammography was used and an 18-month screening interval was strictly adhered to.[37] Evidence from the Swedish Two-County Trial shows that the mortality benefit is smaller and occurs later than in the over-50 age group.[14] There is a study from Japan that has not yet published mortality data, but does demonstrate satisfactory sensitivity in younger women.[44] However, results from the Nijmegen Screening Programme show poor sensitivity in the under-50 age group.[41] While this low sensitivity may be due to increased breast density, it may also be due to rapid tumour growth in young women[45] – hence the necessity for a shorter screening interval. Studies of radiation risk have concluded that the risk of inducing breast cancers from doses used in mammography is extremely small and is greatly outweighed by the reported mortality benefit.[46,47]

The issue of screening younger women is currently being investigated in the UK based Age Trial.[48]

How does screening work?

As neither the causal pathways for breast cancer nor the means of preventing it are known, the only intervention possible at the moment in healthy women to improve mortality from breast cancer is screening. Trials of chemopreventive agents have produced conflicting results. While the American NSABP study has demonstrated a 50% reduction in breast cancer incidence in women taking tamoxifen compared with placebo, these results have not been reproduced in the UK or in Italy.[49] Further follow-up is required to assess the effect on long-term incidence and mortality.

Although treatment, notably chemotherapy and hormonal therapy, has improved, prognosis still deteriorates rapidly with increasing tumour burden. Screening can advance the diagnosis so that the cancer is treated at an earlier stage with more chance of success. This is reflected in the earlier stage of tumours detected in the study group in the Swedish Two-County Trial.[7] The progression of the disease is shown in Figure 1.1.[50] The lead time is the interval between the time when a prevalent case is detected by screening and the time when that case would otherwise have become clinically incident. The longer the lead time for a given case, the better one would expect the prognosis to be. If the cancer is not detected until it becomes clinically detectable, the lead time is zero. The lead time for an individual case is unobservable, but the distribution of lead times is dependent on the distribution of the time spent in the pre-clinical detectable phase (sojourn time). The sojourn time is also unobservable, but may be estimated using the method of Walter and Day. This method will also provide an estimate of the sensitivity of the screen, and this may be used to estimate the optimum screening regime and the potential gains in terms of mortality. For example, if the sojourn time is long, the maximum possible lead time is correspondingly long. If the sojourn time is short, however, the potential benefit from screening is smaller and screening must take place

Table 1.2 **Breast cancer deaths/cases by age group and detection mode and relative risk by detection mode in the Swedish Two-County Trial**

| Detection mode | Breast cancer deaths/cases in age group | | | | | Relative risk |
	40–49	50–59	60–69	70–74	Total	
PSP[a]	32/160	73/315	90/419	40/146	234/1040	1.00
Before screening[b]	1/6	3/5	3/12	1/4	8/27	Not known
First screen	5/39	13/102	20/184	10/101	48/436	0.57
Later screens	9/110	12/156	15/183	6/52	42/501	0.69
Interval 0–11 months	7/32	3/19	2/23	0/2	12/76	0.80
Interval 12–23 months	10/43	7/35	7/36	2/11	26/125	—
Interval 24+ months	6/12	10/32	8/34	2/9	26/87	—
Interval (time not known)	0/4	0/4	0/2	0/0	0/10	—
Refuser	4/10	15/28	20/49	23/50	62/137	1.46
After screening[c]	0/0	0/0	0/0	8/30	8/30	Not known
Total ASP[d]	42/256	3/381	75/523	52/259	232/1419	0.70

[a]Passive study population, i.e. not invited to screening.
[b]Between randomisation and commencement of screening.
[c]In women aged 70–74 after routine screening ceased in this group.
[d]Active study population, i.e. invited to screening.

more frequently to increase the probability that the preclinical disease is detected before it becomes clinically apparent.

Detection status

In a screening trial, breast cancers can be detected in seven different ways: symptomatically in the control group; after randomisation but before screening, at the first (prevalence) screen, at later (incidence) screens, in the intervals between screening, in women who refused screening, or after the trial has finished in the study or the control group. In a routine screening programme, rather than a randomised trial, there are three possible modes of detection: at screening, in the interval between screens, and in refusers. In the Swedish Two-County Trial, a cancer was classified as being in a refuser if it was diagnosed after the woman did not attend a screen to which she was invited but before the invitation to the next. Interval cancers are those that appear symptomatically between screens, after a negative screen. Table 1.2 shows the number of deaths from breast cancer by age and detection mode and also the relative risk of mortality by detection mode in the Swedish Two-County Trial. The cancer detection rate at the first two screens is shown in Table 1.3 by age. The detection rates are also expressed as multiples of the incidence rate in the control group. Detection rates increase steadily with

Table 1.3 **Cancer detection rate in the Swedish Two-County Trial**

Screen	Cancer detection rate/ 1000 women screened	Cancers/ open biopsy
Prevalence	6.1	0.50
First incidence	3.4	0.75

age. Although the detection rate at the prevalence screen was higher, Table 1.2 shows that the relative risk of mortality is lower than for subsequent screens. This is likely to be due to length bias. Many slowly growing cancers, which may have been present for years, will be detected at the first screen and these will have a far better prognosis than the more aggressive rapidly growing tumours. Thus, length bias can be largely eliminated by defining the so-called 'unbiased set' of all tumours diagnosed up to and including the last screen but excluding those diagnosed at the first. The improvement in the cancer-to-biopsy ratio is partly due to increasing expertise as the trial progresses and partly because, at the first screen, more minimally invasive and non-invasive lesions will be picked up.

In younger women, there is a predominance of deaths from interval cancers, whereas in older

Table 1.4 **Control incidence of breast cancer by age at randomisation, with screening prevalence and interval incidence as a percentage of control incidence, by age and by screening round in the Swedish Two-County Trial**

Age group	Control incidence[a]	Interval incidence in year[b]			Screening prevalence[c]
		1	2	≥3	
First interval					*First round*
40–49	1.05	46	53		2.09
50–59	1.87	10	28	52	4.67
60–69	2.50	17	27	57	8.80
70–74	2.99	8	44	48	12.15
Second interval					*Second round*
40–49	As above	66	41		2.65
50–59		19	35	62	3.03
60–69		9	31	43	4.89
70–74					7.50
Third interval					*Third round*
40–49	As above	22	109		2.16
50–59		23	40	85	3.74
60–69		24	22	26	5.07
70–74					
Overall					*Overall*
40–49	As above	45	62		2.30
50–59		17	34	63	3.84
60–69		17	27	46	6.41
70–74		8	44	48	10.13

[a]Incidence per 1000 woman-years.
[b]As a percentage of control incidence; for ages 40–49 only given years 1 and 2+.
[c]Prevalence per 1000 women.

women, there are more deaths in the refuser category. This is due to the fact that interval cancers are more common in younger women and that older women are more likely to be refusers, rather than being due to age variation in case fatalities. A good means for expressing interval cancer rates is to express them as a proportion of the underlying incidence that would be expected in the absence of screening (in a trial, this is given by the control group incidence). The Swedish Two-County Trial proportionate incidence rates for interval cancers are shown in Table 1.4. For women aged over 50, these results have been used to set targets in the UK national programme. The rates for younger women (under 50) are notably higher than for women aged over 50.

Both the lower cancer detection rates and the higher interval cancer rates underline the difficulty of effec-

tive screening for women aged under 50. They provide an explanation of the smaller mortality reduction that is generally seen.

Tumour characteristics

There has been debate in the past as to whether breast cancer is systemic from the outset and size is merely a marker of the age of the tumour or whether it is a progressive disease. It is clear that breast tumours grow and that the lymph nodes become positive with time. What is not clear is whether other features of the tumour, such as grade, DNA ploidy and Anderson type, also change with time. While it is not expected that individual tumour cells change their nature, there do exist tumours that are heterogeneous. It is therefore reasonable to ask if, as time goes on, the more malignant component multiplies faster than the less. There is some evidence to show that the disease is indeed systemic from its inception.[51,52] Fisher,[53] in a study of ipsilateral breast tumour recurrence (IBTR), found that although the frequency of IBTR was reduced when patients treated by lumpectomy also received breast irradiation, the distant disease-free survival was no different from that of those who received lumpectomy alone. The size of the original tumour was an important predictor of distant disease-free survival, but when adjusted for IBTR, this relationship disappeared. Fisher concluded that IBTR and axillary lymph node invasion are merely markers for the risk of developing distant metastases rather than a clinically significant cause of distant disease. He regarded breast cancer as a systemic disease involving a complex spectrum of host–tumour relationships.[53]

There is evidence of progressive disease from the Swedish Two-County Trial[14] and the New York HIP Screening Trial.[8] Both trials show deficits of deaths and advanced stage (by size and lymph node status) in the group invited to screening – a phenomenon that could not be observed if breast cancer were not a progressive disease, which could be influenced by early detection. If we consider the other, more controversial progression hypothesis, namely that of changing grade, and define two populations of tumours – one 'young' (screened) and one 'old' (unscreened) – there is always an excess of grade 3 tumours in the latter group. It may be argued, however, that this is due to length bias. Removal of the prevalence screen largely eliminates the length bias. After doing so in the Swedish Two-County Trial, there was still an excess of grade 3 tumours in the unscreened group, suggesting that this 'phenotypic drift' does indeed occur.

The three prognostic factors of a breast tumour that are most commonly considered are its size, nodal status and an underlying measure of malignant potential such as histological grade. The nodal status is an indication of how far a tumour has spread. If the lymph nodes are negative then the tumour is more likely to be still localised to the breast. If it has spread to the lymph nodes then prognosis will be worse; if distant metastases are present then the prognosis is very poor. Grade is a measure of the aggressiveness of a tumour. Grade 1 tumours have the best prognosis, as they tend to be slow growing (well differentiated), whereas grade 3 tumours are notably more aggressive (poorly differentiated). However, grade is assigned by an individual pathologist and it can be subjective. In the Swedish Two-County Trial, grade was assessed independently by one pathologist in each county and the grade distributions were different. This is

Table 1.5 Estimates of relative hazard based on proportional hazards regression, with each factor adjusted for the others, and for age and county, in the Swedish Two-County Trial

Factors/category	Hazard ratio[a]	
Size (mm)		
1–9	1.00	
10–14	1.57	(0.94–2.63)
15–19	1.84	(1.11–3.07)
20–29	3.23	(1.99–5.23)
30–49	5.35	(3.28–8.74)
≥50	9.97	(6.04–16.4)
Lymph node status		
Negative	1.00	
Positive or distant metastases	3.20	(2.6–3.9)
Histological type		
Others[b]	1.00	
Ductal grade 1	0.75	(0.45–1.27)
Ductal grade 2	1.24	(0.85–1.80)
Ductal grade 3	2.06	(1.44–2.93)
Ductal grade unspecified	1.56	(0.83–2.92)
Lobular	1.19	(0.76–1.86)
Medullary	0.94	(0.50–1.78)
Missing size, lymph node status or type	3.84	(3.21–4.58)

[a]95% confidence interval in parentheses.
[b]Others include ductal carcinoma in situ, mucinous carcinoma, tubular carcinoma and other carcinomas.

more likely to be a reflection of the differences between the two pathologists rather than differences in the tumour populations. However, the effect of grade on prognosis was much the same, suggesting that the pathologists were measuring the same phenomenon but scoring it differently. The prognostic importance of these three factors, when considered together, is given in Table 1.5.[54]

In the same study, detection status was found to be significantly correlated with each of the tumour attributes of size, nodal status and grade. Screen-detected cancers are more likely to be small and have favourable nodal status and grade, all of which indicate a good prognosis. Tumours in the group of refusers are larger, of worse grades and are more likely to have positive nodes or distant metastases. There is no apparent reason to expect cancers in the refusers to have a poorer grade than those detected

Factors/category	Group		Overall
	ASP	**PSP**	
Grade			
1	21.3	16.8	19.3
2	38.7	34.7	36.9
3	40.0	48.5	43.8
No. of cases	600	493	1093
Nodal status			
Negative	68.2	54.5	62.0
Positive	27.6	39.8	33.2
Distant metastases	4.2	5.7	4.8
No. of cases	670	558	1228
Tumour size (mm)			
1–9	18.0	7.1	13.0
10–14	22.4	15.4	19.3
15–19	20.5	19.7	20.0
20–29	23.2	29.0	25.9
30–49	10.5	20.0	14.9
≥50	5.4	8.8	7.0
No. of cases	704	590	1294

Table 1.6 **Percentage distribution of grade, nodal status and size of invasive tumours diagnosed in women aged 40–69 in the active study population (ASP, i.e. invited to screening) and the passive study population (PSP, i.e. not invited to screening) after the prevalence screen in the Swedish Two-County Trial**

at screening unless the grade is not static for each tumour but deteriorates as the tumour grows. This could be explained if tumours have a mixture of poorly and well-differentiated cells; the poorly differentiated cells would be expected to multiply more quickly. In order to test this hypothesis, an unbiased set was required so that a comparison could be made of two groups of tumours whose only major difference was that one was detected at an earlier stage. In the study and control groups, non-invasive (in situ) cancers were excluded, and also those occurring in women aged 70–74 at entry to the trial as they were invited to only two screening rounds. Cancers that occurred before or at the prevalence round were omitted in order to avoid length bias in the study group. The tumour characteristics of the two groups were then compared: these are shown in Table 1.6. The distributions of grade were indeed different in the two groups, indicating that grade does deteriorate as a tumour grows. When grade was controlled for size, however, there was no significant difference between the two groups. One could thus consider the effect of early detection on size to secondarily influence.

Overall, it was found that size, grade and nodal status are significantly and independently related to each other and to detection mode. All three prognostic factors are more favourable in tumours that are detected earlier, but although screen-detected tumours tend to have a lower grade, there are still considerable numbers of high-grade lesions (grade 3). Figures 1.2–1.5 show the survival probabilities plotted against time by nodal status, tumour size, grade and detection status.[6] It is clear that all of these factors have a considerable effect on survival.

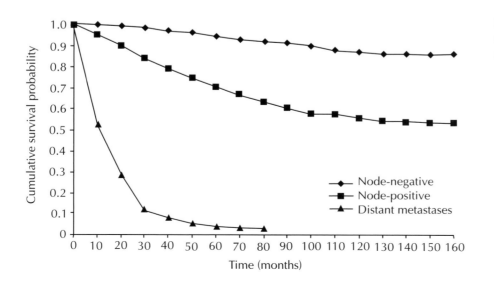

Figure 1.2 Cumulative survival probability by nodal status.

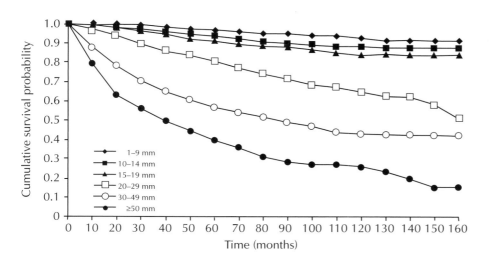

Figure 1.3 Cumulative survival probability by size.

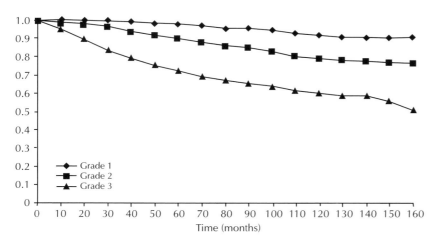

Figure 1.4 Cumulative survival probability by grade.

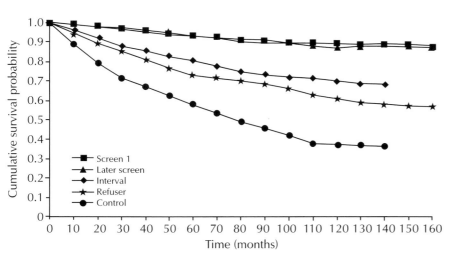

Figure 1.5 Cumulative survival probability by detection status.

Targets and monitoring

In the UK, the NHSBSP is based on the recommendations of the Forrest report.[12] In 1993, the Health of the Nation target was set at 25% reduction in breast cancer mortality, in women of screening age, by the year 2000. Recent data show that mortality from breast cancer has fallen by 21.3% in women aged 55–69 years between 1990 and 1998.[55] Approximately 30% of this reduction is thought to be due to the introduction of screening, although the efficacy of screening was disputed at the time.[56] A more recent International Agency for Research on

Table 1.7 Screening quality targets and achievements 2002–03 (NHSBSP)

Measure	First screen (aged 50–64)		Subsequent screen (aged 50–64)	
	Target	Achievement	Target	Achievement
Acceptance rate at first invitation	≥70.0%	71.8%	—	85.1%
Recall rate	<10%	8.6%	<7.0%	4%
Benign biopsies/1000 women screened	<3.6	2.5	<2.0	0.8
In situ rate/1000 women screened	0.4–0.9	1.9	0.5–1.0	1.3
Invasive cancer detection rate/1000 women screened	>2.7	5.2	≥3.0	5.2
Invasive cancers <15 mm/1000 women screened	≥1.5	2.7	≥1.65	2.8
Non-operative diagnosis rate for cancers	≥70%	84.8%	≥70%	80%
Standardised detection ratio	≥1.0	1.43	≥1.0	1.29
Total no. of women screened for the first time	—	251 178	—	1 041 818

Cancer (IARC) review concluded that many of the criticisms were unsubstantiated.[57] It showed that breast screening of women aged 50–69 results in a 25% reduction in breast cancer mortality; this is estimated to be a 35% reduction in women who actually attend for screening. The review also reported that screening does not significantly reduce mortality in women aged 40–49 (RR 0.81, 95% CI 0.65–1.01).

The expected reduction in mortality may take 10 years to become apparent, so in the meantime progress may be measured using short-term surrogate endpoints. The most relevant trial results for the UK programme are those of the Swedish Two-County Trial. This is because the screening modality used was mammography alone, and the screening interval in the age range of interest (50–64 years) was 33 months, which is close to the UK interval of 3 years. The main indicators of success of the programme are the changes in mortality, the changes in the absolute rate of advanced disease and the parameters of the screening process. These parameters incorporate the screening test and any further diagnostic tests that are performed as a result of the screen. They include sensitivity, specificity, the distributions of lead time and mean sojourn time, and the predictive value for malignancy (i.e. cancer-to-biopsy ratio).

The overall effectiveness of the programme will also depend directly on the proportion of the target population attending for screening. Compliance is therefore another important interim measurement. Every effort must be made to ensure that the population lists used are accurate and that every woman who is invited is both alive and resident in the catchment area. Table 1.7 summarises the target

levels and achievements of the UK programme in 2002/03.[58] It can be seen that the programme is now meeting or exceeding all of the set targets.

Conclusion

The Health of the Nation goal of a 25% reduction in breast cancer mortality rate appears to be on target, given that there was a 21.3% decrease by 1998. The NHSBSP is continually monitored for quality and is now exceeding the standards set from the Swedish Two-County Trial. The programme has now been extended to provide two-view films at all screens and to routinely invite women up to the age of 69. This increase in workload has placed additional strains on the system, which is already facing a national shortage of radiologists and radiographers. In order to meet this demand, new ways are being found to staff the programme using a competency-based approach to achieve a 'skill mix'. State-registered radiographers can now train to become Consultant Practitioners or Advanced Practitioners, who will be qualified either to lead the clinical team or to undertake film reading, breast ultrasound and breast investigative procedures. Underpinning this system will be a new level of Assistant Practitioners who will be trained to carry out mammograms under supervision.

Compliance with invitation to screening is essential to ensure the effectiveness of a breast screening programme. Although nationally the compliance figure exceeds the target of 70%, certain groups have been identified where there are particular needs. Women from minority ethnic groups and those with learning disabilities have particular needs. These issues are the subject of an extensive research project into the needs of these women in order to develop more culturally sensitive information and ways of providing it. It is expected that this project will report in 2007.

References

1. Office for National Statistics. Cancer Statistics Registrations: Registrations of Cancer Diagnosed in 2000. England. Series MBI No. 31. London: National Statistics, 2003.

2. ISD Online: Information and Statistics Division, NHS Scotland, 2003 (www.isdscotland.org).

3. Welsh Cancer Intelligence and Surveillance Unit. Cancer Incidence in Wales 1992–2001. 2002 (www.wales.nhs.uk).

4. Northern Ireland Cancer Registry. Cancer Incidence and Mortality (www.qub.ac.uk/nicr/commoncan.htm).

5. Tubiana M, Koscielny S. Natural history of human breast cancer: recent data and clinical implications. Breast Cancer Res Treat 1991; 18: 125–40.

6. Tabar L, Fagerberg G, Day NE et al. Breast cancer treatment and natural history: new insights from results of screening. Lancet 1992; 339: 412–14.

7. Tabar L, Fagerberg G, Duffy SW et al. Update of the Swedish Two-County Program of Mammographic Screening for Breast Cancer. Radiol Clin North Am 1992; 30: 187–210.

8. Shapiro S. Periodic screening for breast cancer: the HIP randomized controlled trial. Health Insurance Plan. J Natl Cancer Inst Monogr 1997; 22: 27–30.

9. Government Statistical Service. Breast Screening Programme, England: 2003–3. Bulletin 2004/06. 2004.

10. NHSBSP Annual Review 2004 (www.cancerscreening.nhs.uk).

11. Young KC, Burch A. Radiation doses received in the UK Breast Screening Programme in 1997 and 1998. Br J Radiol 2000; 73: 278–87.

12. Forrest APM. Breast cancer screening. Report to the Health Ministers of England, Wales, Scotland and Northern Ireland by a working group chaired by Sir Patrick Forrest. London: HMSO, 1987.

13. Breast Screening Frequency Trial Group. The frequency of breast cancer screening: results from the UKCCCR randomised trial. Eur J Cancer 2002; 38: 1458–64.

14. Tabar L, Vitak B, Chen HH et al. The Swedish Two-County Trial twenty years later. Updated mortality results and new insights from long-term follow-up. Radiol Clin North Am 2000; 38: 625–51.

15. Warren RML, Duffy SW, Bashir S. The value of the second view in screening mammography. Br J Radiol 1996; 69: 105–8.

16. Alexander F, Anderson TJ, Brown HK et al. The Edinburgh Randomised Trial of Breast Cancer Screening: results after 10 years of follow-up. Br J Cancer 1994; 70: 542–8.

17. Shen Y, Zelen M. Screening sensitivity and sojourn time from breast cancer early detection clinical trials: mammograms and physical examinations. J Clin Oncol 2001; 19: 3490–9.

18. Stack JP, Redmond OM, Codd MB et al. Breast disease: tissue characterization with Gd-DTPA enhancement profiles. Radiology 1990; 174: 491–4.

19. Gilles R, Guinebretiere JM, Lucidarme O et al. Nonpalpable breast tumors: diagnosis with contrast-enhanced subtraction dynamic MR imaging. Radiology 1994; 191: 625–31.

20. Orel SG, Schnall MD, Powell CM et al. Staging of suspected breast cancer: effect of MR imaging and MR-guided biopsy. Radiology 1995; 196: 115–22.

21. Allgayer B, Lukas P, Loos W, Kersting-Sommerhoff B. [MRI of the breast with 2D-spin-echo and gradient-echo sequences in diagnostically problematic cases]. Rofo Fortschr Geb Rontgenstr Neuen Bildgeb Verfahr 1993; 158: 423–7.

22. Harms SE, Flamig DP, Hesley KL et al. MR imaging of the breast with rotating delivery of excitation off resonance: clinical experience with pathologic correlation. Radiology 1993; 187: 493–501.

23. Fischer U, von Heyden D, Vosshenrich R et al. [Signal characteristics of malignant and benign lesions in dynamic 2D-MRI of the breast]. Rofo Fortschr Geb Rontgenstr Neuen Bildgeb Verfahr 1993; 158: 287–92.

24. Warner E, Plewes DB, Hill KA et al. Surveillance of BRCA1 and BRCA2 mutation carriers with magnetic resonance imaging, ultrasound, mammography and clinical breast examination. JAMA 2004; 292: 1317–25.

25. Kriege M, Brekelmans CT, Boetes C et al. Efficacy of MRI and mammography for breast cancer screening in women with a familial or genetic predisposition. NEJM 2004; 351: 427–37.

26. UK MRI Breast Screening Study Advisory Group. Rationale for a national multi-centre study of magnetic resonance imaging (MRI) screening in women at genetic risk of breast cancer. Breast 2000; 9: 72–7.

27. Leach MO, Boggis CR, Dixon AK et al. Screening with magnetic resonance imaging and mammography of a UK population at high familial risk of breast cancer: a prospective multicentre cohort study (MARIBS). Lancet 2005; 365: 1769–78.

28. Department of Health Publication 2003/0434 (/www.dh.gov.uk).

29. Andersson I, Aspegren K, Janzon L et al. Mammographic screening and mortality from breast cancer: the Malmö Mammographic Screening Trial. BMJ 1988; 297: 943–8.

30. Alexander FE, Anderson TJ, Brown HK et al. 14 years of follow-up from the Edinburgh Randomised Trial of Breast-Cancer Screening. Lancet 1999; 353: 1903–8.

31. Frisell J, Lidbrink E, Hellstrom L, Rutqvist LE. Follow-up after 11 years – update of mortality results in the Stockholm Mammographic Screening Trial. Breast Cancer Res Treat 1997; 45: 263–70.

32. Miller AB, Baines CJ, To T, Wall C. Canadian National Breast Screening Study: 1. Breast cancer detection and death rates among women aged 40 to 49 years. CMAJ 1992; 147: 1459–75.

33. Miller AB, Baines CJ, To T, Wall C. Canadian National Breast Screening Study: 2. Breast cancer detection and death rates among women aged 50 to 59 years. CMAJ 1992; 147: 1477–88.

34. Baines CJ, Miller AB, Kopans DB et al. Canadian National Breast Screening Study: assessment of technical quality by external review. AJR Am J Roentgenol 1990; 155: 743–7.

35. Bailar JC III, MacMahon B. Randomization in the Canadian National Breast Screening Study: a review for evidence of subversion. CMAJ 1997; 156: 193–9.

36. Nystrom L. Breast cancer screening with mammography: overview of Swedish randomised trials. Lancet 1993; 341: 973–8.

37. Bjurstam N, Bjorneld L, Duffy SW et al. The Gothenburg Breast Screening Trial: first results on mortality, incidence, and mode of detection for women ages 39–49 years at randomization. Cancer 1997; 80: 2091–9.

38. Chen H, Tabar L, Fagerberg G, Duffy SW. Effect of breast cancer screening after age 65. J Med Screen 1995; 2: 10–14.

39. van Dijck JA, Verbeek AL, Beex LV et al. Mammographic screening after the age of 65 years: evidence for a reduction in breast cancer mortality. Int J Cancer 1996; 66: 727–31.

40. Kopans DB. Screening mammography in women over age 65. J Gerontol 1992; 47 (Spec No.): 59–62.

41. Peer PG, Verbeek AL, Straatman H et al. Age-specific sensitivities of mammographic screening for breast cancer. Breast Cancer Res Treat 1996; 38: 153–60.

42. Harris R. Variation of benefits and harms of breast cancer screening with age. J Natl Cancer Inst Monogr 1997; 22: 139–43.

43. Larsson LG, Andersson I, Bjurstam N et al. Updated overview of the Swedish randomized trials on breast cancer screening with mammography: age group 40–49 at randomization. J Natl Cancer Inst Monogr 1997; 22: 57–61.

44. Morimoto T, Sasa M, Yamaguchi T et al. Breast cancer screening by mammography in women aged under 50 years in Japan. Anticancer Res 2000; 20: 3689–94.

45. Kerlikowske K, Grady D, Barclay J et al. Effect of age, breast density, and family history on the sensitivity of first screening mammography. JAMA 1996; 276: 33–8.

46. Feig SA, Hendrick RE. Radiation risk from screening mammography of women aged 40–49 years. J Natl Cancer Inst Monogr 1997; 22: 119–24.

47. Mattsson A, Leitz W, Rutqvist LE. Radiation risk and mammographic screening of women from 40 to 49 years of age: effect on breast cancer rates and years of life. Br J Cancer 2000; 82: 220–6.

48. Moss SM, for the Trial Steering Group. A trial to study the effect on breast cancer mortality of annual mammographic screening in women starting at age 40. J Med Screen 1999; 6: 144–8.

49. Cuzick J. Future possibilities in the prevention of breast cancer: breast cancer prevention trials. Breast Cancer Res 2000; 2: 258–63.

50. Walter SD, Day NE. Estimation of the duration of a pre-clinical disease state using screening data. Am J Epidemiol 1983; 118: 865–86.

51. Connor RJ, Chu KC, Smart CR. Stage-shift cancer screening model. J Clin Epidemiol 1989; 42: 1083–95.

52. Fisher B. Laboratory and Clinical Research in Breast Cancer – A Personal Adventure: The David A Karnofsky Memorial Lecture. Cancer Res 1980; 40: 3863–74.

53. Fisher B, Anderson S, Fisher ER et al. Significance of ipsilateral breast tumour recurrence after lumpectomy. Lancet 1991; 338: 327–31.

54. Tabar L, Fagerberg G, Chen H et al. Tumour development, histology and grade of breast cancers: prognosis and progression. Int J Cancer 1996; 66: 1–7.

55. Blanks RG, Moss SM, McGahan C et al. Effect of NHS Breast Screening Programme on mortality from breast cancer in England and Wales, 1990–8: comparison of observed with predicted mortality. BMJ 2000; 321: 665–9.

56. Olsen O, Gotzsche PC. Cochrane review on screening for breast cancer with mammography. Lancet 2001; 358: 1340–2.

57. International Agency for Research on Cancer (IARC). Efficacy of screening. In: Vainio H, Bianchini F, eds. IARC Handbooks of Cancer Prevention, Volume 7: Breast Cancer Screening. Lyon: IARC Press, 2002: 87–117.

58. NHSBSP Annual Review 2004 (www.cancerscreening.nhs.uk).

2 Mammographic density as an indicator of breast cancer risk

Ruth Warren

The mammogram depicts the constituent tissues of the normal breast, and is taken to show the features of pathology. This technique is now widely used for the early diagnosis of breast cancer by screening of the normal population. The tissues making up the mammographic image can essentially be viewed as those with the radiographic characteristics of water and those of fat. In addition, some pathologies demonstrate calcification, which is always due to an abnormal process, although many of these processes are benign, and of no consequence to the woman. Since the 1970s, starting with observations made by Wolfe, there has been interest in why some women have a greater proportion of dense tissue than others. In 1976, Wolfe[1] proposed four categories for separating women with different amounts of dense tissue and proposed that there was a relationship between the densest mammographic pattern and cancer risk. Figure 2.1 shows a group of four right breast mammograms that illustrate the four Wolfe grades. This hypothesis was debated in the literature for two decades, and was largely not believed by radiologists. In the past few years, greater credence has been given to this hypothesis, and it is now recognised that the densest mammographic patterns express a four to six times increased risk of breast cancer when compared with the least dense.[2,3]

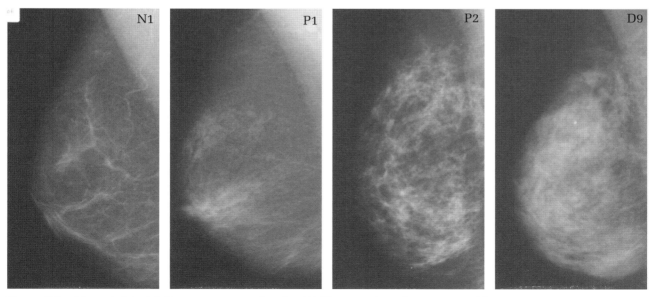

Figure 2.1 Normal right MLO mammograms showing Wolfe parenchymal mammographic patterns.

Relationship between mammographic density and breast cancer risk

Mammographic density has been shown to be one of the most powerful predictors of breast cancer risk, and women with more than 75% density have five times the breast cancer risk (95% confidence interval (CI) 3.6–7.1) of women with fatty breasts, and this relationship holds good for women both before and after the menopause.[4] This relationship is independent of other risk factors. Moreover, the densest pattern is also found to be associated with high-grade (grade 3) tumours and with ductal carcinoma in situ (DCIS).[5] Large tumours are independently associated with the densest pattern, and this is found to be due to a combination of impaired sensitivity and the association with high-grade tumours.[6]

Association between mammographic density and known risk factors for breast cancer

Numerous papers in the literature have explored the relationship between mammographic density and known risk factors for breast cancer. So when mammographic density is studied in relationship to, for example, diet, it is associated with the food constituents that are believed to be risk factors for breast cancer.[7,8] When history of age at menarche, age at menopause, age at first birth and parity are assessed, their relationship to the high-risk patterns (more dense) matches that of the breast cancer risk.[9]

Mammographic density and family history

Research has been undertaken to establish whether there is a genetic component to the density, since genetic factors are clearly involved in some cases of cancer. The relationship of family history to breast density has been incompletely explored to date. Pankow et al[10] studied 1377 women in 258 high-risk families and produced evidence of genetic factors – possibly a dominant inheritance in determining the densest patterns. Further studies exploring this relationship have been described by Kerlikowske, Boyd, Sellers, Chang and their co-workers.[11–14] Hopper and co-workers[15] investigated the density in mono- and dizygotic twins; they showed that there was an association and that approximately 60% of

the density could be accounted for by genetic factors and that the remainder of the determination was due to environmental factors, which may be open to change. Sufficient evidence is available to show that there is a familial relationship determining breast density, but that it is one of several factors, and contributes only in part.

Interrelation with body mass index

Mammographic density shows an inverse relationship with body mass index (BMI); this is not surprising, since as women get more obese the breast becomes permeated with fat, in common with other organs. This is important in the context of the use of these parenchymal patterns as an epidemiological tool. Obesity is a risk factor for breast cancer, and yet mammographic density rather than lucency is associated with breast cancer risk. BMI is then a confounding factor in density estimation, and the calculations must be adjusted for BMI to give a true reading. The relationship between mammographic density and anthropometric measures has been analysed by Sala et al[16] and Boyd et al.[17] Figure 2.2 shows the effect on the appearance of the breast in a woman who had a mammogram at around the time of the menopause, then gained five stones (about 32 kg), which she subsequently lost prior to gallbladder surgery. Figure 2.3 shows a woman who lost several stones in weight due to a debilitating illness, the breasts going from a mixed pattern to smaller but intensely dense.

Mammographic density and its effect on mammographic performance

Dense mammographic patterns are one of the factors that impair mammographic sensitivity, and the radiologist and surgeon will recognise the problem of identifying cancers lying in dense glandular tissue and completely masked by the mammographic density. This is a common situation in young women presenting with symptomatic masses, where the dense mammogram appears to have no valuable part in diagnosis. Magnetic resonance imaging (MRI), breast ultrasound and nuclear medicine studies are all promoted to overcome this shortfall of mammography. The effect on sensitivity in a mammographic screening programme has been documented by Sala et al[18] and by others.[19,20] Hormone replacement therapy (HRT) has the effect in many women of increasing mammographic

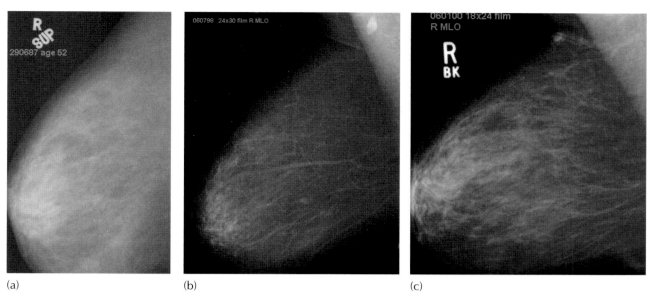

(a) (b) (c)

Figure 2.2 (a) At age 52, P2 pattern. (b) At age 61, P1 pattern – large breast size required larger film. (c) Two years later, after 5 stones (about 32 kg) weight loss for gallbladder surgery, the pattern has returned to an appearance approaching P2.

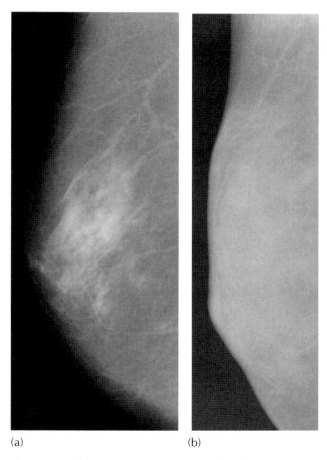

(a) (b)

Figure 2.3 (a) Screening: P1 pattern. (b) Three years later: DY pattern. The diminished breast size and increase in density illustrate the extreme weight loss that has occurred between the two mammograms.

density, and this has been shown to be associated with impaired sensitivity and specificity.[21] This is an important relationship, since many women start to take HRT at the time that they start to attend screening. Thereby the effectiveness of the screening is probably impaired.

Interventions that change mammographic density

HRT

As noted above, HRT has a profound effect on mammographic density in some women. Sala et al[22] demonstrated that this effect was great when the duration of HRT use was prolonged and took place before the menopause. This link with mammographic density was also made by Stomper et al.[23] There has been discussion of the worth of women ceasing to take HRT before their mammography in order to improve sensitivity. There is no adequate evidence-based advice that can be given to women on this subject, and this strategy has not been adopted in clinical screening practice.

Tamoxifen

By contrast, tamoxifen has the effect of reducing mammographic density, as shown in several studies.[24,25] Tamoxifen is used as an adjuvant therapy to prevent recurrence of breast cancer and second primaries in the same or contralateral breast. The reduction in density matches the reduction in risk. One unintended value of this is the beneficial effect that tamoxifen has on mammographic sensitivity, since mammography usually forms part of the surveillance strategy for treated breast cancer.[26] This effect on density is of interest in women taking tamoxifen for prevention, where a beneficial effect on mammography will also be a useful spin-off to the pharmacological effect of the agent.

Density for monitoring interventions in prevention

The recognition that the mammographic parenchymal patterns give a ready reading of risk for breast cancer, together with the extensive use of breast cancer screening by mammography for women at risk of breast cancer (whether by reason of family history or by reason of age (normal population screening)), has prompted the hypothesis that monitoring breast density is an accessible method of monitoring risk.[3,8,27] The proposal that reduction in breast density equates to the reduction in risk is speculative and has not yet been verified by data in the literature. So, when diet or exercise are changed with a view to altering a high-risk woman's propensity to develop cancer, mammographic density may be used to monitor the intervention.[28,29] Likewise, monitoring the effects of pharmacological agents such as tamoxifen and being able to read out the effect on risk will be a valuable tool if it is proven to be a legitimate estimate of risk effect.

Mammographic density as an epidemiological tool

It is being increasingly recognised that mammographic density is a biomarker of risk, and can give useful surrogate information without waiting for the endpoint of the development of cancer, which requires studies of much longer duration.[7,24] Since 1996, there has been a flood of papers in the literature exploring this idea in many different ways, and it is surprising that an observation made in the 1970s should take so long to find its useful development to enhance understanding of cancer. This has driven further work on the methods of measurement of density, particularly with a view to automating the method reliably into a repeatable scientific measurement.

Methods of estimation of mammographic density

Methods of classification were subjected to a meta-analysis by Warner et al[30] in 1992. There have been several descriptions of methods of visual examination of mammograms – the categories described by Wolfe[1] in his original observations comprise four main groups, with the proportion of dense breast tissue plus some morphological features forming the basis of the method. The quantitative aspect was refined by Boyd and co-workers,[30] whose visual method involves allocating the cases to one of six categories based on the estimated proportion of density on the mammogram. Tabar and co-workers[31] devised a method using morphological features, relating them to supposed pathological features. This method is not widely used. Various attempts have been made to apply computer methods to the measurement of breast density – the most widely used is that devised by Boyd's team, and has been refined by others to form their local methods.[32] A study in which the actual volume of fibroglandular and fatty tissue determined by MRI and mammography was compared showed that the two-dimensional area measurements are not real measures of the degree of density, which they tend to overestimate, although this does not detract from the value obtained from density studies in epidemiology.[33] Recently, further automated methods have been explored that estimate the volume of dense tissue; for this, a method of breast thickness is needed, which must be recorded at the time the mammogram is obtained. The mAs (radiation dose) is a surrogate for thickness, and may be used in this situation (Highnam, personal communication).

Conclusion

The importance of mammographic density readings in the estimation of breast cancer risk, and the monitoring of interventions to change it, has become an important epidemiological tool. In due course, better automated measures need to be developed for estimation of this biomarker of risk.

References

1. Wolfe JN. Breast patterns as an index of risk for developing breast cancer. AJR Am J Roentgenol 1976; 126: 1130–7.
2. Byrne C. Studying mammographic density: implications for understanding breast cancer. J Natl Cancer Inst 1997; 89: 531–3.
3. Boyd NF, Lockwood GA, Byng JW et al. Mammographic densities and breast cancer risk. Cancer Epidemiol Biomarkers Prev 1998; 7: 1133–44.
4. Byrne C, Schairer C, Wolfe J et al. Mammographic features and breast cancer risk: effects with time, age, and menopause status. J Natl Cancer Inst 1995; 87: 1622–9.

5. Sala E, Solomon L, Warren R et al. Size, node status, and grade of breast tumours: association with mammographic parenchymal patterns. Eur Radiol 2000; 10: 157–61.

6. Sala E, Warren R, McCann J et al. Mammographic parenchymal patterns and breast cancer natural history – a case–control study. Acta Oncol 2001; 40: 461–5.

7. Sala E, Warren R, Duffy S et al. High risk mammographic parenchymal patterns and diet: a case–control study. Br J Cancer 2000; 83: 121–6.

8. Jakes RW, Duffy SW, Ng FC et al. Mammographic parenchymal patterns and self-reported soy intake in Singapore Chinese women. Cancer Epidemiol Biomarkers Prev 2002; 11: 608–13.

9. Gram IT, Funkhouser E, Tabar L. Reproductive and menstrual factors in relation to mammographic parenchymal patterns among perimenopausal women. Br J Cancer 1995; 71: 647–50.

10. Pankow JS, Vachon CM, Kuni CC et al. Genetic analysis of mammographic breast density in adult women: evidence of a gene effect. J Natl Cancer Inst 1997; 89: 549–56.

11. Kerlikowske K, Grady D, Barclay J et al. Effect of age, breast density, and family history on the sensitivity of first screening mammography. JAMA 1996; 276: 33–8.

12. Boyd NF, Lockwood GA, Martin LJ et al. Mammographic densities and risk of breast cancer among subjects with a family history of this disease. J Natl Cancer Inst 1999; 91: 1404–8.

13. Sellers TA, Anderson VE, Potter JD et al. Epidemiologic and genetic follow-up study of 544 Minnesota breast cancer families: design and methods. Genet Epidemiol 1995; 12: 417–29.

14. Chang J, Yang WT, Choo H. Mammography in Asian patients with BRCA1 mutations. Lancet 1999; 353: 2070–1.

15. Boyd N, Dite G, Stone J et al. Heritability of mammographic density, a risk factor for breast cancer. N Engl J Med 2002; 347: 866.

16. Boyd NF, Lockwood GA, Byng JW et al. The relationship of anthropometric measures to radiological features of the breast in premenopausal women. Br J Cancer 1998; 78: 1233–8.

17. Sala E, Warren R, McCann J et al. High-risk mammographic parenchymal patterns and anthropometric measures: a case–control study. Br J Cancer 1999; 81: 1257–61.

18. Sala E, Warren R, McCann J et al. Mammographic parenchymal patterns and mode of detection: implications for the breast screening programme. J Med Screen 1998; 5: 207–12.

19. Couto E, Harrison D, Duffy S et al. Estimation of disease progression parameters from case-control data: application to mammographic patterns and breast cancer natural history. J Epidemiol Biostatist 2001; 6: 235–42.

20. Mandelson MT, Oestreicher N, Porter PL et al. Breast density as a predictor of mammographic detection: comparison of interval- and screen-detected cancers. J Natl Cancer Inst 2000; 92: 1081–7.

21. Banks E. Hormone replacement therapy and the sensitivity and specificity of breast cancer screening: a review. J Med Screen 2001; 8: 29–34.

22. Sala E, Warren R, McCann J et al. High-risk mammographic parenchymal patterns and hormone replacement therapy: a case–control study. Int J Epidemiol 2000; 29: 629–36.

23. Stomper PC, D'Souza DJ, DiNitto PA, Arredondo MA. Analysis of parenchymal density on mammograms in 1353 women 25–79 years old. AJR Am J Roentgenol 1996; 167: 1261–5.

24. Atkinson C, Warren R, Bingham SA, Day NE. Mammographic patterns as a predictive biomarker of breast cancer risk: effect of tamoxifen. Cancer Epidemiol Biomarkers Prev 1999; 8: 863–6.

25. Brisson J, Brisson B, Cote G et al. Tamoxifen and mammographic breast densities. Cancer Epidemiol Biomarkers Prev 2000; 9: 911–15.

26. Ashkanani F, Sarkar T, Needham G, Coldwells A et al. What is achieved by mammographic surveillance after breast conservation treatment for breast cancer? Am J Surg 2001; 182: 207–10.

27. Boyd NF, Martin LJ, Stone J et al. Mammographic densities as a marker of human breast cancer risk and their use in chemoprevention. Curr Oncol Rep 2001; 3: 314–21.

28. Knight JA, Martin LJ, Greenberg CV et al. Macronutrient intake and change in mammographic density at menopause: results from a randomized trial. Cancer Epidemiol Biomarkers Prev 1999; 8: 123–8.

29. Dirx MJ, Voorrips LE, Goldbohm RA, van den Brandt PA. Baseline recreational physical activity, history of sports participation, and postmenopausal breast carcinoma risk in the Netherlands Cohort Study. Cancer 2001; 92: 1638–49.

30. Warner E, Lockwood G, Tritchler D, Boyd NF. The risk of breast cancer associated with mammographic parenchymal patterns: a meta-analysis of the published literature to examine the effect of method of classification. Cancer Detect Prev 1992; 16: 67–72.

31. Gram IT, Funkhouser E, Tabar L. The Tabar classification of mammographic parenchymal patterns. Eur J Radiol 1997; 24: 131–6.

32. Byng JW, Yaffe MJ, Lockwood GA et al. Automated analysis of mammographic densities and breast carcinoma risk. Cancer 1997; 80: 66–74.

33. Lee N, Rusinek H, Weinreb JC et al. Fatty and fibroglandular tissue volumes in the breasts of women 20–83 years old: comparison of X-ray mammography and computer-assisted MR imaging. AJR Am J Roentgenol 1997; 168: 501–6.

3 Genetics and breast screening

D Gareth Evans

Introduction

Breast cancer is the commonest malignancy affecting women, 1 in 10–12 of whom will develop the disease in their lifetime in the developed world. The annual incidence of breast cancer in England and Wales is 40 000 and 13 000 die each year of this disease (Cancer Research UK Statistics). According to official statistics, the UK has a relatively poor record on survival from breast cancer compared with Continental Europe and the USA. Nonetheless, there has been a 30% reduction in mortality within the UK since the mid-1980s, although minimal improvements in survival have been documented in other parts of the world over the past 30 years. The fall in mortality from breast cancer within the UK can be attributed to the combined impact of breast cancer screening (and earlier detection of the disease) and the introduction of adjuvant systemic therapies, including both chemotherapy and hormonal treatments. In particular, the pioneering work with tamoxifen and the early clinical enthusiasm for this drug may account for the improved mortality figures in the UK (which may become evident in other countries at a future stage).

Prognosis of breast cancer is determined by a combination of tumour size, grade and axillary lymph node status; small tumours (<1 cm) and a favourable histology (grade 1, special types) with no lymph node involvement are associated with a 5-year survival rate in excess of 90%.

Racial and cultural factors appear to influence breast cancer predisposition. The incidence of the disease is relatively low in Chinese and other Asian groups, for whom family history may be more significant.

Risk factors (Table 3.1)

Family history

Family history can be a highly significant factor in predisposition to breast cancer, with about 4–5% of cases being attributed to inheritance of high-risk autosomal dominant genes.[1,2] Hereditary factors may play a role in the remaining sporadic cases, but their contribution is difficult to determine on an individual basis. There is rarely any phenotypic expression of an underlying genetic abnormality that gives rise to an external marker of risk (e.g. Cowden's disease).[3] In order to assess the likelihood of there being a predisposing gene in a family, it is necessary to analyse the cancer pedigree with construction of a family tree. Inheritance of a germline mutation or deletion of a predisposing gene leads to

---

Table 3.1 Factors associated with an increased risk of breast cancer

- Family history
- Early menarche (before 12 years)
- Late first pregnancy (after 28 years)
- Current use of the oral contraceptive pill and for 10 years after
- Nulliparity
- Late menopause
- Prolonged use of hormone replacement therapy (combined)
- Significant weight gain in adult life
- Proliferative breast disease on biopsy (not benign disease such as a fibroadenoma)

development of the disease at a relatively young age and often subsequent occurrence of cancer in the contralateral breast. Some gene mutations may confer susceptibility to other cancers such as carcinomas of the ovary or colon and sarcomas.[4-7] Multiple primary cancers in a single individual or related early-onset cancers in a pedigree are suggestive of a predisposing gene. To illustrate the importance of age, it is estimated that over 25% of breast cancers occurring in women aged under 30 are due to a mutation in a dominant gene, compared with 1% for cases in women aged over 70.[2] The important features in a family tree are therefore:

- age at onset
- bilateral disease
- multiple cases in a family (particularly on one side predominantly)
- other related early-onset tumours
- number of unaffected individuals (large families are more informative)

There are few families for whom a dominant pattern of inheritance can be confidently predicted, but the chance of inheriting this is about 50% when four first-degree relatives with early-onset or bilateral breast cancer exist within a family and a mother or sister is affected. Epidemiological studies have shown that about 80% of individuals with mutations in predisposing genes develop breast cancer in their lifetime. Therefore, unless there is a strong family history involving both maternal and paternal relatives, the maximum risk counselled is 40–45%. Breast cancer genes can be inherited through the paternal line, and a dominant history on the father's side of the family would give at least a 20–25% lifetime risk to his daughters.

Other risk factors

Non-genetic or environmental risk factors relate principally to the hormonal environment of breast tissue. A woman would derive maximal benefit from never ovulating – breast cancer is very uncommon in Turner's (XO) syndrome. A relatively high degree of protection is afforded by minimising the period of ovulation prior to a woman's first pregnancy, and therefore late menarche combined with an early first full-term pregnancy reduces the subsequent risk of breast cancer. Exposure of relatively immature breast tissue to oestrogen (especially unopposed) increases risk, while progesterone associated with pregnancy is protective and may induce terminal differentiation in pluripotential stem cells. Pregnancy transforms breast parenchymal cells into a more stable state where proliferation in the second half of the cycle is less. There is now convincing evidence that current use of the oral contraceptive

pill is associated with a 20% increase in risk and that this persists for 10 years post use.[8] Although the oestrogen component of the oral contraceptive pill suppresses ovulation, proliferation of breast cancer cells is stimulated. The continued rise of incidence of breast cancer may be a consequence of greater numbers of women delaying their first full-term pregnancy, combined with more prolonged use of the oral contraceptive pill. This trend is most apparent in the well-educated professional classes, who may already possess an elevated background risk for breast cancer. Early menopause is protective and reduces cumulative oestrogen exposure. Other factors, such as the number of pregnancies and breast feeding, may have a small protective effect. There is some controversy over the use of hormone replacement therapy (HRT), particularly in breast cancer patients. Prolonged use of HRT for more than 10 years after the menopause is associated with a significant increase in risk. However, a shorter treatment duration may still confer increased risk for individuals with a family history of breast cancer.[9] In a large meta-analysis the risk appeared to increase cumulatively by 1–2% per year, but disappeared within 5 years of cessation.[10] It is becoming clear that the risk from combined oestrogen\progesterone HRT is up to three times greater than for oestrogen only.

Dietary factors play some role in determining breast cancer risk, with epidemiological studies confirming that diets low in animal fats from dairy produce and red meat are associated with marginal risk reductions. Previous breast biopsies revealing proliferative changes such as atypical hyperplasia (lobular or ductal) increase breast cancer risk significantly, and these histopathological changes may be a manifestation of alterations at the genetic level in gene mutation carriers.[11,12]

Risk estimation

In the absence of a dominant family history, risk estimation is based on large epidemiological studies, which have revealed a 1.5- to 3-fold-elevated risk for individuals with a single affected relative.[1,2] It is important to distinguish between lifetime and age-specific risks. For example, some studies quote an increased risk of 9-fold or greater for a first-degree relative with bilateral disease or a personal history of proliferative breast disease. However, in the latter case, risk decreases with increasing time since diagnosis, and with prolonged follow-up eventually returns to normal levels.[11] If cumulative lifetime risk is calculated from these risk estimates multiplied by the overall lifetime incidence of 1 in 12 then some women will apparently have a lifetime risk of breast

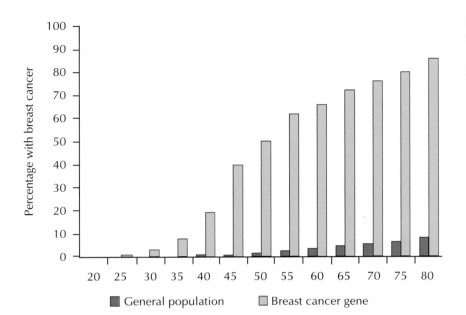

Figure 3.1 Age-specific penetrance for breast cancer in carriers of *BRCA1* or *BRCA2* mutations (adapted from the Breast Cancer Linkage Consortium).

cancer in excess of 100%. Risk estimates for individual factors are not multiplicative and may not be additive in a simple arithmetic manner. Perhaps the most accurate way to assess risk is to define the strongest single factor – which for breast cancer is usually family history. When the level of risk is based on this factor alone, minor adjustments can be made to incorporate other factors. However, it seems unlikely that these additional factors will influence risk to any great extent in the presence of predisposing genes with a high degree of penetrance. Rather than determining the absolute risk of development of breast cancer, they may advance or delay the onset of disease. The effects of non-hereditary elements of risk can only be assumptive rather than calculated in objective terms. Although some studies suggest an increased risk attributable to these non-hereditary factors in family history cases, these may merely represent earlier expression of the gene. Therefore risk assessments will generally range between 40% and 8% (1 in 12) although lower risks are sometimes cited. Higher risks may be applicable when a woman has a 40% genetic risk and is found to have a germline mutation, to have an inherited high-risk allele or to have proliferative breast disease.

Breast cancer genes

The hereditary component of breast cancer is likely to result from several different predisposing genes. Attention is currently focused on two predisposing genes – one on the long arm of chromosome 17

(*BRCA1*)[13] and the other on the long arm of chromosome 13 (*BRCA-2*).[14] These genes have an estimated population frequency of 0.2% and are thought to account for over 80% of highly penetrant inherited breast cancer. The majority of families with a combination of breast and ovarian cancer are linked to *BRCA1*, with mutations of this gene causing the disease. However, up to 20% of families with breast and ovarian cancer may have mutations in *BRCA2*,[15] and mutations in one or other of these two genes account for most, if not all, breast/ovarian cancer predisposition.[15] Furthermore, the occurrence of two or more cases of epithelial ovarian cancer within a family is highly suggestive of *BRCA1* involvement. There is increasing evidence that families with *BRCA1* and *BRCA2* involvement have differential susceptibilities to ovarian cancers. The associated cumulative lifetime risks across all the linked families for mutations of *BRCA1* and *BRCA2* are 85% (breast) and 60% (ovarian)[15,16] and 85% (breast) and 10–20% (ovarian)[15] respectively (Figure 3.1). Two subsets of mutation probably exist, one of which results predominately in ovarian cancer risk while the other confers a relatively low risk of ovarian predisposition.[17] It may transpire that all of these so-called site-specific ovarian cancer families are caused by *BRCA1* mutations. This is supported by evidence from several areas, including (a) long-term follow-up of site-specific families,[18] (b) new cancers in families from the UKCCCR familial ovarian cancer study (B Ponder, personal communication) and (c) linkage and mutation analysis within families.[19,20] Controversy persists over the true cumulative lifetime risk associated with *BRCA1* and *BRCA2* mutations. Although initial studies in

Table 3.2	**Hereditary conditions predisposing to breast cancer**

Disease	Other tumour susceptibilities	Inheritance[a]	Percentage of[b] BC	HPHBC	Location
Familial breast cancer (BRCA1)	Ovary/prostate, bowel	AD	1.7	50	17q
Familial breast cancer (BRCA2)	Ovary/prostate, male breast	AD	1.2	35	13q
Li–Fraumeni syndrome	Sarcoma, leukaemia, brain, adrenal	AD	0.1	1	17p (TP53)
Lynch type 2 syndrome	Bowel (proximal), endometrium, ovary, pancreas, stomach	AD	<1	<1	2p, 3p 7q, 3q
Ataxia telangiectasia	Homozygous (leukaemia, etc.) Heterozygous (?other sites)	AR	0 2	0 0	11q (ATM)
Cowden's disease	Skin, thyroid, bowel	AD	<1	<1	10q (PTEN)
Reifenstein's syndrome	?	?XLR	<1		X
Ha-ras variant		AD	?8	0	11p

[a]AD, autosomal dominant; AR, autosomal recessive; XLR, X-linked recessive.
[b]BC, breast cancer; HPHBC, highly penetrant hereditary breast cancer (e.g. >3 affected relatives).

selected groups revealed high levels of risk, subsequent population studies have shown risks as low as 40%. However, more recent large-scale studies are consistent with higher risk estimates for both genes.[20]

The TP53 (also called p53) gene on chromosome 17p is known to predispose to early breast cancer,[4] and germline mutations of this gene account for over 70% of cases of the Li–Fraumeni syndrome.[21] However the contribution of the Li–Fraumeni syndrome to overall breast cancer incidence is probably minimal. Carriage of the ataxia telangiectasia gene (ATM) is associated with a fivefold increased risk of breast cancer.[22] Although the carrier frequency for mutation of this gene was estimated to be as high as 2%, this was based on five complementation groupings, and the disease is now known to be caused by a single gene on chromosome 11q.[23] The PTEN gene on chromosome 10 is linked to Cowden's disease,[24] but neither this gene nor the ATM gene account for high-risk families. Other genes that might be implicated in breast cancer are being actively sought, and it is likely that several other predisposing genes remain to be identified. Table 3.2 lists known hereditary conditions and locations of genes predisposing to breast cancer.

For the majority of women, it will only be possible to derive an estimate of lifetime risk that will ultimately depend upon whether a gene mutation exists within the family and whether an individual has inherited this. Genetic testing has the potential to significantly modify risk estimates by confirming the presence of or excluding a particular germline mutation. In the latter case, risk is only reduced significantly and confidently by demonstrating the absence of a *known* family mutation.

Communication of risk

Risk can be expressed either as a cumulative lifetime risk or as a risk over a specific period of time. Thus a woman from a breast cancer family with young-onset disease may have a lifetime risk of 40%. However, if she has already reached the age of 60 and remains disease-free, her chance of carrying a gene mutation is only 20%, as more than 60% would have developed breast cancer by the age of 60 in the presence of a genetic predisposition. Moreover, there is only a 10% chance of having an hereditary form of breast cancer in her remaining life, consistent with the gradual equalisation of risk towards normal in patients aged over 60 with a strong family history of breast cancer. Thus communication of risk to women must incorporate these concepts of time dependence and residual lifetime risk. Some women may prefer to have information on annual risk, which is approximately 1% per year from the late 20s for an individual from a dominant family with a 50% chance of inheriting the gene.

Options

The options available for a woman with a significantly increased risk of breast cancer remain limited. Some women ignore this risk and prefer to 'bury their head in the sand' and avoid seeking any professional advice. Others are rendered disillusioned, confused or even sceptical by enthusiastic doctors. While the efficacy of screening young women remains unproven, a degree of circumspection is appropriate when advocating screening for this subgroup of women at higher risk. Nonetheless, many women are prepared to accept any intervention that may be associated with potential benefits in terms of reduction in mortality.

The available options are:
- no action
- try to reduce risk
- early detection of tumours (screening)
- removal of risk

Risk reduction

This may involve:
- planning a family early
- avoiding the use of the oral contraceptive pill and HRT
- adopting a good diet

Some doctors may advocate:
- delaying menarche
- artificial early menopause (oophorectomy)
- anti-oestrogen therapy (tamoxifen)

The identification of a group of women at high risk increases the probability of a sufficient number of events occurring (i.e. development of breast cancer) to justify prevention trials as a worthwhile intervention. There have been three recent major trials of prevention, the principal one being an international collaborative study on tamoxifen in the UK (the IBIS study, which closed in January 2001). Tamoxifen has been shown to reduce the incidence of contralateral breast cancer in treated patients by 30–40%, and in general is well tolerated with few side-effects.[25] It may also confer beneficial effects on the heart and bones, which makes this drug an ideal candidate for prevention trials in which it is administered to otherwise fit and healthy volunteers. Results from these prevention trials to date are conflicting; the largest study conducted by the US National Surgical Adjuvant Breast and Bowel Project (NSABP) showed a 50% reduction in incidence of both invasive and in situ carcinoma,[26] but two smaller European studies showed no significant reduction.[27,28] However, a larger study, IBIS1, showed a 30–40% reduction in breast cancer risk, but a rise in all-cause mortality. Interestingly, the Royal Marsden trial recruited patients on the basis of a strong family history of breast cancer, but subset analysis of patients within the NSABP P-1 trial who are likely carriers of BRCA1 and BRCA2 mutations confirms a chemopreventive effect of tamoxifen in this higher-risk subgroup. Furthermore, results from the IBIS-1 trial[29] involving more than 7000 women showed a significant reduction in breast cancer risk that was of comparable magnitude to those reported in the NSABP P-1 study: 32% reduction in both invasive and non-invasive disease (95% confidence interval (CI) 8–50%). A more recent overview of four tamoxifen prevention trials showed an overall reduction of 38% in breast cancer incidence (95% CI 28–46%; $p<0.001$).[30] An increase in thromboembolic events in the tamoxifen arms was witnessed in all trials (relative risk 1.9; 95% CI 1.4–2.6%; $p<0.0001$), together with more frequent requirement for hysterectomy and oophorectomy (increased incidence of endometrial cancer, endometrial polyps, endometrial thickening and ovarian cyts). The overall risk-to-benefit ratio for tamoxifen in the preventative setting remains unclear, but its use may be justified in a very high-risk subgroup with a sufficiently high annual incidence rate and thus an absolute benefit from risk reduction interventions.[30]

Other studies being undertaken involve dietary modification with reduction of fat intake (Canada), administration of retinoids (Italy) and trials comparing tamoxifen with raloxifene (the STAR trial). A trial is being piloted in the UK and Australia involving switching off the ovaries with goserelin and protecting the bones and breasts with raloxifene (the RAZOR trial). Variations of this theme are the basis of further trials in the USA and Continental Europe.

Early detection (screening)

This may involve:
- regular self-examination
- annual mammography screening from age 35 or 5 years before the earliest cancer in the family.

The latter may be partly replaced by:
- annual ultrasound
- magnetic resonance imaging (MRI) scanning (part of a UK Medical Research Council (MRC)-funded study)

Annual screening should have the capacity to identify over 60% of cancers in young women,[31] but interval cancers still occur. The breast tissue of younger women is denser and more difficult to interpret. However, as the relative risk at age 35 compared with the general population may be as high as 40-fold, this group demands special consideration. Although evidence is now beginning to emerge for a significant survival advantage for general population screening under age 50,[32,33] the incidence of disease within this age group is probably too low to render screening a cost-effective exercise. Nonetheless, we have shown that small impalpable lesions are detected in the 35–49 age group and that detection rates comparable to those reported by the NHS Breast Screening Programme (NHSBSP) are attainable by targeted screening.[34] Mammography may eventually be superseded by other imaging modalities with greater sensitivity, such as MRI,[35] but these newer techniques are currently too expensive and of restricted availability to be of practical use beyond screening of very high-risk groups. The minimal doses of radiation associated with mammography carry only a small theoretical risk of inducing breast cancer.[36] The cumulative exposure from regular screening is unlikely to cause more than 1 additional cancer per 10 000 women screened. This is a negligible risk compared with a 40% lifetime risk. Some individuals with specific gene mutations are more susceptible to radiation induced damage including carriers of the *ATM* gene and possibly *BRCA2* carriers. The BRCA2 protein has been found to interact with a protein involved in DNA repair (RAD51), and mutation carriers may have reduced potential for DNA repair and maintenance of genomic integrity. A proportion of women undergoing screening will have radiological abnormalities that necessitate either percutaneous or open biopsy and are subsequently proven benign. This aspect of screening is associated with a degree of psychological as well as physical morbidity, but with the advent of image-guided biopsy techniques (fine-needle aspiration cytology or core biopsy), the number of open surgical biopsies for benign lesions is small.[37]

Removal of risk

Prophylactic mastectomy, which is often perceived as a rather drastic measure, has been more commonly practised in the USA than in Europe. For those women with a particularly high risk, this option for risk reduction should be considered and discussed sensitively with the patient. The usual procedure undertaken for prophylaxis has been a subcutaneous mastectomy that preserves the nipple–areola complex and therefore leaves behind a small amount of sub-areolar breast tissue, in which there is a risk of subsequent tumour development,[38] although the placement of implants within a subpectoral muscular pocket not only greatly improves cosmetic results but also ensures that any residual breast tissue lies anterior to the prosthesis (which may otherwise mask any tumour). From an oncological point of view, a more appropriate surgical procedure may be a complete mastectomy preserving most of the breast envelope but sacrificing the nipple areola complex (a skin-sparing mastectomy). Nonetheless, there is evidence from a study involving almost 1000 women carried out at the Mayo Clinic that breast cancer risk can be reduced by 90% when subcutaneous mastectomy is undertaken as a prophylactic procedure.[39] Further studies are under way to confirm the benefits of surgical prophylaxis in *BRCA1* and *BRCA2* mutation carriers.[40] It remains unclear whether there are any long-term sequelae of preventive surgery; it is essential that women be prepared psychologically for bilateral prophylactic mastectomy and have realistic expectations of cosmetic results, which may not always be satisfactory to any individual woman. The attendant risks of general anaesthesia (especially if there are concomitant medical problems) and surgery must be taken into account when making a final decision about prophylactic mastectomy. Significant reductions in levels of anxiety in cancer-related worry have been found in women opting for prophylactic mastectomy compared with those who do not.[41] In the UK, women at high risk are increasingly opting for prophylactic mastectomy, and it is important that comprehensive protocols that include psychological assessment be available to prepare women prior to surgery.[42] As genetic testing becomes more widely available, allowing the identification of women whose lifetime risk approaches 80–90%, the demand for prophylactic mastectomy is likely to increase. Reports from our own group and from a Dutch group indicate uptake rates of around 50% in unaffected mutation carriers.[43,44] High-risk women are more likely to choose prophylactic surgery than prevention trials.[44]

The subpopulation of women who might benefit from presymptomatic genetic testing is difficult to define. Any individual could, in principle, undergo mutation testing for either *BRCA1* or *BRCA2* (or both), but the detection rate of mutations would be very low unless those individuals were identified as being at increased risk for a genetic fault and hence breast cancer in the first place. Those individuals without any family history of breast or ovarian cancer would have no alteration to their lifetime risk from a negative screen. Furthermore, these women would not be in screening programmes outside the NHSBSP where screening commences at age 50. It is doubtful whether those individuals with one or two relatives with breast cancer would benefit much in terms of reassurance from a negative genetic screen. Currently, the target population is at-risk relatives and families with four or more cases of breast cancer under age 60 or ovarian cancer at any age. There must be an affected family member alive who is willing to provide a blood sample for mutation screening. These criteria will eventually be extended to allow for testing of much smaller aggregations of breast cancer cases. It is estimated that only 1 in every 1000 individuals come from families suitable for genetic testing at present and 3% at most of breast cancer cases could be prevented by testing for *BRCA1* and *BRCA2* mutations. There may be potential cost savings from withdrawal of women who test negative from existing surveillance programmes.

The genetic testing programme

The majority of work currently being undertaken in the field of cancer predisposition is research-funded and includes not only laboratory-based activity but also family history clinics. Therefore who should be offered genetic testing and how should this be carried out? Clearly testing cannot be offered on demand to all individuals requesting screening for *BRCA1* or *BRCA2* mutations. This would entail a significant expansion of current laboratory services together with the peritest counselling that is a crucial aspect of genetic screening. A more realistic approach is to offer testing to those individuals with a family history of breast or ovarian cancer. Approximately 1 in 10 women develop breast cancer in their lifetime, and thus many women will have some family history of the disease. Even if access were restricted to those with a more significant history, there would be a potentially huge demand.

What will a positive or negative screen mean for a woman? Those individuals in the general population without a family history have a less than 0.1% chance of carrying a mutation in the *BRCA1* gene. Therefore a negative screen would not reduce their breast cancer risk even if the sensitivity of the test were 100%. An individual with a first-degree relative with breast cancer at age 45 whose lifetime risk is 1

in 6 would derive no meaningful reduction in their chance of developing breast cancer. Even where there is a strong family history of breast and ovarian cancer, mutation testing at 90% sensitivity would not lead to a risk reduction that justifies cessation of screening or prophylactic intervention (D Easton, personal communication). It therefore would appear logical to offer a predictive test only when a mutation has been identified in a family and has been shown to be relevant to disease causation. This will allow those family members without a mutation to be completely reassured and permit the provision of informed risk estimates of breast and ovarian cancer to those with a mutation. However, in a small nuclear family, it may be difficult to assess whether a mutation confers a high (80%) or low (10–20%) risk of ovarian cancer.[17] Evidence from the International Linkage Consortium (ILC) suggests that although *BRCA1* and *BRCA2* account for the great majority of families with four or more affected cases under age 60 with breast and/or ovarian cancer, they account for much less of the predicted hereditary component of smaller families.[15] Thus a family with two affected sisters under age 50 would have more than a 50% chance of a genetic disposition, yet *BRCA1* and *BRCA2* mutations account for only about 15% of these families.[15] A large number of population studies have attempted to determine the proportion of early-onset breast cancer[45,46] and ovarian[20,47] cancer caused by *BRCA1* mutations (assuming a sensitivity of mutation detection as low as 70%). However, several populations exhibit a significant 'founder' effect whereby a limited number of mutations account for a large proportion of hereditary disease.[48] This is particular true for Ashkenazi Jews, among whom three distinct mutations are found in 2.5% of the entire population.[49] Were the population frequency of other *BRCA1* and *BRCA2* mutations to be the same as in the non-Jewish population (0.2%) then testing for three mutations would account for over 90% of highly penetrant families. We have shown that a significant proportion of the smaller aggregations are due to these founder mutations.[50] Population testing is therefore likely to have a higher predictive value in the Jewish community, and because of the relatively high frequency of mutations within this group, testing of unaffected individuals without a known family history of breast cancer is feasible.

In the main, however, research laboratories will be carrying out mutation testing in those families with affected individuals with a high probability of a *BRCA1* mutation. This would include (a) families linked with a previously identified *BRCA1* mutation, (b) families with several cases of breast and/or ovarian cancer, or (c) families where an individual has developed either disease at a young age or has more than one primary tumour.

Table 3.3	Summary of potential problems in identifying an appropriate target population

- Too much demand for too little yield
- Residual risk (population risk or still above) for women who test negative
- Unknown psychological sequelae
- Economic cost benefit only if management is changed

Once a mutation has been found this will usually be passed on to a service laboratory for verification and further testing will be instituted of the extended family. When research grants become exhausted, alternative sources of funding must be earmarked for initial identification of mutations in service laboratories. Early surveys indicated that approximately 60% of women would accept the offer of *BRCA1* gene testing.[51–54] This figure came from our preliminary data based on 75 individuals distributed among five families,[54] in addition to population studies and a clinical survey.[55] Evidence to date suggests that techniques such as gene sequencing and DHPLC will be capable of detecting 80–85% of *BRCA1* mutations. Should these techniques become widely available, expansion of the number of genetic counsellors and appropriately trained clinicians will be essential if at-risk individuals are to be adequately prepared for predictive testing. Funding will have to be made available not only to carry out testing but also to make provision for the consequences of genetic testing.

The potential problems arising in the identification of an appropriate target population for testing are summarised in Table 3.3.

Uptake of genetic testing and outcome

Approximately 60% of eligible women undergo genetic testing for breast cancer predisposition[43,51,52,54] and theoretical surveys of women with a low probability of *BRCA1* or *BRCA2* carriage suggest a similarly high uptake.[55] However, when the poor predictive value of testing unaffected relatives is explained to individuals, the uptake may prove to be much lower. In practice, the uptake in tested families remains much lower than predicted from surveys, and testing should be extended to families that have not yet been contaminated by involvement in large-scale research. The large number of families in whom mutations have been found (approximately

800 in the UK) will facilitate these broader studies and uptake of genetic testing. Although limited information is available on the outcome of testing, early data suggest that individuals obtain significant benefit psychologically from a low-risk result and may not be adversely affected by a high-risk result. From the perspective of health economics, it is essential to know what options women will choose. If more than 50% opt for prophylactic surgery then additional provision with increased operating capacity will be necessary. However, in the longer term, preventive surgery may result in economic benefits from the reduction in the number of women requiring chemotherapy for metastatic disease.

Genetic testing is difficult to cost; commercial laboratories in the USA such as MYRIAD charge a total of $2975 for initial complete screening of the *BRCA1* and *BRCA2* genes. Once a specific mutation has been identified for that family, subsequent tests are charged at a much lower rate of about $350. In the UK the equivalent costs are £800 for a complete screen of *BRCA1/2* and £42 for subsequent testing. Screening for family mutations is relatively cheaper. Thus it costs approximately £42 to screen for the three common mutations (185 del AG, 5382 ins C and 6174 del T) within the Ashkenazi Jewish population, which is potentially cost-effective. A cost analysis that we have undertaken for the non-Jewish population has also shown a significant cost benefit if over 40% of women choose prophylactic surgery and those individuals deemed to be at low risk are discharged from screening (60% uptake of testing).

Cost savings will only be forthcoming if management is changed as a consequence of genetic testing. This is unlikely to be the case for women outside families with proven *BRCA1* or *BRCA2* mutations, and testing unaffected women without knowledge of the family mutation (if one exists) may not alter their breast cancer risk in a practically meaningful way. An exception to this in the non-Jewish population would be a woman contemplating prophylactic mastectomy who may be sufficiently reassured by a negative *BRCA1/BRCA2* test to abandon surgery. Even within the Jewish population, exclusion of the three common mutations does not equate with minimal risk. Although a large proportion of hereditary risk is excluded, a family history of breast cancer still confers an increased risk and new mutations can occur within the Jewish population.

Conclusion

Cancer genetics has emerged as a new speciality over the last decade, with familial risk clinics being established across Europe and North America. Categorisation of individuals into high-, moderate- and average- (low)-risk groups has permitted genetic testing to be targeted to those most likely to benefit.[56]

Genetic testing is likely to become more widely available with improvements in molecular biological techniques and the discovery of the remaining genes that predispose to breast cancer.

References

1. Newman B, Austin MA, Lee, M, King M. Inheritance of human breast cancer: Evidence for autosomal dominant transmission in high-risk families. Proc Natl Acad Sci 1988; 85: 3044–8.

2. Claus EB, Risch N, Thompson WD. Autosomal dominant inheritance of early onset breast cancer. Cancer 1994; 73: 643–51.

3. Nelen MR, Padberg GW, Peeters EAJ et al. Localisation of the gene for Cowden disease to chromosome l0q22–23. Nat Genet 1996: 13: 114–16.

4. Malkin D, Li FP, Strong LC et al. Germline p53 mutations in cancer families. Science 1990; 250: 1233–8.

5. Leach FS, Nicolaides NC, Papadopoulos N et al. Mutation of a mut S homolog in hereditary non polyposis colorectal cancer. Cell 1993; 75: 1215–25.

6. Papadopoulos N, Nicolaides NC, Wei Y-F et al. Mutation of a Mut L homolog in hereditary colon cancer. Science 1994; 263: 1625–9

7. Nicolaides NC, Papadopoulos N, Liu B et al. Mutation of two PMS homologs in hereditary non polyposis colorectal cancer. Nature 1994; 371: 75–80.

8. Breast cancer and hormonal contraceptives: collaborative reanalysis of individual data on 53,297 women with breast cancer and 100,239 women without breast cancer from 54 epidemiological studies. Lancet 1996; 347: 1713–27.

9. Steinberg KK, Thacker SB, Smith J et al. A meta-analysis of the effect of oestrogen replacement therapy on the risk of breast cancer. JAMA 1991; 1985–90.

10. Collaborative group on hormonal factors in breast cancer. Breast cancer and hormone replacement therapy: collaborative reanalysis of data from 51 epidemiological studies of 52,705 women with breast cancer and 108,411 women without breast cancer. Lancet 1997; 350: 1047–59.

11. Dupont WD, Page DL. Relative risk of breast cancer varies with time since diagnosis of atypical hyperplasia. Hum Pathol 1989; 20: 723–5.

12. Scolnick MH, Cannon-Albright LA, Goldgar DE et al. Inheritance of proliferative breast disease in breast cancer kindreds. Science 1990; 250: 1715–21.

13. Miki Y, Swensen J, Shattuck-Eidens D et al. A strong candidate for the breast and ovarian cancer gene BRCA1. Science 1994; 266: 66–71.

14. Wooster R, Bignell G, Lancaster J et al. Identification of the breast cancer susceptibility gene BRCA2. Nature 1995: 378; 789–92.

15. Ford D, Easton M, Stratton S et al. Genetic heterogeneity and penetrance analysis of the BRCA1 and BRCA2 genes in breast cancer families. Am J Hum Genet 1998; 62: 676–89.

16. Easton DF, Ford D, Bishop DT. Breast and ovarian cancer incidence in BRCA1 mutation carriers. Am J Hum Genet 1994; 56: 265–71.

17. Gayther SA, Mangion J, Russell P. Variations of risks of breast and ovarian cancer associated with different germline mutations of the BRCA2 gene. Nat Genet 1997; 15: 103–5.

18. Evans DGR, Donnai D, Ribeiro G, Warrell D. Ovarian cancer family and prophylactic choices. J Med Genet 1992; 29: 416–18.

19. Steichen-Gersdorf E, Gallion HH, Ford D et al. Familial site specific ovarian cancer is linked to BRCA1 on 17q12–21. Am J Hum Genet 1994; 55: 870–5.

20. Risch HA, McLaughlin JR, Cole DEC et al. Prevalence and penetrance of germline BRCA1 and BRCA2 mutations in a population series of 649 women with ovarian cancer. Am J Hum Genet 2001; 68: 700–10.

21. Varley JM, Evans DGR, Birch JM. Li–Fraumeni syndrome – a molecular and clinical review. Br J Cancer 1997; 76: 1–14.

22. Swift ML, Reitnauer PJ, Morrell D, Chase CL. Breast and other cancers in families with ataxia telangiectasia. N Engl J Med 1987; 316: 1289–94.

23. Savitsky K, Bar-Shira A, Gilad S et al. A single ataxia telangectasia gene with a product similar to PI-3 kinase. Science 1995; 268: 1749–53.

24. Liaw D, Marsh DJ, Li J et al. Germline mutations of the PTEN gene in Cowden disease, an inherited breast and thyroid cancer syndrome. Nat Genet 1997; 16: 64–7.

25. Powles TJ, Tillyer CR, Jones AL et al. Prevention of breast cancer with tamoxifen: an update on the Royal Marsden Hospital pilot programme. Eur J Cancer 1990; 26: 680–4.

26. Fisher B, Constantino JP, Wickerham DL et al. Tamoxifen for prevention of breast cancer: report of the National Surgical Adjuvant Breast and Bowel Project P-1 study. J Natl Cancer Inst 1998; 90: 1371–87.

27. Powles TJ, Eeles R, Ashley S et al. Interim analysis of the incidence of breast cancer in the Royal Marsden Hospital tamoxifen randomised chemoprevention trial. Lancet 1998; 352: 98–101.

28. Veronesi U, Maisonneuve P, Costa A et al. Prevention of breast cancer with tamoxifen: preliminary findings from the Italian randomised trial among hysterectomised women. Lancet 1998; 352: 93–7.

29. IBIS Investigators. First results from the International Breast Cancer Intervention Study (IBIS-1): a randomised prevention trial. Lancet 2002; 360: 817–24.

30. Cuzick J, Powles T, Veronesi U et al. Overview of the main outcomes in breast cancer prevention. Lancet 2003; 361: 296–300.

31. Tabar L, Faberberg G, Day NE, Holmberg L. What is the optimum interval between mammographic screening

examinations? An analysis based on the Swedish Two County Breast Cancer Screening Trial. Br J Cancer 1987; 56: 547–51.

32. Tabar L, Fagerberg G, Chen HH et al. efficacy of breast cancer screening by age. Cancer 1995; 75: 2507–17.

33. Report of the Coordinating Group for Breast Cancer Screening, Falun Meeting, Falun, Sweden. Breast screening with mammography in women 40–49 years. Int J Cancer 1996; 68: 693–9.

34. Lalloo F, Boggis CRM, Evans DGR et al. Screening by mammography women with a family history of breast cancer. Eur J Cancer 1998; 34: 937–40.

35. Brown J, Buckley D, Coulthard A et al. Magnetic resonance imaging screening in women at genetic risk of breast cancer: imaging and analysis protocol for the UK Multicentre study. Br J Radiol 2000: 73: 123–32.

36. Law J. Cancers detected and induced in mammographic screening: new screening schedules and younger women with family history. Br J Radiol 1997; 70: 62–70.

37. Moller P, Evans G, Maehle L et al. Use of cytology to diagnose hereditary breast cancer. Dis Markers 1999; 15: 212–16.

38. Goodnight JE, Quagliani JM, Morton DL. Failure of subcutaneous mastectomy to prevent the development of breast cancer. J Surg Oncol 1984; 26: 198–201.

39. Hartmann LC, Schaid DJ, Woods JE et al. Efficacy of bilateral prophylactic mastectomy in women with a family history of breast cancer. N Engl J Med 1999; 340: 77–84.

40. Meijers-Heijboer EJ, van Geel B, van Putten WLJ et al. Breast cancer after prophylactic bilateral mastectomy in women with a BRCA1 or BRCA2 mutation. N Engl J Med 2001; 345: 159–64.

41. Hatcher MB, Falowfield L, A'Hern B. The psychosocial impact of bilateral prophylactic mastectomy: prospective study using questionnaires and semistructured interviews. BMJ 2001; 322: 1–7.

42. Lalloo F, Baildam A, Brain A et al. Preventative mastectomy for women at high risk of breast cancer. Eur J Surg Oncol 2000; 26: 711–13.

43. Meijers-Heijboer EJ, Verhoog LC, Brekelmans CTM et al. Presymptomatic DNA testing and prophylactic surgery in families with a BRCA1 or BRCA2 mutation. Lancet 2000; 355: 2015–20.

44. Evans DGR, Lalloo F, Shenton A, et al. Uptake of screening and prevention trials in women at very high risk of breast cancer. Lancet 2001; 358: 889–900.

45. Fitzgerald MG, MacDonald DJ, Krainer M et al. Germline BRCA1 mutations in Jewish and non-Jewish women with early onset breast cancer. N Engl J Med 1996; 334: 143–9.

46. Langston AA, Malone KE, Thompson JD et al. BRCA1 mutations in a population based sample of young women with breast cancer. N Engl J Med 1996; 334: 137–42.

47. Stratton J, Gayther SA, Russell P et al. Contribution of BRCA1 mutations to ovarian cancer. N Engl J Med 1997; 336: 1125–30.

48. Thorlacius S, Olafsdottir G, Tryggvadottir L et al. A single BRCA2 mutation in male and female breast cancer families from Iceland with varied cancer phenotypes. Nat Genet 1996; 13: 117–19.

49. Tonin P, Weber B, Proffit K et al. Frequency of recurrent BRCA1 and BRCA2 mutations in the Ashkenazi Jewish breast cancer families. Nat Med 1996; 11: 1179–83.

50. Lalloo F, Cochrane S, Bulman B et al. An evaluation of common breast cancer mutations within a population of Ashkenazi Jews. J Med Genet 1998; 35: 10–12.

51. Watson M, Murday V, Lloyd S et al. Genetic testing in breast/ovarian cancer (BRCA1) families. Lancet 1995; 346: 583.

52. Lerman C, Narod S, Schulman K et al. BRCA1 testing in families with hereditary breast ovarian cancer. A prospective study of patient decision making and outcomes. JAMA 1996; 275: 1928–9.

53. Binchy A, Craufurd D, Evans DGR et al. Uptake of predictive testing for BRCA1. 2001; submitted.

54. Lerman C, Daly M, Masny A, Bashem A. Attitudes about genetic testing for breast ovarian cancer susceptibility. J Clin Oncol 1994; 12: 843–50.

55. Mohammed S, Barnes C, Watts S et al. Attitudes to predictive testing for BRCA1. J Med Genet 1995; 32: 140A.

56. Eccles DM, Evans DGR, Mackay J. Guidelines for a genetic risk based approach to advising women with a family history of breast cancer. J Med Genet 2000: 37: 203–9.

4 Endocrine prevention of breast cancer

Trevor J Powles, Jenny Chang

Introduction

Breast cancer is a particularly attractive target for prevention in view of the importance of oestrogen in the development of the disease[1-3] and because there are well-established and effective anti-oestrogenic treatments, such as tamoxifen.[4] Furthermore, when used as adjuvant therapy for treatment of patients with operable breast cancer, tamoxifen has been shown to almost halve the risk of developing new contralateral breast cancer.[4]

On this basis, prevention trials were started in 1986 using tamoxifen in healthy women at increased risk of breast cancer based on a variety of risk factors.[5] These trials showed that tamoxifen had a spectrum of oestrogenic and anti-oestrogenic activity on normal tissues, including conservation of bone in postmenopausal women,[5] and tamoxifen and related triphenylethylenes are therefore now classified as selective oestrogen receptor modulators (SERMs). Around this time, another SERM, raloxifene, was under investigation for prevention of osteoporotic fractures, and in the MORE trial (see below), breast cancer incidence was included as a secondary endpoint. These early trials are nearing completion with encouraging results, and further trials have been initiated to evaluate a variety of anti-oestrogenic agents in the chemopreventive setting.

This chapter will review the original four tamoxifen trials together with those involving raloxifene and comment on new trials that are either underway or are planned.

The National Surgical Adjuvant Breast and Bowel Project (NSABP) P-1 trial

Eligibility for this trial included women with an estimated risk of breast cancer of at least 1.66 per 100 women per 5 years determined by the Gail model.[6] This incorporates age, number of previous benign breast biopsies, age at menarche and first live birth, and number of first-degree relatives with breast cancer, but excludes some details of family history. In 1998, the results of this trial were published[7] and the observed risk reduction of breast cancer, by 49% ($p = 0.0001$), was considered so striking that the trial was prematurely closed and unblinded before a full evaluation of the overall clinical benefits and risks (including mortality) could be made. This decision meant that no further randomised data from longer follow-up could be obtained from this trial, and the crucial question of whether it was better to reduce risk rather than treat as the disease arose remained uncertain.

This was particularly so because most of the 85 cancers that had not occurred in the women on tamoxifen compared with placebo were likely to be small, node-negative and oestrogen receptor (ER)-positive cancers, which would be potentially curable if they had subsequently developed. Furthermore, the toxicity of tamoxifen among the 6700 healthy women who received the drug for a total duration in excess of 3 years was more than had been anticipated, with documented increases in endometrial pathology (cancer, polyps and cysts), thromboembolism, cataracts and vasomotor symptoms.

A mathematical model was developed in an attempt to balance the observed risk reduction against the toxicity.[8] Those who gained most risk reduction appeared to be younger women who had benign pathology associated with higher-risk lesions such as lobular carcinoma in situ (LCIS) or atypical ductal hyperplasia (ADH). It was recommended that younger women at particular risk or older hysterectomised women might gain most overall benefit. However, the trial failed to show that prescribing tamoxifen for healthy women to prevent development of breast cancer was better than treating the cancers as they arose – i.e. that prevention is better than cure. Based on the results of this trial, tamoxifen was approved by the US Food and Drug Administration (FDA) for risk reduction of breast cancer in women who have a Gail risk assessment score of 1.66 per 100 women per 5 years. Such approval was not granted in Europe, where tamoxifen should only be considered for risk reduction in women with ADH or LCIS.

The Italian National Trial (INT)

Healthy women who had previously undergone a hysterectomy but otherwise possessed no special risk factors for breast cancer were eligible for this trial (74% of them had concomitant oophorectomy). Initial results were reported in 1998,[9] with an update in 2002,[10] and showed no significant overall risk reduction for breast cancer. However, there was a risk reduction for those women who had used hormone replacement therapy (HRT). Because most women had received ovarian ablation, the risk of breast cancer was generally low, which may have reduced the impact of any subsequent tamoxifen risk reduction (unless the women were also users of HRT).

The Royal Marsden Hospital Trial (RMHT)

This trial was initiated in 1986 as a pilot study. Because of the potential toxicity and side-effects of tamoxifen in healthy women, eligibility was restricted to those women deemed to be at high risk because of a strong family history of breast cancer. Trial participants were therefore younger than the average age in the other trials. Moreover, the age-corrected risk for breast cancer was about fourfold, which was higher than risk levels for women in other trials. Women with high-risk benign lesions such as LCIS or ADH were excluded. Results of this trial were reported in 1998 and showed that no risk reduction for breast cancer was conferred by tamoxifen.[11]

The International Breast Intervention Study I (IBIS-I)

Over 7000 women were randomised in this trial. The age-corrected risk for breast cancer was approximately 2–3 based on family history and other risk factors.[12] Results showed an overall risk reduction for breast cancer of about 32%, but significance was

lost when non-invasive cancers were excluded. A total of 64 invasive cancers developed in patients on tamoxifen versus 85 for those receiving placebo (relative risk (RR) 0.75 with a 95% confidence interval (CI) of 0.54–1.04). The 21 fewer invasive breast cancers that failed to occur in women on tamoxifen were estimated to be ER-positive, and mostly axillary lymph node-negative (<2 cm in diameter). If they had been allowed to develop, these tumours would mostly have been curable. The toxicity levels for this trial were comparable to those reported for the NSABP P-1 trial, raising doubts about the net clinical benefit of using tamoxifen for breast cancer risk reduction in healthy women. This is particularly important in the context of this trial, because there was a significant ($p = 0.01$) increase in overall mortality for women on tamoxifen.

The Multiple Outcomes of Raloxifene Evaluation (MORE trial)

This trial involved almost 8000 postmenopausal women with a mean age of 66.5 years. It was a requirement of the trial that women had no family history of breast cancer or a personal history of endometrial cancer. After 30 months of follow up there was a 76% reduction in the incidence of breast cancer[13,14] associated with a significant reduction in the incidence of osteoporotic fractures in the spine,[15] in serum cholesterol,[16] and in cardiac events in women at increased risk of heart disease.[17] However, there was an increase in thromboembolism and vasomotor symptoms, but no evidence of an increase in the risk of endometrial cancer, polyps, cysts or endometrial thickening. Unlike tamoxifen, raloxifene is not uterotrophic, indicating that its oestrogenic activity is relatively impeded.[18] This could account for the greater risk reduction for breast cancer in this trial compared with those observed in the tamoxifen prevention trials, with the implication that raloxifene may be more effective than tamoxifen for breast cancer risk reduction.[19] These two agents are being compared 'head to head' in the NSABP P-2 (STAR) trial, which will accrue 22 000 women with a similar Gail score to the women in the P-1 trial. If this confirms that raloxifene is the more effective agent then the next set of trials will involve a comparison of raloxifene with an aromatase inhibitor.

Overview of tamoxifen trials

A meta-analysis of outcomes from the four tamoxifen breast cancer prevention trials has been published[20] and reveals an overall risk reduction for breast cancer of 38% (95% CI 28–46%; p = 0.001). This meta-analysis addressed primary outcome (breast cancer incidence) as well as secondary outcomes (endometrial cancer incidence, vascular events and mortality).

Both endometrial cancer (RR 2.4, 95% CI 1.5–4.0) and thromboembolic events (RR 1.9, 95% CI 1.4–2.6) were increased, but cardiovascular events were similar in the two groups and there was no significant effect on mortality (RR 0.91, 95% CI 0.70–1.18). These data, together with extensive data from adjuvant tamoxifen trials,[4] suggest that mortality is not increased by tamoxifen.

Figures for breast cancer risk reduction in the four tamoxifen prevention trials are only just statistically compatible, indicating that factors other than statistical variation may account for the differences in results. It is likely that individual risk factor profiles for women in these trials are important in determining response to tamoxifen. Some risk factors are oestrogen-based while others are not. For example, in the P-1 trial, younger women with either ADH or LCIS were eligible for inclusion. These risk factors are known to be oestrogen-sensitive and could have accounted for a greater chemopreventative effect in this group of women. By contrast, in the RMHT, women with these higher-risk benign lesions were excluded. However, a high proportion of younger women who were likely to be carrying high-risk breast cancer predisposing genes were included in this trial, and it is possible that these women were more likely to develop tamoxifen-resistant cancers. The risk criteria for women in the IBIS trial were intermediate between those for the P-1 trial and the RMHT.

A 40% risk reduction for development of breast cancer attributable to tamoxifen is probably a realistic figure and is encouraging. However, the absolute number of women for whom breast cancer is prevented is modest, in comparison with the large numbers of healthy women who would need prolonged, potentially toxic treatment to achieve this.

In order for prevention of breast cancer to be worthwhile (as a clinical intervention), the efficacy of treatment must be maximised and toxicity minimised. One approach to improving overall benefit of chemoprevention is to define individual risk factors that identify those women at increased risk who are likely to gain most benefit from the use of chemopreventative agents. If those women who are unlikely to derive benefit from anti-oestrogenic intervention are eliminated from future trials, the efficacy and risk–benefit ratio for these agents will improve.

Alternatively, novel agents could be developed that are more effective and less toxic than tamoxifen. These could be used either as single agents or as combination therapy, based on a biological rationale.

Oestrogenic risk factors

The growth of most breast cancers is promoted by oestrogen, and many of the risk factors for breast cancer are likely to be oestrogen-based. These include factors such as increasing age, early menarche, late menopause, nulliparity, non-lactation, cellular atypia and LCIS, together with plasma hormone levels.[21]

As an example of an oestrogenic risk factor, high mammographic breast density is of special interest, because it does appear to be predominantly genetically determined[22–24] and is, in part, associated with increased circulating levels of oestrogen[24] or the use of HRT.[25] Furthermore, breast density is reduced by use of tamoxifen,[22,23] and this factor could be used to identify and monitor women who are suitable targets for breast cancer risk reduction using anti-oestrogens.

Ideally, a model is required that is based on independent endocrine risk factors. These include (a) breast density, (b) bone density, (c) circulating oestrogen levels, (d) menstrual, obstetric and lactational history, (e) ER-positive high-risk pathological lesions such as ADH or LCIS, and (f) the use of oral contraceptives or HRT and any other factors that may have an oestrogenic basis.

New agents

The results of the ATAC (Arimidex, Tamoxifen Alone or in Combination) trial have shown that anastrozole (Arimidex) is more effective than tamoxifen or a combination of tamoxifen and anastrozole for reducing locoregional relapse and more importantly in the prevention setting for reducing the incidence of contralateral breast cancer.[26] These results indicate that the anti-oestrogenic efficacy of tamoxifen is blunted in part by its partial agonist activity, and that a pure anti-oestrogenic intervention using an aromatase inhibitor might be more effective for risk reduction of breast cancer in healthy women. However, the very low levels of oestrogen induced by these agents might cause toxicity to normal tissues, such as bone loss with increased risk of fractures, and such sequelae have already been reported.[26] The IBIS-II multicentre trial has been initiated and is recruiting healthy women at increased risk of breast cancer for randomisation to anastrozole or placebo. Other aromatase inhibitors such as letrozole and exemestane are also likely to be considered for breast cancer prevention trials.

Alternatively, SERMs other than tamoxifen may have less oestrogenic activity due to differences in their chemical structure that may confer greater efficacy for breast cancer risk reduction. For example, tamoxifen is oestrogenic for uterine tissue, whereas raloxifene, which has a side-chain that masks a critical part of the oestrogen receptor, is not stimulatory to the uterus[18] and may be more effective for breast cancer risk reduction.[19] The encouraging results from the MORE trial support this hypothesis. The MORE trial has now continued follow-up for 8 years with use of raloxifene and results will be reported shortly. Other SERMs such as lasofoxifene are being evaluated within osteoporosis trials to determine their potential for breast cancer risk reduction.

If raloxifene proves superior to tamoxifen in the P-2 trial, a back-to-back comparison of raloxifene with anastrozole to directly compare efficacy and toxicity will be essential. As a general principle, the development of a SERM that combines enhanced risk reduction for breast cancer (less uterotrophic activity) with additional benefits in other tissues seems likely to be a more promising strategy than the use of aromatase inhibitors. The latter produce severe oestrogen depletion and are likely to have detrimental anti-oestrogenic side-effects. The complexities of 'add-on' prevention to minimise the complications of aromatase inhibitors (such as the use of bisphosphonates to prevent fractures) detracts from a preventative strategy in the context of healthy women.

Conclusions

The next generation of trials for endocrine prevention of breast cancer need to be more focused. Risk factor algorithms should be devised that identify women with a high risk for development of oestrogen-dependent cancers. Such individuals should be recruited into trials to assess the next generation of potentially more active agents. These further trials should help clarify whether there is real clinical benefit from risk reduction of breast cancer.

It is essential that these trials of chemoprevention evaluate adverse as well as favourable outcomes in order to identify longer-term overall clinical benefit. Within these prevention trials, absolute benefits are likely to be relatively small and the attendant risks

involved with large numbers of healthy women are potentially great. It should be remembered that the majority of women in these trials will never develop breast cancer.

The results of chemoprevention trials to date indicate that it may be possible in the future to effectively prevent breast cancer in a well-defined high-risk group who may receive other incidental clinical benefits with acceptable long-term toxicity. Future prevention trials of newer SERMs and aromatase inhibitors will aid in the identification of risk factors and optimal chemopreventative agents. In the meantime, the use of tamoxifen for breast cancer risk reduction in healthy women should be confined to those women who have biopsy-proven pathological changes of ADH or LCIS.

References

1. Lacassagne A. Hormonal pathogenesis of adenocarcinoma of the breast. Am J Cancer 1936; 27: 217–25.
2. Clemons M, Goss P. Estrogen and the risk of breast cancer. N Engl J Med 2001; 344: 276–85.
3. Cauley J, Lucas F, Kuller L. Elevated serum estradiol and testosterone concentrations are associated with a high risk for breast cancer: Study of Osteoporotic Fractures Research Group. Ann Intern Med 1999; 130: 270–7.
4. Early Breast Cancer Triallists' Collaborative Group. Tamoxifen for early breast cancer: an overview of the randomised trials. Lancet 1998; 351: 1451–67.
5. Powles T, Hardy JR, Ashley SE et al. A pilot trial to evaluate the acute toxicity and feasibility of tamoxifen for prevention of breast cancer. Br J Cancer 1989; 60: 126–31.
6. Gail M, Brinton LA, Byar DP et al. Projecting individualised probabilities of developing breast cancer for white females who are examined annually. J Natl Cancer Inst 1989; 81: 1879–86.
7. Fisher B, Costantino JP, Wickerham DL et al. Tamoxifen for prevention of breast cancer: report of the National Surgical Adjuvant Breast and Bowel Project P-1 Study. J Natl Cancer Inst 1998; 90: 1371–88.
8. Gail M, Costantino JP, Bryant J et al. Weighing the risks and benefits of tamoxifen treatment for preventing breast cancer. J Natl Cancer Inst 1999; 91: 1829–46.
9. Veronesi U, Maisonneure P, Costa A et al. Prevention of breast cancer with tamoxifen: preliminary findings from the Italian randomised trial among hysterectomised women. Lancet 1998; 352: 93–7.
10. Veronesi U, Maisonneure P, Sacchini V et al. Tamoxifen for breast cancer among hysterectomised women. Lancet 2002; 359: 1122–4.
11. Powles T, Eeles R, Ashley S et al. Interim analysis of the incidence of breast cancer in the Royal Marsden

Hospital tamoxifen randomised chemoprevention trial. Lancet 1998; 352: 98–101.

12. IBIS Investigators. First results from the International Breast Cancer Intervention Study (IBIS-1): a randomised prevention trial. Lancet 2002; 360: 817–24.

13. Cummings S, Eckert S, Krueger KA et al. The effect of raloxifene on risk of breast cancer in postmenopausal women. Results from the MORE randomized trial. JAMA 1999; 281: 2189–97.

14. Cauley J, Norton L, Lippman LE et al. Continued breast cancer risk reduction in postmenopausal women treated with raloxifene: 4 year results from the MORE trial: Multiple Outcomes of Raloxifene Evaluation. Breast Cancer Res Treat 2001; 65: 125–34.

15. Ettinger B, Black DM, Mitlak BH et al. Reduction of vertebral fracture risk in postmenopausal women with osteoporosis treated with raloxifene: results from a 3-year randomized clinical trial. Multiple Outcomes of Raloxifene Evaluation (MORE) Investigators. JAMA 1999; 282: 637–45.

16. Walsh B, Kuller LH, Wild RA et al. Effects of raloxifene on serum lipids and coagulation factors in healthy postmenopausal women. JAMA 1998; 279: 1445–51.

17. Barrett-Connor E, Grady D, Sashegyi A. Raloxifene and cardiovascular events in osteoporotic postmenopausal women: four-year results from the MORE (Multiple Outcomes of Raloxifene Evaluation) randomized trial. JAMA 2002; 287: 847–57.

18. Shang Y, Brown M. Molecular determinants for the tissue specificity of SERMs. Science 2002; 295: 2465–8.

19. Powles T. Anti-oestrogenic prevention of breast cancer – the make or break point. Nat Rev Cancer 2002; 2: 787–94.

20. Cuzick J, Powles T, Veronesi U et al. Overview of the main outcomes in the breast cancer prevention trials. Lancet 2003; 361: 296–300.

21. Powles TJ. Anti-oestrogenic chemoprevention of breast cancer – the need to progress. Eur J Cancer 2003; 39: 572–9.

22. Ursin G, Pike MC, Spicer DV et al. Can mammographic densities predict effects of tamoxifen on the breast? J Natl Cancer Inst 1996; 88: 128–9.

23. Atkinson C, Warren R, Bingham SA, Day NE. Mammographic patterns as a predictive biomarker of breast cancer risk: effect of tamoxifen. Cancer Epidemiol Biomarkers Prev 1999; 8: 863–6.

24. Boyd N, Dite GS, Stone J et al. Heritability of mammographic density, a risk factor for breast cancer. N Engl J Med 2002; 347: 886–94.

25. Ursin G, Astrahan M, Salane M. The detection of changes in mammographic densities. Cancer Epidemiol Biomarkers Prev 1998; 7: 43–7.

26. ATAC Trialists' Group. Anastrozole alone or in combination with tamoxifen versus tamoxifen alone for adjuvant treatment of postmenopausal women with early breast cancer: first results of the ATAC randomised trial. Lancet 2002; 359: 2131–9.

5 The biological basis for breast cancer screening and relevance to treatment

John R Benson

Introduction

The principles of screening were enunciated by the World Health Organization (WHO) in 1968[1] and formed the basis for breast screening programmes designed to detect disease before it becomes clinically apparent. The aims of screening are to prevent, delay or reduce the clinical impact of a target disease. Included amongst the preconditions for effective population screening was the assumption that the natural history of the disease in question should be 'well understood', with a recognisable early stage for which treatment initiation would lead to enhanced outcome compared with later stages. Thus there should be a preclinical phase with a consistent abnormality that is easily detectable with affordable, non-invasive methods.

Randomised controlled trials of breast cancer screening have now confirmed the efficacy of screening in women aged over 50, for whom reductions in breast cancer mortality of between 25% and 30% are attainable.[2–5] A meta-analysis of five Swedish trials revealed relative risk reductions of 29% in the 50–69 age group using mammography alone, and these are sustained after longer term follow up.[6,7] A more modest impact on mortality (a 10–18% risk reduction) is evident in women aged 40–49, but becomes apparent only after prolonged follow-up of more than 12 years.[8,9] Screening within this age group remains controversial due to compromises in planning strategies and the vagaries of statistical interpretation. The latter introduce potential biases that may either mask or create any mortality benefit.[5,10] However, despite the apparent success of screening as judged by the endpoint of population mortality, it could be argued that the aforementioned screening criteria have not been fully satisfied in relation to breast cancer. For this reason, the underlying mechanism and extent by which advancing the time of diagnosis improves the overall survival of a screened population remains unclear. Breast cancer is a heterogeneous disease, in terms both of variation among different tumours and of cellular composition within any individual tumour. This biological heterogeneity confers a variable natural history upon breast cancer, and may ultimately undermine and limit the potential impact not only of screening programmes but also of treatment schedules for breast cancer. Conservative estimates reveal a broad range of individual tumour growth rates,[11–13] with stochastic models being most applicable to breast cancer growth.[14] This limits the breadth of predictions about the growth of mammary tumours, and may hinder the design and planning of optimum schedules for breast cancer screening, where there are often 'trade-offs' between the generalisability of screening outcomes and the validity of individual trials.[5]

Biological models of breast cancer

The essence of breast cancer screening is to detect malignant lesions at an earlier stage in their natural developmental history for which instigation of appropriate therapies will lead to mortality reduction. Detection of a lesion at a smaller size per se will not necessarily impact on mortality; diagnosis of disease at an earlier chronological stage will only translate into improved outcomes if effective therapies can be instituted at this time. Otherwise, increased survival will be ascribed to 'lead time' bias, and individuals merely acquire advanced knowledge of their disease, with their date of death and hence mortality remaining unchanged.

For screening to produce a genuine improvement in survival and reduction of cause-specific mortality, there must be an event in the natural history of the disease beyond which prognosis is adversely affected, and for which there is a threshold effect reflected in the size of a detectable lesion. If a lesion progressively increased in size without any such concomitant 'event' then it would be of no consequence whether this was excised at size x or $x + 1$ provided that excision was complete.

There are two events that may occur in the natural history and progression of malignant breast lesions that could account for the efficacy of screening and provide a biological rationale for early detection strategies: (a) early dissemination and (b) phenotypic progression. Should one or both of these events occur at some stage in neoplastic development that is dependent upon tumour size then earlier detection and intervention may pre-empt the formation of micrometastases and/or a more biologically aggressive primary tumour and so lead to improved prognosis.[15] Stochastic models of tumour growth imply that such an event could occur relatively suddenly during tumour development due to a random growth 'spurt'.[14] Concepts of orderly progression may be deceptive – tumours can disseminate prior to reaching thresholds of either mammographic detection or clinical presentation.[13,16]

There are two dominant paradigms of breast cancer biology that have governed the management of breast cancer over the past century: the Halstedian paradigm and that of biological predeterminism. Although the latter has become pre-eminent in recent years, both are relevant to the philosophy of breast screening, and indeed an intermediate paradigm may be most appropriate contemporaneously.

Halstedian paradigm

Virchow proposed a centrifugal theory for the dissemination of breast cancer in which a tumour was considered initially to invade local tissues and subsequently spread in a progressive, sequential and predictable manner upon ever more distant structures that lay in anatomical continuity.[17,18] The lymph nodes were thought to act as mechanical filters that formed a circumferential line of defence against such centrifugal dissemination and temporarily impeded the spread of cancer. However, once this filtration capacity was exhausted, cancer cells would then pass into efferent lymphatics and thence to more distant sites. This model provided the rationale for the Halsted radical mastectomy, in

which an en bloc resection of tumour and loco-regional tissues was performed.[19] As a tumour was believed to spread in a sequential manner with successive involvement of structures in anatomical continuity, such en bloc resection was considered to offer the best chance of 'cure'. Although the operation of radical mastectomy provided high rates of local disease control,[20] there was no evidence for improved survival relative to lesser surgical procedures.[21] This implied that some 'event' had occurred prior to mastectomy that predetermined survival and was unaffected by surgical intervention per se. Analysis of survival data for patients undergoing radical mastectomy revealed that fewer than a quarter of these patients shared a similar hazard ratio as an age-matched control population.[22] Therefore radical mastectomy could not be hailed as a general curative procedure for breast cancer, and fostered some doubt in the underlying paradigm.

Biological predeterminism

Fisher[23] proposed an alternative paradigm that challenged the concept of progressive centrifugal spread according to anatomical and mechanical criteria. Instead, breast cancer was considered to be largely a systemic disease at the outset as a consequence of cancer cells entering the bloodstream at an early stage in tumour development. In particular, such haematogenous dissemination was not conditional upon lymph node involvement, and regional lymph nodes were not viewed as the instigators of distant metastases. Rather, they reflected a tumour–host relationship that favoured dissemination. Experimental models were employed to demonstrate transnodal passage of tumour cells[24] together with destruction of tumour cells by lymph nodes. These findings repudiated the concept of lymph nodes as passive filters,[25,26] and showed that cancer cells could pass not only directly into efferent lymphatics, but also into the bloodstream via lymphaticovenous communications. Furthermore, animal models had shown that dormant tumour cells could develop into overt metastases under appropriate conditions. These experimental observations formed the basis for an alternative paradigm of biological predeterminism in which cancer is viewed as a predominantly systemic disease at inception, with clinical outcome being predetermined by micrometastases present at the time of diagnosis. Prognosis is ultimately determined by the propensity for these micrometastases to develop into overt metastatic disease.

There are important consequences of this hypothesis that have implications both for the potential efficacy of any screening programme and for treatment strategies. In terms of therapeutic sequelae, this paradigm of biological predeterminism would predict that the extent of primary surgery does not influence overall survival, as the latter is dependent upon micrometastases that are present in all patients irrespective of surgical treatment. Trials of breast conservation surgery have confirmed that lesser surgical resections do not compromise overall survival, although they are associated with higher rates of local recurrence.[27–30] The Guy's Hospital trial showed that for patients with stage I disease, overall survival was similar in patients undergoing radical mastectomy and chest wall irradiation compared with wide local excision with breast irradiation. However, stage II patients had a higher incidence of distant metastases and a corresponding reduced survival.[27] Subsequent trials found no difference in overall survival for either stage I or II disease. Fisher's group compared total mastectomy with lumpectomy either with or without breast irradiation. Although survival rates were similar in all groups, local relapse was much higher in the non-irradiated breast conservation group.[28] Veronesi et al[29] compared mastectomy with quadrantectomy, axillary dissection and radiotherapy (QUART) for small tumours (≤2.5 cm). Once again, this trial and other smaller ones[30] confirmed that overall survival rates were not influenced by the extent of primary surgery, and supported the notion of predeterminism based on subclinical dissemination of micrometastases.

The second therapeutic sequela of this hypothesis is that initiation of systemic therapies that could destroy these putative micrometastases should improve prognosis. This aspect of treatment would therefore be complementary to locoregional therapy

(surgery with or without radiotherapy). Clinical trials of adjuvant therapy for breast cancer have provided corroborative evidence for the second prediction of this alternative paradigm.[31] In 1992, the Early Breast Cancer Trialists Collaborative Group (EBCTCG) published the results of a 10-year overview of adjuvant trials of endocrine and chemotherapy involving a total of 75 000 women.[32] Adjuvant polychemotherapy reduced the annual risk of disease recurrence by 28% and mortality by 17% in an unselected group of breast cancer patients. Similarly, adjuvant tamoxifen therapy was most effective in the over-50 age group, where the risk of local recurrence was reduced by 30% and mortality by 19%. The most recent overview of trials of adjuvant tamoxifen therapy has revealed that the proportional reductions in local recurrence and mortality are principally dependent upon oestrogen receptor (ER) status, with benefits being largely confined to ER-positive (and ER-unknown) tumours and irrespective of age, menopausal and nodal status[33] (see Figure 5.1).

Application of models to breast screening

The above evidence, together with data on the clinical outcome of stage I and II breast cancer, indicates that micrometastases are present in over 50% of cases of 'early' breast cancer at the time of clinical diagnosis. If one adopts the philosophy that all breast cancer is systemic at the outset, then any screening programme is doomed to failure, as earlier detection and treatment of a primary lesion will not reduce mortality if survival has already been predetermined by early dissemination and the presence of micrometastatic disease at the time of preclinical detection of breast cancer.

To date, there is no conclusive evidence for any subgroup of breast cancer patients who have been 'cured' as defined by either statistical or clinical criteria[34]. Statistical cure[35] can only be claimed if after prolonged follow-up a subgroup of patients are found to have an annual death rate from all causes that is identical to an age-matched control population. Several studies, including that of Brinkley and Haybittle,[36] have identified subgroups whose survival approximates to that of a control group, but in none of these has the ratio of observed to expected deaths been unity.[36–38] Similarly, there is no evidence for a clinically cured group who are deemed to have no increased relative risk of subsequently dying from breast cancer. Most studies reveal that all groups of treated patients remain at relatively increased risk of death from breast cancer and also of developing a contralateral cancer.[36,37,39]

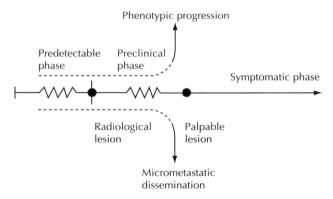

Figure 5.1 Schematic representation of sequential development of a tumour through pre-detectable, pre-clinical and symptomatic phases. Though these are time dependent and a function of absolute tumour size, formation of distant metastases and phenotypic progression have an unpredictable and non-obligate relationship to size and therefore phase of neoplastic development. When these two processes occur in the pre-clinical phase (after radiological detection) then screening offers the potential for mortality reduction.

Although 'cure' cannot so far be claimed on strict statistical criteria, there are reports that purport to define subgroups with a highly favourable prognosis who may be effectively cured. This particularly applies to small tumours and may have some bearing on screening. Thus Hayward has analysed long-term follow-up of stage I and II patients treated at Guy's Hospital by mastectomy.[40] Some of these have attained hazard ratios approaching, although not identical to, those of an age-matched control population. Similarly, patients with a Nottingham Prognostic Index (NPI)[41] of less than or equal to 3 have been declared to have equivalent survival to a control population. Sigurdsson and colleagues[42] analysed prognostic factors (percentage S phase, progesterone receptor (PgR) and tumour size) in stage I patients within a screening programme and described a subgroup of approximately 30% who would have a calculated relative survival of 100%.

Notwithstanding the pre-eminence of biological predeterminism, it is implicit from a breast screening programme that a substantial proportion of patients are potentially curable by earlier detection. If it is believed that screening can genuinely reduce mortality then it probably has to be accepted that all breast cancer is not systemic at the outset. Nonetheless, it is assumed that dissemination and establishment of viable micrometastases can occur during the preclinical phase when a breast cancer is mammographically detectable. The crucial question is what proportion of tumours disseminate between the time of radiological detection and clinical presentation. In other words, what proportion of cancers can be successfully detected mammographically *before* any development of micrometastases? Is there a threshold of tumour size above which dissemination occurs? As breast cancer is a heterogeneous disease, the answer to this question is unlikely to be consensual, with a range of sizes rather than a single threshold value. This issue of the stage at which microscopic dissemination occurs is embodied in the emerging concept of an 'intermediate' paradigm; some tumours behave in a Halstedian manner and can be 'cured' by locoregional treatment. The chances of cure are enhanced by earlier detection, and these tumours would benefit from screening. Other tumours tend to disseminate early and become systemic during either the preclinical or predetection phases of growth. Screening strategies will only be successful if detection occurs prior to the development of micrometastases. A tumour requires a blood supply to grow beyond the size of a million cells (a few cubic millimetres),[43] but it is quite feasible to propose that a tumour can possess an established vasculature without necessarily showing vascular invasion at these early stages of tumour development. Furthermore, cancer cells could travel to the regional lymph nodes and remain there without entering the circulation via lymphaticovenous communications. In both of these scenarios, cure could theoretically be achieved by excision of tumour and regional nodes. Patients with microscopic nodal deposits on conventional H&E criteria have been reported to have a similar prognosis to node-negative cases, although this remains a controversial area.[44–48]

Even if tumour cells gain access to the circulation at a very early stage, these may not necessarily develop into viable micrometastatic foci. The host immune system can destroy rogue cancer cells within the bloodstream, and successful establishment of micrometastases will depend upon innate biological properties of the tumour cells, as well as local host factors. From a clinical perspective, it is of greater significance to ascertain the earliest stage in tumour development at which viable metastatic foci can form. Screening programmes would aim to maximize radiological sensitivity and specificity and hence the capacity to detect lesions before this clinical dissemination occurred. The smallest lesion that can be detected mammographically with state-of-the-art technology is approximately 2–3 mm. By the time a tumour has attained this size, it will probably contain over 1 million cells and therefore have already entered the vascular phase of growth.[49] In experimental models, tumours reach a maximum size of only 1–2 mm in the absence of vascularisation, although growth rapidly accelerates upon induction of a vasculature that provides nutritional support for the tumour cells.[43] Despite the tendency for new blood vessels to be 'leaky',[50] it does not follow that vascular invasion is an obligate phenomenon once neovascularisation has occurred. The downregulation of integrin expression and alterations in the cellular profile of other cell adhesion molecules (CAMs) will determine not only the tendency of cells to break away from the tumour bolus and enter the circulation, but also for these self-same cells to harbour at distant sites with formation of micrometastatic foci.[51] Therefore detection by screening of smaller tumours that are in the vascular phase of growth could still precede systemic dissemination. Ideally, screening should pick up tumours while they are still in the prevascular phase where growth is relatively slower and there is no opportunity for haematogenous spread. However, such lesions are unlikely to have any radiological 'signature', which is dependent upon induction of a stromal response in the vicinity of tumour cells.

It was stated in the introductory section that the efficacy of screening could be accounted for by two possible mechanisms. In addition to detection of tumours prior to any systemic dissemination, screening might also pick up tumours with a more favourable grade and biological credentials. There is some evidence that the malignant phenotype evolves and becomes more 'aggressive' as a tumour grows,[52] although this remains controversial and unproven.[53] If cancers can progress to less well-differentiated forms then screening might improve prognosis if it permitted detection and removal of lesions prior to any histological progression.

Relationship between reduction of mortality and changes in size and stage distribution of screen-detected tumours

So to what extent can screening reduce tumour size, and is such a reduction in the size of tumours per se related to prognosis? Screening is associated with a reduction in the proportion of larger tumours and metastatic lesions.[4,54,55] This section examines how improvements in survival among patients with screen-detected cancers can be accounted for by changes in conventional prognostic indices and whether screening can detect lesions prior to any dissemination.

Lymph node status remains the most accurate prognostic indicator for breast cancer,[56,57] and has yet to be succeeded by newer biological indices such as ploidy, percentage S phase and abnormal gene expression. Survival is closely correlated with the number of lymph nodes infiltrated by tumour. If there is no axillary nodal involvement then 5-year survival rates are of the order of 80–90%, falling to approximately 65% if up to three nodes are positive and 30% if four or more nodes are affected. Prognosis is particularly poor if more than 10 nodes are positive.[57] By implication, lymph node status is an indirect indicator of the likelihood of micrometastatic foci pre-existing at the time of primary surgery. Tumour size is related both to lymph node status and to the risk of distant metastases,[58–60] and there is provisional evidence that a similar relationship appertains to screen-detected lesions.[55]

In the Swedish Two-County Trial,[61] there was a significant reduction in both size and nodal status of screen-detected invasive cancers. More than half of the tumours were less than 15 mm in diameter and 80% were node-negative. Comparison of tumour size with the control group revealed a 26% reduction in tumours more than 20 mm in size and a 40% reduction in those over 30 mm. The observed incidence of node negativity represented a 24% reduction in the proportion of patients with positive nodes. This reduction in tumour size and node

positivity was paralleled by an improved survival, presumably reflecting a lower incidence of micrometastases in these screened breast cancer patients.

Hatschek and colleagues reported a very favourable reduction of node positivity for invasive tumours detected in incidence screens from 40% (controls) to 18%, and an increase in small tumours (≤20 mm) from 59% to 85%.[62] Of interest, in the Edinburgh trial, the node positivity rate remained high for the incidence rounds (28%) and only half of invasive tumours detected were 20 mm or smaller. As might be expected, this study found more favourable effects on tumour size, lymph node status and histology in the prevalence round, but this was not sustained for the incidence round.[63] Prevalence screens are innately biased towards tumours with better prognostic indices,[64] and there has been some criticism of studies based exclusively on prevalence data.[65,66] Crisp and colleagues[66] reported a higher proportion of smaller tumours with less lymph node involvement in a population of 131 screen-detected compared with clinical tumours (7.4 tumours per 1000 women screened). Furthermore, these authors translated these data into predictions of survival using the NPI and concluded that screening conferred a survival advantage of 26.5% at 5 years, consistent with the 30% reduction in mortality.

These data suggest that screening can lead to a change in the stage distribution of invasive breast cancers. This so-called 'stage drift' may represent detection of cancers at an earlier biological stage. However, the relationship between reduction in tumour size and lymph node positivity may be more complex in the context of screen-detected lesions; an increased proportion of smaller tumours may not necessarily be accompanied by predicted changes in nodal status based on data from clinical tumours. Following the introduction of a mass screening programme in Colorado involving over 15 000 patients, Abernathy and colleagues[67] reported that there was an increase of approximately 20% in the fraction of tumours smaller than 2 cm. However, an interesting finding of this study was an increase in the proportion of tumours between 2 cm and 5 cm with positive lymph nodes. At first, this anomalous result might appear to indicate a reversed stage drift! The authors have suggested that screening detects lesions at a smaller size, and facilitates their removal before they can develop into node-negative tumours within this size range. This implies that increasing tumour size does not invariably lead to a stage shift involving a progression to node positivity. Screening will tend to be biased towards these node-negative tumours because they are likely to be slower growing – i.e. length time bias. Therefore the effects of screening on nodal status and hence precise stage distribution may be inherently more complex than previously thought.

Even if there is a genuine stage shift,[68] screening methods must ultimately be capable of detecting lesions prior to any haematogenous dissemination; node negativity does not equate with absence of micrometastases, but rather reflects a relationship between tumour and host in which the chances of dissemination are minimised.[23] The goal of screening practice is therefore not to achieve stage I status per se, but to detect tumours at a size that precedes the threshold for haematogenous dissemination. The fundamental problem is that this threshold size will vary between tumours, and the precise proportion of lesions that are detected at this predissemination stage will be dictated not only by the natural history of individual tumours, but also by technical nuances of mammographic screening. There are no specific mammographic features that correlate with the biological behaviour of an invasive tumour and its propensity to metastasize, although some correlation between mammographic densities and increased risk of non-invasive proliferative lesions has been reported.[69] Screening provides information on the size and local extent of a tumour only. Techniques, including DNA microarrays, are currently being developed to extract maximal prognostic information from tissue biopsy samples, and these may help predict which screen-detected lesions are likely to have already metastasised.

The above studies on screen-detected lesions have revealed changes in distribution not only of tumour size and nodal status, but also of histological type and grade. Some studies claiming that breast screening detects less-aggressive cancers have been confined to prevalence screens only, and should perhaps be interpreted with caution.[65] Nonetheless, others have found a persistent change in the histological grade and 'malignant potential' of incidence screen-detected tumours.[61,63,66,70,71] Indeed, in the Swedish Two-County Trial referred to above, improved survival could not entirely be accounted for by reductions in tumour size and the proportion of node-positive tumours. Screen-detected tumours were also of more favourable histological grade, and when taken together with these other two factors, differences in survival between screened and control groups could be fully accounted for.[72]

Most studies have revealed a significantly higher proportion of special tumour types among screen-detected lesions compared with symptomatic cancers.[63,66,71,73] Approximately 8% of the latter are of special histological type, while these have constituted between 12.5% and 25% of screen-detected invasive lesions. The value of 12.5% reported by Crisp and colleagues[67] is significantly lower than others quoted, which are on average approximately 20%.[63,74] Of interest, in an analysis of breast cancer histology and age, Wicks and colleagues[74] found the highest incidence of tubular carcinomas in the age group corresponding to the screened population (50–69 years). Anderson and colleagues[63] found a difference in the proportion of special and variant tumours compared with 'no special type' (or not otherwise specified, NOS) in prevalence versus incidence screens, and surmised that this might reflect a natural progression of lesions to less well-differentiated forms. In their analysis of the Swedish Two-County Trial, Duffy and colleagues[52] noted a much lower proportion of high-grade (III) tumours among smaller screen-detected lesions. By comparing size and grade of malignancy in the control and 'unbiased' screen-detected groups, the expected distribution corresponded with the observed, demonstrating that any differences in grade distribution were attributable to size only – an effect therefore independent of length bias. These authors concluded that malignancy grade evolves (i.e. worsens) as a tumour enlarges. Grade of malignancy was considered to represent an underlying variable that faithfully reflected 'malignant potential'. However, grade is a surrogate marker for the latter, which ideally should be measured by some biological index relating directly to proliferative activity.

The concept of phenotypic progression is supported by the known heterogeneity of tumours. Thus different cell populations within a single tumour would have variable biological behaviour and growth characteristics. Up to one-third of breast cancers have foci of more than one histological type.[75] Variations in nuclear grade and degrees of pleiomorphism are frequently observed within the same tumour. Furthermore, in vitro studies with thymidine labelling have revealed a wide variation in indices of proliferative potential between cells derived from a single tumour.[76] Curiously, Ponten and colleagues[77] carried out extensive DNA ploidy studies on incidence screen-detected cancers and reported no differences in ploidy profiles between screen-detected and clinical cancers. However, DNA ploidy has been reported to display less intra-tumoral variation than these other proliferative indices.[78] Hakama and colleagues[53] analysed the aggressiveness of cancers among a screened population using DNA index (ploidy) and S-phase fraction. On these criteria of proliferative indices alone (and not inclusive of histological data), cancers detected in the prevalence round were of lower malignant potential. However, in subsequent incidence rounds, the level of aggressiveness was similar in control and screened groups, suggesting that 'biological aggressiveness' did not increase during the preclinical phase of tumour development. By contrast, screen-detected lesions in this study were of smaller size and more favourable stage than controls, this being predictive of a future reduction in mortality from population screening.[53]

Patterns of growth in the preclinical phase

The concept of malignant progression during the preclinical phase when lesions are impalpable yet detectable mammographically is attractive, and offers a further explanation for the potential efficacy of breast screening programmes in reducing mortality. To some extent, this phenomenon is related to the issue of preclinical dissemination; tumours with greater malignant potential are more likely to metastasize. The proportion of cells within a tumour with the capacity to invade blood vessels, travel in the circulation and establish viable micrometastases will increase with progression to a more malignant phenotype. The latter may be manifest by enhanced activity at several steps in the process of invasion and metastasis.

Therefore screening could improve prognosis by detecting lesions of smaller size that are better differentiated, of lower metastatic potential and less likely to have already disseminated. Such lesions could be cured by appropriate locoregional treatment, and systemic therapy would not be indicated, as micrometastases would theoretically be non-existent.

The issue of whether a subgroup of patients with truly localised breast cancer exists is controversial. Moreover, such a subgroup may only represent a small proportion of all screen-detected lesions and therefore have little impact overall on the screened population as a whole. The locoregional containment of disease in some patients is supported by the results of two randomised trials investigating the value of postoperative radiotherapy in patients undergoing mastectomy and adjuvant chemotherapy. The selective use of radiotherapy in a subgroup of premenopausal node-positive women is associated with gains in overall survival of approximately one-third, which compares favourably with the relative benefits of adjuvant systemic therapies and breast cancer screening.[79,80] Effective irradiation of locoregional disease at the time of primary treatment may prevent any persistent disease, or 'oligometastases' becoming the source of distant disease.[81]

In view of the apparent efficacy of screening programmes to date, it might be argued that screening detects not only those lesions that are predissemination, but also some that have already metastasised with a minimal micrometastatic load. Results of adjuvant systemic therapy trials reveal that absolute benefits from such therapies are relatively modest, being of the order of 5–10%. However, in a preclinical setting with a small primary tumour, adjuvant therapies may be much more effective against a lighter micrometastatic burden, and complete elimination of all distant foci of disease may be possible. Thus efficacy of screening may not be confined to strictly 'Halstedian' tumours, but may be effective in a subgroup of systemic or 'Fisherian' tumours that have a minimal micrometastatic component. Micrometastases demonstrate a Gompertzian pattern of growth, with an inverse relationship between rates of cell division and size. By virtue of higher rates of cell cycling, these smaller foci of micrometastases are more sensitive to the effects of chemotherapy, and total eradication is more likely.[14,82] Animal tumour models confirm this quantitative relationship between tumour burden and the efficacy of chemotherapy, with tumour doubling times ranging from 2 to 10 days, depending on the size of micrometastases.[83] A Gompertzian model appears consistent with the clinical impression that smaller tumours grow more rapidly and rates of growth decrease progressively as a tumour enlarges. Nonetheless, Speer and colleagues[14] have proposed an amended stochastic model for breast cancer growth; tumours are considered to grow in 'spurts' with random, spontaneous changes in growth rate from time to time. A series of random episodes of mini-Gompertzian growth results cumulatively in a stepwise pattern of growth with an average predetection growth period of 8 years. The random nature of these events accounts for the heterogeneity of breast cancer and a broad spectrum of 'sojourn periods'. Furthermore, during periods of reduced proliferative activity, tumours would be relatively resistant to adjuvant chemotherapy due to lower rates of cell cycling.[14]

As mentioned above, screening is inherently biased towards slowly growing, less aggressive tumours. These have a longer sojourn period and hence are less likely to grow to clinically detectable size prior to screen detection. There is much natural variance in the growth rates of breast cancer within the preclinical phase. Innate rates of growth are a critical aspect of the natural history of this disease and are determined by a combination of time-dependent processes, including cell cycle time, nutritional factors (vascular supply) and host immune response. Heuser and colleagues[84] detected measurable growth in 23 out of 32 primary breast cancers on serial mammograms spaced 88–730 days apart. Of interest, the remaining nine tumours showed no measurable growth on the basis of changes in tumour nucleus shadows identified retrospectively. Estimates of tumour volume doubling times ranged from 109 days to 944 days, with a mean of 325 days, when calculated from serial mammograms on the assumption that tumours are oblate spheroids. The authors concluded that tumour growth rates were dichotomised into slowly and rapidly growing subsets, with the latter being more likely to be associated with node-positive disease (34%) than slowly growing tumours (16%). This difference was statistically significant, suggesting that a more malignant phenotype is ascribable to rapidly growing tumours.[84] Within the slowly growing subset, some tumours would grow so slowly that they would never reach a clinically significant size in the patient's lifetime, while a proportion of the rapidly growing lesions would surface within 12 months of a previous negative screening mammogram – i.e. an interval cancer. Thus screening programmes would tend to be skewed in favour of more slowly growing tumours – so-called length bias. These tumour doubling times were calculated for tumours that were mammographically detectable although still in the preclinical phase of growth. The 'sojourn period' usually refers to the time interval between a tumour being detected mammographically and its symptomatic presentation. The sojourn period has also been considered to represent the predetectable phase of growth, i.e. from tumour induction as a single cell to the point of actual mammographic detection.[13] This period is perhaps more appropriately referred to as the 'presojourn' period and is a theoretical time interval that cannot be measured for any individual tumour. However, Spratt and colleagues[13] attempted to estimate growth rates within this predetectable phase of growth using a modified definition of sojourn time – the time between a tumour first becoming mammographically visible (assuming a patient to be screened just as a tumour reached a threshold size for detection) and the moment when the tumour was actually detected mammographically. These estimates of sojourn times could be derived from the ratio of prevalence to incidence rates within the Breast Cancer Detection and Demonstration Project (BCDDP), and values ranged from 365 to 1383 days within the age group 35–74 years. Tumour doubling times could be calculated by dividing sojourn times by the number of net cell doublings required for growth from a threshold to size at mammographic detection. Doubling times were variable and dependent upon both stage at detection and age of the patient, ranging from approximately 50 days in the age range 35–39 years to 150 days by age 70 years.[13] These tumour doubling times are significantly shorter than estimates for tumours in the preclinical phase,[84] and therefore doubling times for tumours that are large enough to be mammographically detectable are longer than estimated doubling times in the predetection phase. Thus many cancers appear to grow more rapidly in the pre-detectable phase of growth and some will inevitably present clinically as interval cancers between screens.

Moreover, these variable rates of growth and proliferative activity in the predetectable phase of breast cancer development portends that some tumours have properties that favour early dissemination and/or phenotypic progression prior to the threshold size for radiological detection.

Interval cancers

These variable growth rates of breast cancer are of relevance to interval cancers, which constitute a heterogeneous group of lesions. These cancers are by definition detected within 24 months of a negative mammogram, and a distinction must be made between cancers present but missed for whatever reason and rapidly growing cancers that were not mammographically detectable at the time of the last screen. The overall proportion of cancers missed on screening mammograms (total interval cancer rate) ranges from 10% to 30% after the first year of screening,[85–87] and within the NHS Breast Screening Programme (NHSBSP) they represent more than 80% of cancers detected in the third year of screening.[88]

There are three reasons why a cancer may not have been evident on a previous mammogram. First, some cancers are missed due to errors of interpretation or suboptimal technical quality (approximately 30%).[89–91] Secondly, there is a group of 'masked' cancers that are mammographically occult due either to patient factors such as age or breast density or to tumour characteristics such as particular histological types. Thus lobular tumours spread diffusely and elicit minimal stromal reaction while mucinous tumours contain lakes of mucin that are poorly imaged with mammography.[90,92,93] Finally, there are true interval cancers that appear to be rapidly growing and have arisen de novo since the last screen.[94] These cancers would be expected to be more aggressive and fatal than screen-detected lesions, and their failure to be detected at an earlier stage by screening could undermine the potential for screening programmes to reduce mortality. The term 'de novo' in this context refers to a tumour that was either non-existent (preinduction) or in a mammographically undetectable phase of growth at the time of a previous screen. In the latter scenario, although tumour induction has occurred and growth rates are relatively high, the tumour bolus remains small due to there being few net cell doublings and there is no radiological correlate. Often masked lesions are classified with true interval cancers, as the distinction can be blurred. Both lesions are invisible on mammography, but true interval cancers are below the threshold size for detection (2 mm) while masked lesions are larger than this. The true interval cancer rate varies from 3% to 17%[94–96] and is the number of interval cancers expressed as a proportion of the total cancers detected during a screening interval. In their analysis of tumour growth rates, Spratt and colleagues[11] estimated that more than 4% of cancers could grow from a threshold size of 2 mm to a clinically palpable size of 10 mm in a 12-month period and hence present as interval surfacing cancers within a year of a negative mammogram. Porter and others[96–98] have concluded that 'true' interval cancers represented 65–75% of interval surfacing cancers. Furthermore, there is now evidence that true interval cancers are biologically more aggressive than screen-detected lesions, with higher intrinsic growth rates and proliferative indices when adjustments for size and age are made.[97,99,100] Thus interval cancers are more likely to be of higher histological[96,101] and nuclear grade,[96] to be ER- and PgR-negative, and to be associated with increased proliferative indices such as percentage S phase fraction,[53,96,97,99,102] aneuploidy,[53,99,102] Ki67[96] and mitotic counts.[96] Measurements of proliferative activity per se should be interpreted with caution, as these only apply to a single time point and rates for any individual tumour are variable (stochastic growth). When time to diagnosis is taken into account and adjustment made for tumour size, interval cancers are no more likely to be node-positive than their screen-detected counterparts.

The implication of these studies comparing histological and prognostic features of interval and screen-detected lesions is that the former represent a group of biologically aggressive tumours that arise following previous screening and grow rapidly between screens. There is evidence that these histological features per se may reduce radiological detectability.[103] Thus a proportion of these true interval cancers may indeed be 'masked' lesions and may actually be present at the time of previous mammography rather than genuinely arising de novo (see above). Nonetheless, they possess the innate properties of rapid growth and propensity to metastasise and tend to be more common in younger women.[101] These interval cancers constitute a significant proportion of mammographic failures and the balance of evidence is that they have a poorer outcome.[72,104] This relatively high frequency coupled with a worse prognosis may limit the impact of screening on mortality reduction.[105,106]

Prospects for further reductions of mortality from breast cancer screening

An increased frequency of screening could increase the proportion of screen-detected cancers and possibly reduce the numbers of rapidly growing interval cancers, although of necessity those growing most rapidly will be the last to be detected as the screening interval is reduced. Mortality reductions may therefore be correspondingly limited. Moreover, the prognosis of these rapidly growing tumours is probably more dependent upon innate biological parameters than earlier detection at a smaller size. Many of these tumours may indeed be aggressive from the outset, rather than as a consequence of any phenotypic drift. More frequent screening would reduce the average size of screen-detected tumours, which in turn increases the chance of detecting lesions prior to both systemic dissemination and any progression to a more aggressive phenotype. Further clinical trials are required to clarify the relative benefits of reducing the screening interval to establish 'equipoise' with maximal sensitivity and specificity of mammography and optimal cost-effectiveness of screening programmes.[107] Screening schedules and even modality may have to be modified depending on patient characteristics; mammography is of lower sensitivity in younger women and those with a positive family history of breast cancer.[108,109] Interestingly, a small study has suggested that palpable tumours in BRCA1 mutation carriers are less readily detectable on mammography.[110] This may also apply to impalpable lesions in BRCA1 carriers and would accord with the lower sensitivity of mammography in patients with a family history of breast cancer. Furthermore, interval cancers share a similar histological phenotype to tumours arising in BRCA1 and BRCA2 carriers,[111] and these features may render mammographic detection more difficult.[112] There is indirect evidence that hormone replacement therapy (HRT) usage may reduce the sensitivity of screening mammography, with a resultant increase in the numbers of missed cancers. A higher proportion of patients developing interval cancers within the first round of screening were reported to be current users of HRT (33%) compared with those women with screen-detected cancers (16%).[113] An increasing number of women in Western societies are now taking HRT (30–35%), and this may impact on the efficacy of screening programmes.

Carcinoma in situ

Discussion has hitherto been restricted to invasive forms of breast cancer, as these are ultimately responsible for mortality. However, with the advent of breast cancer screening, non-invasive disease has acquired increasing prominence, with ductal carcinoma in situ (DCIS), alone or in association with micro-invasion, now representing approximately 20–25% of all screen-detected cancers.[114] By contrast, in the prescreening era, only 2–5% of clinical (symptomatic) cancers represented DCIS, while 14% of all new cases of breast cancer are now exclusively in situ disease.[115]

Although screening is effective at detecting DCIS on account of commonly associated microcalcification, it is currently unknown to what extent this will influence trends in mortality. Not all cases of DCIS will progress to invasive disease, and estimates for this proportion range from 25% to 50%, depending partly on the grade of the lesion.[116] Reports on the incidence of DCIS in routine autopsy studies (15–39%)[117,118] suggest that some non-invasive lesions that are detected mammographically and subsequently excised with either complete or partial mastectomy would have been of no clinical consequence to the patient during their lifetime. This raises the issue of 'non-obligate progression' and the resulting uncertainties,[119] and poses problems in terms of both the biological behaviour of non-invasive disease and clinical management. Screening programmes might effectively result in a 'reservoir' of indolent non-progressive DCIS being tapped into mammographically.[120] Once detected, clinicians are obliged to treat this disease – and herein lies the predicament, as this is almost invariably (99%) treated surgically.[121] Undoubtedly, some patients with low-grade DCIS will undergo surgery for a condition that would not have progressed pathologically to clinical significance. This so-called 'pseudodisease' could potentially lead to overdiagnosis within a screening programme and undermine its overall benefits.[122] This applies particularly to women in the age group 40–49 years, where DCIS constitutes a higher proportion of all newly diagnosed breast cancers. However, this may result in a delayed mortality reduction in older age groups, in whom there will be a reduction in the number of cases of invasive disease that have progressed from earlier DCIS lesions (higher grade) that have been appropriately treated. By implication, if only 25–50% of DCIS progress to invasive disease then 50–75% of cases fail to do so and therefore pose no clinical threat to patients. Furthermore, within the older age group, life expectancy is likely to be determined not by a diagnosis of DCIS but by competing causes (e.g. atherosclerotic disease).[123]

Evidence to date suggests that screening programmes have not encouraged overdiagnosis when analysis is confined to invasive tumours. However, until more is learnt about carcinoma in situ and its relationship to the natural history of breast cancer, this claim cannot be extended to non-invasive disease. As DCIS may constitute up to a quarter of all screen-detected lesions, this justifies some concern regarding both overdiagnosis and 'excessive' treatment.[122] Insight into the natural history of DCIS can only be gleaned from limited data derived from retrospective studies. Techniques such as genetic fingerprinting may help predict the biological behaviour of individual tumours and permit the identification of cases that are of clinical consequence.

Conclusion

This chapter has discussed the scientific rationale for breast screening in the context of proposed paradigms of breast cancer biology. Ironically, the philosophy of screening is something of an anathema to the paradigm of biological predeterminism according to its strictly orthodox dictates. A screening programme cannot be applied to a disease that is invariably systemic at the outset.

If it is accepted that screening is effective in reducing mortality in certain age groups then there must be a finite growth period for breast cancers during which disease is localised to the breast with no haematogenous dissemination. A corollary of this is that development of micrometastases can occur between the time of screen detection and the clinical presentation of a cancer.

Analysis of survival curves for breast cancer patients over prolonged periods of follow-up has revealed no evidence for a 'cure' in any subgroup according to statistical criteria. However, just as adjuvant treatment can extend life for patients with clinical breast cancer, so too may early detection by screening achieve a 'personal cure' whereby disease-free survival is prolonged to a point at which a patient dies of a concomitant condition unrelated to breast cancer. Even if cure is not achieved in the statistical sense, this would be of no consequence to individual patients under these circumstances.

The capacity of any screening modality to reduce mortality is dependent upon the frequency of screening. A crucial consideration with breast cancer screening programmes is the potential for improving prognosis as the screening interval is contracted. An increased frequency of screening will reduce the average size of tumours, but it is difficult to predict how this will translate into a reduction in mortality consequent to removal of a lesion prior to microscopic dissemination and phenotypic progression. Interval cancers can be minimised, although not eliminated from a screening programme, and those that are refractory to manipulation of screening schedules are likely to be have the highest growth rates and to be of worse prognosis. Conversely, up to 15% of tumours exhibit such slow growth kinetics that mammographic detection at a smaller size would confer no survival gain.[11] This extreme variability in growth rates of breast cancers, coupled with the stochastic character of tumour growth, may fundamentally limit the impact of screening strategies. Furthermore, any clinical benefits must be balanced against financial constraints in order to retain a cost-effective screening programme for the population as a whole.

However cogent are theories that offer a biological rationale, breast cancer screening remains an issue of contention with the fundamental assertions of screening having been challenged.[124,125] Although some of these criticisms are flawed,[7,126] the case for indefinite mass screening in terms of overall clinical efficacy relative to cost remains unproven.[127–129]

References

1. Wilson JMG, Junger G. Principles and Practice of Screening for Disease (Public Health Paper No. 34). Geneva: World Health Organization, 1968.

2. Shapiro S, Venet W, Strax P et al. Ten- to fourteen-year effect of screening on breast cancer mortality. J Natl Cancer Inst 1982; 69: 349.

3. Tabar L, Fagerberg CJG, Gad A et al. Reduction in mortality from breast cancer after mass screening with mammography. Lancet 1985; i: 829.

4. Fletcher SW, Black W, Harris R et al. Report of the International Workshop on Screening for Breast Cancer. J Natl Cancer Inst 1993; 85: 1644–56.

5. Humphrey LL, Helfand M, Chan BKS, Woolf SH. Breast cancer screening: a summary of the evidence for the U.S. Preventive Services Task Force. Ann Intern Med 2002; 137: 347–60.

6. Nystrom L, Rutqvist LE, Walls S et al. Breast screening with mammography: overview of Swedish randomised trials. Lancet 1993; 341: 973–8.

7. Nystrom L, Andersson NB, Frisell J et al. Long-term effects of mammography screening: updated overview of the Swedish randomized trials. Lancet 2002; 359: 909–19.

8. Kerlikowske K, Grady D, Barclay J et al. Effect of age, breast density and family history on the sensitivity of first screening mammography. JAMA 1996; 276: 33–8.

9. Hendrick RE, Smith RA, Rutledge JH et al. Benefit of screening mammography in women ages 40–49; a new meta-analysis of randomised controlled trials. J Natl Cancer Inst Monograph 1997; 22: 87–92.

10. Kopans DB. Screening for breast cancer. In: Singletary SE, Robb GL, eds. Advanced Therapy of Breast Disease. Hamilton, Ontario: BC Decker, 2000: 1–8.

11. Spratt JA, von Fournier D, Spratt JS, Weber E. Mammographic assessment of human breast cancer growth and duration. Cancer 1993; 71: 2020–6.

12. Wette R, Katz IN, Rodin EY. Stochastic processes for solid tumor kinetics: I. Surface regulated growth. Math Biosci 1974; 19: 231–55.

13. Spratt JS, Greenberg RA, Heuser LS. Geometry, growth rates and duration of cancer and carcinoma in situ of the breast before detection by screening. Cancer Res 1986; 46: 970–4.

14. Speer JF, Petrosky VE, Retsky MW, Wardwell RH. A stochastic numerical model of breast cancer growth that stimulates clinical data. Cancer Res 1984; 44: 4124–30.

15. Holmberg L, Ekbom A, Zack M. Do screen-detected invasive breast cancers have a natural history of their own? Eur J Cancer 1992; 28A: 920–3.

16. Hellman K. Angiogenesis: tumour size is no guide to malignancy. Lancet Oncol 2001; 2: 259–60.

17. Virchow R. Cellular Pathology (Chance F, transl). Philadelphia: Lippincott, 1863.

18. Virchow R. Die Krankhaften Geschwulste. Berlin: A Hirschwald, 1863–1873.

19. Halsted WS. The radical operation for the cure of carcinoma of the breast. Johns Hopkins Hosp Rep 1898; 28: 557.

20. Halsted WS. The results of operations for the cure of cancer of the breast performed at The Johns Hopkins Hospital from June, 1889 to January, 1894. Johns Hopkins Hosp Rep 1894–5; 4: 297–350.

21. Baum M. The history of breast cancer. In: Forbes JF, ed. Breast Disease. Edinburgh: Churchill Livingston, 1986: 95–105.

22. Brinkley D, Haybittle JL. The curability of breast cancer. Lancet 1973; ii: 95–8.

23. Fisher B. Laboratory and Clinical Research in Breast Cancer – A Personal Adventure: The David A Karnofsky Memorial Lecture. Cancer Res 1980; 40: 3863–74.

24. Fisher B, Fisher ER. Transmigration of lymph nodes by tumour cells. Science 1966; 152: 1397–8.

25. Fisher B, Fisher ER. Barrier function of lymph node to tumour cells and erythrocytes I. Normal nodes. Cancer 1967; 20: 1907–13.

26. Fisher B, Fisher ER. Barrier function of lymph node to tumour cells and erythrocytes II. Effect of X-ray, inflammation, sensitisation and tumour growth. Cancer 1967; 20: 1914–19.

27. Atkins H, Hayward JL, Klugman DJ, Wayte AB. Treatment of early breast cancer: A report after 10 years of a clinical trial. BMJ 1972; ii: 423–9.

28. Fisher B, Redmond C, Poisson R et al. Eight year results of a randomised clinical trial comparing total mastectomy and lumpectomy with or without irradiation in the treatment of breast cancer. N Engl J Med 1989; 320: 822–7.

29. Veronesi U, Saccozzi R, Del Vecchio M et al. Comparing radical mastectomy with quadrantectomy, axillary dissection and radiotherapy in patients with small cancers of the breast. N Engl J Med 1981; 305: 6–11.

30. Sarrazin D, Dewar JA, Arriagada R et al. Conservative management of breast cancer. Br J Surg 1986; 73: 604–6.

31. Fisher B, Slack N, Katrych D et al Ten-year follow up results of patients with carcinoma of the breast in a cooperative clinical trial evaluating surgical adjuvant chemotherapy. Surg Gynaecol Obstet 1975; 140: 528–34.

32. Early Breast Cancer Trialists Collaborative Group.

Systemic treatment of early breast cancer by hormonal, cytotoxic or immune therapy. 133 randomised trials involving 31,000 recurrences and 24,000 deaths among 75,000 women. Lancet 1992; 339: 1–15, 71–5.

33. Early Breast Cancer Trialists Collaborative Group. Tamoxifen for early breast cancer: an overview of randomised trials. Lancet 1998; 351: 1451–67.

34. Haybittle JL. Curability of breast cancer. Br Med Bull 1990; 47: 319–23.

35. Berkson J, Harrington SW, Clagett OT et al. Mortality and survival in surgically treated breast cancer: a statistical summary of some experience of the Mayo Clinic. Proc Staff Meet Mayo Clin 1957; 32: 645.

36. Brinkley D, Haybittle JL. Long-term survival of women with breast cancer. Lancet 1984; i: 1118; ii: 353.

37. Le MG, Hill C, Rezvani A et al. Long-term survival of women with breast cancer. Lancet 1984; ii: 922.

38. Langlands AO, Pocock SJ, Kerr GR, Gore SM. Long-term survival of patients with breast cancer: A study of the curability of the disease. BMJ 1979; ii: 1247.

39. Adair F, Berg J, Lourdes J, Robbins GF. Long-term follow up of breast cancer patients: the 30-year report. Cancer 1974; 33: 1145.

40. Hayward J, Caleffi M. The significance of local control in the primary treatment of breast cancer. Arch Surg 1987; 122: 1244.

41. Todd JH, Dowle C, Williams MR et al. Confirmation of a prognostic index in primary breast cancer. Br J Cancer 1987; 56: 489–92.

42. Sigurdsson H, Baldetorp B, Borg A et al. Indicators of prognosis in node-negative breast cancer. N Engl J Med 1990; 322: 1045–53.

43. Folkman J. What is the evidence that tumours are angiogenesis dependent? J Natl Cancer Inst 1990; 82: 4–6.

44. Pickren JW. Significance of occult metastases. Cancer 1961; 14: 1266–71.

45. Fisher ER, Swamidoss S, Lee CH et al. Detection and significance of occult axillary node metastases in patients with invasive breast cancer. Cancer 1978; 45: 2025–31.

46. de Mascerel I, Bonichon F, Coindre JM, Trojani M. Prognostic significance of breast cancer axillary lymph node micro-metastases assessed by two special techniques: re-evaluation with longer follow up. Br J Cancer 1992; 66: 303–6.

47. Trojani M, de Mascerel I, Bonichon F et al. Micro-metastases to axillary lymph nodes from carcinoma of breast: detection by immunohistochemistry and prognostic significance. Br J Cancer 1987; 55: 303–6.

48. International (Ludwig) Breast Cancer Study Group. Prognostic importance of occult axillary lymph node micrometastases from breast cancer. Lancet 1990; 335: 1565–8.

49. Weidner N, Semple JP, Welch WR, Folkman J. Tumour angiogenesis and metastasis – correlation in invasive breast carcinoma. N Engl J Med 1991; 324: 1–8.

50. Liotta L, Kleinerman J, Saidel G. Quantitative relationships of intravascular tumour cells, tumour vessels and pulmonary metastases following tumor implantation. Cancer Res 1974; 34: 997–1004.

51. Rosfjord EC, Dickson RB. Role of integrins in the development and malignancy of the breast. In: Bowcock A, ed. Breast Cancer: Molecular Genetics, Pathogenesis and Therapeutics. New Jersey: Humana Press, 1999: 285–304.

52. Duffy SW, Tabar L, Fagerberg G et al. Breast screening, prognostic factors and survival – results from the Swedish two county study. Br J Cancer 1991; 64: 1133–8.

53. Hakama M, Holli K, Isola J et al. Aggressiveness of screen-detected breast cancer. Lancet 1995; 345: 221–4.

54. Fagerberg CJG, Baldetorp L, Grontoft O et al. Effects of repeated mammographic screening on breast cancer stage distribution. Acta Radiol (Oncol) 1985; 24: 465.

55. Tabar L, Duffy SW, Krusemo UB. Detection method, tumour size and node metastases in breast cancers diagnosed during a trial of breast cancer screening. Eur J Cancer 1987; 23: 959–62.

56. Fisher B, Ravdin RG, Ausman RK et al. Surgical adjuvant chemotherapy in cancer of the breast. Results of a decade of co-operative investigation. Ann Surg 1968; 168: 337–56.

57. Salvadori B, Greco M, Clemente C et al. Prognostic factors in operable breast cancer. Tumori 1983; 69: 477–84.

58. Fisher B, Slack NH, Bross IDJ et al. Cancer of the breast: size of neoplasm and prognosis. Cancer 1969; 24: 1071–80.

59. Haagensen CD. Diseases of the Breast, 3rd edn. Philadelphia: Saunders, 1986: 659.

60. Nemoto T, Vanna J, Bedwani RN et al. Management and survival of female breast cancer: results of a national survey by the American College of Surgeons. Cancer 1984; 45: 2917–24.

61. Tabar L, Fagerberg CJG, South MC et al. The Swedish Two County Trial of mammographic screening for breast cancer: recent results on mortality and tumour characteristics. In: Miller AB, Chamberlain J, Day NE, eds. Screening for Cancer. Bern: Hans Huber, 1991.

62. Hatschek T, Fagerberg G, Olle S et al. Cytometric characterisation and clinical course of breast cancer diagnosed in a population-based screening program. Cancer 1989; 64: 1074–81.

63. Anderson TJ, Lamb J, Donnan P et al. Comparative pathology of breast cancer in a randomised trial of screening. Br J Cancer 1991; 64: 108–13.

64. Cole P, Morrison AS. Basic issues in population screeing for cancer. J Natl Cancer Inst 1980; 65: 1263.

65. Klemi PJ, Joensuu H, Toikkanen J et al. Aggressiveness of breast cancers found with and without screening. BMJ 1992; 304: 467–9.

66. Crisp WJ, Higgs MJ, Cowan WK et al. Screening for breast cancer detects tumours at an earlier biological stage. Br J Surg 1993; 80: 863–5.

67. Abernathy CM, Hedegaard H, Weger N. Screening for breast cancer detects tumours at an earlier biological stage. Lancet 1994; 81: 922.

68. Bull A, Mountney L, Sanderson H. Stage distribution of breast cancer: a basis for the evaluation of breast screening programmes. Br J Radiol 1991; 64: 516–19.

69. Boyd NF, Jensen HM, Cooke G, Lee Han H. Relationship between mammographic and histological risk factors for breast cancer. J Natl Cancer Inst 1992; 1170–9.

70. Bennet IC, McCaffrey JF, Baker CA et al. Changing patterns in the presentation of breast cancer over 25 years. Aust NZ J Surg 1990; 60: 665–71.

71. Rajakariar R, Walker RA. The biological nature of screen-detected invasive breast cancer. J Pathol 1993; 170 (Suppl): 387A.

72. Day NE. Screening for breast cancer. Br Med Bull 1991; 47: 400–15.

73. Nicholson S, Webb AJ, Coghlan B et al. Will screening for breast cancer reduce mortality? Evidence from the first year of screening in Avon. Ann R Coll Surg 1993; 75: 8–12.

74. Wicks K, Fisher CJ, Fentimen IS, Millis RR. Breast cancer histology and age (meeting abstract). J Pathol 1992; 167 (Suppl): 139A.

75. Fisher B, Saffer E, Fisher ER. Studies concerning the regional nodes in cancer IV. Tumour inhibition by regional lymph node cells. Cancer 1974; 33: 631–6.

76. Fisher B, Saffer E, Fisher ER. Studies concerning the regional nodes in cancer VII. Thymidine uptake by cells from nodes of breast cancer patients. Cancer 1974; 33: 271–9.

77. Ponten J, Holmberg L, Trichopoulos D. Biology and natural history of breast cancer. Int J Cancer 1990; 5: 1–21.

78. Meyer JS, Witliff JL. Regional heterogeneity in breast carcinoma: thymidine labelling index, steroid hormone receptors, DNA ploidy. Int J Cancer 1991; 47: 213.

79. Ragaz J, Jackson SM, Le N et al. Adjuvant radiotherapy and chemotherapy in node-positive pre-menopausal women with breast cancer. N Engl J Med 1997; 337: 956–62.

80. Overgaard M, Hansen PS, Overgaard J et al. Post-operative radiotherapy in high risk pre-menopausal women with breast cancer who receive adjuvant chemotherapy. N Engl J Med 1997; 337: 949–55.

81. Hellman S. Stopping metastases at their source (editorial). N Engl J Med 1997; 337: 996–7.

82. Salmon S. Kinetic rationale for adjuvant chemotherapy of cancer. In: Salmon S, Jones S, eds. Adjuvant Chemotherapy of Cancer. Amsterdam: Elsevier/North-Holland Biomedical Press, 1977: 15–27.

83. Skipper H, Schabel F Jr. Quantitative and cytokinetic studies in experimental tumor systems. In: Holland JF, Frei E III, eds. Cancer Medicine, 2nd edn. Philadelphia: Lea and Febiger, 1982: 636–48.

84. Heuser L, Spratt JS, Polk HC Jr. Growth rates of primary breast cancers. Cancer 1979; 43: 1888–94.

85. Moskowitz M. Breast cancer: age specific growth rates and screening strategies. Radiology 1986; 161: 37–41.

86. Holland R, Mravunac M, Hendriks JHCL, Bekekr BV. So-called interval cancers of the breasts: pathologic and radiologic analysis of sixty four cases. Cancer 1982; 49: 2527–33.

87. Heuser L, Spratt JS, Polk HC Jr, Buchanan J. Relation between mammary cancer growth kinetics and the intervals between screenings. Cancer 1979; 43: 857–62.

88. Woodman CBJ, Threlfall AG, Boggis CRM, Prior P. Is the three year breast screening interval too long? Occurrence of interval cancers in NHS Screening Programme's Northwestern Region. BMJ 1995; 310: 224–6.

89. Martin JE, Moskowitz M, Milbrath JR. Breast cancer missed by mammography. AJR Am J Roentgenol 1979; 132: 737–9.

90. Holland R, Hendriks JH, Mravunac M. Mammographically occult breast cancer. A pathologic and radiologic study. Cancer 1983; 52: 1810–19.

91. Frisell J, Eklund G, Hellstrom L, Somell A. Analysis of interval breast carcinomas in a randomised screening trial in Stockholm. Breast Cancer Res Treat 1987; 9: 219–25.

92. Ma L, Fishell J, Wright B et al. Case–control study of factors associated with failure to detect breast cancer by mammography. J Natl Cancer Inst 1992; 84: 781–5.

93. Ikeda D, Andersson I, Wattsgard C et al. Interval cancers in the Malmö Mammographic Screening Trial: radiographic appearance and prognostic considerations. AJR Am J Roentgenol 1992; 159: 287–94.

94. Heuser LS, Spratt JS, Kuhns JG et al. The association of pathologic and mammographic characteristics of primary human breast cancers with 'slow' and 'fast' growth rates and with axillary lymph node metastases. Cancer 1984; 53: 96–8.

95. von Fournier D, Abel U, Spratt JS, Anton H. Growth rate of breast cancer, implication for early detection and therapeutic effects. Geburtshilfe Frauenheilkde 1994; 54: 286–90.

96. Porter PL, El-Bastawissi AY, Mandelson MT et al. Breast tumor characteristics as predictors of mammographic detection: comparison of interval and screen-detected cancers. J Natl Cancer Inst 1999; 91: 2020–8.

97. Brekelmans CT, van Gorp JM, Peeters PH, Collette HJ. Histopathology and growth rate of interval breast carcinoma. Characterization of different subgroups. Cancer 1996; 78: 1220–8.

98. Frisell J, von Rosen A, Wiege M et al. Interval cancer and survival in a randomised breast cancer screening trial in Stockholm. Breast Cancer Res Treat 1992; 24: 11–16.

99. Klemi PJ, Toikkanen S, Rasanen O et al. Mammography screening interval and the frequency of interval cancers in a population-based screening. Br J Cancer 1997; 75: 762–6.

100. Hatschek T, Fagerberg G, Stal O et al. Cytometric characterization and clinical course of breast cancer diagnosed in a population-based screening program. Cancer 1990; 64: 1074–81.

101. Gilliland FD, Joste N, Stauber PM et al. Biologic characteristics of interval and screen-detected breast cancers. J Natl Cancer Inst 2000; 92: 743–9.

102. Arnerlov C, Emdin SO, Lundgren B et al. Breast

carcinoma growth rate described by mammographic doubling time and S-phase fraction. Correlations to clinical and histopathologic factors in a screened population. Cancer 1992; 70: 1928–34.

103. Narod SA, Dube M-P. Biologic characteristics of interval and screen-detected breast cancers. J Natl Cancer Inst 2001; 93: 151.

104. Andersson I, Aspegren K, Janzon L et al. Effect of mammographic screening on breast cancer mortality in an urban population in Sweden. Results from the Malmö Mammographic Screening Trial (MMST). BMJ 1988; 297: 943–8.

105. Vitak B. Invasive interval cancers in the Ostergotland Mammographic Screening Programme: radiological analysis. Eur Radiol 1998; 8: 639–46.

106. Day N, McCann J, Camilleri-Ferrante C et al. Monitoring interval cancers in breast screening programmes: the East Anglian experience. Quality Assurance Management Group of the East Anglian Breast Screening Programme. J Med Screen 1995; 2: 180–5.

107. Benson JR, Purushotham A, Warren R. Screening and litigation – the rate of interval cancers is too high. BMJ 2000; 321: 760–1.

108. Kerlikowski K, Grady D, Barclay J et al. Effect of age, breast density and family history on the sensitivity of first screening mammography. JAMA 1996; 276: 33–8.

109. Tabar L, Fagerberg G, Chen HH et al. Screening for breast cancer in women aged under 50: mode of detection, incidence, fatality and histology. J Med Screen 1995; 2: 94–8.

110. Chang J, Yang WT, Choo HF. Mammography in Asian patients with *BRCA-1* mutations. Lancet 1999; 353: 2070–1.

111. Phillips KA, Andrulis IL, Goodwin PJ. Breast carcinomas arising in carriers of mutations in *BRCA-1* and *BRCA-2*: are they prognostically different? J Clin Oncol 1999; 17: 3653–63.

112. Phillips KA. Biologic characteristics of interval and screen-detected breast cancers. J Natl Cancer Inst 2001; 93: 151–2.

113. Hole D, Stallard S. Breast cancer after HRT. Presented at 3rd Milan Breast Cancer Conference, Milan, Italy, June 2001.

114. Roberts MM, Alexander FE, Anderson TJ et al. Edinburgh trial of screening for breast cancer: mortality at seven years. Lancet 1990; i: 241–6.

115. Surveillance, Epidemiology and End Results (SEER) Program Cancer Statistics Review (1973–1995). Bethesda, MD: National Cancer Institute, Division of Cancer Prevention and Control, Surveillance Program, Cancer Statistics Branch, 1998.

116. Rosen PP, Braun DW, Kinne DE. The clinical significance of pre-invasive breast cancer. Cancer 1980; 46: 919–25.

117. Anderson J, Nielsen M, Christensen L. New aspects of the natural history of in situ and invasive carcinoma in the female breast: results from autopsy investigations. Verh Dtsch Ges Pathol 1985; 69: 88–95.

118. Welch HG, Black WC. Using autopsy series to estimate the disease 'reservoir' for ductal carcinoma in situ of the breast: How much more breast cancer can we find? Ann Intern Med 1997; 127: 1023–8.

119. Anderson TJ. Genesis and source of breast cancer. Br Med Bull 1991; 47: 305–18.

120. Black WC, Welch HG. Screening for disease. AJR Am J Roentgenol 1997; 168: 3–11.

121. Kerlikowski K, Salzman P, Philips KA et al. Continuing screening mammography in women aged 70–79 yrs: impact on life expectancy and cost-effectiveness. JAMA 1999; 282: 2156–63.

122. Satariano WA, Ragland DR. The effect of co-morbidity on 3 year survival of women with primary breast cancer. Ann Intern Med 1994; 120: 104–10.

123. Gotzsche PC, Olsen O. Is screening for breat cancer with mammography justifiable? Lancet 2000; 355: 129–34.

124. Sjonell G, Stahle L. Halsokontrollermed mammografi minskar inte dodligher i brostcancer. Lakartidningen 1999; 96: 904–13.

125. Duffy SW. Interpretation of the breast screening trials: a commentary on the recent paper by Gotzsche and Olsen. Breast 2001; 10: 209–12.

126. Wright CJ, Muller CB. Screening mammography and public health policy: the need for perspective. Lancet 1995; 346: 29–32.

127. Baum M. Screening for breast cancer, time to think – and stop? Lancet 1995; 346: 436.

128. Querci della Rovere G, Benson JR, Warren R. Screening for breast cancer, time to think – and stop? Lancet 1995; 346: 437.

129. Baum M. Commentary: false premises, false promises and false positives – the case against mammographic screening for breast cancer. Int J Epidemiol 2004: 33: 66–7.

6 Interval carcinomas

Ruth Warren, Guidubaldo Querci della Rovere, Lynda Bobrow

Introduction

A feature of all forms of screening for cancer is the occurrence of cases between the screening events. This is a group of cancers of particular interest, as these cases may be the ones missed by the screening examination. They represent a valuable tool in the assessment of screening quality and can be compared between different programmes as an audit of screening effectiveness. These cancers may also include the more rapidly growing cases that reach the size of clinical detection in the screening interval, and so prognostic factors such as size, grade and nodal status may be different from those of the screen-detected group. Mammographic examinations allow us to observe tumour growth, and to understand tumour biology, in a way that is not possible for most cases presenting clinically. Sadly, these cases are also a source of complaint and litigation by patients and their relatives. Screening mammography, like other radiological and pathological material, provides the evidence of failed diagnosis, and erroneous interpretation.

This chapter will explore the extensive literature on this topic. In the past two decades, there have been many publications exploring various aspects of interval cancers. They have come from the major randomised trials of breast screening, and also now from the various regional and national screening programmes set up as a consequence of the trials. The literature has provided critiques of different operational aspects of screening, which are relevant because of the limitations of this public health intervention in reducing mortality from breast cancer. It is also a window on the behaviour of tumours. The mammographic characteristics of the tumours can be observed over successive years' examinations, and can be correlated with pathological features and other prognostic factors.

Classification of cancers

If, as indicated above, the interval cancer rate is to be used to monitor screening performance and as a surrogate predictor of screening effectiveness then it is essential to define the terms used and the categories of cancers that are to be considered. In the UK National Health Service Breast Screening Programme (NHSBSP), considerable work has been undertaken to provide clear definitions, and this material is available in a publication to guide the units of the national programme.[1] As a result, it has been possible to give an early analysis of the first adverse signs of screening performance that have emerged, and to put in place changes that will improve outcomes.

In this NHSBSP publication,[1] the following categories have been identified in relation to a screening programme:

- *Cancers in non-attenders:* in women who have failed to attend, following an invitation for screening.
- *Cancers in lapsed attenders:* in women who have attended for screening and who, either by their own choice or because they have exceeded the recommended age, do not attend.
- *Cancers in the uninvited:* in women who have not yet been invited, who have been suspended from screening or who have not been called because of inaccuracy of the population register.
- *Interval cancers:* in women who have been screened, and whose cancer arises clinically before the next invitation for screening. The rates will be affected by the woman's age and the screening interval.
- *Programme-provoked presentation:* a few women present clinically after receiving an invitation for screening, or after screening and before

assessment, and are difficult to categorise under the headings above. It is likely that the screening invitation triggers clinical presentation in a woman who suspects she has a breast lump.

Categories of interval cancer

For audit of radiology to be useful, interval cancers are categorised. For the NHSBSP, the following categories have been defined:

- *True interval cancers:* which developed in the screening interval.
- *False negatives:* for legal reasons, these are not termed missed cancers.
- *Minor signs:* cancers where the lesion can be identified with hindsight, but where it was not possible to diagnose it prospectively due to non-specific features that can occur in normal breasts.
- *Mammographically occult:* cancers not visible on the mammogram at clinical presentation.
- *Cancers in follow-up non-attenders.*
- *Unclassifiable:* cases where there is no mammogram at the time of clinical presentation for comparison with the screening mammogram.

This categorisation is standard to the NHSBSP. Initially, it differed from some of the international publications in the literature. Many of the papers recognise a minor signs group, considered so subtle as to be reasonably overlooked. 'Missed with minor signs' is one description of this situation. From 1996, the NHSBSP added such a category.[2,3]

The ways in which the definitions of interval cancer in the different screening programmes are applied determine whether their results will be comparable. In some publications, the definitions include cancers arising within a year of a negative screen, which is an appropriate definition for a screening programme offered annually, as happens in many parts of the USA. In the UK, with a 3-year screening round, the definition includes those cancers that arise within 36 months of a negative screen. When the screening round length is above what it should be, cancers may occur at 38 or 40 months from the last screen, and would be excluded by the definition. The screening programme as a whole is failing to meet its objectives. Faux et al[4] have questioned whether the definition masks underperformance. Radiologists will not wish these to be included, because interval cancers for them reflect poor detection. Yet such cancers arising after a prolonged interval may contribute to early death.

Some definitions include those invasive cancers that present clinically, but not those found on an incidental mammogram. In situ carcinoma may be specifically excluded.[5]

The effect of the screening interval

From what has been said in the previous section, it is evident that one factor affecting the number of interval cancers is the screening interval. When the original trials were designed, the appropriate screening interval was not known, and an interval of up to 3 years was used. For example, the Canadian trial[6,7] used mammography and clinical examination in alternate years. The Swedish Two-County Trial used three years for the older age group.[8] From these trials, and subsequent service screening, further information has become available about the effectiveness resulting from different screening intervals. The screening interval has an effect on the number of interval cancers. It may also have an effect on tumour size and nodal status. If tumours dedifferentiate with time, it will also have an effect on grade and other markers of tumour growth.[9] As a result of the interval cancer rates found in the UK in 1995, the question was asked whether the 3-year screening interval was too long.[10,11] Comparisons between the UK and Dutch programmes have been made, but the difference in screening cycles limits comparison.[12] Several authors have discussed the need for a shorter screening cycle in younger women owing to the relatively higher rates of interval cancers in premenopausal woman.[13-17] Interval cancers in relation to age are discussed later in this chapter.

Interval cancers as a means of monitoring screening performance

In setting up a breast screening programme, national governments require evidence of effectiveness.[18] The analysis of interval cancer rates is one of the measures by which screening quality can be judged.[2] Randomised screening trials form the benchmark against which such comparisons can be made. A series of publications represent the performance in the various screening trials.[19-24] As the new screening programmes attempt to evaluate whether their performance matches the trials, publications offer comparisons with these trial results. For example in the UK, the North West region and East Anglia were among the first to report robust data.[5,10] The results showed higher rates of interval cancers than the Swedish Two-County Trial, and there was anxiety whether trial results could be replicated,[25] or whether changes in the programme were necessary.[10,26,27] Subsequently, interval cancers were reported from other UK units,[11,28–30] from European centres,[12,15] and from North America and Australia.[20,31,32] Although there is some repetition in these publications, they are very important, and it is reassuring that results are comparable between the different services. They lie within the range performance of many of the screening trials. The introduction of breast screening to tackle one of the dominant causes of death of the female population in middle years is a major drain on a nation's health resources. The effectiveness of this intervention has often been questioned.[33–35] Proof that screening centres can achieve the desired targets given in the publicly accessible scientific literature is essential,[36] before unequivocal evidence is provided that the expected mortality reduction has been achieved.[37]

Radiological features of interval cancers

Methods of review

In order to achieve better screen detection of cancers, it is of value to observe the radiological features of the cases that arise in the screening interval. This may be done by retrospective review of the screening films of the cancers that subsequently present symptomatically in the interval. The method of review has been extensively discussed because it has a large effect on the number of cases assigned to the categories listed above.[31,38] It has been reported that about 25% of cancers presenting in the screening interval will be visible with hindsight on the original mammograms.[39] This is confirmed by experimental psychology of the subject, which uses the phenomenon of vigilance. The false-negative cases found at screening mammography occurred at rates predictable from previously published vigilance experiments.[40] Methods in which the review cases are mixed with normal screening films, so that the rereading exercise is undertaken in ignorance of which cases subsequently developed cancer, have been described.[29,41] This not surprisingly has an effect on the proportion of cases categorised as false-negative. Other authors have used methods that did not mix the interval cancers with normal films.[42–44] Comparison between blind and informed reviews showed that the false-negative rates were lower when the films were pooled with studies subsequently proven to be free from cancer.[45–47]

Radiological signs

It is rather surprising how few of these papers have analysed the radiological features of the various cancer types, but some have recorded the signs that are found on false-negative screening studies. A pictorial review of false-negative mammograms, including issues of film quality that may result in a cancer being missed on film reading, is available.[48] The signs that may be missed on the first round of screening and can be seen with hindsight at the next screen are ill-defined masses (52%), architectural distortion (20%), asymmetrical densities (16%), enlarged lymph nodes (8%) and well-defined lesions (4%).[49,50] However, a prospective review of 3184 of these minor radiological signs showed that very few turned out to be cancer-related.[51] Radiopathological review of features of interval cancers has shown that they present more often as architectural distortion, are larger, are of higher grade and are more likely to have lymph node metastases than screen-detected tumours; they resemble symptomatic cancers.[16,30]

Radiological site

Only two articles have recorded the site in the breast where the subtle signs of interval cancers were found.[49,52] About 50% present in the breast parenchyma and 50% in the four review areas:[49] area 1, top of the breast–axillary tail; area 2, behind the breast disc; area 3, retroareolar area; area 4, inframammary angle.[53]

Radiological assessment of lesions

Few papers have considered interval cancers arising following radiographic assessment of lesions. One study examined 40 such cases.[54] In 12 of these, the lesion for which the patient was recalled was not the same as the definitive carcinoma. The 28 cases where the assessment failed to diagnose a cancer were analysed. In 12 of these, microcalcifications were wrongly assigned, and only 5 of these were biopsied. Of 16 women with mammographic lesions, 10 had normal ultrasound.

Interval cancers and risk factors for breast cancer

Mammographic density

In 1976, Wolfe[55] suggested that there was a relationship between mammographic density and the risk of developing breast cancer. This relationship has had a chequered course in the literature, but there is ample confirmation of a real relationship between density and cancer risk. There is now good evidence that interval cancers are more likely to develop in dense breasts and that dense breasts mask mammographic detection.[16,20,42,47,56] This will be a factor in the finding of more interval cancers in women screened at a young age, since breast density is inversely related to age. This relationship has been studied in depth.[57–60] Breast density is the cause of poor sensitivity and is also related to the more rapidly growing and higher-grade cancers, which develop in the screening interval. In 1981, one of the first studies of interval cancers from Nijmegen identified the association with mammographic density, and recommended a more frequent screening regime for these women.[61]

Age

Screening programmes permit greater understanding of tumour biology and growth, and this is outstandingly demonstrated by results from the Swedish Two-County Trial.[14] An extensive study of the tumours from the trial has given us real understanding of the differences between the cancers that occur in women aged under 50 and those occurring in women over 50. In younger women, cancers feature more often as interval cancers, and this seems to be due to faster tumour growth. In consequence, a shorter screening interval is required. The cancers occur in women with a greater proportion of dense breasts, which hamper cancer detection by mammography. The importance of age in the consideration of interval cancers has featured in many papers.[13,15,16,24,27,43,56,57,59,60,62–66] It is the presence of high rates of interval cancers, and therefore of a greater proportion overall of poor-prognosis tumours, that has led to the widely accepted view that if screening is to be offered to women under 50 then it needs to be frequent (yearly) to be effective. The prognostic features of the tumours at diagnosis will then be good. This can be expected to have a beneficial effect on mortality. The effect can be expected to be less than in postmenopausal women.

Hormone replacement therapy

A number of publications have analysed the effects of hormone replacement therapy (HRT) on screening effectiveness – both sensitivity and specificity. Poorer sensitivity of mammography and increased rate of interval cancers in women taking HRT is well established.[57,59,62,67,68] There is a relationship between breast density and HRT use; this is most marked in women who take such hormones for a prolonged period before the menopause.[69] A review of the sensitivity of 183 134 screening examinations showed impaired sensitivity in women who both had dense breasts and were users of HRT.[59] In a further study of the histopathological characteristics of interval cancers, it was shown that HRT is a factor affecting sensitivity.[62]

Anthropometric risk factors

In a single study, women with interval cancers were found to be more likely to have previous benign breast disease, to have had an artificial menopause, to be taller and to be heavier than women with screen-detected cancer. This may suggest some difference in cancer causation between the two groups.[24]

Histological features of interval cancers

In many of the studies where interval cancers have been reviewed, analysis of histological types has been undertaken to see whether particular ones occur more frequently in the screening interval. In 1982, Holland et al[61] noted that invasive lobular histology resulted in masking of the cancer, due to the poorly outlined tumour mass. In 1983, de Groote et al[70] identified interval cancers as a more aggressive subset of tumours, with a higher incidence of involvement of axillary nodes, more grade 3 cancers and mortality curves showing that these were bad-prognosis tumours. Since then, many further reports have been made, and the evidence is not so bleak as results of de Groote et al[70] suggest. As there is diversity in the screening regimes, we may expect that the cancers may not be similar. Where screening is intensive – yearly with clinical examination, two views of each breast and two radiologists reporting the films – the findings may well be quite different from minimal screening at a 3-year interval with one mammographic view of each breast. Moreover, age will be a further factor, and this is analysed in material from the Two County Trial:[13] there was a greater proportion of grade 3 tumours and medullary carcinomas in younger women than in those aged over 50, and many of these presented in the interval period.

Later analyses of interval cancers have reinforced these findings: there is an excess of lobular carcinomas among the false-negative tumours;[63,71,72] there are fewer tubular cancers among the interval cancers than the screen-detected group, and more grade 3 tumours and tumours with vascular invasion in the symptomatic and interval group.[72] Interval cancers are therefore similar to the symptomatic group and differ from the screen-detected group.[30]

Markers of tumour growth

Following through from the hypothesis of de Groote et al[70] that interval cancers are a more aggressive group associated with more malignant cellular behaviour and poorer survival, a series of pathological studies have been undertaken that examine cytochemical characteristics associated with more rapid tumour growth. In 1985, von Rosen et al[73] examined 42 cancers for DNA content, histological differentiation and estrogen receptor (ER), and found that the 8 most aggressive tumours were true interval cancers, but that others had low malignancy potential. In a further study in 1992,[74] they found overrepresentation of tumours with aneuploid features among the true interval cancers. Looking at size, axillary nodal involvement, ER and progesterone receptor (PgR) status, DNA ploidy, and S-phase fraction (SPF), in screen-detected and control cancers from the normal population, it has been observed that there are features of less metastatic potential and less cancer cell proliferation in the screen-detected cases.[15,75] Similar results have been confirmed by other authors.[17,62,63,72,76]

Missed breast cancers (false negatives), on the other hand, showed significantly higher proportions of grade 1, low-SPF, ER-positive tumours.[63] Mammography preferentially identifies tumours with favourable prognostic features, in contrast with clinical breast examination (CBE).[77]

However, analysis of the relationships between factors of chronology and biology in the cancers of the Edinburgh study, taking into account interval, never-screened, incidence-screened and prevalence-screened groups, has led to the conclusion that favourable characteristics of screen-detected cases are often due to the effect of length bias on biological factors and fail to show that current local screening practice has succeeded in advancing the diagnosis of breast cancer to a less aggressive phase.[9] This is in conflict with the findings of the Two County Trial, whose 17-year figures indicate better prognostic indices as a result of screening.[37]

The content of the last two sections is summarised in Table 6.1, and Figures 6.1–6.8 illustrate the pathological material described above.

Consequences of the findings about growth and prognostic factors

Do interval cancers grow faster than screen-detected and clinically diagnosed cancers?

From what has been said above regarding histology and markers of tumour growth, it can be seen that the literature is not fully consistent in the reply to this question. In many of the series, there is a subset of cancer with bad prognostic features on the basis of size, grade and nodal status and by other tests, which would suggest that a poor outcome would ensue. In others, the difference is less clear-cut, and perhaps this illustrates how interval cancers in both number and nature may indicate the effectiveness of the screening process. Among those cancers missed at mammography are also some with good prognosis.[63]

What is the metastatic potential of interval cancers?

Holmberg et al[78] showed that interval cancers have greater metastatic potential than screen-detected cancers, and resemble the control cancers in the trial. The method of detection of breast cancer also appears to affect metastatic potential; cancers detected by mammography or CBE had a lower probability of recurrence than those detected by self-examination,[79] and these findings were statistically significant. Interval cancers were not analysed in this study. Disease-free survival is not an endpoint that has been reported in the interval literature. Most of the information that we have comes either from pathologic prognostic indices or from survival analysis.

Survival of interval cancer patients

It has been suggested that interval cancers have a poorer prognosis and observed survival.[70] In trials, interval cancers showed incidence of distant metastatic disease and survival that matched the controls, but were not more aggressive than the latter. Both groups, however, had a more adverse clinical course than the screen-detected cancers.[78,80] Comparison of outcomes between interval cancers and controls showed that interval cases fared better than the control group, but there was no difference between the interval cancers considered to be missed and those called true interval cancers.[23] In the Two County Trial figures, with respect to women screened aged 40–49, the interval cancers had survival curves that lay between those of the screen-detected cancers and those of the controls. The authors considered that the high incidence of interval cancers was an adverse feature in the screening of younger women. They recommended yearly screening at this age to mitigate this high rate.[13] The Nijmegen team found no statistical difference in survival between interval and screen-detected cases, but both groups fared better than unscreened women who were clinically detected.[81] In the North West of the UK, women with interval cancers were found to have survival no worse than those outside the screening programme, and so the screening programme was not affecting the women

Table 6.1 Summary of publications which analyse the prognostic features of interval cancer. (In some of these there are comparisons with screen detected or symptomatic cases.)

Ref	Year	Place	No. of cases	Interval	Screen-detected	Sympto-matic	Size[a]	Grade 1[b]	Stage II or more[c]	Axillary node-positive[d]	NPI <3.4[e]	ER-positive[g]	PgR-positive[g]	SPF >6[h]	c-erbB2-positive	p53-positive	Ki67	DNA ploidy	Statistical analysis[i]
61	1982	Nijmegen	275	64	209		+			+									No
70	1983	Newark, NJ	120	21	99		22.6/19.3		24/19	68/32									Some
73	1985	Stockholm	42	42	–	–		+		+		+						+	No
74	1992	Stockholm	125	125	–	–		+		+								+	No
30	1996	Nottingham	804	87	267	450	*60/89	13/42	+	30/16	30/71								Yes
15	1997	Turku	347	45	250	52	*61/78	19/38	55/33	36/20				63/38>6.0				68/55 aneuploid (NS)	Yes
56	1997	Linköping	843	496	262	85	21.1/16.7		65/49	44/35		65/76		9.1/6.8				63/56	Yes
63	1999	Linköping	455	455	–	–	*61>2 cm	14	61	45		44		72%>5.0					
76	1999	Newcastle	135	51	84	–	20.5/17.7	10/42		51/40		35/60	30/40		19/5	40/16			Yes
62	1999	Seattle	329	150	279	–	*69/84	30/43	49/26	28/17.6		74.3/86.8	70.3/76.8	–	18.5/20.7	37.8/34.8	15/30.7		Yes
72	2000	Gateshead/Newcastle	336	112	112	112	19.5/14.8	23/45		32/24	24/46	#	#		#	#	#		
17	2000	Los Angeles	127	64	63	84	26.8/29.8	21/25				73.1/76.9	69.2/69.2		35/15.9		51/52.3		Yes
77	2001	Toronto	727	–	643	84	21/16			34/20									Yes

[a]Mean size interval/mean size screen detected or * % <2 cm for intervals/% <2 cm for screen-detected.
[b]% grade 1 tumours interval/% grade 1 tumours screen-detected.
[c]% stage II or more interval/% stage II or more screen-detected.
[d]% axillary node-positive interval/% axillary node-positive screen-detected.
[e]%Nottingham Prognostic Index (NPI) <3.4 interval/%NPI <3.4 screen-detected.
[f]%vascular invasion present interval/% vascular invasion present screen-detected.
[g]% ER- or PR-positive interval/% ER- or PR-positive screen-detected.
[h]% S-phase fraction (SPF) > 6 interval/% SPF > 6 screen-detected.
[i]Any statistical analysis of results.
Some results but cannot be presented in a comparable way.

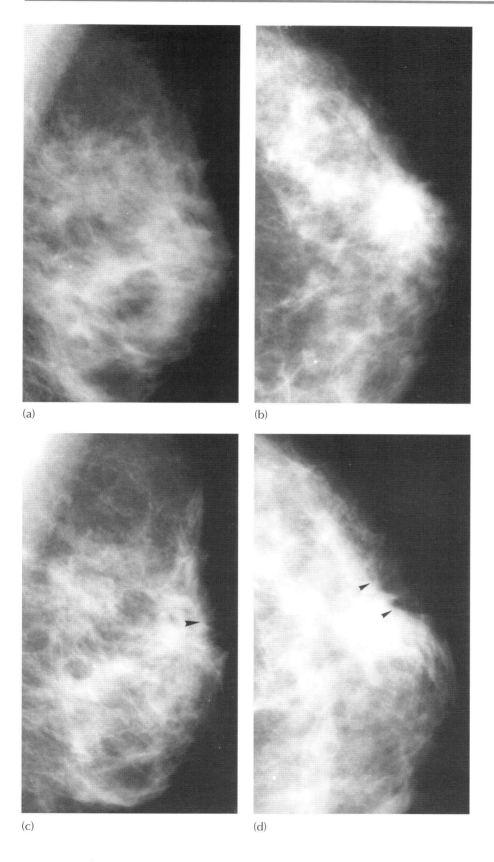

(a)

(b)

(c)

(d)

Figure 6.1 Patient aged 55; false-negative interval cancer, 8 months after screening; 10 mm, grade 2 invasive lobular carcinoma with lobular carcinoma in situ, 1 out of 12 nodes involved. (a) MLO view, normal film, 12 December 1989. (b) CC view, film, 12 December 1989, which is probably abnormal with hindsight, but the features are very subtle. (c) MLO view at diagnosis, 23 August 1990; the cancer is marked with an arrow. (d) CC view at diagnosis, 23 August 1990; the cancer is marked with arrows.

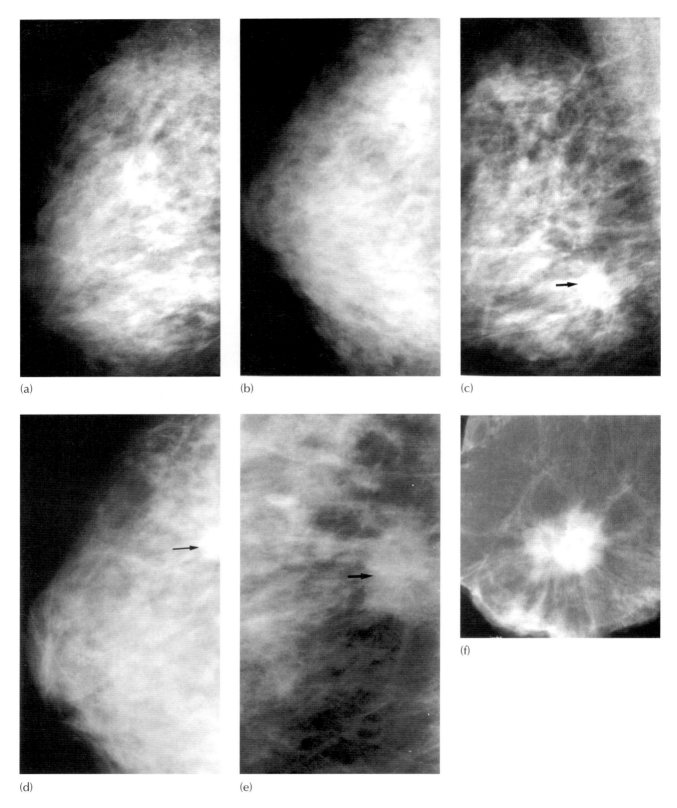

(a) (b) (c)

(d) (e) (f)

Figure 6.2 Patient aged 62; true interval cancer 17 months from screening; grade 2, invasive ductal carcinoma, 15 mm diameter, no nodal involvement. (a) MLO view, 28 June 1988; normal examination. (b) CC view, 28 June 1988, normal examination. (c) MLO view, 16 November 1989, at diagnosis. (d) CC view, 16 November 1989, at diagnosis. (e) MLO magnification view, 16 November 1989. (f) Specimen mammogram.

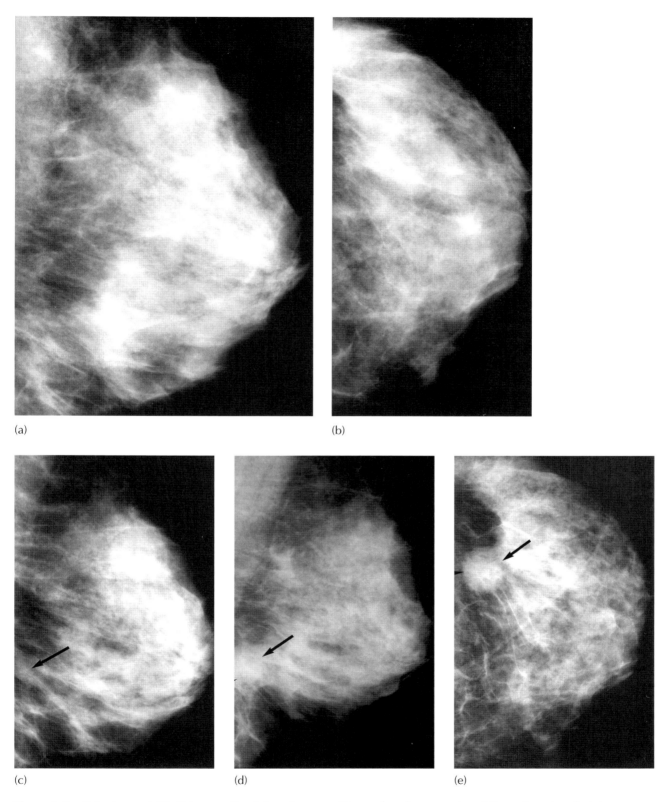

Figure 6.3 Patients aged 62. False-negative interval cancer 22 months after screening; 15 mm invasive ductal carcinoma with 3 out of 8 lymph nodes involved. (a) MLO screening film, 28 June 1989. (b) CC screening film, 28 June 1989. (c) MLO screening film, 26 May 1992; the arrow shows the small tumour visible with hindsight. (d) MLO diagnostic film, 9 March 1994. (e) CC diagnostic film, 9 March 1994.

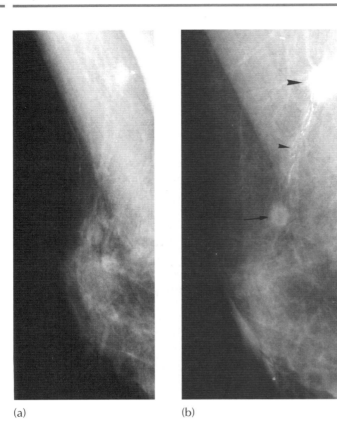

(a)   (b)

Figure 6.4 Patient aged 56. False-negative interval cancer 24 months from screening; this 8 mm tumour was of invasive ductal type with 1 lymph node out of 14 involved. The small tumour can be seen with hindsight and has been misinterpreted as a small normal lymph node on the original screening examination. Its position in this woman with tiny breasts rendered detection by the patient at a small size possible. (a) MLO screening film, 13 June 1990. (b) MLO diagnostic film, 18 June 1992; the black arrowheads indicate the small tumour mass and the line of calcification; the arrow indicates a lymph node, probably involved by tumour.

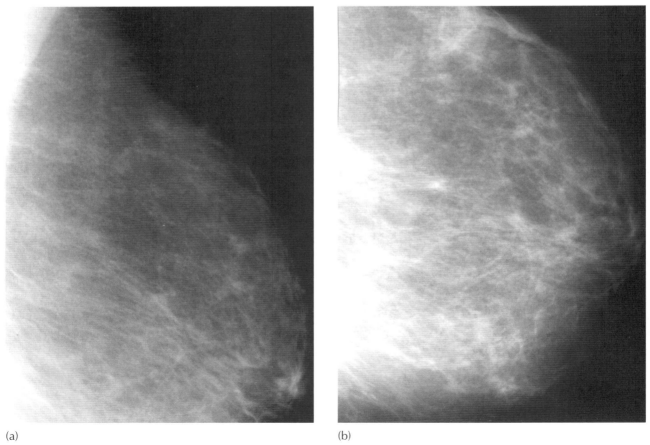

(a)   (b)

Figure 6.5 Patient aged 52. True interval cancer 17 months from screening; a tumour of 20 mm diameter, a grade 2 lobular carcinoma with 2 out of 11 lymph nodes involved. (a) Upper MLO of left breast, screening film, 3 April 1990. (b) Lower MLO of left breast, screening film, 3 April 1990.

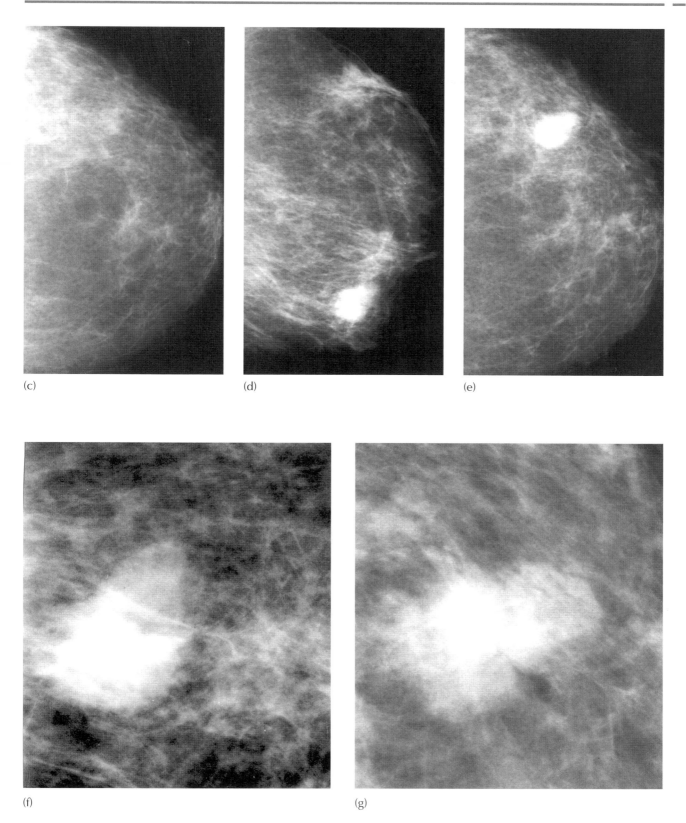

Figure 6.5 continued (c) CC view, 3 April 1990. (d) MLO view, diagnostic film, 16 September 1991. (e) CC view, 6 September 1991. (f) Magnification view of tumour, MLO. (g) Magnification view of tumour, CC projection.

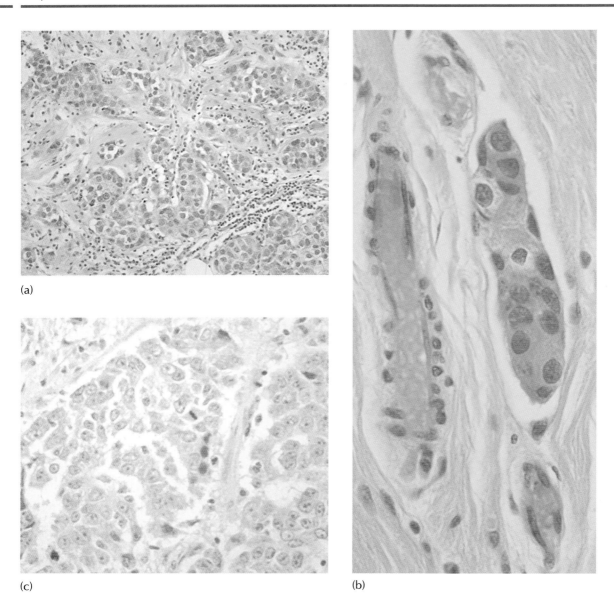

(a)

(c)

(b)

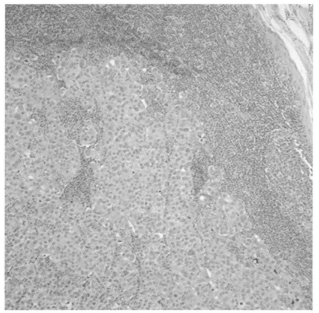

(d)

Figure 6.6   (a) Medium-power view of a grade 3 infiltrating ductal carcinoma. (b) High-power view showing vascular invasion by grade 3 invasive ductal carcinoma cells. (c) Very high-power view of this grade 3 invasive ductal carcinoma to show frequent mitoses, which indicate a high proliferation rate. (d) Medium-power view showing a lymph node containing a metastasis from this same grade 3 carcinoma.

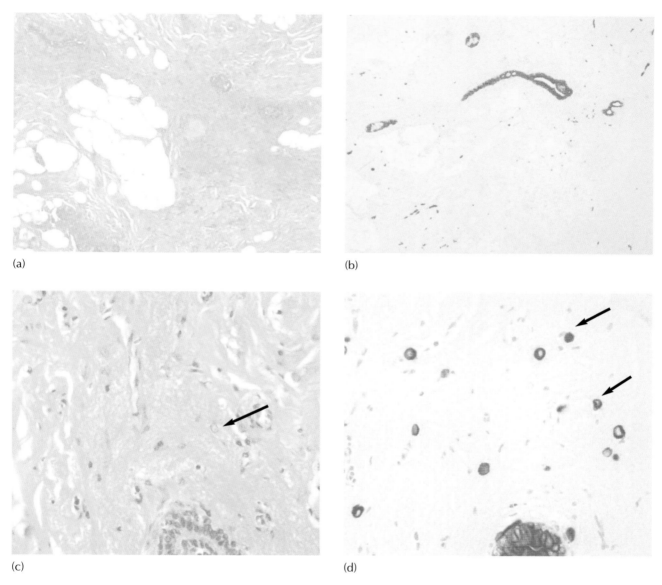

Figure 6.7 (a) Low-power view of haematoxylin and eosin (H&E)-stained specimen of subtle infiltrating lobular carcinoma around normal breast structures. (b) The same field of view as stained with low-molecular-weight cytokeratin (CAM5.2) to highlight infiltrating carcinoma cells around normal structures. (c) High-power H&E-stained specimen of breast with subtle infiltrating lobular carcinoma cells. (d) The same field of view as (c), stained with CAM5.2 to highlight infiltrating carcinoma cells.

adversely despite interval rates above Two County Trial levels.[82] Tabar et al[14] showed that interval cancers follow a course with poorer survival than the screen-detected and control groups, but better than non-attenders (Figure 6.9).

Interval breast cancer, delayed diagnosis and litigation

From the patient's perspective, it is not surprising that when screening seems to have failed, women wish to apportion blame. Patients and lawyers take action in the courts to obtain financial restitution for this wrong. This may be fuelled by the anger that many patients feel when they have cancer and ask 'Why me?' – anger directed against their disease but acted out against their doctor. But the content of this chapter tells a story that shows that every screening programme and every radiologist has missed cases. Whether humans or machines report the films, that will always be the case. We treat individuals, and the woman and her lawyer look only at the particular case and not at the results of the whole programme. The injustice that this represents for

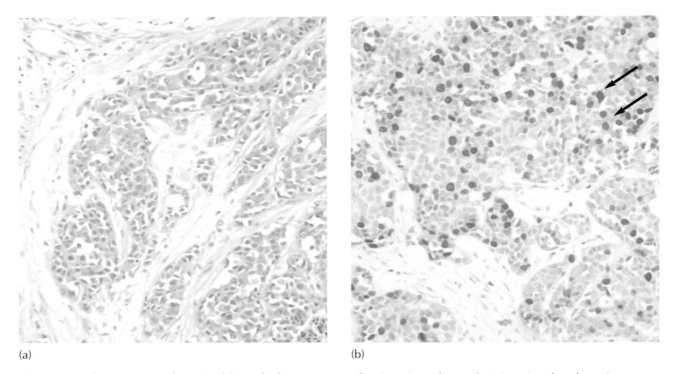

(a)   (b)

Figure 6.8   The H&E-stained section (a) is a high-power magnification view of a grade 3 invasive ductal carcinoma. The adjacent serial section (b) at the same magnification has been stained with an antibody to Ki67. The latter is an antigen expressed by cells undergoing cell division. The positive nuclear stain is dark brown. The large number of cells in mitosis is indicative of a rapidly proliferating tumour.

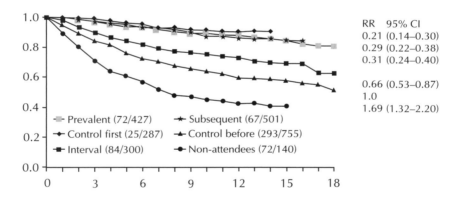

Figure 6.9   Cumulative survival by detection mode. Women aged 40–74 Swedish Two-County Trial, years since operation to 31 December 1996. (RR, relative risk; 95% confidence interval (CI)). This shows that women who have cancers diagnosed at screening (top three curves) at prevalent, incident or first round of screening have an equally good outlook, and that interval cancers from screening have better survival than the original unscreened control group and non-attendees, but worse than all screen-detected cancers. Reprinted with permission from Tabar L, Duffy SW, Vitak B, et al. The natural history of breast carcinoma: What have we learned from screening? cancer 1999; 86: 449–62.

doctors becomes a potential source of failure of screening. Early diagnosis and mortality reduction by screening may not be available to women because doctors will not participate in screening.[83] This topic has its own evolving literature, and although there is a chapter in this book on litigation in breast

cancer care, a brief mention of the radiological literature on this topic is of value and pertinent to any discussion of interval cancers.

There is dispute as to whether delay in diagnosis will cause adverse outcomes. In 1999, the Lancet published two major articles on whether delay caused adverse outcome. Sainsbury et al[84] looked at 36 222 cases in Yorkshire and showed no evidence of a survival disadvantage in delays of three months or more. In the same issue of the Lancet, Richards et al[85] conducted a systematic review, and concluded that delays of 3–6 months were associated with lower survival. This latter group also analysed cases treated at Guy's Hospital, London between 1975 and 1990 (2964 women), and concluded that there was an adverse effect from delay.[86] In a systematic review, Ramirez et al[87] looked at the reasons for delay in presentation, and called for urgent primary research on this topic. These unresolved issues are key to the award of large sums in damages to women whose cancers were not diagnosed by screening. The legal system and the emotional atmosphere in the Courts when a patient with metastatic disease is the plaintiff make the refusal of damages unlikely.

Much of the radiological literature on this topic comes from the USA, and the comments have gradually changed down the years as litigation has changed.[88–93] Lawyers adapt their approach to be effective in achieving high settlements for their clients. In 1996, Wolverton and Sickles[94] contributed usefully to this literature by undertaking a prospective study that determined the outcomes of the many small queries raised by radiologists as they question whether a small abnormality is present. Wolverton and Sickles showed that, in 543 findings in 382 women, no unsuspected cancers were found. They questioned the appropriateness of malpractice claims when such minor lesions are viewed with hindsight. The UK is fast following down the same route of litigation, although screening is a government intervention under heavy central control. Limited by financial constraints, the screening programme was introduced with one view only of each breast, and an interval of 3 years between screens. It is this government service that pays the medical indemnity. The service is based on effectiveness advice of health economists that fails to include the indemnity settlements in the calculations. Moreover in a government directive in 2001, instructions were given that when a medical audit, designed to monitor and improve the programme, detects a cancer that has been missed, the patient must be informed – the standard set for doctors is therefore 100% detection. The reason for this directive is the patient's 'right to know', and typifies a new style of openness in UK healthcare. One may anticipate that litigation will soar, and radiologists will cease to wish to be involved in screening.

A US editorial[95] has called for an educational drive to make women realise that mammography will not provide 100% detection. It is merely the current best but imperfect test for early diagnosis of cancer, and there will inevitably be missed cases.[96] Some countries have a no-fault system of compensation, and thus avoid the cost and adversarial atmosphere of litigation. This may be appropriate for population screening, where decisions that benefit whole communities may not give the best result for the individual. This surely must be the solution to the need for openness if the UK national programme is to survive. Such a system is in place in New Zealand.[97]

Can we draw conclusions?

This chapter has demonstrated the importance of interval cases in understanding the diversity of breast cancer. Interval cancers give understanding also of the screening process, the screeners and the service in which they work. They are a disappointment to the women who attend screening, as much as to the radiologists who have to discuss with them their shortfalls. While mammography remains the mainstay of early diagnosis for breast cancer, interval cancers will occur. Even if a chemical or genetic test is invented to supersede mammography, interval cancers will still occur, since no medical test is 100% effective. Doctors must teach the public to understand the limited capabilities of diagnostic tests, who in turn must revise the nature of their trust in medicine and doctors. Careful informed consent and open honest communication will be the key to a more mature partnership between patient and doctor.

References

1. Patnick J, Muir Gray J. Guidelines in the Collection and Use of Breast Cancer Data. Sheffield: NHSBSP, January 1993, Rep No. 26.
2. Day N, Williams D, Khaw K. Breast cancer screening programmes: the development of a monitoring and evaluation system. Br J Cancer 1989; 59: 954–8.
3. Moss S, Blanks R, Group ICW. Calculating appropriate target cancer detection rates and expected interval cancer rates for the UK NHS Breast Screening Programme. J Epidemiol Comm Health 1998; 52: 111–15.
4. Faux AM, Richardson DC, Lawrence GM, et al. Interval breast cancers in the NHS Breast Screening Programme: Does the current definition exclude too many? J Med Screen 1997; 4: 169–73.
5. Day N, McCann J, Camilleri-Ferrante C, et al. Monitoring interval cancers in breast screening programmes: the East Anglian experience. J Med Screen 1995; 2: 180–5.
6. Miller AB, Baines CJ, To T, Wall C. Canadian National Breast Screening Study: 2. Breast cancer detection and

death rates among women aged 50 to 59 years. CMAJ 1992; 147: 1477–88 [erratum 1993; 148: 718].

7. Miller AB, Baines CJ, To T, Wall C. Canadian National Breast Screening Study: 1. Breast cancer detection and death rates among women aged 40 to 49 years. CMAJ 1992; 147: 1459–76 [erratum 1993; 148: 718].

8. Tabar L, Fagerberg G, Duffy SW, et al. Update of the Swedish Two-County Program of mammographic screening for breast cancer. Radiol Clin North Am 1992; 30: 187–210.

9. Alexander FE, Anderson TJ, Hubbard AL. Screening status in relation to biological and chronological characteristics of breast cancers: a cross sectional survey. J Med Screen 1997; 4: 152–7.

10. Woodman C, Threlfall A, Boggis C, Prior P. Is the three year breast screening interval too long? Occurrence of interval cancers in NHS Breast Screening Programme's North Western Region. BMJ 1995; 310: 224–6.

11. Everington D, Gilbert FJ, Tyack C, Warner J. The Scottish Breast Screening Programme's experience of monitoring interval cancers. J Med Screen 1999; 6: 21–7.

12. Fracheboud J, de Koning HJ, Beemsterboer PM, et al. Interval cancers in the Dutch Breast Cancer Screening Programme. Br J Cancer 1999; 81: 912–17.

13. Tabar L, Fagerberg G, Chen H, et al. Screening for breast cancer in women aged under 50: mode of detection, incidence, fatality and histology. J Med Screen 1995; 2: 94–8.

14. Tabar L, Duffy SW, Vitak B, et al. The natural history of breast carcinoma: What have we learned from screening? Cancer 1999; 86: 449–62.

15. Klemi P, Toikkanen S, Rasanen O, et al. Mammography screening interval and the frequency of interval cancers in a population-based screening. Br J Cancer 1997; 75: 762–6.

16. Vitak B. Invasive interval cancers in the Ostergotland Mammographic Screening Programme: radiological analysis. Eur Radiol 1998; 8: 639–46.

17. Gilliland FD, Joste N, Stauber PM, et al. Biologic characteristics of interval and screen-detected breast cancers. J Natl Cancer Inst 2000; 92: 743–9.

18. de Koning HJ. Assessment of nationwide cancer-screening programmes. Lancet 2000; 355: 80–1.

19. Tabar L, Chen HH, Fagerberg G, et al. Recent results from the Swedish Two-County Trial: the effects of age, histologic type, and mode of detection on the efficacy of breast cancer screening. J Natl Cancer Inst Monogr 1997; 22: 43–7.

20. Ma L, Fishell E, Wright B, et al. Case–control study of factors associated with failure to detect breast cancer by mammography. J Natl Cancer Inst 1992; 84: 781–5.

21. Moss S, Coleman D, Ellman R, et al. Interval cancers and sensitivity in the screening centres of the UK Trial of Early Detection of Breast Cancer. Eur J Cancer 1993; 29A: 255–8.

22. Ikeda D, Andersson I, Watsgard C, et al. Interval cancers in the Malmö mammographic screening trial: radiographic appearance and prognostic considerations. AJR Am J Roentgenol 1992; 159: 287–94.

23. Frisell J, von Rosen A, Wiege M, et al. Interval cancer and survival in a randomised breast cancer screening trial in Stockholm. Breast Cancer Res Treat 1992; 24: 11–16.

24. Brekelmans C, Peeters P, Faber J, et al. The epidemiological profile of women with an interval cancer in the DOM programme. Breast Cancer Res Treat 1994; 30: 223–32.

25. Field S, Michell M, Wallis M, Wilson A. What should be done about interval breast cancers? BMJ 1995; 310: 203–4.

26. Asbury D, Boggis CR, Sheals D, et al. NHS Breast Screening Programme: Is the high incidence of interval cancers inevitable? BMJ 1996; 313: 1369–70.

27. Threlfall AG, Woodman CB, Prior P. Breast screening programme: Should the interval between tests depend on age? Lancet 1997; 349: 472.

28. Warren R, Duffy S. Interval cancers as an indicator of performance in breast screening. Breast Cancer 2000; 7: 6–18.

29. Simpson W, Neilson F, Young J, et al. The identification of false negatives in a population of interval cancers: a method for audit of screening mammography. Breast 1995; 4: 183–8.

30. Burrell HC, Sibbering DM, Wilson AR, et al. Screening interval breast cancers: mammographic features and prognosis factors. Radiology 1996; 19: 811–17.

31. Bird R, Wallace T, Yankaskas B. Analysis of cancers missed at screening mammography. Radiology 1992; 184: 613–17.

32. Burhenne HJ, Burhenne LW, Goldberg F, et al. Interval breast cancers in the Screening Mammography Program of British Columbia: analysis and classification. AJR Am J Roentgenol 1994; 162: 1067–71; discussion 1072–5.

33. Baum M. Survival and reduction in mortality from breast cancer. Impact of mammographic screening is not clear. BMJ 2000; 321: 1470; discussion 1471–2.

34. Gotzsche PC, Olsen O. Is screening for breast cancer with mammography justifiable? Lancet 2000; 355: 129–34.

35. Roberts MM. Breast screening: time for a rethink? BMJ 1989; 299: 1153–5.

36. Sickles EA, Ominsky SH, Sollitto RA, et al. Medical audit of a rapid-throughput mammography screening practice: methodology and results of 27,114 examinations. Radiology 1990; 175: 323–7.

37. Tabar L, Vitak B, Tony HH, et al. Beyond randomized controlled trials: organized mammographic screening substantially reduces breast carcinoma mortality. Cancer 2001; 91: 1724–31.

38. van Dijck JA, Verbeek AL, Hendriks JH, Holland R. The current detectability of breast cancer in a mammographic screening program. A review of the previous mammograms of interval and screen-detected cancers. Cancer 1993; 72: 1933–8.

39. Kopans DB. Accuracy of mammographic interpretation. N Engl J Med 1994; 331: 1521–2.

40. Laming D, Warren R. Improving the detection of cancer in the screening of mammograms. J Med Screen 2000; 7: 24–30.

41. Duncan A, Wallis M. Classifying interval cancers. Clin Radiol 1995; 50: 774–7.

42. Saarenmaa I, Salminen T, Geiger U, et al. The visibility of cancer on earlier mammograms in a population-based screening programme. Eur J Cancer 1999; 35: 1118–22.

43. Saarenmaa I, Salminen T, Geiger U, et al. The visibility of cancer on previous mammograms in retrospective review. Clin Radiol 2001; 56: 40–3.

44. Britton PD, McCann J, O'Driscoll D, et al. Interval cancer peer review in East Anglia: implications for monitoring doctors as well as the NHS Breast Screening Programme. Clin Radiol 2001; 56: 44–9.

45. Harvey JA, Fajardo LL, Innis CA. Previous mammograms in patients with impalpable breast carcinoma: retrospective vs blinded interpretation. 1993 ARRS President's Award. AJR Am J Roentgenol 1993; 161: 1167–72.

46. Moberg K, Grundstrom H, Tornberg S, et al. Two models for radiological reviewing of interval cancers. J Med Screen 1999; 6: 35–9.

47. de Rijke JM, Schouten LJ, Schreutelkamp JL, et al. A blind review and an informed review of interval breast cancer cases in the Limburg Screening Programme, The Netherlands. J Med Screen 2000; 7: 19–23.

48. Huynh PT, Jarolimek AM, Daye S. The false-negative mammogram. Radiographics 1998; 18: 1137–54; quiz 1243–4.

49. Daly CA, Apthorp L, Field S. Second round cancers: How many were visible on the first round of the UK National Breast Screening Programme, three years earlier? Clin Radiol 1998; 53: 25–8.

50. Duncan KA, Needham G, Gilbert FJ, Deans HE. Incident round cancers: What lessons can we learn? Clin Radiol 1998; 53: 29–32.

51. Sickles EA. Periodic mammographic follow-up of probably benign lesions: results in 3,184 consecutive cases. Radiology 1991; 179: 463–8.

52. Brown M, Eccles C, Wallis M. Geographical distribution of breast cancers on the mammogram: an interval cancer database. Br J Radiol 2001; 74: 317–322.

53. Tabar L, Dean P. Teaching Atlas of Mammography, 2nd edn. Stuttgart: Georg Thieme Verlag, 1985.

54. Burrell HC, Evans A, Wilson AR, Pinder SE. False-negative breast screening assessment. What lessons can we learn? Clin Radiol 2001; 56: 385–8.

55. Wolfe JN. Breast patterns as an index of risk for developing breast cancer. AJR Am J Roentgenol 1976; 126: 1130–7.

56. Vitak B, Stal O, Manson JC, et al. Interval cancers and cancers in non-attenders in the Ostergotland Mammographic Screening Programme. Duration between screening and diagnosis, S-phase fraction and distant recurrence. Eur J Cancer 1997; 33: 1453–60.

57. Mandelson MT, Oestreicher N, Porter PL, et al. Breast density as a predictor of mammographic detection: comparison of interval- and screen-detected cancers. J Natl Cancer Inst 2000; 92: 1081–7.

58. Sala E, Warren R, McCann J, et al. Mammographic parenchymal patterns and mode of detection: implications for the breast screening programme. J Med Screen 1998; 5: 207–12.

59. Rosenberg RD, Hunt WC, Williamson MR, et al. Effects of age, breast density, ethnicity, and estrogen replacement therapy on screening mammographic sensitivity and cancer stage at diagnosis: review of 183,134 screening mammograms in Albuquerque, New Mexico. Radiology 1998; 209: 511–18.

60. Kerlikowske K, Grady D, Barclay J, et al. Effect of age, breast density, and family history on the sensitivity of first screening mammography. JAMA 1996; 276: 33–8.

61. Holland R, Mravunac M, Hendriks J, Bekker B. So-called interval cancers of the breast. Cancer 1982; 49: 2527–33.

62. Porter PL, El-Bastawissi AY, Mandelson MT, et al. Breast tumor characteristics as predictors of mammographic detection: comparison of interval- and screen-detected cancers. J Natl Cancer Inst 1999; 91: 2020–8.

63. Vitak B, Olsen K, Manson J, et al. Tumour characteristics and survival in patients with invasive interval breast cancer classified according to mammographic findings at the latest screening: a comparison of true interval and missed interval cancers. Eur Radiol 1999; 9: 460–9.

64. Kavanagh AM, Mitchell H, Farrugia H, Giles GG. Monitoring interval cancers in an Australian mammographic screening programme. J Med Screen 1999; 6: 139–43.

65. Brekelmans C, Colette H, Colette C, et al. Breast cancer after a negative screen: follow-up of women participating in the DOM screening programme. Eur J Cancer 1992; 28A: 893–5.

66. Peer PG, Verbeek AL, Straatman H, et al. Age-specific sensitivities of mammographic screening for breast cancer. Breast Cancer Res Treat 1996; 38: 153–60.

67. Litherland JC, Stallard S, Hole D, Cordiner C. The effect of hormone replacement therapy on the sensitivity of screening mammograms. Clin Radiol 1999; 54: 285–8.

68. Stallard S, Litherland JC, Cordiner CM, et al. Effect of hormone replacement therapy on the pathological stage of breast cancer: population based, cross sectional study. BMJ 2000; 320: 348–9.

69. Sala E, Warren R, McCann J, et al. High-risk mammographic parenchymal patterns and hormone replacement therapy: a case–control study. Int J Epidemiol 2000; 29: 629–36.

70. de Groote R, Milazzo J, Warden M, Rocko J. Interval breast cancer: a more aggressive subset of breast neoplasias. Surgery 1983; 94: 543–7.

71. Maxwell AJ. Breast cancers missed in the prevalent screening round: effect upon the size distribution of incident round detected cancers. J Med Screen 1999; 6: 28–9.

72. Cowan WK, Angus B, Gray JC, et al. A study of interval breast cancer within the NHS Breast Screening Programme. J Clin Pathol 2000; 53: 140–6.

73. von Rosen A, Erhardt K, Hellstrom L, et al. Assessment of malignancy potential in so-called interval mammary carcinomas. Breast Cancer Res Treat 1985; 6: 221–7.

74. von Rosen A, Frisell J, Nilsson R, et al. Histopathological and cytochemical characteristics of interval breast carcinomas from the Stockholm Mammography Screening Project. Acta Oncol 1992; 31: 399–402.

75. Klemi P, Joensuu H, Toikkanen S, et al. Aggressiveness of breast cancers found with and without screening. BMJ 1992; 304: 467–9.

76. Crosier M, Scott D, Wilson RG, et al. Differences in Ki67 and c-erbB2 expression between screen-detected and true interval breast cancers. Clin Cancer Res 1999; 5: 2682–8.

77. Narod SA, Dube MP. Re: Biologic characteristics of interval and screen-detected breast cancers. J Natl Cancer Inst 2001; 93: 151–2.

78. Holmberg L, Tabar L, Adami H, Bergstrom R. Survival in breast cancer diagnosed between screening examinations. Lancet 1986; ii: 27–8.

79. Senie R, Lesser M, Kinne D, Rosen P. Method of tumor detection influences disease-free survival of women with breast carcinoma. Cancer 1993; 73: 1666–72.

80. Brekelmans C, Peeters P, Deurenberg J, Clete H. Survival in interval breast cancer in the DOM screening programme. Eur J Cancer 1995; 31A: 1830–5.

81. Schroen AA, Wobbes T, van der Sluis RF. Interval carcinomas of the breast: a group with intermediate outcome. J Surg Oncol 1996; 63: 141–4.

82. Collins S, Woodman CB, Threlfall A, Prior P. Survival rates from interval cancer in NHS Breast Screening Programme. BMJ 1998; 316: 832–3.

83. Austin R, McLendon W. The Papanicolau smear. Medicine's most successful cancer screening procedure is threatened. JAMA 1997; 277: 754–55.

84. Sainsbury R, Johnston C, Haward B. Effect on survival of delays in referral of patients with breast-cancer symptoms: a retrospective analysis. Lancet 1999; 353: 1132–5.

85. Richards MA, Westcombe AM, Love SB, et al. Influence of delay on survival in patients with breast cancer: a systematic review. Lancet 1999; 353: 1119–26.

86. Richards MA, Smith P, Ramirez AJ, et al. The influence on survival of delay in the presentation and treatment of symptomatic breast cancer. Br J Cancer 1999; 79: 858–64.

87. Ramirez AJ, Westcombe AM, Burgess CC, et al. Factors predicting delayed presentation of symptomatic breast cancer: a systematic review. Lancet 1999; 353: 1127–31.

88. Potchen EJ, Bisesi MA, Sierra AE, Potchen JE. Mammography and malpractice. AJR Am J Roentgenol 1991; 156: 475–80.

89. Brenner RJ. Mammography and malpractice litigation: current status, lessons, and admonitions. AJR Am J Roentgenol 1993; 161: 931–5.

90. Brenner R. Medicolegal aspects of breast imaging. Radiol Clin North Am 1992; 30: 277–86.

91. Brenner RJ, Lucey LL, Smith JJ, Saunders R. Radiology and medical malpractice claims: a report on the Practice Standards Claims Survey of the Physician Insurers Association of America and the American College of Radiology. AJR Am J Roentgenol 1998; 171: 19–22.

92. Brenner RJ. False-negative mammograms. Medical, legal, and risk management implications. Radiol Clin North Am 2000; 38: 741–57.

93. Brenner RJ, Berlin L. Evaluation of the mammographic abnormality. AJR Am J Roentgenol 1996; 167: 17–19.

94. Wolverton D, Sickles E. Clinical outcome of doubtful mammographic findings. Am J Roentgenol 1996; 167: 1041–5.

95. Berlin L. The missed breast cancer redux: time for educating the public about the limitations of mammography. AJR Am J Roentgenol 2001; 176: 1131–4.

96. Berlin L. Dot size, lead time, fallibility, and impact on survival: continuing controversies in mammography. AJR Am J Roentgenol 2001; 176: 1123–30.

97. Lewis A. No-fault liability – twenty years experience in New Zealand. Med Law 1996; 15: 425–8.

7 Mammography screening for women under 50

Ismail Jatoi and Michael Baum

Introduction

During the last two decades, mammography screening for women under age 50 has been one of the most intensely debated topics in medicine. Although common practice in the USA, it is generally not recommended in Europe.[1] After reviewing the same evidence, many experts and medical organisations have often arrived at opposite conclusions concerning its merits. For example, in February 1993, the American Cancer Society (ACS) and the European Society of Mastology (EUSOMA) met in New York and Paris respectively to review the results of mammography screening trials. After reviewing the same data, the two organisations arrived at opposite conclusions: the ACS reaffirmed its long-standing recommendations of screening women starting at age 40, while EUSOMA recommended that screening be reserved for women above age 50.[2]

In more recent years, several mammography screening trials have reported updated results. Recent meta-analyses of these results now seem to suggest that a significant benefit to screening younger women emerges after long-term follow-up. This has led some organisations to alter their recommendations concerning mammography screening for younger women. The US Preventive Services Task Force (USPSTF), for instance, reviewed the evidence concerning mammography screening for women below age 50 in 1996.[2] At that time, the USPSTF found insufficient evidence to recommend for or against routine screening in younger women. In 2002, they reviewed the updated results from the screening trials and concluded that there was now fair evidence that mammography screening every 1–2 years could significantly reduce breast cancer mortality for women aged 40 and older.[3] However, others have argued that the 'delayed benefit' of

mammography screening in younger women (as suggested by the clinical trials) can simply be attributed to screening these women after age 50, and that the potential risks of screening younger women ought to be carefully considered. In this review, we discuss the ongoing controversy concerning screening in younger women, and present our views on this issue.

Biases of clinical studies

More is known about screening for breast cancer than screening for any other type of cancer. Over the past four decades, various studies have been undertaken to determine the efficacy of mammography screening: case–control studies, retrospective analyses and prospective studies. There are three biases pertinent to many of these studies: lead-time, length and selection.[1] An understanding of these biases is necessary before discussing the merits of mammography screening. Ultimately, the success of mammography screening should be measured by its ability to reduce mortality, rather than its ability to improve survival.

Survival refers to the period of time from cancer diagnosis to death. Lead-time bias refers to the interval between diagnosis of cancer by screening and usual clinical detection. Lead-time bias may make it appear that screening prolongs survival, when, in fact, it simply extends the period of time over which the disease is observed. As screening advances the time of breast cancer diagnosis, patients with screen-detected cancers will inevitably have better survival rates than those with clinically detected cancers, even if screening does nothing to delay the time of death. Thus retrospective studies comparing survival between screened and unscreened populations fail to account for lead-time bias, and are flawed.

Length bias relates to the fact that screening tends to detect tumors with a better prognosis. More slowly growing tumours (those with a better prognosis) exist for a longer period in the preclinical phase and are therefore more likely to be diagnosed by mammography screening. In contrast, more rapidly growing tumours exist for a shorter period of time in the preclinical phase, and are more likely to be detected in the intervals between screening sessions. Thus length bias invalidates comparisons of tumours detected by screening mammography with those detected by physical examination. The impact of length bias is best seen when cancers detected by screening are compared with interval cancers (cancers detected between screening sessions).[4] Interval cancers generally carry a poorer prognosis than screen-detected cancers.

Selection bias refers to the fact that women who volunteer for screening are more likely to be health-conscious, and have a lower mortality from all causes. In general, women who volunteer for screening are more likely to eat nutritional foods, exercise regularly and maintain a healthy lifestyle. This is sometimes also referred to as the 'healthy-screenee effect'. The impact of selection bias was illustrated in a case–control evaluation of the effect of breast cancer screening in the UK, comparing attenders and non-attenders for screening.[5] By comparing populations from two separate districts (one a breast cancer screening district and the other a comparison district), breast cancer mortality was found to be relatively higher among non-attenders in the screening district. This finding was attributed to selection bias.

Randomised prospective studies

All of these biases can be excluded by comparing screened and unscreened populations in a randomised study with all-cause mortality as the endpoint and cause-specific mortality as a questionable surrogate endpoint. There have been eight randomised prospective trials designed to evaluate the efficacy of mammography screening, and of these seven have evaluated its impact on mortality reduction in women younger than 50: the Health Insurance Plan (HIP), the Swedish Two-County Trial, the Malmo, Stockholm, Gothenburg and Edinburgh studies, and the first Canadian National Breast Screening Study (CNBSS-I) (Table 7.1).[6] Only CNBSS-I was specifically designed to evaluate mammography screening in women under age 50, while the others evaluated the impact of screening in women of a broad age range.

The HIP was the first randomised controlled trial of mammography screening for breast cancer, initiated

Table 7.1 The mammography screening trials that included women below age 50

Screening trial	Age at entry	Screening modality[a]
Health Insurance Plan (HIP)	40–64	MM + CBE
Swedish Two-County	40–74	MM
Malmo	45–69	MM
Stockholm	40–64	MM
Gothenburg	40–59	MM
Edinburgh	45–64	MM + CBE
Canadian (CNBSS-I)	40–49	MM + CBE

MM, mammography; CBE, clinical breast examination.

in 1963.[7] The study involved 62 000 women between the ages of 40 and 64 from the HIP medical insurance scheme of New York, who were randomly assigned to either a study or a control group of 31 000 women each. However, the HIP was not designed specifically to assess the potential benefits of screening younger women. Among women aged 40–49 at the start of the study, after a median follow-up of 14 years, there was a non-significant reduction in breast cancer mortality in the screened group, the relative risk being 0.78 (95% confidence interval (CI) 0.56–1.08). It is also important to note that in the HIP study screening was carried out with clinical breast examinations (CBE) as well as mammography. Ultimately, only 19% of breast cancers in women of all ages were detected exclusively by mammography, and the majority (57%) were detected by CBE alone. Thus the HIP does not necessarily justify mammography screening for any age group. If anything, it suggests that CBE may have an important role to play as a screening modality.

There have been four screening mammography trials undertaken in Sweden: the Stockholm, Gothenburg and Malmo studies and the Two-County Trial.[8,9] For women aged 40–49 at entry, these trials have had median follow-ups of 14.3, 12.7, 13.3 and 13 years, respectively. For each of these trials, the relative risk of breast cancer death in the screened group in comparison with the control group was 1.52 (95% CI 0.8–2.88), 0.58 (95% CI 0.35–0.96), 0.73 (95% CI 0.51–1.04), and 0.87 (95% CI 0.54–1.41) respectively. Each of these trials examined the efficacy of mammography screening alone. CBE was not utilised as a screening modality in any of these trials.

The Edinburgh trial was a randomized clinical trial involving 45 130 women between the ages of 45 and

64, initiated in 1979.[10] Women in the study group received screening mammography and CBE, while the control group received usual care. There were only 5913 women younger than 50 enrolled in the study. After a median follow-up of 13 years, the relative risk of breast cancer death among women below age 50 in the screened group was 0.75 (95% CI 0.48–1.18).

CNBSS-I is the only trial specifically designed to assess the efficacy of screening for women between the ages of 40 and 49.[11] The total number of women enrolled in CNBSS-I was 50 430. It was designed with sufficient statistical power to detect at least a 40% reduction in mortality by screening. The screened group received mammography and CBE on an annual basis for four or five examinations, while the control group received an initial CBE upon entry and thereafter follow-up by mail. After 7 years, there was a non-significant excess in mortality in the screened group, the relative risk in the screened group being 1.36 (95% CI 0.84–2.21). However, after a median follow-up of 13 years, the relative risk of breast cancer deaths in the screened group was 0.97 (95% CI 0.74–1.27).

Thus far, CNBSS-I is the only trial specifically designed to assess the efficacy of screening for women between the ages of 40 and 49 to have reported results. It has received far greater scrutiny than any of the other mammography screening trials, and has withstood this scrutiny. Its critics have charged that in the first 2 years of the study, over 50% of the mammograms were technically inadequate, and that neither the equipment nor the training of the radiologists was properly standardised.[12] However, it should seem apparent that in a large study such as this, total standardisation would be impractical and that CNBSS-I represented the true technology and skills of the radiologists of the communities at the time the study was undertaken. We also note with irony that no such criticisms were levelled against the HIP study, which used techniques and standards now considered obsolete, suggesting a double standard for those only willing to reinforce their prejudice!

CNBSS-I has also been criticised on the grounds that there was contamination of the control group: about 26% of the unscreened population had 'diagnostic' mammograms to evaluate palpable breast masses.[13] The critics argue that mammography is not particularly useful as a 'diagnostic' procedure, and that in a symptomatic woman, the benefit comes from screening the ipsilateral and contralateral breast for clinically occult cancer. Thus some believe that CNBSS-I in fact compared screened women with other screened women, and that this might account for the lack of mortality reduction in the study

group. However, it seems unlikely that such mammograms would serve to change significantly the outcome of such a large study. Given the standard practice of medicine in the world today, it would be impossible to run a trial in which women presenting with palpable breast masses were denied mammography, and proceeded directly with excisional biopsy. Finally, there have been charges that CNBSS-I may have failed to demonstrate lower rates of breast cancer deaths among women assigned to the mammography arm because the randomisation of enrolled women was compromised.[14] These concerns were raised because the mammography group in CNBSS-I contained considerably more women with four or more positive axillary nodes than the control group. Independent reviewers were therefore asked to review the randomisation strategy in CNBSS-I, and no subversion of the randomisation process was ever found.[15]

Perhaps the most definitive evidence on the impact of mammography screening in younger women will come from a large randomised controlled trial now underway in the UK.[16] In this study, women will be aged 40–41 at entry. A study group of 65 000 women will be offered mammography at the first visit and annually thereafter for seven or eight rounds, while a comparison group of 135 000 women will be offered the usual care with no screening. Upon reaching the age of 50, both groups will be offered regular screening. A follow-up of 14–15 years is planned, and the study has been designed to give 80% power to detect a mortality reduction of 20%, assuming that 70% of the women accept the offer to undergo screening.

In addition to the results of the individual trials mentioned above, several meta-analyses of mammography screening trials have now been published. Many of these indicate that, after long-term follow-up, a statistically significant benefit to screening women under age 50 does indeed emerge. For example, in their meta-analysis of all eight trials, Hendrick et al[17] and Smart et al[18] have reported a significant decrease in breast cancer mortality in the screened group after 12.7 years of follow-up, the relative risk being 0.82 (95% CI 0.71–0.95). In a meta-analysis of the eight trials, after a median follow-up of about 12 years, Kerlikowske[19] reported that the relative risk of breast cancer deaths in the screened group was 0.84 (95% CI 0.71–0.99). In a more recent meta-analysis, Humphrey et al[3] excluded the Edinburgh trial (which they considered of poor quality), and found, after 14 years of follow-up, that the relative risk of death for women under 50, in the screened group, was 0.85 (95% CI 0.73–0.99). However, Olsen and Gotzsche[20] have argued that six of the mammography screening trials are flawed or of poor quality. In their meta-analysis, they included only the Canadian and Malmö trials, and found, after 13 years of follow-up, no benefit to screening women below age 50, the relative risk of breast cancer deaths in the screened group being 1.03 (95% CI 0.77–1.38).

Thus, with the exception of the results of Olsen and Gotzsche,[20] the various meta-analyses generally suggest that, after long-term follow-up, a benefit to mammography screening for younger women does eventually emerge. Overviews of the randomised trials suggest that mammography screening reduces breast cancer mortality by about 25% in women over age 50, and that the benefit emerges after 7–9 years of follow-up. In contrast, mammography screening in women below age 50 reduces breast cancer mortality by only 16–18%, and it takes 12–14 years for that benefit to emerge.[21]

Biological considerations

Why should it take longer to see a benefit for women who are below age 50 at the start of mammography screening trials? This question remains open to speculation, but there are several possible explanations. One possibility is that screening may detect very slowly growing (indolent) tumours in younger women, so that a reduction in breast cancer mortality may take longer to emerge. However, Kerlikowske[19] has argued that if this is indeed the case then detecting these slowly growing tumours after age 50 could perhaps produce the same reduction in risk of breast cancer deaths. Yet another possibility is that mammography screening in younger women is less effective. Thus the delayed benefit of screening women below age 50 might actually be attributed to screening these women after age 50. deKonig et al[22] addressed this possibility with a computer simulation model known as MISCAN (microsimulation screening analysis). Their study suggested that most of the reduction in breast cancer mortality for women who were between the ages of 40 and 49 at the start of the screening trials was, in fact, the result of screening these women beyond the age of 50.

Another important question is why the efficacy of mammography screening should abruptly change at age 50. Indeed, some investigators have argued that there is no rational basis for such an abrupt change. Yet, age 50 corresponds approximately to the age at menopause, and the epidemiology and biology of breast cancer differ between pre- and post-menopausal women. There are, for example, changes in the incidence of breast cancer that occur in most populations around the time of the menopause: a steep rise in incidence occurs until

about age 45–55, followed by a less rapid increase thereafter.[23] Changes in tumour characteristics are also apparent, with tumours of younger women having a lower proportion of oestrogen receptor (ER)-positive tumors and a higher labelling index.[24] There are also differences in risk factors between pre- and postmenopausal women. In many studies, obesity is associated with a higher risk of postmenopausal breast cancer but a lower risk of premenopausal cancer.[25] Thus the results of mammography screening trials are consistent with the results of other studies showing differences in the epidemiology and biology of pre- and post-menopausal breast cancer.

Finally, one might ask why mammography screening might be less effective in premenopausal women than in postmenopausal women. Again, there are several possible explanations. It is important to remember that the real benefit of screening is not early detection, but rather early treatment. As screening advances the time of breast cancer diagnosis, it allows for the early initiation of therapy. Thus the results from the screening trials may suggest that premenopausal women benefit less from early therapy than do postmenopausal women. Alternatively, the results of the screening trials may also be largely attributable to the fact that the sensitivity of mammography is lower in premenopausal women, making it a less effective screening test in younger women.[26]

However, breast cancer is much less common in women below age 50 than it is in women above that age, and Kopans[27] has argued that there are insufficient numbers of women under the age of 50 in the world's screening trials to show an immediate mortality benefit to screening. Thus one might argue that the delayed benefit of mammography screening in younger women is attributable to the fact that breast cancer is much less common in this age group, and it takes longer to accrue sufficient numbers of deaths in the trials to see a statistically significant benefit to screening younger women. Indeed, Kopans[27] has estimated that a trial that could prove a 25% mortality reduction at 5 years for women between the ages of 40 and 49 would require about 500 000 women. Proponents of screening for younger women also argue that technology has improved over the years, and that mammography equipment today is better able to detect earlier breast tumours. Thus they argue that the trials of the past are not indicative of what can be achieved using the more modern technology of today.[28] However, it would be very difficult to conduct a screening trial involving such a large number of women as proposed by Kopans. The biggest trial to date has been the Canadian study, involving over 50 000 women, and a trial involving 10 times this number of women is unlikely ever to be conducted. And, with regard to the technology issue, one might argue that technology is constantly improving and it would be impractical to conduct a new trial every time there is an improvement in mammography technology. Furthermore, in the face of the potential hazards of screening (to be described in the next section), the onus of proof should rest on the proponents of screening, who would have us accept this intervention on trust alone.

Hazards of screening

If there is no clear evidence that mammography screening reduces breast cancer mortality in younger women then is it justifiable to continue to recommend screening for these women? It would seem not, because there are at least five harmful effects of mammography screening: cost, lead time, radiation exposure, false positives and overdiagnosis (Table 7.2).

Cost

In recent years, healthcare costs have increased dramatically, and governments around the world are attempting to reduce those costs. In the light of these constraints, attention has focused on the cost of mammography screening in younger women, particularly as the efficacy of screening in this age group is not clearly established. Kattlove et al[29] analysed the expense and benefits of mammography screening in a hypothetical American healthcare organisation in which 360 new cases of breast cancer are diagnosed each year. They concluded that the most cost-effective guideline for such a healthcare organization would be to restrict screening to women aged 50–69. Salzmann et al[30] have argued that screening mammography is relatively cost-ineffective among women aged 40–49 because mammography is less efficacious in women of this age group, and the incidence of breast cancer is lower than in older age groups.

Lead time

Mammography screening detects breast cancer earlier, but if this is not accompanied by a reduction in breast cancer mortality then the patient is given advanced notice of impending death, with no tangible gain. This has an adverse effect on the quality of life. This 'lead time' is probably in the range of 2–4 years, meaning that many women will suffer needless worry and anxiety during this period.[1]

Table 7.2	**Hazards of screening younger women**
Harmful effect	**Consequences**
Cost	Increased expenditure on intervention of no proven value
Lead time	Advanced notice of impending death
Radiation exposure	Increased risk of breast cancer in women who carry the gene for ataxia telangiectasia (ATM)
False positives	Unnecessary breast biopsies
Overdiagnosis	Financial/emotional consequences of being falsely labelled as a cancer patient

Radiation exposure

Mammography screening results in exposure to low-dose radiation, and this may actually induce breast cancer. Beemsterboer et al[31] developed a computer simulation model of a mammography screening programme to calculate breast cancer deaths induced by exposure to low-dose radiation and the number of lives saved. Their estimates were based on data from the Swedish screening mammography trials and the Netherlands breast cancer screening programme. In their model, they assumed a 2-year screening interval and a mean glandular dose of 4 mGy to each breast from a two-view mammogram. They calculated that the ratio between the number of breast cancer deaths prevented and those induced as a result of mammography screening for women aged 50–69 is 242:1. When mammography screening is expanded to include screening women aged 40–49 every 2 years, the ratio becomes 97:1. Thus their model suggests that the potential hazards of low-dose radiation are greatly increased if screening is initiated before age 50. Additionally, Swift et al[32] have suggested that heterozygous carriers of the gene for ataxia telangiectasia (ATM) are at increased risk for developing breast cancer after exposure to low-dose radiation. An estimated 1.4% of the general population are heterozygous carriers of the ATM gene, and they may have a sixfold increased risk of developing breast cancer after exposure to low-dose radiation.

False positives

Elmore et al[33] have shown that after 10 screening mammograms, a woman has about a 49% cumulative risk of a false-positive result. Furthermore, the risk of false positives is dependent on age. Thus, for women between the ages of 40 and 49, the risk is about 56%, while for women aged 50–79, the cumulative risk of a false-positive result after 10 mammograms is about 47%. False positives have a very detrimental effect on quality of life, resulting in unnecessary anxiety, unnecessary surgery and additional costs.

In the USA, where litigation is of paramount concern, the incidence of false positives has historically been higher than in Europe, probably due to the unwillingness of radiologists to commit themselves to a benign diagnosis. Analysis of data from the American Breast Cancer Detection Demonstration Project (BCDDP) suggested that the positive predictive value of mammography screening was only 10%, meaning that nine women had a false-positive result on screening for every cancer found.[34] In contrast, European studies during the same time period indicated positive predictive values ranging from 30% to 60%.[35] These figures represent the positive predictive value of screening in all age groups. If women below the age of 50 were considered alone, the incidence of false positives would be higher.

Overdiagnosis

Overdiagnosis of breast cancer is a very serious adverse consequence of mammography screening, and one that profoundly affects quality of life. Peeters et al[36] define overdiagnosis as 'a histologically established diagnosis of invasive or intraductal breast cancer that would never have developed into a clinically manifest tumor during the patient's normal life expectancy if no screening examination had been carried out'. Following the introduction of mammography screening, there has been an increase in the incidence of breast cancer, particularly a sharp increase in that of ductal carcinoma in situ (DCIS).[37] DCIS is almost exclusively detected by screening mammography, and very rarely by palpation. Prior to screening mammography, DCIS accounted for only 1–2% of all breast cancers, but today accounts for 12% of all such cancers and for 30% of those detected by screening.

There is ample evidence to suggest that most DCIS detected by mammography would not progress to invasive cancer during a woman's lifetime. Several years ago, Nielsen et al[38] reported the results of 110 medicolegal autopsies of women between the ages of 20 and 54 dying of accidents. DCIS was detected in 15%, which is a prevalence four to five times greater than the number of overt cancers expected to develop over 20 years.

Additionally, in autopsies of women diagnosed with breast cancer, Alpers and Wellings[39] have found DCIS in 48% of the contralateral breasts, even though only 12% of all breast cancer patients develop contralateral breast cancer after 20 years of follow-up. And in two separate studies, Rosen et al[40] and Page et al[41] reviewed benign breast biopsies and found several instances where DCIS had been overlooked by the pathologist. Only a small number of these women developed clinically manifest tumors after 15–18 years of follow-up. All of these studies suggest that not all DCIS progresses to invasive cancer, and most of the increase in incidence of DCIS may in fact represent overdiagnosis.

However, the consequences of overdiagnosis can be devastating. Women with DCIS are generally classified as cancer patients, and, in the USA may sometimes face denial of life insurance or dramatically increased health insurance costs.[42] In addition, they are subjected to treatments that would have been unnecessary if the lesion had not been detected by screening.

Conclusion

Since the 1970s, the USA has been the only major industrialized country to encourage mammography screening for women below the age of 50. However, age-adjusted breast cancer mortality rates in the USA continue to mirror those of other western countries, suggesting that screening younger women has had little effect in altering overall population-based mortality trends.[43] Thus any long-term mortality benefits of mammography screening in younger women (as suggested by some of the meta-analyses) do not translate into any real benefits in population-based statistics.

In the debate concerning the efficacy of mammography screening for younger women, the potential harm of screening has largely been ignored. Given the doubts concerning the efficacy of mammography screening in younger women and the potential for harm outlined above, we believe that it is unethical to screen women under age 50 without first obtaining proper informed consent.[44] Thus informed consent should be viewed as the middle ground in the continuing debate over whether or not to screen women under the age of 50.

References

1. Jatoi I, Baum M. American and European recommendations for screening mammography in

younger women: a cultural divide? BMJ 1993; 307: 1481–3.

2. US Preventive Services Task Force. Guide to Clinical Preventive Services, 2nd edn. Washington, DC: Office of Disease Prevention and Health Promotion, 1996.

3. Humphrey LL, Helfand M, Chan BKS, Woolf SH. Breast cancer screening: a summary of the evidence for the U.S. Preventive Services Task Force. Ann Intern Med 2002; 137: 347–60.

4. Miller AB. Mammography in women under 50. Hematol Oncol Clin North Am 1994; 8: 165–77.

5. Moss SM, Summerley ME, Thomas BJ et al. A case–control evaluation of the effect of breast cancer screening in the United Kingdom trial of early detection of breast cancer. J Epidemiol Comm Health 1992; 46: 362–4.

6. Jatoi I. Breast cancer screening. Am J Surg 1999; 177: 518–24.

7. Shapiro S. Periodic screening for breast cancer: the HIP randomized controlled trial. Health Insurance Plan. J Natl Cancer Inst Monogr 1997; 22: 27–30.

8. Nystrom L, Anderson I, Bjurstam N et al. Long-term effects of mammography screening: updated overview of the Swedish randomized trials. Lancet 2002; 359: 909–19.

9. Tabar L, Vitak B, Chen HH et al. The Swedish Two-County Trial twenty years later: updated mortality results and new insights from long-term follow-up. Radiol Clin North Am 2000; 38: 625–51.

10. Alexander FE, Anderson TJ, Brown HK et al. 14 years of follow-up from the Edinburgh randomized trial of breast cancer screening. Lancet 1999; 353: 1903–8.

11. Miller AB, To T, Baines CJ, Wall C. The Canadian National Breast Screening Study-I, breast cancer mortality after 11–16 years of follow-up in women age 40–49. Ann Intern Med 2002; 137: 305–12.

12. Canadian study of breast screening under 50. Lancet 1992; 339: 1473–4.

13. Kopans DB. Screening for breast cancer and mortality reduction among women 40–49 years of age. Cancer 1994; 74: 311–22.

14. Tarone RE. The excess of patients with advanced breast cancer in young women screened with mammography in the Canadian National Breast Screening Study. Cancer 1995; 75: 997–1003.

15. Bailar JC, MacMahon B. Randomization in the Canadian National Breast Screening Study: a review for evidence of subversion. CMAJ 1997; 156: 193–9.

16. Breast screening in women under 50. Lancet 1991; 337: 1575–6.

17. Hendrick RE, Smith RA, Rutledge JH III, Smart CR. Benefit of screening mammography in women aged 40–49: a new meta-analysis of randomized controlled trials. J Natl Cancer Inst Monogr 1997; 22: 87–92.

18. Smart CR, Hendrick RE, Rutledge JH III, Smith RA. Benefit of mammography screening in women ages 40 to 49 years: current evidence from randomized controlled trials. Cancer 1995; 75: 1619–26.

19. Kerlikowske K. Efficacy of screening mammography among women aged 40 to 49 years and 50 to 69 years: comparison of relative and absolute benefit. J Natl Cancer Inst Monogr 1997; 22: 79–86.

20. Olsen O, Gotzsche PC. Cochrane review on screening for breast cancer with mammography. Lancet 2001; 358: 1340–2.

21. Kerlikowske K, Grady D, Rubin SM et al. Efficacy of screening mammography. A meta-analysis. JAMA 1995; 273: 149–54.

22. deKonig HJ, Boer R, Warmerdam PG et al. Quantitative interpretations of age-specific mortality reductions from the Swedish breast cancer screening trials. J Natl Cancer Inst 1995; 87: 1217–23.

23. Clemmensen J. Carcinoma of the breat. Results from statistical research. Br J Radiol 1948; 21: 583.

24. Henderson IC. Biologic variations of tumors. Cancer 1992; 69: 1888–95.

25. Willett W. Nutritional Epidemiology. New York: Oxford University Press, 1990.

26. Buist DSM, Porter PL, Lehman C, Taplin SH, White E. Factors contributing to mammography failure in women aged 40–49 years. J Natl Cancer Inst 2004; 96: 1432–40.

27. Kopans DB. Screening for breast cancer and mortality reduction among women 40–49 years of age. Cancer 1994; 74: 311–22.

28. Sickles EA, Kopans DB. Deficiencies in the analysis of breast cancer screening data. J Natl Cancer Inst 1993; 85: 1621–4.

29. Kattlove H, Liberati A, Keeler E, Brook RH. Benefits and costs of screening and treatment for early breast cancer. Development of a basic benefit package. JAMA 1995; 273: 142–8.

30. Salzmann P, Kerlikowske K, Phillips K. Cost-effectiveness of extending screening mammography guidelines to include women 40 to 49 years of age. Ann Intern Med 1997; 127: 955–65.

31. Beemsterboer PM, Warmerdam PG, Boer R, de Koning HJ. Radiation risk of mammography related to benefit in screening programmes: a favourable balance? J Med Screen 1998; 5: 81–7.

32. Swift M, Morrell D, Massey RB, Chase CL. Incidence of cancer in 161 families affected by ataxia-telangiectasia. N Engl J Med 1991; 325: 1831–6.

33. Elmore JG, Barton MB, Moceri VM et al. Ten-year risk of false positive screening mammograms and clinical breast examinations. N Engl J Med 1998; 338: 1089–96.

34. Baker LH. Breast cancer detection demonstration project: 5–year summary report. CA Cancer J Clin 1982; 42: 1–35.

35. Reidy J, Hoskins O. Controversy over mammography screening. BMJ 1988; 297: 932–3.

36. Peeters PHM, Verbeek ALM, Straatman H et al. Evaluation of overdiagnosis of breast cancer in screening with mammography: results of the Nijmegen programme. Int J Epidemiol 1989; 18: 295–9.

37. Ernster VL, Barclay J, Kerlikowske K et al. Incidence of and treatment for ductal carcinoma in situ of the breast. JAMA 1996; 275: 913–18.

38. Nielsen M, Thomsen JL, Primdahl S et al. Breast cancer

and atypia among young and middle aged women: a study of 110 medicolegal autopsies. Br J Cancer 1987; 56: 814–19.

39. Alpers CE, Wellings SR. The prevalence of carcinoma in situ in normal and cancer-associated breasts. Hum Pathol 1985; 16: 796–807.

40. Rosen PR, Braum DW Jr, Kinne DE. The clinical significance of pre-invasive breast carcinoma. Cancer 1980; 46: 919–25.

41. Page DL, Dupont WD, Rogers LW, Landenberger M.

Intraductal carcinoma of the breast: followup after biopsy only. Cancer 1982; 49: 751–8.

42. Jatoi I, Baum M. Mammographically detected ductal carcinoma in situ: Are we over diagnosing breast cancer? Surgery 1995; 118: 118–20.

43. Jatoi I, Miller AB. Why is breast cancer mortality declining? Lancet Oncol 2003; 4: 251–4.

44. Baum M. Commentary: false premises, false promises and false positives – the case against mammographic screening for breast cancer. Int J Epidemiol 2004; 33: 66–7.

8 A critical appraisal of breast cancer screening for women aged 50 and over*

Sue Moss

Introduction

The association between prognosis and stage at diagnosis of breast cancer suggests that there is a potential for screening to diagnose breast cancer while it is still asymptomatic in order to reduce mortality from the disease, and a number of research studies have been conducted to investigate this. Despite recent controversy, it is generally accepted that research findings support the conclusion that screening by mammography reduces the risk of death from breast cancer in women aged between 50 and 69 at first invitation to screening. However, debate continues about whether the reduction in the risk of death is sufficient to outweigh the potential physical and psychological disadvantages inherent in the screening of well women, and the substantial resource costs of public health screening programmes. This chapter reviews these issues and discusses the current policies adopted in various countries.

Size of benefit shown in research trials

The most valid way of assessing the reduction in risk of death achieved by screening is to compare the subsequent cancer death rate in a population for whom screening has been provided with that in a control population without a screening programme.[1,2] However, the development of prognostic indicators combining information on tumour size, node status, grade and histological characteristics has led to increased use of surrogate outcome measures to predict mortality.[3] Such analyses nevertheless need careful planning in order to avoid potential biases. Ideally, comparison of mortality should be the endpoint of a randomised controlled trial in which eligible disease-free subjects are randomly allocated to an offer of screening or to a control group, both groups being followed up for a number of years to record all subsequent deaths. A number of such trials of breast cancer screening have been conducted during the past 40 years.

The Health Insurance Plan trial

This study, devised by Shapiro and his colleagues[4] and started in 1963, was a model for population-based randomised controlled trials of preventive medical intervention, and similar methodologies, although differing in organisational details, have been followed in many subsequent trials of breast cancer screening. A total of 62 000 women aged 40–64 who were insured for comprehensive healthcare with the Health Insurance Plan (HIP) of New York were randomly allocated to an intervention group or a control group.[4] Women in the intervention group were invited to attend a screening clinic, where they underwent two-view mammography and physical examination of the breasts. Repeat invitations were sent annually for 3 successive years, after which screening ceased. Two-thirds of women invited accepted the first screen, falling to 45% at the final screen. Women in the control group received their normal medical care. Details of all breast cancers, all breast cancer deaths and all other deaths were recorded in both intervention group and control group over an 18-year period.

---

*This chapter updates the chapter by Professor Jocelyn Chamberlain in the 1st edition.

Within 5 years of the women's entry to the trial, a reduction in breast cancer mortality was observed in the intervention group relative to the control group. After 10 years of follow-up, the reduction in breast cancer deaths was concentrated mainly among women aged 50 or over at entry, although subsequently a suggestion of benefit also appeared in the younger age group. By 18 years, the risk of breast cancer death in the intervention group relative to the control group was 0.79 (95% confidence interval (CI) 0.62–0.99). In women aged 50 and over at entry to the trial, the relative risk (RR) was 0.80 (95% CI 0.59–1.08).

The Swedish Two-County Trial

This study, which started in the late 1970s, studied the effect on breast cancer mortality of screening using only a single mediolateral oblique-view mammogram with no physical examination.[5] In this trial, 135 000 women aged 40 and over and resident in Kopparberg and Östergotland counties were randomly allocated by cluster according to the parish in which they lived to an intervention group (78 000) or a control group (57 000). Women aged 50 and over in the intervention group were invited for routine screening at average intervals of 33 months. In women aged 40–74, the average acceptance of screening was 89%, and mortality analyses are restricted to this age group. After 13 years of follow-up, the odds ratio of dying from breast cancer for women aged 50–74 at entry in the intervention group relative to the control group was 0.66 (95% CI 0.46–0.93).[6]

The Malmo trial

At about the same time, a further trial was started in Malmo, Sweden, in which 42 000 women aged 45–69 were randomised by birth cohort to an intervention group offered screening by two-view mammography at 18–24 month intervals or to a control group; 74% of women in the intervention group accepted screening.[7] In the analyses, women are divided into those above and below age 55 at entry to the trial. In those aged 55 and over, there was a non-significant mortality reduction RR 0.79, 95% CI 0.51–1.24) after 9 years. Approximately 25% of control group women were known to have had mammography during the course of the trial.

The Stockholm trial

In 1981, a further trial was started in Stockholm in which 60 000 women aged 40–64 were randomised by birth cohort into an intervention group (40 000), who were invited for single-view mammography at 2-yearly intervals, or to a control group (20 000). Compliance with the screening invitation was 80%. After an average of 11.4 years, among women aged 50–64 at entry, the risk of breast cancer death in the intervention group relative to the control group was 0.62 (95% CI 0.38–1.00).[8]

The Gothenburg trial

Another Swedish trial, in the city of Gothenburg, started in 1982 and randomised 50 000 women aged 40–59 to an intervention group of 21 000 offered screening by two-view mammography at 18-month intervals or to a control group of 29 000. The results of this trial have been included in the overview of all Swedish trials. Among women aged 50–59 at entry, the risk of breast cancer mortality in the intervention group relative to the control group after 13.2 years of follow-up was 0.94 (95% CI 0.62–1.43).[9]

The Edinburgh trial

This trial started in 1979 and randomised 45 000 women aged 45–64, according to the general practitioner with whom they were registered, into an intervention group of 23 000 and a control group of 22 000. Women in the intervention group were invited for screening every year for 7 years. Screening was by mammography and physical examination every 2 years, with physical examination only in the intervening years. Sixty-one percent of women accepted the first invitation to screening and non-responders were not reinvited in subsequent years. After 14 years of follow-up the overall reduction in the risk of breast cancer death was 13% (RR 0.87, 95% CI 0.70–1.16).[10] In women aged 50–64 at entry, the reduction at 10 years of follow-up was 15% (RR 0.85, 95% CI 0.62–1.15).[11] Analysis of this trial has been hampered by a bias in socioeconomic status between the intervention and control groups, which became apparent when all-cause mortality was considered. Adjustment for this bias results in a lower relative risk of breast cancer mortality in the intervention group.

Meta-analyses

The findings of those individual trials for women aged 50 or over at entry are summarised in Table 8.1. There are a number of differences between the trials that affect their interpretation, including differences in screening methods, available technology, frequency of screening, quality of screening, compliance, contamination by screening in the control group, duration of observation and sample size.[12]

Table 8.1 **Randomised trials of breast screening by mammography**

Study	Screening Interval (months)	CBE[a] included	No. of women	Length of follow-up (years)	Relative risk[b] in women aged 50 and over
HIP	12	Yes	62 000	10	0.68 (0.49–0.96)
Two-County Trial	24–33	No	133 000	13	0.66 (0.54–0.81)
Malmo	18–24	No	42 300	8	0.79[d] (0.51–1.24)
Gothenburg	18	No	52 000		0.94 (06.2–1.43)
Stockholm	30	No	60 300	11.4	0.62 (0.38–1.00)
Edinburgh	24	Yes (annual)	50 000	10	0.85 (0.62–1.15)
NBSS-2[c]	12	Yes	39 400	13	1.02 (0.78–1.33)

[a]CBE, Clinical breast examination.
[b]Relative risk of breast cancer mortality in intervention arm. 95% confidence interval in parentheses.
[c]Mammography plus CBE versus CBE alone.
[d]Age 55+.

A number of meta-analyses have been published in recent years. An overview of all the Swedish trials assessed breast cancer mortality by linking the identification details of all women enrolled in the trials with Swedish national mortality statistics. An independent committee reviewed the case notes of all women with breast cancer who had died without knowledge of whether each woman was in the intervention group or control group. The most recent results from this overview, which do not include the Kopparberg part of the Two-County Trial, show an overall reduction of 21% (RR 0.79, 95% CI 0.70–0.89) at a median 15.8 years of follow-up, with the greatest reduction (33%) being in women aged 60–69 at entry, and only a small effect in women aged 50–54 at entry.[9]

A meta-analysis performed in 1995, which also included the Edinburgh, HIP and Canadian trials found a mortality reduction of 23% (RR 0.77, 95% CI 0.69–0.87) in women aged 50–74 at entry.[13] Summary estimates did not vary with screening interval (12 months vs 18–33 months) or length of follow-up (7–9 years vs 10–12 years).

A Cochrane review and a more extensive publication[14] have criticised a number of the randomised trials on the grounds of potential bias in randomisation, and have also cast doubt on the validity of breast cancer mortality as an outcome measure. Including only the two trials with 'medium-quality' data according to their criteria (the Malmö trial and the Canadian NBSS) gave a relative risk of breast cancer mortality in women aged 50 and over of 0.97 (95% CI 0.82–1.14) after 13 years of follow-up. The authors concluded that the available evidence 'does

not show a survival benefit of mass screening for breast cancer', and also that screening leads to overdiagnosis and increased use of more aggressive treatment.

However, an expert group convened by the World Health Organization (WHO) in March 2002 dismissed these conclusions, and other experts have also refuted this analysis. It seems clear from the available evidence that breast cancer mortality can be reduced by one-quarter to one-third among women aged 50–69 invited to regular routine breast screening by mammography who are free from the disease at time of invitation. It should be noted that this estimate of overall reduction in breast cancer mortality includes deaths in women who did not accept invitation to screening. While it is necessary to include these women for an unbiased comparison, it is clear that the proportionate reduction among women who accept screening must be greater. Thus the statistical estimate of risk reduction in these trials gives a measure of the public health benefit that screening would confer on population mortality risk; the benefit to an individual screened women would be greater than this. Day[16] has estimated that the risk reduction in a women aged over 50 who accepts screening is 39%.

Screening by physical examination

While it is clear from the Swedish trials that mammography alone is effective in reducing mortality, there remains a question as to whether physical examination alone could produce a similar benefit.[17]

This is a most important question for developing countries, in many of which the risk of breast cancer mortality is increasing but which may not have the necessary resources for population screening by mammography. In the HIP trial, 45% of screen-detected cancers were found by physical examination alone, and it is therefore reasonable to conclude that some of the observed benefit was achieved by this means. However, advances in mammography since the 1960s have improved its sensitivity such that in the Edinburgh trial only 6% of screen-detected cancers were found by physical examination alone.[18]

The only trial published so far that has addressed the question of the effectiveness of physical examination is the Canadian National Breast Screening Study.[19] Among women aged 50–59, the aim of the trial was not to assess whether screening had any benefit but rather to measure the size of any incremental mortality reduction conferred by the addition of mammography to physical examination. Here, 39 500 women who had volunteered to take part in the trial were randomly allocated to a group offered annual screening by mammography plus physical examination or to a group offered annual screening by physical examination alone. Despite the fact that the incidence of interval cancers was lower in the mammographic arm of the trial, after 11 years of follow-up there was no significant difference in breast cancer mortality between the two groups (RR 1.14, 95% CI 0.83–1.6).[20] This particular trial has been criticised on a number of grounds, including poor mammographic quality and small sample size. In addition, the fact that the subjects in this trial were volunteers resulted in a lower underlying breast cancer mortality than the average Canadian population, meaning that longer follow-up was necessary to give the trial statistical power.

Evidence on the disadvantages of screening

Like many preventive medical interventions, breast screening has a number of unwanted side-effects that will mainly affect those people who do not benefit from screening, i.e. women who in the absence of screening would not develop or die from breast cancer. The disadvantages may be subdivided into those inherent to the screening procedure itself, those resulting from false-positive test results, those resulting from overdiagnosis of borderline lesions of little biological significance, those resulting from false-negative test results and finally the opportunity costs of screening.

Disadvantages of the screening procedure

Psychological effects
It has been postulated that inviting women to be screened increases anxiety both by increasing awareness of breast cancer and by inducing feelings of guilt in those who do not accept the invitation. However, there is little if any evidence to support these hypotheses.

One study, using a well-validated psychological questionnaire, found no difference in psychiatric morbidity between women attending for screening and an age-matched sample of the general population.[21] Similarly, no difference in psychiatric morbidity has been found between attenders and non-attenders for screening.[22] More recent studies found no difference between anxiety levels in attenders immediately before and immediately after screening in those screened negative.[23,24]

Discomfort
The compression of the breast needed in order to obtain a clear mammographic picture of the whole breast causes discomfort in some women. Early studies of screened women in the USA[25] and the UK[26] suggested that around one-third of women experience some discomfort, but that in only 5% or less did this amount to pain.

Some more recent studies have reported higher levels; in a study in the Netherlands, 72.9% of women described mammography as 'mild to severely painful',[27] and in a Finnish study, 61% reported painful mammograms.[28] There is little evidence that experience of pain acts as a deterrent to attendance for future screening, but these findings do have implications for staff responsible for providing information to women and those directly involved in the screening process.

Radiogenic induction of cancer
The potential of mammography to induce cancer by radiation exposure has caused considerable concern. Estimates of the likely rate of induction of breast cancer are obtained by extrapolating from data on excess incidence of breast cancer in women who have received very high doses of radiation either due to medical irradiation or as nuclear bomb survivors. Based on the latest estimates for the mean dose in the UK Breast Screening Programme, using two-view mammography, it has been calculated that for women aged 50–64 the ratio of cancers detected by screening to cancers induced ranges from 104 to 182, and that even for a small subgroup with a much larger dose level, benefit is likely to exceed radiological risk by a substantial margin.[29]

Disadvantages of false-positive test results

Women who are recalled for further assessment following a positive screening test will inevitably experience some anxiety and will have to undergo further medical investigation, some of which will entail physical morbidity. For those women eventually found not to have cancer, this psychological and physical morbidity will have been unnecessary. In the UK Trial of Early Detection of Breast Cancer conducted in the 1980s, for example, it was shown that the absolute rate of benign biopsies in a population offered screening was 7 times greater than in a control population during the prevalence screening period, falling to 1.5 times greater during later screening rounds. However, benign biopsy rates have been reduced considerably since then by the increased use of non-operative diagnostic techniques.

There are many anecdotes about extreme anxiety caused to women recalled for further tests. While a number of studies using validated methods suggest that increased anxiety in these women is short-lived[30,31] or have found that anxiety is lower in women referred from screening than in symptomatic women,[32,33] others have reported more sustained anxiety.[24]

Overdiagnosis

An unknown proportion of women with screen-detected cancer would not otherwise have been diagnosed with the disease in their lifetime. Up to 20% of screen-detected cancers are ductal carcinomas in situ (DCIS), whose natural history remains unclear. Autopsy studies of women who have died of other causes have shown that DCIS and even some cases of invasive cancer may be undiagnosed during a woman's lifetime. A review of seven autopsy series of women not known to have had breast cancer during life found a median prevalence of invasive breast cancer of 1.3% (range 0–1.8%) and a median prevalence of DCIS of 8.9% (range 0–14.7%).[30] However, follow-up of untreated (misdiagnosed) DCIS has shown that over a period of 10 years, one-quarter will go on to develop invasive, sometimes metastatic, breast cancer.[34] There is therefore a dilemma of knowing how to manage patients with a condition that may progress or remain latent. To label such women as breast cancer patients will bring with it the physical morbidity of treatment and the psychological morbidity of anxiety in themselves and their family, as well as other potential disbenefits such as inability to obtain insurance. While these side-effects apply to some extent for all women with screen-detected cancer, one study of psychological morbidity in breast cancer patients who were disease-free 1 year or more after diagnosis found that there was less anxiety and depression among breast cancer patients than among age-matched control women from the same population.[35]

False-negative screening results

False-negative screening results in women who subsequently present with interval cancers are a serious disadvantage to any screening programme. Some of these will have been present at the time of screening, and it is sometimes postulated that because the woman concerned has had the reassurance of an earlier negative screen, she may ignore symptoms, and present with a cancer that is more advanced at diagnosis than it would have been in the absence of screening. However, in controlled trials of screening, there was little evidence that the prognosis of interval cancers is any different from that of control group breast cancers.

Resource costs of screening programmes

While the cost of screening in the private sector is eventually controlled by what an individual is prepared to pay, public health screening programmes use limited public funds. which would otherwise be available to spend on other healthcare or alternative projects. These are the so-called opportunity costs of breast screening programmes and have been the cause of much debate.

Several countries have made estimates of the costs of their public screening programmes, but even if these are all expressed in a standard currency, it is difficult to compare them because of differences in national healthcare organisation, funding and salaries. A UK estimate derived from earlier research, and updated to 1999/2000 prices, suggests that the average cost per woman screened, including the cost of an invitation and recall system, the cost of screening and the cost of providing diagnostic assessment to those screened positive, is £22.36 and the cost per cancer detected is £4124.59 for women aged 50–64.[36]

Implementation and quality assurance

Population-based breast screening programmes have now been introduced in a number of countries,[36] and most of these have acknowledged the need to achieve the same quality standards as those obtained in research trials in order to obtain the same level of benefit. To this end, targets of interim indicators of screening performance have been set, and information systems have been established to enable the performance of the programmes to be monitored.

Quality assurance of any screening programme is essential in order to maintain maximum benefit and minimum harm from the programme.

Quality assurance also includes measures to reduce anxiety and improve consumer satisfaction, monitoring of radiological equipment and radiation dose, and provision of dedicated and efficient staff in screening clinics.

Routine monitoring of outcome measures of the screening programme will assist in identifying areas where there are potential problems and that need further investigation. Likewise, continued analysis of potential changes to the programme may identify areas where improvements may be made. In the Netherlands, results from the period 1990–95 showed that targets for attendance and for detection rates and stage distribution of cancers at initial screens were being met, but that cancer detection rates at subsequent screens were lower than expected.[37]

In the UK, the National Health Service Breast Screening Programme (NHSBSP) was set up following the recommendations of an expert advisory group that examined the evidence on breast cancer screening becoming available in the mid-1980s.[38] This group drew largely on the findings of the Swedish Two-County Trial, and recommended that all women between ages 50 and 64 should be routinely invited for screening by single-oblique-view mammography every 3 years. The initial targets set in the UK included a participation rate of at least 70%, a referral rate at first screening of no more than 7% and a breast cancer detection rate of at least 5 per 1000. These targets have subsequently been revised, and new targets have been set to include outcome measures at routine rescreening[39] and expected rates of interval cancers. Results for the programme up to 1999 showed that considerable advances in performance had been made since its inception in 1988, with uptake and age-standardised cancer detection rates in excess of targets by 1999.[40] However, as the time since the introduction of screening increases, it becomes increasingly difficult to estimate the underlying incidence rates that are used to calculate standards.

There are a number of trade-offs that need to be born in mind when assessing the performance of the screening programme. Ensuring a high participation rate of the eligible population will maximise the benefit in terms of reduction of breast cancer deaths. However, this needs to be balanced against the need for sufficient information to be given to women on both the potential benefits and disadvantages of screening to enable an informed choice to be made. Maximising specificity will decrease the disbenefits by reducing the number of false positives, but there is a trade-off between sensitivity and specificity, and a certain level of referral for further assessments may be necessary in order to maintain high sensitivity for screen-detected cancers.[41] It is often found that a change that will enhance benefit may have an unwanted side-effect in increasing disbenefit or cost. A notable exception to this is the finding from a randomised controlled trial that the use of two-view mammography instead of single-view not only improves sensitivity, increasing the percentage of screen-detected cancers by 24%, but also improves specificity, reducing the false-positive rate by 15%.[42] In this case, the increased cost of two-view screening was almost counterbalanced by the reduction in costs of further investigation of false positives.

Effect of population screening on breast cancer mortality

Even given that the findings of the randomised trials are widely accepted as proving a benefit of screening, there is considerable interest internationally in whether a similar effect can be demonstrated from population-based screening programmes. It is important to appreciate that, for two main reasons, the effect of such programmes will take some time to be observed. Firstly, the results of the randomised trials studied those women free from breast cancer at time of entry to the trials, whereas, without detailed record linkage, these cases will be included in population mortality rates from breast cancer, and will dilute any observed effect from screening for a number of years. Secondly, even in the randomised trials, the difference between intervention and control groups took between 3 and 5 years to emerge. In most countries, the introduction of population screening has been spread over a number of years. For example in the UK, the first units began screening in 1988, but it was not until 1994 that full coverage of the population was achieved. It will therefore be a number of years after the first introduction of screening before any benefit should be expected, and a number of critics of population screening programmes have merely been expecting a benefit to become apparent too early.

In some countries where record linkage is possible, researchers have studied so-called 'refined' breast cancer mortality, excluding those deaths in cases diagnosed before the start of screening. In Finland, where screening was introduced in different years for different birth cohorts, a reduction in refined breast cancer mortality was observed between the first cohort that was invited and the so-called control population during the first 5 years of follow up.[43] Similar studies in Sweden have estimated a non-significant 20% reduction in refined breast cancer mortality in women aged 50–69 after a mean follow-up of 10.6 years after the start of screening.[44] In the Netherlands, the MISCAN simulation model has been used to predict the expected breast cancer mortality both in the absence of screening and with the screening programme as being carried out; the observed breast cancer mortality is being tracked against these predicted rates. In the UK, an analysis has attempted to estimate the effect of screening on population mortality by comparing the reduction in mortality rates in the age group affected by screening with the reduction where mortality is likely to have been affected only by other factors – primarily changes in treatment. This analysis estimated that in 1998, of the 21% observed mortality reduction in women aged 55–69, approximately one-third of this was due directly to screening.[45]

Conclusions

Many expert groups advising national policy makers in developed countries have concluded that regular mammographic screening for women aged 50 and over is a priority area, and many national, provincial or pilot programmes now exist.

The cost-effectiveness of breast screening in different countries will vary according to the breast cancer mortality rate. For example, using the MISCAN simulation model, it has been estimated that the cost per life-year gained by screening women in Spain would be more than twice that gained by screening women in the Netherlands or the UK.[46]

Those disagreeing with the provision of breast cancer screening voice concerns on the psychological and physical harm incurred, both in women with false-positive results, and as a result of overdiagnosis, particularly of ductal carcinoma in situ.

However, the main argument against screening remains the use of resources that could be employed elsewhere, and the question of whether population-based screening programmes will achieve the same level of mortality reduction as that shown in randomised trials. Changes in breast cancer mortality due to other factors such as changes in incidence and improved outcomes from therapy will also be occurring and need to be taken into consideration. It is only by continued monitoring and evaluation of screening that the true effect in practice can be measured.

References

1. Chamberlain J. Evaluation of screening for cancer. In: Veronesi U, Peckham M, eds. Oxford Textbook of Oncology. Oxford: Oxford University Press, 1995: 185–98.

2. Chamberlain J. Breast cancer screening in the UK. In: Shapiro S, Greberman M, Kessler L, Prorok PC, eds. Hans Huber, 1995.

3. Day NE, Duffy SW. Trial design based on surrogate end points – application to comparison of different breast screening frequencies. J R Statist Soc 1996; 159: 49–60.

4. Shapiro S, Venet W, Strax P, Venet L. Periodic screening for breast cancer. In: The Health Insurance Plan Project and its sequelae, 1963–1986. Baltimore: Johns Hopkins University Press, 1988.

5. Tabar L, Fagerberg G, Duffy SW et al. Update of the Swedish Two-County Program of Mammographic Screening for Breast Cancer. Radiol Clin North Am 1992; 30: 187–210.

6. Tabar L, Fagerberg G, Chen HH et al. Efficacy of breast cancer screening by age. New results from the Swedish Two-County Trial. Cancer 1995; 75: 2507–17.

7. Andersson I, Aspegren K, Janzon L et al. Mammographic screening and mortality from breast cancer: the Malmö mammographic screening trial. BMJ 1988; 297: 943–8.

8. Frisell J, Lidbrink E, Hellstrom L, Rutqvist L-E. Follow up after 11 years – update of mortality results in the Stockholm mammographic screening trial. Breast Cancer Res Treat 1997; 45: 263–70.

9. Nystrom L, Andersson I, Bjurstam N, Frisell J, Nordenskjold B. Long-term effects of mammography screening: updated overview of the Swedish randomised trials. Lancet 2002; 359: 909–19.

10. Alexander FE, Anderson TJ, Brown HK et al. 14 years of follow-up from the Edinburgh randomised trial of breast-cancer screening. Lancet 1999; 353: 1903–8.

11. Alexander FE, Anderson TJ, Brown HK et al. The Edinburgh randomised trial of breast cancer screening: results after 10 years of follow-up. Br J Cancer 1994; 70: 542–8.

12. Morrison AS. Screening for cancer of the breast. Epidemiol Rev 1993; 15: 244–55.

13. Kerlikowske K, Grady D, Rubin SM et al. Efficacy of screening mammography. A meta-analysis. JAMA 1995; 273: 149–54.

14. Gotzche PC, Olsen O. Is screening for breast cancer with mammography justified? Lancet 2000; 355: 129–34.

15. Kmietowicz Z. WHO insists screening can cut breast cancer rates. BMJ 2002; 324: 695.

16. Day NE. Screening for breast cancer. Br Med Bull 1991; 47: 400–15.

17. Mittra I, Baum M, Thornton H, Houghton J. Is clinical breast examination an acceptable alternative to mammographic screening? BMJ 2000; 321: 1071–3.

18. Moss SM. Breast cancer screening. Br J Hosp Med 1992;48:178–81.

19. Miller AB, Howe GR, Wall C. The National Study of

Breast Cancer Screening. Protocol for a Canadian randomized controlled trial of screening for breast cancer in women. Clin Invest Med 1981; 4: 227–58.

20. Miller AB. Effect of screening programme on mortality from breast cancer. Benefit of 30% may be substantial overestimate. BMJ 2000; 321: 1527.

21. Dean C, Roberts MM, French K, Robinson S. Psychiatric morbidity after screening for breast cancer. J Epidemiol Community Health 1986; 40: 71–5.

22. Hunt SM, Alexander F, Roberts MM. Attenders and non-attenders at a breast screening clinic: a comparative study. Public Health 1988; 102: 3–10.

23. Sutton S, Saidi G, Bickler G, Hunter J. Does routine screening for breast cancer raise anxiety? Results from a three wave prospective study in England. J Epidemiol Comm Health 1995; 49: 413–18.

24. Meystre-Agustoni G, Paccaud F, Jeannin A, Dubois-Arber F. Anxiety in a cohort of Swiss women participating in a mammographic screening programme. J Med Screen 2001; 8: 213–9.

25. Stomper PC, Kopans DB, Sadowsky NL et al. Is mammography painful? A multicentre patient survey. Arch Intern Med 1988; 148: 521–4.

26. Rutter DR, Calnan M, Vaile MSB et al. Discomfort and pain during mammography: description, prediction and prevention. BMJ 1992; 305: 443–5.

27. Keemers-Gels ME, Groenendijk RP, van den Heuvel HJ et al. Pain experienced by women attending breast cancer screening. Breast Cancer Res Treat 2000; 60: 235–40.

28. Aro AR, Absetz-Ylostalo P, Eerola T et al. Pain and discomfort during mammography. Eur J Cancer 1995; 32A: 1674–9.

29. Law J, Faulkner K. Cancers detected and induced, and associated risk and benefit, in a breast screening programme. Br J Radiol 2001; 74: 1121–7.

30. Welch GH, Black WC. Using autopsy series to estimate the disease 'reservoir' for ductal carcinoma in situ of the breast: How much more breast cancer can we find? Ann Intern Med 1997; 127: 1023–8.

31. Scaf-Klomp W, Sanderman R, van de Wiel HBM et al. Distressed or relieved? Psychological side effects of breast cancer screening in the Netherlands. J Epidemiol Comm Health 1997; 51: 705–10.

32. Ellman R, Angeli N, Christians A et al. Psychiatric morbidity associated with screening for breast cancer. Br J Cancer 1989; 60: 781–4.

33. Bull AR, Campbell MJ. Assessment of the psychological impact of a breast screening programme. Br J Radiol 1991; 64: 510–15.

34. Dupont WD, Page DL. Breast cancer risk associated with proliferative disease, age at first birth a family history of breast cancer. Am J Epidemiol 1987; 125: 769–79.

35. Fracheboud J, de Koning HJ, Beemsterboer PM et al. Nation-wide breast cancer screening in the Netherlands: results of initial and subsequent screening 1990–1995. Int J Cancer 1998; 75: 694–8.

36. Blanks RG, Moss SM, Wallis MG. Monitoring and evaluating the UK National Health Service Breast Screening Programme: evaluating the variation in radiological performance between individual programmes using PPV-referral diagrams. J Med Screen 2001; 8: 24–8.

37. Shapiro S, Coleman EA, Broeders M et al, for the International Breast Cancer Screening Network (IBSN) and the European Network of Pilot Projects for Breast Cancer Screening. Breast cancer screening programmes in 22 countries: current policies, administration and guidelines. Int J Epidemiol 1998; 27: 735–42.

38. Forrest APM. Breast Cancer Screening: Report to the Health Ministers of England, Wales, Scotland and Northern Ireland. London: HMSO, 1986.

39. Moss S, Blanks R, for the Interval Cancer Working Group. Calculating appropriate target cancer detection rates and expected interval cancer rates for the UK NHS Breast Screening Programme. J Epidemiol Comm Health 1998; 52: 111–15.

40. Blanks RG, Moss SM, Patnick J. Results from the UK NHS Breast Screening Programme 1994–1999. J Med Screen 2000; 7: 195–8.

41. Blanks RG, Moss SM. Breast cancer screening sensitivity in the NHSBSP: recent results and implications. Breast 1999; 8: 301–2.

42. Wald NJ, Murphy P, Major P et al. UKCCCR multicentre randomised controlled trial of one and two view mammography in breast cancer screening. BMJ 1995; 311: 1189–93.

43. Hakama M, Pukkala E, Heikkila, Kallio M. Effectiveness of the public health policy for breast cancer screening in Finland: population based cohort study. BMJ 1997; 314: 864–7.

44. Jonsson E, Banta HD, Schersten T. Health technology assessment and screening in Sweden. Int J Technol Assess Health Care 2001; 17: 380–8.

45. Blanks RG, Moss SM, McGahan CE et al. Effect of NHS breast screening programme on mortality from breast cancer in England and Wales, 1990–8: comparison of observed with predicted mortality. BMJ 2000; 321: 665–9.

46. van Ineveld BM, van Oortmarssen GJ, de Koning HJ et al. How cost-effective is breast cancer screening in different EC countries? Eur J Cancer 1993; 12: 1663–8.

9 The organisation of breast screening

Julietta Patnick

Introduction

The value of breast screening in preventing deaths from breast cancer was first investigated by the Health Improvement Plan (HIP) of Greater New York in the early 1960s using annual mammography and clinical breast examination. This study showed benefit to women, with a 30% reduction in mortality from breast cancer.[1,2] It was followed in the 1970s by the Swedish Two-Counties Study, which used mammography only and showed comparable results.[3,4] Several other studies investigating the value of breast cancer screening were subsequently initiated.[5] By the late 1980s, mammographically based breast screening programmes were being introduced in many European countries and opportunistic breast screening was becoming part of routine healthcare for women in other developed countries.

Meta-analyses have amalgamated evidence from all published trials and have concluded that mammographic breast screening is protective.[6] It has generally been accepted that for women aged 50–69 (and probably up to age 74) the death rate from breast cancer amongst regular attenders for screening can be reduced by as much as 35%. This view has been echoed by the International Agency for Research on Cancer (IARC).[7] Indeed, for women aged 50–69, it stated that 'there is sufficient evidence from randomised trials that inviting women 50–69 years of age to screening with mammography reduces their mortality from breast cancer'. There is inadequate evidence on the value of screening beyond age 69, but there is some belief that it may benefit women who are otherwise well and have a life expectancy of 10 years or more.

Controversy still exists about screening of women aged under 50, particularly those of average risk and who are between the ages of 40 and 49. The US National Cancer Institute (NCI) recommends mammography from age 40,[8] but the European guidelines advocate screening from age 50.[9] The British Age Trial, which is assessing annual mammography from age 40, may resolve this issue when it reports its findings around 2006. Frequency of screening is another area of controversy and uncertainty; the NCI recommends mammography every 1–2 years, but European organisations suggest a minimum frequency of every 3 years.[8,9] An international overview revealed a variety of target age groups and screening frequencies in existence around the world.[10] The World Health Organization (WHO), through the IARC, concluded that there was limited evidence of benefit for women aged 40–49 and that a screening frequency more than 3-yearly yielded only a marginal benefit.[7]

The role of clinical examination in breast screening is a subject that has generated much debate. Clinical examination was a component of the UK Trial of Early Detection of Breast Cancer,[11] and later Canadian researchers attempted to address specifically the relative contribution of clinical examination.[12] This latter trial has proved to be highly controversial; although the results are within the overall range that might be expected for a screening trial, criticisms have been made of both the target population and the quality of mammography employed, particularly early on in the trial. The UK, together with most of its European neighbours, does not include clinical examination as a component of its screening programme. Indeed, the UK specifically recommends that clinical examination of the breast should not be undertaken on asymptomatic women.[13] There is inadequate evidence demonstrating that clinical examination, whether alone or in addition to screening mammography, reduces the death rate from breast cancer.

An overview from researchers at the Nordic Cochrane Centre claimed that the efficacy of mammographic screening has not been proven, due to innate flaws in the design of the original screening trials.[14] This analysis triggered great debate within the international screening community on the true benefits or otherwise of breast screening. An update on the Swedish trials was subsequently published and, following much deliberation, the IARC declared that many of these criticisms of the original trials were unfounded and that those that were upheld did not invalidate the overall conclusion that mammographic screening reduces deaths from breast cancer.[7,15]

When assessing the effectiveness of mammographic screening, it should be emphasised that its impact will be dependent upon the quality of the service delivered. This variation in effectiveness due to quality issues may be considered a weakness of screening programmes. Furthermore, the effects of quality variation will become apparent only after several years have passed. In the original trials of breast screening, benefits emerged after 4 years and the full impact was seen only with more prolonged follow-up. In service screening, even longer periods are necessary, because populations targeted for service screening (unlike 'clean' trial populations), include many women with a pre-existent breast cancer diagnosis. In addition, these women are living longer than previously due to improvements in treatment, namely the introduction of hormonal therapy and improved use of chemotherapy.

The initial effects of screening have been demonstrated in Finland,[16] the Netherlands[17] and the UK,[18] although it will take time before the full impact of introducing breast screening into a population becomes apparent. For this reason, those involved in the organisation of screening programmes must remain as committed as the early enthusiasts to the delivery of high-quality programmes to women in the local populations. The challenge is to ensure that these service programmes deliver on the expectation of trial results. This chapter discusses the organisation of screening programmes for defined populations of women at average risk. It does not consider women with a family history or screening for known breast cancer genes (see Chapter 3). However, many of the principles outlined for population screening will have general application.

Essential components of a breast screening programme

Breast screening takes place within a range of different healthcare systems. At one extreme, screening may be at the complete discretion of an individual woman and her clinician. Breast cancer mortality rates are highest in the developed world, where most countries have screening policies, reflecting a professional consensus about age, frequency and quality of mammography. Organised population breast screening is considered to be more efficient than opportunistic screening, and is particularly appropriate where a suitable population can be defined and targeted. Under these circumstances, there are several essential components of a screening programme including:

- support for a screening service within the population as a whole
- resources
- clear protocols underpinned by training and quality assurance
- evaluation
- information systems and database
- public information and recruitment

Support within the population as a whole

Wilson and Jungner,[19] on behalf of the WHO, stipulated that a disease for which population screening takes place should be recognised as 'an important public health problem'. In the absence of such recognition, there will be no financial support from funders, clinicians will neither recommend nor participate in a screening programme and attendance is likely to be poor among the target population.

Breast cancer is a leading cause of cancer death in developed countries, second only to lung cancer. However, it is the commonest malignancy among women, and in recognition of this significant health problem there is both political and financial support for management of this disease, with funding coming from central government and insurance companies. It is essential that these sources of funding incorporate provision for treatment of cancers detected at screening. Screening without appropriate follow-up treatment would be unethical.

Professional support for a breast screening programme is crucial in order that clinicians will encourage women to participate and to enable the recruitment and retention of staff. Breast screening can sometimes be perceived as a repetitive and rather tedious activity. However, the many subtle radiological signs present a considerable challenge and film reading demands constant vigilance if abnormalities are not to be missed. Finally, there must be support from the population targeted for screening. Strategies to maximise recruitment of women will be discussed later in this chapter, but it is important that women within the target population recognise screening to be an effective tool in the fight against breast cancer, as this will help engage the population.

Resources

Staff

Breast screening is an image-driven programme, so a major resource is the image reader and his or her visual skills. Computer-aided devices for the reading of mammograms are coming into use, but have yet to supplant the interpretational ability of the human brain, generally due to limited specificity. Radiologists prefer double reading of films, and a minimum amount of regular mammogram reporting is needed to develop and maintain expertise.[20] Thus many countries set a minimum number of mammograms to be reported; in the UK, a radiologist must report at least 5000 sets of films per year. Obtaining good-quality images requires a level of skill that should not be underestimated. The requisite qualifications to undertake this task vary around the world. Mammography has traditionally been undertaken in the UK by state registered radiographers, but recently a programme to train lay persons without any background in imaging to take mammograms has been established. These alternative imaging practices are proving very successful.

By employing non-state-registered practitioners to carry out mammography, radiographers have been released to undertake advanced tasks previously undertaken by medical staff. These include mammography reading and interpretation, ultrasound examinations, and image-guided biopsies. Breast clinicians who are neither specialist surgeons nor radiologists are also a valuable component of the screening scene, with their role varying according to innate skills and local service requirements.

Following initial imaging, further investigation may be required to make a complete diagnostic assessment. Women should undergo triple assessment (clinical, radiological and pathological), although for screen-detected lesions there is often no clinical correlate to the radiological abnormality. This involves a multidisciplinary team composed not only of imaging staff, but also of a pathologist with a special interest in breast disease, a breast surgeon and a breast care nurse trained in counselling. The precise role of the surgeon in the management of screen-detected lesions is often debated, but while the majority of these can now be diagnosed non-operatively with percutaneous biopsy techniques (91% in the NHS Breast Screening Programme, NHSBSP[21]), there remains a proportion of women who require a surgical opinion and will proceed to an open surgical biopsy to establish a definitive diagnosis.

Many women value and appreciate the support of a breast care nurse along the screening pathway. This might involve discussion of possible procedures prior to attending the assessment clinic or further explanation and clarification following diagnosis of cancer. Although breast care nurses are accustomed to dealing with newly diagnosed breast cancer patients and explaining treatment options, a woman diagnosed through screening presents additional challenges, having been previously asymptomatic. She has had little time to contemplate the possibility of having cancer, which can prove to be an additional burden when coping initially with a diagnosis of breast cancer. Under these circumstances, an experienced and understanding nurse can be of great assistance. Close teamwork between the various professional disciplines is essential.

Facilities

The quality of X-ray imaging equipment is of primary importance to a screening programme. Full-field digital mammography is being developed and some hardware is available for use. However, this technology is expensive and yet to be a standard replacement for the latest film/screen technology. Standard analogue mammography equipment for basic screening will be relatively uncomplicated, but a set-up that permits full diagnostic work-up will have additional facilities for magnification and stereotaxis. All equipment should enable both 18 mm × 24 mm and 24 mm × 30 mm images to be taken, which will ensure that larger breasts can be encompassed in a single exposure, thus minimising radiation dose.

Dedicated film handling and processing equipment is available for use both in a hospital setting and in some mobile units. Specimen radiography equipment should also be available and within easy reach of the theatre to ensure that excised lesions can be radiographed to check that the identified radiological abnormality is contained within the specimen. Ultrasound equipment is an integral component of a full breast screening service. It reliably distinguishes between solid and cystic lesions, and permits aspiration of cysts and biopsy of solid masses under image guidance. A range of equipment and needles are available for percutaneous biopsy procedures, and although these may appear expensive, these costs should be considered in comparison with the physical, psychological and financial costs of an open surgical biopsy. The ready availability of these techniques compared with operative biopsy may have contributed to the improvements in the cancer detection rate within the NHSBSP and have certainly contributed to the high rate of non-operative diagnosis.

Prone biopsy tables have been introduced into a few screening units, and are said to improve the accuracy of biopsy techniques with greater convenience for both the practitioner and women who require diagnostic evaluation of a suspicious radiological lesion. However, these units are expensive, and, in most cases, equally satisfactory biopsies can be obtained using conventional equipment. Availability may therefore be restricted to specialist centres to which appropriate cases will be referred.

Breast screening is carried out on well women, and the general atmosphere and physical ambience of a screening unit should not be ignored. When women attend for screening, they should find themselves in as pleasant and relaxing an environment as possible. Mobile screening units have proved very popular in many countries, including the UK, and acceptability is higher for a mobile unit than for a hospital department.[22] However, mobile units are only suitable for basic screening activity, and more comprehensive diagnostic work-up must be undertaken in a hospital setting. It must be remembered that most of the women do not have breast cancer and care should be taken to ensure they are kept separated from cancer patients or from women presenting symptomatically. In effect, they should be treated as well women, as the majority are just this.

Finance

The finance required to operate a breast screening service will clearly vary with context. Different countries in the developed world have adopted different approaches to the funding of national screening programmes, which generally depend on central funding or reimbursement or a combination. The cost-effectiveness evidence supporting the use of breast screening is dependent on studies that have examined not only the overall cost-effectiveness of screening, but also aspects of screening technique such as the number of views, reports, frequency and the age band exposed to screening.

The above comments on the multifactorial nature of attainment of high quality and effectiveness in breast screening illustrate why it is essential that the funding be sufficient to support the chosen regimen. Moreover, a screening programme should not be embarked upon where women who are diagnosed with cancer are unable to access appropriate treatment. This is true across any particular health system as a whole and for individual women.

Protocols, training and quality assurance

Population screening for breast cancer has certain parallels with a production line, whereby a single

hospital clinic or doctor is capable of screening thousands of women per year, the vast majority of whom will not have cancer. In order to cope with the volume of work and minimise psychological distress to the majority of women without cancer, standard protocols must be developed and adhered to. These should encompass a broad remit, including the administrative aspects of dealing with large numbers of women, the optimum methods for imaging women in different circumstances and how radiologically suspicious abnormalities should be assessed to obtain diagnostic clarification. In the latter situation, the screening process becomes more focused, with women receiving more individual attention.

Clinical protocols are outlined in medical texts and often discussed at scientific meetings. With experience, a multidisciplinary team will derive its own detailed protocols, reflecting the skill mix and knowledge available locally, and reach a consensus on which protocols should be applied to women under their care.[23] Once this point is reached, professional training programmes can be set up to ensure that minimum standards of practice are guaranteed for that community and to encourage inflow of skilled personnel into the community with dissemination of knowledge and skills relating to new techniques.

Breast screening is a high-risk activity in a medicolegal context and, from a clinical perspective, has the potential to cause harm to women. Screening involves large numbers of healthy women, and relatively minor aberrations can affect large numbers of women in a very short space of time. Quality assurance measures must be applied to every step of the process to ensure that any minor faults or problems are quickly identified and promptly corrected. All units should have written protocols and audits undertaken to ensure that protocols are adhered to. Protocols should be regularly reviewed and updated in the light of changes in hospital procedures and advances in knowledge and techniques. Audits and quality assurance may expose an area where further training is needed or where the protocols need amending. The audit loop involves constant monitoring and quality improvement. Protocols, training and quality assurance are important elements of all aspects of breast screening and increase the chances that women participating in screening will ultimately derive more benefit than harm.

Evaluation

Evaluation of screening is most conveniently considered within two timescales – the short term, which deals with the process of screening, and the long term, where the outcome of screening is examined. Long-term outcomes inevitably reflect screening practices and activity dating back several years when they may have been suboptimal compared with current practice. Short-term indicators of performance are therefore important in the early identification of problems and minimising the chance of doing harm rather than good.

Short-term process indicators will reflect current screening practice. They will include the uptake and cancer detection rates, the proportion of women found to have a radiological abnormality requiring further assessment, and the positive predictive value of these investigations. The histopathological features of individual tumours detected will be predictive of the future outcome of current screening methods and practice. In addition to overall programme indicators, each speciality within breast screening will have its own criteria for assessment of current professional practice. Radiographers, for example, will be particularly interested in the technical repeat rate and the pathologist in the predictive values of reports issued.

The ultimate long-term outcome indicator for a breast screening programme is the mortality rate. Breast cancer mortality is falling worldwide, which is partly due to improvements in adjuvant therapy in recent years. The precise proportion of the mortality reduction attributable to screening per se is difficult to determine.[18]

Measurements of survival might provide another potential long-term outcome indicator, with improved survival among screen-detected compared with symptomatic cancers. There is evidence emerging from the NHSBSP that this is the case.[21] However, these data can be difficult to interpret because of the phenomena of lead-time and selection biases. More favourable tumours may be overdiagnosed in a screening programme.

The interval cancer rate can be useful for longer-term evaluation of a breast screening programme. There is no evidence to suggest that women who develop interval cancers have a worse prognosis than women who present symptomatically. In particular, there is no evidence that presentation is delayed as a consequence of 'false reassurance' from a negative screen. Nonetheless, much can be learned from the occurrence of interval cancers, as they represent an element of failure and are by definition 'the ones that got away'. Comparison of current with previous screening films can be instructive, with some interval cancers being apparent in retrospect on the previous screen. The proportion of cancers that present as interval cases compared with the

underlying incidence should be minimal in order to maximise the effectiveness of the screening programme (see Chapters 5 and 6).

Interval cancers can be notoriously difficult to monitor and obtain information about. Screening programmes that have low rates of interval cases must ensure that appropriate efforts have been made to identify all such cases and thus for the quoted rates to be accurate rather than there existing much missing data with a resultant overoptimistic impression of efficacy.

Information systems and database

A robust and reliable information system is essential for any screening service, whether this is run by an individual clinician or is a formal population screening programme. With regular screening, serial films are built up and provide a useful documentation of personal screening history. The timing and results of previous episodes should be available at the time of the current screen and previous films available for comparison.

When screening is adopted as a public health policy, the service must be accessible to the entire population. If this is to be achieved then a reliable database of the population providing a minimum of age, sex and address is mandatory. This facilitates the process of sending invitations: the proportion of women in the population who have recently been screened (the coverage rate) can be calculated; those women who have not been screened can be identified and targeted, and population demographics can be kept under review for planning purposes.

How these population databases or registers are compiled varies from one health system to another. The UK has almost complete registration of the population with the NHS, which has allowed a universal invitation system to be introduced relatively easily. Other countries have been able to use the electoral or fiscal registers as a starting point. In some countries, there has been no access to any kind of pre-existing database, which has led to registers being built up as women are recruited. The variations between systems often reflect the data protection legislation pertaining to each country.

Information systems should ideally hold or have access to all relevant data about an individual woman within a screening programme. Recorded information should include if and when a woman was invited for screening, and her acceptance or otherwise. In addition, the outcome of an attendance should be clearly documented. If cancer is detected, information relevant to referral for further investigation and management should be recorded, together with the prognostic details about the cancer, such as size, grade and lymph node status. Collating data for each individual screened will provide an overall picture of the effectiveness of the screening programme and its effect in the screened population.

Information systems such as this are complicated in design, but they should be as easy to use as possible for doctors, nurses, radiographers and administrative staff in order that data be as accurate and complete as possible. It is essential that all users of the system be well trained and comfortable with its use. It is advantageous for staff to be able to enter the data for which they are directly responsible themselves, and thus transcription, with its attendant faults, is avoided.

Public information and recruitment

Hand in hand with the introduction of a screening programme is the provision of information to the public. This should include basic information such as for whom the programme is intended and how women may access its services. Various strategies can be employed to encourage general awareness of the programme and raise the public profile. These include contact with local and national print and broadcast media, liaison with charities and other women's organisations, and advertising campaigns. When a woman is invited for screening, she needs more specific information. She not only needs to know where and when to go for screening, but must also have some understanding of the process involved and the likely benefits and potential harms from screening. In the early days of breast cancer screening, there was a tendency to underplay the disadvantages and potential adverse effects of screening. For example, women were often not informed that mammography might be uncomfortable or that screening is not guaranteed to identify all cancers present at the time of screening. Today, however, women are encouraged to make an informed choice about whether or not to attend for screening, rather than being persuaded to attend even if they have an element of doubt or reluctance. It is quite unacceptable to attempt to convince non-attenders that they have made an unwise or even foolish decision and try to persuade them to attend after all. There are always some women who are difficult to reach with invitations and information. These are often women without a fixed address who relocate regularly and/or who are without a 'usual care provider' (e.g. a general practitioner). In addition, this group of women are likely to have poor literary skills and may find it difficult to grasp the issues presented with the intention of helping them make an 'informed choice'. Immigrants whose command of the host language and culture is weak present a particular challenge, as do women who have disabilities. Several strategies have been adopted to improve uptake of screening among these 'hard to reach' groups of women. Community health educators have worked successfully with women from ethnic minority groups,[24] and special materials are available for women with learning disabilities.[25] Opening screening clinics in the evenings and weekends has not proved successful in raising rates of attendance. Studies are regularly undertaken to examine the reasons for non-attendance, but this is a heterogeneous group of women and the development of a range of novel strategies is required to ensure that these individuals have access to and consent to screening.

Conclusion

Mammographic screening of women aged 50–69 has been shown to reduce mortality from breast cancer. There may be benefits from screening women outside this age group (40–49 and over 70), although this remains unproven. The success and effectiveness of a screening programme depends on a combination of organisation, ability to recruit women from the target population and the quality of the mammography and diagnostic processes. Successful screening programmes can play a significant part in the continued reduction in the mortality rates from breast cancer.

References

1. Shapiro S, Strax P, Venet L et al. Periodic breast cancer screening in reducing mortality from breast cancer. JAMA 1971; 215: 1777–85.
2. Shapiro S, Venet W, Strax P et al. 10 to 14 year effect of breast cancer screening on mortality. J Natl Cancer Inst 1982; 69: 349–55.
3. Tabar L, Fagerberg CJG, Gad A et al. Reduction in mortality from breast cancer after mass screening with mammography: randomised trial from the Breast Cancer Screening Working Group of the Swedish National Board of Health and Welfare. Lancet 1985; i: 829–32.
4. Tabar L, Vitak B, Chen H-H et al. The Swedish 2 County Trial 20 years later: updated mortality results and new insights from long term follow up. Radiol Clin North Am 2000; 38: 625–51.
5. Nystrom L, Rutqvist L E, Wall S et al. Breast cancer screening with mammography: overview of Swedish randomised studies. Lancet 1993; 341: 973–8.
6. Kerlikowske K, Gray DD, Rubin SM et al. Efficacy of screening mammography. A meta-analysis. JAMA 1995; 273: 149–54.

7. International Agency for Research on Cancer, Handbook of Cancer Protection no 7: Breast Cancer Screening. IARC Lyon 2002.

8. National Cancer Institute. NCI Statement on Mammography Screening, updated February 21, 2002 (www.nci.nih.gov/cancer_information).

9. Lynge E, Patnick J, Tornberg S et al, Position paper: Recommendations on cancer screening in the European Union. In: European Guidelines for Quality Assurance in Mammography Screening, 3rd edn. Terry N, Broeders M, DeWolf C et al, eds. Luxembourg, European Commission, 2001.

10. Ballard-Barbash R, Klabunde C, Paci E et al. Breast cancer screening in 21 countries: delivery of services, notification of results and outcomes assessment. Eur J Cancer Prev 1999; 9: 417–26.

11. Moss SM, Coleman DA, Ellman R et al. Interval cancers and sensitivity in the screening centres of the UK Trial of Early Detection of Breast Cancer. Eur J Cancer 1993; 29a: 255–8.

12. Miller AB, To T, Baines CJ, Wall C. Canadian National Breast Screening Study – 2: 13 year results of a randomised trial in women aged 50–59. J Natl Cancer Inst 2000; 92: 1490–9.

13. Chief Medical Officer and Chief Nursing Officer. Clinical Examination of the Breast, PL/CMO/98/1 and PL/CNO/98/1. London: Department of Health, 1998.

14. Olsen O, Gotzsche PC. Cochrane review on screening for breast cancer with mammography. Lancet 2001; 358: 340–2.

15. Nystrom L, Andersson I, Bjurstam N et al. Long term effects of mammography screening: updated overview of the Swedish randomised trials. Lancet 2002; 359: 909–19.

16. Hakama M, Pukkala E, Kallio M, Heikkila M. Effectiveness of the public health policy for breast cancer screening in Finland: population based cohort study. BMJ 1997; 314: 864–7.

17. van den Akker-van Marle E, de Koning H, Boer R, van der Maas T. Reduction in breast cancer mortality due to the introduction of mass screening in the Netherlands: comparison with the United Kingdom. J Med Screen 1999; 6: 30–4.

18. Blanks RG, Moss SM, McGahan CE et al. Effect of the Breast Screening Programme on mortality from breast cancer in England and Wales, 1990–98. Comparison of observed with predictive mortality. BMJ 2000; 321: 663–9.

19. Wilson JMG, Jungner G. Principles and Practice of Screening for Disease. WHO Public Health Paper 34. Geneva: World Health Organisation, 1968.

20. Esserman L, Cowley H, Eberle C et al. Improving the accuracy of mammography: volume and outcome relationships. J Natl Cancer Inst 2002; 94: 369–75.

21. Association of Breast Surgery at the British Association of Surgical Oncology (BASO). An Audit of Screen Detected Breast Cancers for the Year of Screening, April 2002–March 2003 (www.cancerscreening.nhs.uk).

22. Chamberlain J. Breast Screening Acceptability: Research and Practice. NHSBSP Publication 28. Sheffield: NHS Breast Screening programme, 1993.

23. Wilson R, Liston J (eds). Clinical Guidelines for Breast Cancer Screening Assessment. NHSBSP Publication 49. Second edition. Sheffield: NHS Breast Screening Programme, 2001.

24. Chiu LF. Straight Talking: Communicating Breast Screening Information in Primary Care. Training Pack for Hard to Reach Groups. Nuffield Institute for Health, University of Leeds, 2002.

25. Good Practice in Breast and Cervical Screening for Women with Learning Difficulties. NHSBSP Publication 46. Sheffield: NHS Breast Screening Programme, 2000.

10 Quality assurance and evaluation in the NHS Breast Screening Programme

Gill Lawrence

Introduction

The UK National Health Service Breast Screening Programme (NHSBSP) was set up in 1988 in response to the recommendations of the Forrest Report published in 1986.[1] Based on the results of the Swedish Three-County Randomised Control Trial,[2] it was anticipated that the introduction of organised breast cancer screening should lead to a significant reduction in mortality from breast cancer in the UK. This belief was further reinforced by the inclusion in 1992 in the 'Health of the Nation' white paper[3] of a target to reduce by 25% breast cancer mortality in women aged 50–69 by the year 2000. This target was subsequently amended to apply to women aged 55–69. Given the long-term nature of the improvements expected to result from screening, it was necessary to identify a number of key proxy measures against which standards of performance could be monitored in order to gauge progress towards the NHSBSP's ultimate aim. One of the prime purposes of quality assurance (QA), which has been an integral part of the NHSBSP since its inception, is to monitor performance against these key national standards and to work with screening programmes to identify and address the reasons for underperformance.

Key elements of breast screening quality assurance

QA structures, policies and standards

The key elements of the breast screening QA programme are summarised in Table 10.1. Policies and standards are set by the National Coordination Team with advice from national coordinating groups for each of the professions involved in the NHSBSP. These are published by the NHSBSP in a series of guidelines that are regularly reviewed and updated.[4–11] At regional level, the cornerstones of the QA service are the QA teams and the analytical and administrative support staff in the QA Reference Centres (QARCs). Each regional QA team is composed of professional coordinators for each of the areas covered by the screening programme and is led by a Regional Director of Breast Screening Quality Assurance, who is directly accountable to the Regional Director of Public Health (RDPH).[12] The areas covered by the professional coordinators include screening office management (in the screening unit and at the primary care trust (PCT) where call/recall registers are held), radiography, medical physics, radiology, pathology, surgery and breast care nursing. Each coordinator is nominated by their peers and is formally appointed to their role. Service level agreements with the QARC specify the service that will be provided in return for payments received by the coordinators' employers. The regional coordinators meet regularly with their professional counterparts at national level and with their professional colleagues at regional level, forming an important communication channel between the NHSBSP's national office and local professionals.

Data collection, audit and dissemination of results

Data concerning the performance of individual screening services are collected each year via standard contract data set returns submitted to the Department of Health (DH) by screening services (KC62 returns) and PCTs running call/recall registers (KC63 returns). These data are published each year

Table 10.1   The key elements of a successful quality assurance (QA) programme

Key element	Detail
Set up a structure within which to carry out quality assurance	• Establish multidisciplinary professional QA teams at national and regional level • Establish regional QA reference centres to provide administrative and analytical support for the QA teams • Provide funding to pump prime regional and local QA initiatives that can be disseminated more widely if they are successful
Set policies and standards	• Set policies and standards against which to judge performance • Ensure that standards are consistent across the programme being monitored and preferably also in different countries offering similar programmes to facilitate evaluation of outcomes • Involve professional groups in the development of policies and standards to ensure ownership
Implementation	• Use a multidisciplinary team approach • Set up standard data collection and analysis procedures, emphasising structured reporting and data quality • Seek out champions to win the hearts and minds of peer groups to provide pressure for change
Audit the process	• Establish local audit to encourage critical analysis of the service by those who provide it • Carry out national and regional comparative audits to demonstrate performance relative to other services • Undertake peer review via QA team visits to individual services using standardised proforma for each professional area, supported by routine performance data for each aspect of the service
Disseminate the results	• Provide services and host trust management with detailed QA team visit reports containing clear recommendations with deadlines for completion • Inform commissioners of services, cancer networks and the national office of the recommendations made at QA team visits and the points of good practice noted • Organise workshops at cancer network, regional and national level to discuss performance against standards and to share good practice
Encourage improvements in performance	• Work with each professional group and each screening service to look for the reasons for poor performance against standards • Ensure that QA team visit reports are considered by host trust and service commissioner executive teams and clinical governance committees • Follow up recommendations at regular intervals, involving service commissioners and performance management staff as necessary
Target investment	• Work with clinicians and commissioners of services to ensure that limited resources are targeted at areas of most clinical need using evidence collected during the QA process
All-important overall approach	• Carry out QA in a non-confrontational environment • Develop a climate of mutual trust and honesty • Look for the reasons for failure rather than apportioning blame

by the NHSBSP in an annual review of the programme[13] and by the DH in an NHSBSP Statistical Bulletin.[14] Selected data concerned with radiological performance are analysed each year by the National Radiology Coordinating Group with the assistance of the Cancer Screening Evaluation Unit (CSEU) and are disseminated at regional level via regional radiology coordinators. Since 1997, surgical performance data have been collected and analysed at national level through a joint NHSBSP–

Association of Breast Surgery at the British Association of Surgical Oncology (BASO) Audit (NHSBSP–BASO Audit). These data are published each year[15] and are presented for discussion at the annual meeting of the Association of Breast Surgery at BASO. In each region, the Surgical QA Coordinator, QA Director and QA Coordinator work together to ensure that the data are collected from their breast screening services. Lead surgeons in each breast screening unit are responsible for making sure that the data are made available and are complete. The identification of people responsible for ensuring that data are gathered and are a true reflection of surgical work is intended to encourage ownership of the information for this audit. As with the radiology outcome data distributed by the Radiology Coordinating Group, ownership of the information is essential if a need for change is highlighted that must be accepted and implemented.

One of the key functions of the QARCs is to preprocess the KC62, KC63 and NHSBSP–BASO Audit data and to liaise with their local screening services and PCTs to resolve data quality problems. QARCs can then combine these data with information obtained from the computer systems in their screening units using standard cowriter reports (e.g. round length, screen-to-results and screen-to-assessment times, and cytology and histology data) or other sources (e.g. medical physics external survey data and customer satisfaction surveys) to produce regional outcome data summarising the overall performance of their screening units. In the West Midlands Region, these data are disseminated locally in an Annual Outcomes Booklet (in paper and electronic form). Selected measures are also included in the Breast Screening QA module of the West Midlands Cancer Intelligence Unit's (WMCIU) electronic Cancer Information Service, which is available to all organisations in the West Midlands that are connected to the NHS Net. In addition, key outcome data for each screening service are presented at the annual regional QA study day and more detailed analyses at workshops for each professional group. In one of the latter workshops, surgical and pathological outcome data for the screening programme are presented alongside data for symptomatic women obtained via the cancer registration function of the WMCIU.

QA team visits, recommendations and performance management

Peer review QA team visits to the NHS trusts acting as hosts for screening services and to the PCTs providing the call/recall service are carried out by the regional QA team each year.[11] Every screening service is visited at least once every 3 years.

Additional visits, either by the whole QA team or by selected professional coordinators, may be instituted if a formal review of the annual outcome data identifies areas of concern for a particular screening service. QA team visits provide an opportunity for the QA team to look at the whole screening service, to visit the facilities and to meet with all the staff. Prior to a QA team visit, the QA team reviews the outcome data for each component of the service to identify areas of concern. Standardised proforma are also completed in advance of the QA team visit by staff leading each element of the service. These are discussed with the professional coordinators during one-to-one discussions with their counterparts that cover outcome data, policies and procedures, qualifications and training, and participation in external QA (EQA) schemes. The QA team visit also provides an opportunity for formal reviews of interval cancers by the Radiology Coordinator, of selected slides by the Pathology Coordinator, of internal radiographic quality control data and external survey results by the Medical Physics Coordinator and a formal audit by the Administrative and Clerical Coordinator of the patient records maintained in the screening office. The Radiography QA Coordinator may also take this opportunity to lead a formal review of film quality by carrying out a PGMI assessment exercise with the radiographers.

In recent years, a multidisciplinary case review session has been introduced into QA team visits by many QA teams. In the West Midlands Region, cases for discussion are selected jointly by the QARC and the screening service. All benign open biopsies are included, as are selected interval cancers and early recall cases. Other interesting or discordant cases are chosen by the QARC on the basis of data submitted to the annual NHSBSP–BASO Audit and in the annual KC62 returns. All of the cases are reviewed by the Pathology Coordinator as part of the latter's slide review session. Because treatment options are frequently discussed in the multidisciplinary case review sessions, breast screening services are requested to ask their lead oncologist to attend this part of the QA team visit. Another feature that may form part of a QA team visit is a 'patient journey' during which a member of the QA team attempts to find and attend the screening service's assessment clinic in response to a standard recall-to-assessment letter.

One of the key features of a QA team visit is the feedback of the findings to the screening service, the host NHS trust and other interested parties. This generally begins with a verbal feedback session during the QA team visit to which all screening staff and representatives from the host trust management, commissioners and cancer network(s) are invited. In this session, feedback is provided on each aspect of the service either by each professional coordinator or by the QA Director, and areas of good practice and recommendations for improvement are identified. In the West Midlands, QA team visit recommendations are identified for immediate action, for action with a 3-month deadline and for longer-term action. The latter are followed up at 6-monthly intervals. The 3-month recommendations are confirmed in writing to the screening service and its commissioners within 1 week of the QA team visit. Details of the longer-term recommendations are provided in a full report, which is available within one month of the QA team visit. This report also highlights areas of good practice.

At the end of the QA team visit, it is helpful to include a management meeting where the recommendations can be discussed and action plans initiated. Experience in the West Midlands has demonstrated that if the host trust's chief executive or another member of their senior management team is present at the verbal feedback session and the management meeting, more progress tends to be made in achieving the recommendations from the QA team visit. It is also beneficial if service commissioners are present so that they can appreciate the context in which recommendations with cost implications have been made, as this greater understanding often results in appropriate investments being made.

Local ownership is further increased if the report of the QA team visit is considered formally by the executive boards and clinical governance committees of the host trust and the service commissioner as recommended by the Commission for Health Improvement's report on the West of London Breast Screening Service.[16] The importance of engaging host trust management in the QA process cannot be overemphasised, as the implementation and maintenance of reliable internal quality management systems must be the major means by which service quality is assured rather than through the external QA provided by the regional QA team. The QA team, for its part, must ensure that recommendations from QA team visits are followed up tenaciously and that appropriate measures be taken if areas of difficulty arise. These may initially take the form of further meetings with screening staff and/or host trust chief executives, but may eventually require the involvement of service commissioners, cancer networks or performance management/clinical governance leads at the strategic health authority.

Quality assurance standards

QA standards for each professional area contributing to the NHSBSP are published in a series of NHSBSP guidelines.[4–11] Of these, a small number of key standards have been identified through which to monitor the performance of the NHSBSP. These are listed in Table 10.2, where they have been divided into those designed to minimise risk and those designed to maximise benefit. The importance of minimising unnecessary risk is an important feature of screening QA, since the majority of those invited for screening will be free from disease and will thus receive little benefit (other than reassurance) from the screening process. It is also important in this context to find the right balance of sensitivity and specificity – a policy that will inevitably mean that the screening process cannot be 'perfect' and that unnecessary stress is caused to some women who are recalled to assessment only to be placed on normal recall.

One major area of risk is the danger from excess radiation exposure due to faulty equipment. This is minimised through routine quality control measurements undertaken by radiographers and regular surveys carried out by external medical physics services, which can lead to equipment being suspended from use. Excess radiation exposure is also minimised by setting a standard limiting the number of women who have to have additional mammograms because of technical errors. A second area of concern is the frequency of unnecessary surgical treatment and the risks associated with general anaesthesia. This is minimised by monitoring preoperative diagnosis and benign open biopsy rates. Finally, it is also important to take into account the stress that may be caused to women as a result of the screening process. Upper limits on the proportion of women recalled for assessment or placed on early recall, together with process standards measuring time to results, time to assessment, time between the first assessment appointment and surgical assessment, and waiting times for therapeutic surgery, attempt to minimise this type of risk.

Of the standards included to maximise the benefits of screening, the most important are cancer detection rates (particularly for small cancers less than 15 mm diameter), uptake rates, screening round length and interval cancer rates. Cancer detection rates are now usually expressed as age-standardised detection ratios (SDRs), which compare the sensitivity for the detection of invasive cancers with the equivalent that would have been achieved by the Swedish Two-Counties Trial.[2,17] Detection of small cancers that, being at an early stage, will respond well to treatment is vital. Uptake (attendance) rates are important because if only a small proportion of eligible women attend for screening, high cancer detection rates will have little influence on overall cancer mortality and survival of women in the screening age band. As underlying breast cancer incidence is higher in the

Table 10.2 Key NHSBSP quality assurance standards (for women aged 50–64)

Objective	Criteria	Minimum standard	Target
(a) Standards designed to minimise risk			
1. To achieve optimum image quality	(a) High-contrast spatial resolution		
	(b) Minimal detectable contrast	≥12 lp/mm	
	5–6 mm detail	≤1.2%	≤0.8%
	0.5 mm detail	≤5%	≤3%
	0.25 mm detail	≤8%	≤5%
	(c) Standard film density	1.5–1.9	
2. To limit radiation dose	Mean glandular dose per film to standard breast using a grid	≤2.5 mGy	
3. To minimise the number of women undergoing repeat examinations	Number of repeat examinations	<3% of total examinations	<2% of total examinations
4. To ensure that the majority of cancers, both palpable and impalpable, receive a non-operative tissue diagnosis of cancer	Percentage of women who have a non-operative diagnosis of cancer by cytology or needle histology	≥80%	≥90%
5. To minimise the number of unnecessary operative procedures	Rate of benign biopsies	Prevalent round <3.6 per 1000 Incident round <2.0 per 1000	Prevalent round <1.8 per 1000 Incident round <1.0 per 1000
6. To minimise the number of women screened who are referred for further tests	(a) The percentage of women who are referred for assessment	Prevalent screen <10% Incident screen <7%	Prevalent screen <7% Incident screen <5%
	(b) The percentage of women screened who are placed on short-term recall	<0.5%	≤0.25%
7. To minimise anxiety for women who are awaiting the results of screening	Percentage of women who are sent their result within 2 weeks	≥90%	100%
8. To minimise the interval from the screening mammogram to assessment	The percentage of women who attend an assessment centre within three weeks of attendance for the screening mammogram	≥90%	100%
9. To minimise the delay for women who require surgical assessment	Proportion of women for whom the time interval between the decision to refer to a surgeon and surgical assessment is one week or less	≥90%	100%
10. To minimise any delay for women who require treatment for screen-deteted breast cancer	The percentage of women who are admitted for treatment within two months of their first assessment visit	≥90%	100%
(b) Standards designed to maximise benefit			
11. To maximise the number of cancers detected	(a) The rate of invasive cancers detected in eligible women invited and screened	Prevalent screen ≥2.7 per 1000 Incident screen ≥3.0 per 1000	Prevalent screen ≥3.6 per 1000 Incident screen ≥4.0 per 1000
	(b) The rate of cancers detected that are in situ carcinoma	Prevalent screen ≥0.4 to ≤0.9 per 1000 Incident screen ≥0.5 to ≤1.0 per 1000	
	(c) Standardised detection ratio (SDR)	≥0.85	≥1.0

Table 10.2	Key NHSBSP quality assurance standards (for women aged 50–64) – continued		
12. To maximise the number of small invasive cancers detected	Rate of invasive cancers <15 mm in diameter detected in eligible women invited and screened	Prevalent screen ≥1.5 per 1000 Incident screen ≥1.65 per 1000	Prevalent screen ≥2.0 per 1000 Incident screen ≥2.2 per 1000
14. To maximise the number of eligible women who attend for screening	Percentage of eligible women who attend for screening	≥70% of invited women to attend for screening	80%
15. To ensure that women are recalled for screening at appropriate intervals	Percentage of eligible women whose first offered appointment is within 36 months of their previous screen	≥90%	100%
16. To minimise the number of cancers in the women screened presenting between screening episodes	The rate of cancers presenting in screened women: (a) In the 2 years following a normal screening episode (b) In the 3rd year following a normal screening episode	Expected standard: 1.2 per 1000 women screened in the first 2 years 1.3 women per 1000 women screened in the 3rd year	

most affluent women who are the most likely to attend for screening, breast screening services in areas with relatively low uptake rates may need to take attendance and socio-economic status into account when using SDRs to monitor performance. Joint studies with the local cancer registry to determine screening histories for all women in the screening age band diagnosed with breast cancer may provide additional insights into the efficacy of the screening programme through the calculation of mortality and survival rates in non-attenders and in women with screen-detected cancer.

The screening round length standard monitors the proportion of women who receive a subsequent appointment for screening within 36 months of their last screen and gives an indication of whether or not the programme is running on schedule. If the screening round length is too long then more cancers may develop between screens, and the cancers detected may be of a later stage and therefore less likely to respond successfully to treatment. Interval cancer rates are important because they measure the number of cancers that are diagnosed symptomatically between screens and hence give an indication of the total number of cancers that might have been detected had the NHSBSP been more effective. It must be recognised, however, that with the current technology and screening round length, some interval cancers are inevitable. Thus some cancers are radiologically occult and as such are not visible on mammograms, and 'true' interval cancers are not visible on previous screens, having developed between 3-year screening rounds.

Using quality assurance to encourage improved performance and changes in practice

Peer review QA visits and the sharing of comparative outcome data at regional and national level to enable professionals to see and discuss their performance relative to that of their peers coupled with constructive discussion concerning the reasons for poor outcomes are key features of QA. These processes must be carried out in a non-confrontational environment, and a climate of mutual trust and honesty is essential if service improvement is to be achieved. The main purpose of QA should not be to allocate blame, but rather to work with service providers to find the reasons for failure to meet national standards and to agree mechanisms for improvement. The success of this approach is illustrated by the gradual improvements in outcome measures that have been recorded since the introduction of the NHSBSP, some of which are illustrated in Figures 10.1–10.3 and in Tables 10.3 and 10.4.

Improved data quality

If meaningful outcome measures are to be calculated then data quality is of paramount importance. The data collected by the NHSBSP are now recognised to be among the most complete and most accurate in the UK. This has been achieved by having a small

Table 10.3	Improvements in the recording of nodal information for invasive breast cancers recorded at national level between 1992/93 and 2002/03 in the NHSBSP–BASO Audit

Year of data collection	Percentage with nodal information
1992/93[a]	58
1993/94[a]	62
1994/95[a]	69
1995/96[a]	72
1996/97	81
1997/98	87
1998/99[a,b]	90
1999/00	93
2000/01	93
2001/02	94
2002/03	95
2003/04	94

[a]Data from Scotland are absent in 1992/93–1995/96 and 1998/99.
[b]Data from Northern Ireland are absent in 1998/99.

The data are obtained directly from screening office computer systems, access to which is gained via the NHS Net. If a screening service has failed to meet the 90% minimum standard (see item 15 in Table 10.2), an explanation is requested by the QARC. Comparative data for the region and trend data for each service are fed back to screening services each quarter and reasons for under-performance are discussed at QA visits. Figure 10.1 illustrates the improvements in screening round length that have occurred at regional level in the West Midlands between 1998/99 and 2002/03. Thus, the percentage of women invited for screening within 36 months of their previous screening appointment has risen from only 71% in 1998/99 to 84% in 2001/02. The slight decrease to 81% in 2002/03 is related to the increased pressure put on the breast screening services by the introduction of two-view screening for all women and the extension of the NHSBSP to include women aged 65–70 as part of the NHS Cancer Plan. Figure 10.1 also shows that although the region has not succeeded in meeting the round length minimum standard, the slippage has never been more than 2 months as 90% of women have been invited for screening within 38 months of their previous screening appointment throughout the 5-year period.

number of standardised computer software systems on which to collect the data and by ensuring that screening office staff are fully trained in their use. In addition, the introduction of standard reporting forms for pathology and surgery has markedly enhanced the quality of the diagnostic and treatment data. Further improvements have resulted from the involvement of regional QARCs in the preprocessing of KC62 and KC63 returns prior to their submission to the DH to ensure that the information on screening unit computer systems is accurately and completely recorded. By feeding these collated comparative data back to screening services, QARCs can then stimulate local discussion about the efficacy of data transfer to the screening office computer system and highlight deficiencies in the recording of clinical details in patient notes or on the NHSBSP's structured reporting forms. The improvements in data quality that these processes have brought about are particularly well illustrated by the nodal status data summarised in Table 10.3. Thus, whereas in 1992/93, nodal status was known for only 58% of invasive cancers, in 2003/04, 94% of invasive cancers had known nodal status.

Round length

In the West Midlands Region, quarterly round length data are collected on a routine basis by the QARC.

Preoperative diagnosis and open biopsies

As well as having a significant impact at local and regional level, screening QA initiatives have brought about changes in practice at national level. One of the best examples of this is the gradual increase in the preoperative diagnosis of screen-detected breast cancers that has been demonstrated by the joint audit carried out by the NHSBSP and BASO. Figure 10.2 illustrates the 50% improvement in preoperative diagnosis rate recorded in the UK in 8 years of the audit. It is generally agreed that the major reason for this improvement is the introduction of wide-bore needle biopsy as a preoperative diagnostic technique, although there remain in the UK a small number of screening services that achieve very high preoperative diagnosis rates using cytology alone. The audit data also show that, as illustrated in Table 10.4, benign and malignant open biopsy rates have decreased as preoperative diagnosis rates have increased. The decrease in the malignant open biopsy rate has, however, been far greater, with the result that as preoperative diagnosis rates have increased from 62% to 93%, the benign-to-malignant biopsy ratio has also increased from 0.74 to 1.93. This is not an unexpected finding, as it suggests that the majority of malignant cases are being picked up preoperatively, leaving behind a residue of difficult cases where a definitive diagnosis can only be obtained from a surgical excision specimen.

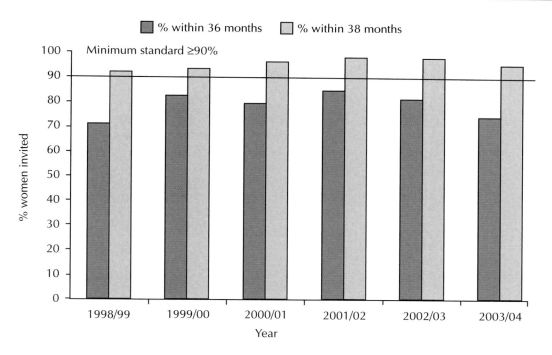

Figure 10.1
Improvements in screening round length recorded in the West Midlands region between 1998/99 and 2002/03.

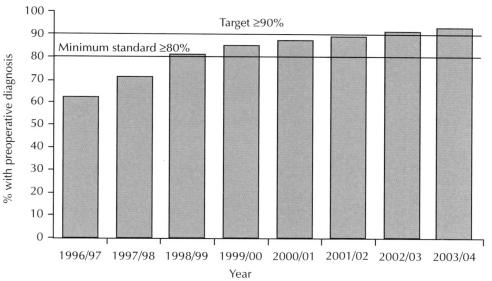

Figure 10.2
Improvements in the preoperative diagnosis rate recorded in the UK since the NHSBSP–BASO Audit of screen-detected breast cancer started in 1996/97.

Standardised detection ratios

Standardised detection ratios (SDRs) for the NHSBSP as a whole and for individual screening programmes are produced each year for the National Radiology Coordinating Group by the CSEU. Figure 10.3 illustrates the improvements in SDRs for cancers of all sizes that occurred in the NHSBSP during the 8-year period between 1993/94 and 2001/02. Prevalent SDRs increased by 57%, incident SDRs by 34% and total SDRs by 45%.

Surgical specialisation

One of the underlying principles fundamental to the NHSBSP is the importance of specialised training

and the need for all staff to undertake continuous professional development. Women should thus receive their mammograms from certified radiographers; their films should be read by specialist radiologists who participate in PERFORMS; their slides should be examined by specialist pathologists who participate in EQA; and their operations should be performed by specialist breast surgeons. The NHSBSP–BASO Audit has examined the proportion of women who receive their surgery from specialist breast surgeons (defined as those treating more than 30 screen-detected cancers per year) and has demonstrated that this increased from 63% in 1996/97 to 72% in 2002/03. The Calman–Hine Report published in 1995[18] recommended that the principle of surgical site specialisation that forms such an important part

Table 10.4   Changes in benign and malignant open biopsy rates and benign-to-malignant open biopsy ratios recorded at national level between 1992/93 and 2002/03 in the NHSBSP–BASO Audit

Year of data collection	No. of women screened	No. of benign open biopsies	No. of malignant open biopsies	Benign open biopsy rate per 1000 women screened	Malignant open biopsy rate per 1000 women screened	Benign-to-malignant open biopsy ratio
1996/97	1 340 175	2015	2734	1.50	2.04	0.74
1997/98	1 419 287	2251	2349	1.59	1.66	0.96
1998/99[a]	1 308 751	1830	1553	1.40	1.19	1.18
1999/00	1 429 905	1838	1316	1.29	0.92	1.40
2000/01	1 535 019	2042	1304	1.33	0.85	1.56
2001/02	1 507 987	2018	1148	1.34	0.76	1.76
2002/03	1 582 269	1901	1018	1.20	0.64	1.88
2003/04	1 685 661	1825	952	1.08	0.56	1.93

[a]Data from Scotland and Northern Ireland are absent in 1998/99.

of the ethos of the NHSBSP should be introduced for all cancers. A decade on, it is interesting to examine the extent to which this surgical specialisation has been implemented. Figure 10.4, which was derived using cancer registration data for the West Midlands Region, shows that whereas major changes occurred for breast cancer, between 1994 and 1999, there was little movement towards surgical specialisation for colorectal cancer. Data for colon cancer cases diagnosed in 2002 are very similar to those for cases diagnosed in 1999, with much less site specialisation evident than for breast cancer. Part of the reason for the lack of change in colorectal cancer is the need to provide cover for emergency admissions, but it is tempting to believe that the NHSBSP has had a major

positive influence on surgical specialisation for breast cancer.

Waiting times

Although QA encourages enhanced practice, it is not always possible to achieve improvements in outcomes if large-scale organisational change is required. This is illustrated in Table 10.5, which shows the proportion of women diagnosed with screen-detected breast cancer who were offered therapeutic surgery within the standard timescale set by the NHSBSP. These data show that, even taking patient choice and clinical decision into

Table 10.5   Waiting time for therapeutic surgery in the NHSBSP recorded at a national level between 1996/97 and 1999/00 in the NHSBSP–BASO Audit

Year	No. of cases in sample	% admitted within 21 days	% admitted within 21 days allowing for clinical decision and patient choice
1996/97	1245	77	82
1997/98	1516	74	81
1998/99	1748	74	80
1999/00	2092	70	77

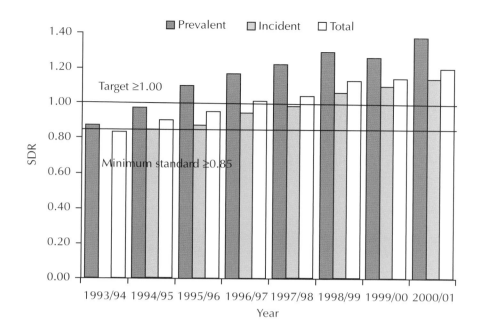

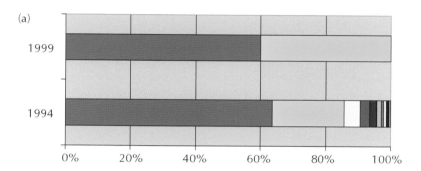

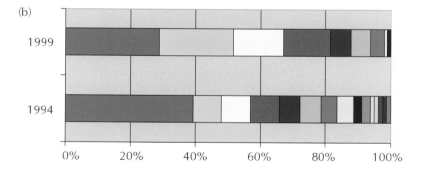

Figure 10.3 Improvements in the standardised detection rate (SDR) for cancers of all sizes recorded in the UK during the period 1993/94–2000/01.

Figure 10.4 Changes in (a) breast cancer and (b) colorectal cancer surgical specialisation recorded in a hospital in the West Midlands between 1994 and 1999. Each band represents the proportion of the total number of cases treated by an individual surgeon.

account, between 1996/97 and 1999/2000 this standard was never achieved at a national level. In 1999/2000, the main reasons given for the failure to meet the standard were lack of theatre time (in 33% of cases) and lack of staff or bed availability (in 18% of cases).[19] Clearly, these issues cannot be addressed solely by working with individual clinicians to bring about changes in practice, and the standard will only be achieved if detailed analyses of cancer patient pathways are carried out to identify where

structural and organisational re-engineering and investment can best be introduced.

Conclusions

It is now generally agreed that breast cancer screening,[20] and the NHSBSP in particular,[21] can significantly affect breast cancer mortality in women in the screening age band. Steadily improving SDRs suggest that the influence of the NHSBSP on breast cancer mortality rates should increase in the future. QA has contributed to this success by encouraging improvements in performance and changes in practice through peer review and the sharing of comparative outcome data between the professional groups providing the screening service. Many of the principles of breast screening QA are now being adopted in policies designed to improve the general quality of the UK's health services. The introduction within the NHS Cancer Plan[22] of the concept of clinical governance and the encouragement of the development of a 'no-blame culture' in which organisations can learn from their experiences[23,24] are both extensions of these principles. It will be important over the next few years to ensure that these similarities are recognised and that the wealth of expertise developed by those working within breast screening QA is shared with and built upon by those in the wider health services community.

References

1. Breast Cancer Screening. Report to the Health Ministers of England, Wales, Scotland and Northern Ireland by a Working Group Chaired by Professor Sir Patrick Forrest. London: Department of Health and Social Security, 1986.

2. Tabar L, Fagerberg CJ, Gad A et al. Reduction in mortality from breast cancer after mass screening with mammography. Randomised trial from the Breast Cancer Screening Working Group of the Swedish National Board of Health and Welfare. Lancet 1985; i: 829–32.

3. Department of Health. The Health of the Nation: A Strategy for Health in England. London: HMSO, 1992.

4. Quality Assurance Guidelines for Administrative and Clerical Staff. NHSBSP Publication 47. Sheffield: NHS Cancer Screening Programmes, 2000.

5. Quality Assurance Guidelines for Radiographers. NHSBSP Publication 30. Sheffield: NHS Cancer Screening Programmes, 2000.

6. Quality Assurance Guidelines for Medical Physics Services. NHSBSP Publication 33. Sheffield: NHS Cancer Screening Programmes, 1995.

7. Quality Assurance Guidelines for Radiology. NHSBSP Publication 59. Sheffield: NHS Cancer Screening Programmes, 2005.

8. Guidelines for Breast Pathology Services. NHSBSP Publication 2. Sheffield: NHS Cancer Screening Programmes, 1997.

9. Quality Assurance Guidelines for Surgeons in Breast Cancer Screening. NHSBSP Publication 20. Sheffield: NHS Cancer Screening Programmes, 2003.

10. Guidelines for Nurses in Breast Cancer Screening. NHSBSP Publication 29. Sheffield: NHS Cancer Screening Programmes, 2002.

11. Guidelines on Quality Assurance Visits. 2nd edn. NHSBSP Publication 40. Sheffield: NHS Cancer Screening Programmes, 2000.

12. EL(97)67. Cancer Screening: Quality Assurance and Management. London: NHS Executive, 1997.

13. NHS Breast Screening Programme. Informing Choice in Breast Screening: Breast Screening Programme Annual Review. Sheffield: NHS Cancer Screening Programmes, 2001.

14. Department of Health. Statistical Bulletin: Breast Screening Programme, England: 2003/04. London: Department of Health, 2005.

15. An Audit of Screen Detected Breast Cancers for the Year of Screening April 2003 to March 2004. Association of Breast Surgery at the British Association of Surgical Oncology and the NHS Breast Screening Programme, 2005.

16. Investigation into the West of London Breast Screening Service at Hammersmith Hospitals NHS Trust. London: Commission for Health Improvement, 2002.

17. Blanks RG, Day NE, Moss SM. Monitoring the performance of breast screening programmes: use of indirect standardisation in evaluating the invasive cancer detection rate. J Med Screen 1996; 3: 79–81.

18. Expert Advisory Group on Cancer. A Policy Framework for Commissioning Cancer Services: A report to the Chief Medical Officers of England and Wales. London: Department of Health, 1995.

19. An Audit of Screen Detected Breast Cancers for the Year of Screening April 1999 to March 2000. UK: British Association of Surgical Oncology and NHS Breast Screening Programme, 2001.

20. Nystrom L, Andersson I, Bjurstam N et al. Long-term effects of mammography screening: updated overview of the Swedish randomised trials. Lancet 2002; 359: 909–19.

21. Blanks RG, Moss SM, McGahan CE et al. Effect of NHS Breast Screening Programme on mortality from breast cancer in England and Wales, 1990–8: comparison of observed with predicted mortality. BMJ 2000; 321: 665–9.

22. The NHS Cancer Plan: A Plan for Investment, a Plan for Reform. London: Department of Health, 2000.

23. An Organisation with a Memory: Report of an Expert Group on Learning from Adverse Events in the NHS Chaired by the Chief Medical Officer. London: Department of Health, 2000.

24. Building a Safer NHS for Patients: Implementing an Organisation with a Memory. London: Department of Health, 2001.

11 Film reading and recall of patients in screening and symptomatic mammography

Ruth Warren, Erika Denton

Symptomatic mammography reporting

The symptomatic mammogram request is like any other radiological referral, an instruction to the radiographer and radiologist for a radiological examination. A report is required in response to a clinical problem. The report should stand alone when the films are not available, and it is usual for the text of the report to respond to the query in the request in quite specific ways. Commonly in the UK, the report is descriptive; free text describing the appearance of the mammogram, some quasipathological description of the stroma, and a description of any lesions, including whether they are likely to be of clinical significance. This is followed by, if the report is to be useful at all, some clear comment on whether or not features indicative of cancer are present. There may also be advice on additional tests, such as further mammographic views, ultrasound or biopsy, that may be useful.

Reports of this sort can be quite confusing to those not familiar with the complexities of breast disease, such as the general practitioner, and may, without intending to do so, generate doubt and the need for additional tests. In the UK, the Royal College of Radiologists has published guidelines suggesting that requests for breast imaging not be made by general practitioners but rather by hospital doctors with a primary interest in breast disease.[1] Kopans[2] has recommended standardised mammography reporting to remove doubts associated with such descriptive communications. In many centres, a standard format is developed after discussion within the multidisciplinary diagnostic team so that all requesting clinicians receive comparable reports. An initial statement may give a description of mammographic density, such as the Wolfe pattern[3] and note implants where relevant. The two breasts are reported separately, and only striking or symptomatic benign features are described. It is understood that the critical judgement is whether features suggesting cancer are present or absent from each breast. The report may conclude with a score, often for the two breasts individually and usually out of 5, where 1 is normal; 2 abnormal, definitely benign; 3 indeterminate; 4 abnormal, probably malignant; and 5 abnormal, definitely malignant. Scores of 3 or above necessitate further action. This generates a report that is less cluttered with difficult terms, contains a clear comment on the clinical relevance of benign or malignant lesions described, and recommends further tests (or no action) that helps clinicians advise the patient appropriately. The American College of Radiologists has devised standardised reporting terminology for symptomatic mammogram reporting, BIRADS (Breast Imaging Reporting and Data System).[4] This is detailed and designed to bring uniformity to the description of mammographic findings so that reports from different radiologists can be more easily compared. It is designed to be used with a breast-imaging database. It is not routinely used by radiologists in the UK, as it is felt by many to be time-consuming and unwieldy for use when reporting large numbers of cases, as is common in British practice.

Screening mammography reporting

In the screening situation, an even simpler format is required to avoid the false alarms for which screening has been criticised.[5–8] The result is often communicated to the woman without her doctor as intermediary, and so clear-cut reassurance must be given for a normal result, or for one containing an innocent benign feature. In the screening situation, the result may be generated by a computer in the form of a letter that is of standard format. Recalls for additional investigation may be addressed to the woman herself, and will probably not contain details of why further assessment is needed. The content of these letters must be acceptable to women, readily understood by the vast majority and designed so that panic is not caused. Additional tests must be arranged to take place within a few days of receipt of a letter advising further investigations. In order to produce reports of this sort, it is common to use computer codes, or even barcode readers, which record results directly into the computer, which then automatically generates the appropriate letter to each woman.

Reading mammograms: how?

In the symptomatic service, or where small numbers of films are read at a time, the films may be viewed on standard radiographic viewing boxes. It is important that the boxes be sufficiently bright and not have scratched surfaces. The films should be mounted in a standard format so that errors of side or position of a lesion are not made. In order to make this easy, standard radiographic procedures must be adopted for marking the medial and lateral sides and for the position of the identity label. In this way, a lesion can be localised at a glance by an experienced radiologist.

Calcification and other features critical to cancer diagnosis may be very small, approaching the grain size of the film, and so the use of some form of magnification by lenses is almost universal. This can take the form of a large hand lens held close to the film, or a binocular viewer of about 2 dioptres strength (Figure 11.1). Such a binocular viewer also masks the brightness from extraneous areas of the viewing box. When a hand lens is used, it may be useful to mask bright uncovered parts of the viewing box with black card or film. It is usual to read the films initially at a distance for bold features such as contour deformities or asymmetry between the two sides, and then close up to observe fine detail such as calcification. After specialist training in mammography reporting, each film reader develops his or her own scanning pathway around mammogram films.[9] There are, however, standard review areas studied to avoid missing subtle abnormalities. These include, in the mediolateral oblique film, the inframammary fold, the retro-areolar area and the tissues overlying the pectoralis, and in the craniocaudal view, the medial aspect of the breast.[10]

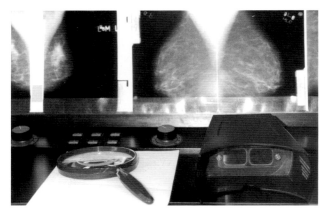

Figure 11.1 A hand lens of the type available for reading mammograms and the binocular viewer designed for use in mammography film editing.

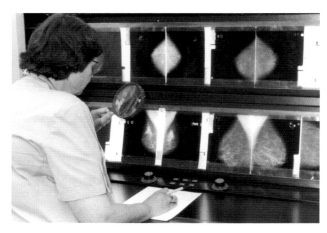

Figure 11.2 A radiologist reading films on one format of the multiviewer systems available for reading large numbers of mammograms. The transparent bands holding the films can be moved horizontally, so that the films are rolled up around drums at each end. The slight slope of the lower bank of films places them in the ideal position for film interpretation. Up to 800 films of 24 × 30 format can be accommodated on the viewer.

For reporting large numbers of mammograms, multiviewers have been developed so that the films can be loaded for reading. Such viewers (Figure 11.2) can carry the films of 100 or more examinations in a position designed for the comfort of the reading radiologist. Attempts are being made to devise digital readers for reporting mammograms, but they are not yet in a useful stage of development for reading large numbers of films at any speed.

When reporting both symptomatic and screening mammograms, it is important, whenever possible, to have any previous mammograms available for direct comparison.[11] This avoids unnecessary further assessment of benign lesions such as long-standing glandular asymmetry or unchanged benign mass lesions.

Reading mammograms: who and how many readers?

Mammography is traditionally a radiological technique, and so from the time of its development, the natural person to generate a mammogram report was the consultant radiologist. The majority of symptomatic mammograms continue to be reported by consultant radiologists. With the onset of large screening programmes on a national basis, and the difficulties that have ensued in finding trained radiologists willing to report the large numbers of screening films, consideration has been given to whether radiographers, breast physicians, obstetricians or nurses could be trained to read the screening mammograms. Any of these groups can achieve good film reading results after appropriate training, and increasingly in the UK National Health Service Breast Screening Programme (NHSBSP), trained radiographers read screening mammograms. This has enabled many individual centres to double-read screening films despite a shortage of radiological staff.[12,13]

Conventionally, radiological examinations are read by one radiologist only, except in teaching departments, where double checking of trainee radiologists' work may be required. In the clinical setting, a referring clinician may examine films in addition to the radiologist. In screening mammography, large numbers of repetitive films are read, there is no referring clinician who routinely sees the films at a later date, and it is recognised that inattention may result in missed cancers.[14] Many centres now double-read screening mammograms. This matter has been scientifically examined by several groups, and the use of double reading has resulted in between 9% and 15% more cancers being diagnosed.[15,16] It is becoming the norm for a well-run screening service to employ two radiologists to report mammograms in order to achieve maximum sensitivity. Studies of the cost-effectiveness of this additional staffing requirement are now available from France,[15] Finland[17] and the UK.[18] When it is not possible to use two trained radiologists, other doctors (e.g. breast physicians or surgeons in breast surgery or obstetrics and gynaecology), nurses or radiographers can all be trained to read mammograms, provided that they submit themselves to suitable training programmes and performance tests, and undertake appropriate follow-up of the cases to gain ongoing experience.[12,13]

Radiologists have several advantages: firstly, they are trained for many years in a speciality where visual acumen is developed in pattern recognition to a sophisticated level; they are familiar with the faults and artefacts that may occur in the complex chain involved in the production of a radiograph, and in the use of the equipment to maximise technical quality of the film; and they will work in a natural way with the technician for constant improvement in the technical quality of the film, which is so critical an issue in mammography.

In order to maintain high sensitivity and specificity in mammography reporting, specialist training is required. For a high-quality screening programme, personnel must be skilled in both image interpretation and radiopathological correlation of the images. Knowledge must be gained from following positive cases through the diagnostic and therapeutic processes. It is also necessary to review cases where a cancer has presented some time after screening, to view with hindsight the features of small cancers. Diagnosis of these small cancers prospectively is essential to obtain reductions in mortality from a screening programme. Learning for both the individual and the team goes on over a much longer period than might be expected.[19]

Methods have been devised for monitoring the performance of radiologists reading screening mammograms by using test films, and these can be used on sequential occasions to demonstrate improvement.[20–22] While physical performance of the radiographic chain is critical in achieving good outcomes, the quality of interpretation of the mammogram is probably the most important factor in diagnosing small invasive cancers, which ultimately determine the success of screening.

For screening units operating a policy of double reading, a decision must be made whether to recall every query raised, to reach a consensus, or to use the opinion of the most experienced person or that of a third reader – arbitration. These different strategies can give rise to very different recall rates, and it is essential that the benefit in improved sensitivity gained by the second report be accrued without unnecessary recalls and a reduction in specificity. Studies have shown that the highest cancer detection rates without inappropriately high recall rates are to be found in screening units using double reading with arbitration.[23] Obviously, to maintain this protocol necessitates units being staffed by three trained film readers at all times.

Computer-aided detection

The use of computer-generated prompts in reporting symptomatic mammograms has become commonplace in the USA and is being evaluated for use

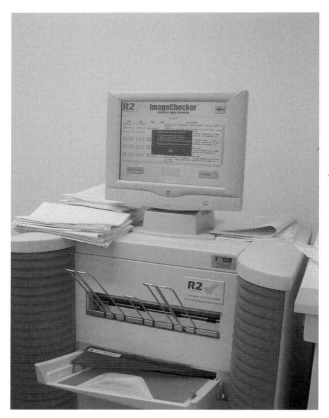

(a)

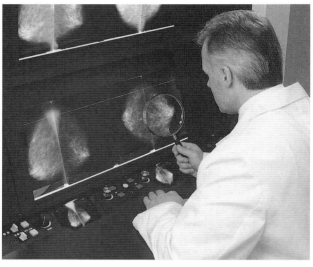

(b)

Figure 11.3 Computer-aided diagnosis: (a) image digitiser into which mammograms are fed to be analysed, for the computer-aided detection system to generate images with prompts. (Photograph courtesy of Dr Ros Given Wilson and Dr Mamatha Reddy of St George's Hospital, London). (b) The radiologist reviews the mammogram films first and then rechecks suspicious areas identified by the R2 ImageChecker system. (Photograph courtesy of R2 Technology, Inc.)

when reporting large numbers of screening mammograms. Mammographic images are digitised then subjected to computer-based analysis, which is designed to detect calcification, masses and asymmetry between the two breasts (Figure 11.3). The threshold at which the computer generates a prompt must be adequate to detect most abnormalities without resulting in a high false-prompt rate likely to distract the reporting radiologist. The prompts may be in the form of a paper printout of the mammographic images with areas of concern marked or as a computer screen with digital images displayed, including prompts.[24–26] It may be that computer-aided diagnosis for mammography offers similar gains in sensitivity to a second reader. Studies evaluating this are awaited. Figures 11.4 and 11.5 show the image prompts given by a computer-aided detection device.

Recalling women with abnormal mammograms

After the films have been reported, a selected group of women must be recalled for further tests. High-quality office procedures must be adopted, particularly when large numbers of women are screened, in order to ensure that every minor query raised by the radiologist or film reader is acted upon.[27] This has been an issue in cervical cytology in the UK where failed recall procedures have given rise to missed cancers.

When a woman is recalled after undergoing mammography, whether in a screening programme or after presenting with symptoms, she will automatically jump to the conclusion that a cancer has been found. Depending on the recall rate of a particular centre, the probability of a cancer diagnosis for a woman recalled from screening is between 1 in 6 and 1 in 20. Being recalled is therefore likely to give rise to anxiety, which is disproportionate for the majority of women. It is very important that the time between notifying a recall and arranging further tests be as short as practically possible, that the wording of the letter be well thought out and that those conducting the additional tests be sensitive to the anxieties that this process engenders for women. Honesty, in the context of recognisable caring, of all involved in the diagnostic and therapeutic pathways for these women is paramount. Psychological studies have been undertaken to assess the effect of screening on women.[6,28]

A 'one-stop' or rapid-diagnosis clinic is the ideal diagnostic scenario.[29] All the tests are done in one visit to hospital and a final report is often given at

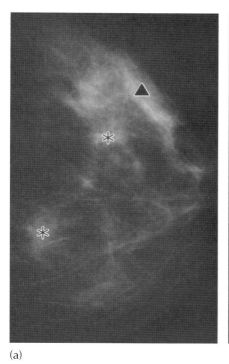
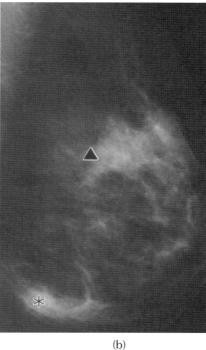

(a) (b)

Figure 11.4 Digital mammograms obtained on GE equipment used with the R2 ImageChecker computer-aided detection (CAD) system. The patient was aged 46 and presented with a mass lateral to the nipple. This was identified by the CAD equipment on the craniocaudal (CC) view (a), and, in addition, a further lesion is seen medial to the nipple. Both of these lesions were confirmed by ultrasound to be malignant masses. The CAD also highlighted with a triangle a calcification of no clinical consequence on the CC view and a mass of no consequence on the mediolateral oblique (MLO) view (b). (This case was kindly contributed by Dr Nick Perry and Mrs Sue Milner of the Princess Grace Hospital, London.)

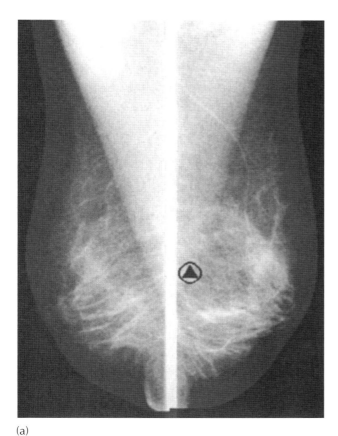
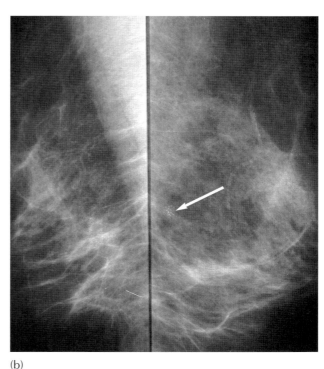

(a) (b)

Figure 11.5 (a) A calcification identified by the R2 ImageChecker system on a scanned film mammogram. This is a CAD-prompted image with emphasis marked on the cluster of suspicious microcalcification. (b) Bilateral mammograms with a cluster of microcalcification (arrow) in the left breast centrally and posteriorly, corresponding to the site of the computer prompt. (This case was kindly contributed by Dr Ros Given Wilson and Dr Mamatha Reddy of St George's Hospital, London.)

the end of the clinic, particularly for those who are to be reassured. In the case of patients found to have cancer, it is sometimes too heavy an emotional impact to give all the information necessary at one visit, and some form of phasing (but in a context of honesty) may be helpful. The presence of a trained breast care nurse counsellor is extremely beneficial. When there is a delay between the mammogram and additional tests, it is especially important to communicate the final conclusion as soon and as clearly as possible to the woman.

Conclusion

This short chapter has highlighted one of the most important aspects of breast cancer care. The early diagnosis of cancer by mammography at a size smaller than that possible by clinical examination is believed to be one of the reasons for the reduction in mortality from breast cancer observed in recent years.[30] This early diagnosis will have been partly brought about by formal screening of asymptomatic cases, and also by the routine use of mammography in women who consult with breast problems. It is for this reason that film interpretation has been the subject of intense research efforts in recent years.

References

1. Making the Best Use of a Department of Clinical Radiology; Guidelines for Doctors, 4th edn. London: Royal College of Radiologists, 1998.
2. Kopans DB. Standardized mammography reporting. Radiol Clin North Am 1992; 30: 257–64.
3. Wolfe JN. Breast patterns as an index of risk for developing breast cancer. AJR Am J Roentgenol 1976; 126: 1130–7.
4. D'Orsi CJ, Kopans DB. Mammography interpretation: the BI-RADS method. Am Fam Physician 1997; 55: 1548–50, 1552.
5. Ong G, Austoker J, Brett J. Breast screening: adverse psychological consequences one month after placing women on early recall because of a diagnostic uncertainty. A multicentre study. J Med Screen 1997; 4: 158–68.
6. Gilbert FJ, Cordiner CM, Affleck IR et al. Breast screening: the psychological sequelae of false-positive recall in women with and without a family history of breast cancer. Eur J Cancer 1998; 34: 2010–14.
7. Olsson P, Armelius K, Nordahl G et al. Women with false positive screening mammograms: How do they cope? J Med Screen 1999; 6: 89–93.
8. Tobias IS, Baum M. False positive findings of mammography will have psychological consequences. BMJ 1996; 312: 1227.
9. Noton D, Stark L. Eye movements and visual perception. Sci Am 1971; 224: 35–43.
10. Daly CA, Apthorp L, Field S. Second round cancers: How many were visible on the first round of the UK National Breast Screening Programme, three years earlier? Clin Radiol 1998; 53: 25–8.
11. Callaway MP, Boggis CR, Astley SA, Hutt I. The influence of previous films on screening mammographic interpretation and detection of breast carcinoma. Clin Radiol 1997; 52: 527–9.
12. Pauli R, Hammond S, Cooke J, Ansell J. Radiographers as film readers in screening mammography: an assessment of competence under test and screening conditions. Br J Radiol 1996; 69: 10–14.
13. Tonita JM, Hillis JP, Lim CH. Medical radiologic technologist review: effects on a population-based breast cancer screening program. Radiology 1999; 211: 529–33.
14. Laming D, Warren R. Improving the detection of cancer in the screening of mammograms. J Med Screen 2000; 7: 24–30.
15. Seradour B, Wait S, Jacquemier J et al. [Modalities of reading of detection mammographies of the programme in the Bouches-du-Rhone. Results and costs 1990–1995]. J Radiol 1997; 78: 49–54.
16. Warren R, Duffy S. Comparison of single reading with double reading of mammograms and change in effectiveness with experience. Br J Radiol 1995; 68: 958–62.
17. Leivo T, Salminen T, Sintonen H et al. Incremental cost-effectiveness of double-reading mammograms. Breast Cancer Res Treat 1999; 54: 261–7.
18. Brown J, Bryan S, Warren R. Mammography screening: an incremental cost effectiveness analysis of double versus single reading of mammograms. BMJ 1996; 312: 809–12.
19. Warren R. Team learning and breast cancer screening. Lancet 1991; 338: 514.
20. Gale A, Wilson A. Evaluation of radiologists' performance in reading mammograms. Br J Radiol 1991; 64: 476.
21. Gale A, Wilson A, Roebuck E. Mammographic performance: radiological performance as a precursor to image processing. In: Acharya R, Goldof D, eds. Biomedical Image Processing and Biomedical Visualisation; 1993. Proc SPIE 1993: 458–64.
22. Goddard C, Gilbert F, Needham G, Deans H. Routine receiver operating characteristic analysis in mammography as a measure of radiologist's performance. Br J Radiol 1998; 71: 1012–17.
23. Blanks RG, Wallis MG, Moss SM. A comparison of cancer detection rates achieved by breast cancer screening programmes by number of readers, for one and two view mammography: results from the UK National Health Service Breast Screening Programme. J Med Screen 1998; 5: 195–201.
24. Birdwell RL, Ikeda DM, O'Shaughnessy KF, Sickles EA. Mammographic characteristics of 115 missed cancers later detected with screening mammography and the potential utility of computer-aided detection. Radiology 2001; 219: 192–202.

25. Warren Burhenne LJ, Wood SA, D'Orsi CJ et al. Potential contribution of computer-aided detection to the sensitivity of screening mammography. Radiology 2000; 215: 554–62.

26. Boggis CR, Astley SM. Computer-assisted mammographic imaging. Breast Cancer Res 2000; 2: 392–5.

27. Warren R. Breast screening applies for BS5750/ISO9002. Br J Radiol 1992; 65: 84.

28. Brett J, Austoker J, Ong G. Do women who undergo further investigation for breast screening suffer adverse psychological consequences? A multi-centre follow-up study comparing different breast screening result groups five months after their last breast screening appointment. J Public Health Med 1998; 20: 396–403.

29. Gui GP, Allum WH, Perry NM et al. One-stop diagnosis for symptomatic breast disease. Ann R Coll Surg Engl 1995; 77: 24–7.

30. Peto R, Boreham J, Clarke M et al. UK and USA breast cancer deaths down 25% in year 2000 at ages 20–69 years. Lancet 2000; 355: 1822.

12 Radiology of the normal breast and differential diagnosis of benign breast lesions

Stefano Ciatto, Daniela Ambrogetti

The normal breast

The mammographic appearance of the normal breast varies with age and individual characteristics. Before the menopause, the parenchyma is well represented and usually occupies about half of the breast volume, being localised in the subareolar and upper outer regions (Figure 12.1). The amount and distribution of parenchyma is quite variable, especially before the menopause, when changes are possible even in the same subject under special circumstances (e.g. pregnancy or lactation).

The opacity of breast parenchyma is a determinant of mammographic sensitivity. The normal parenchyma is opaque enough to mask the limited density of a small carcinoma. So far, this is the most convincing explanation for the failure in reducing mortality in women aged 40–49 by mammographic screening.

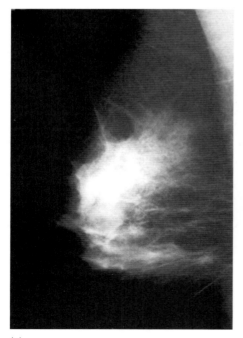

(a)

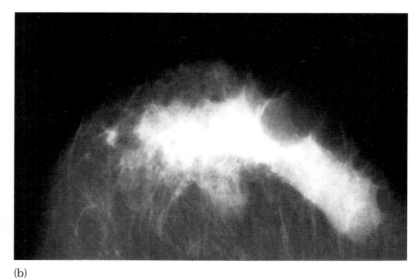

(b)

Figure 12.1 Normal premenopausal breast: breast parenchyma is depicted as a large opacity occupying about half of the breast volume, localised in the subareolar and upper outer region of the breast. (a) Mediolateral oblique view. (b) Craniocaudal view.

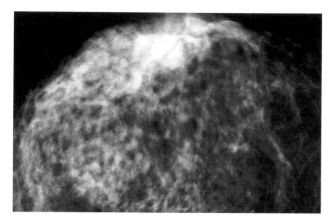

Figure 12.2 Normal breast: breast parenchyma with micronodular opacities (Wolfe's pattern or P2).

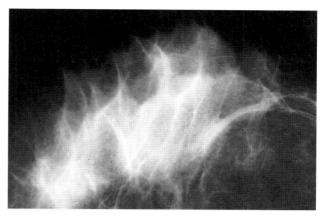

Figure 12.3 Normal breast: breast parenchyma with sheet-like large opacities (Wolfe's pattern DY).

Epithelial and connective tissues are depicted as densities of variable size, from small nodular (Figure 12.2) to large sheet-like homogeneous opacities (Figure 12.3). These two dominant patterns have been proposed by Wolfe[1] to classify the normal breast into four categories of increasing density, associated with a progressively increasing risk of subsequent breast cancer. Parenchymal patterns have been studied by several authors, but none of them was able to reproduce Wolfe's original results (Table 12.1). Although there is general agreement that denser breasts (P2-DY patterns) are associated with a slightly higher risk of breast cancer, it is unclear whether parenchymal patterns are really indicative of an intrinsic increased risk, or denser breasts are simply masking the presence of minimal

cancer[3] that will surface during the subsequent follow-up. In fact, parenchymal patterns are not currently used for clinical purposes (e.g. selecting women for different surveillance regimens). After the menopause, parenchymal densities gradually disappear, until the breast is essentially made of fat and fibrous tissue (Figure 12.4).

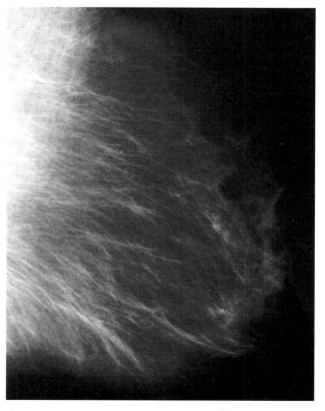

Figure 12.4 Normal postmenopausal breast: the parenchymal opacity has regressed completely, and only radiolucent fat tissue is left.

Table 12.1 Relative risk of developing breast cancer according to mammographic parenchymal pattern[a]

Authors	Cases	Relative risk by mammographic pattern			
		N1	P1	P2	DY
Wolfe	76	1.0	2.6	12.0	30.7
Ciatto	61	1.0	1.0	1.9	1.9
Ciatto	279	1.0	3.7	5.4	8.3
Wilkinson	42	1.0	2.1	2.1	5.8
Hainline	171	1.0	1.5	2.7	7.2
Egan	385	1.0	2.3	2.0	10.0
Krook	67	1.0	2.5	4.0	6.8

[a]Modified from Rosselli del Turco et al.[2]

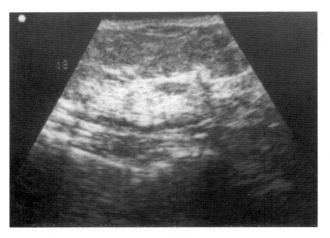

Figure 12.5 Normal breast: ultrasonography (10 MHz) shows a hyperechoic island of parenchyma surrounded by hypo-echoic fat.

This regression is variable in time and extent, depending on individual characteristics (e.g. endogenous extraovarian production of oestrogens or hormone replacement therapy), and fibroadipose or dense breasts will occasionally be seen in young or older women respectively. The sonographic features of the normal breast are also strictly correlated with the amount and distribution of the epithelial and connective tissue with respect to the surrounding fat. Fat is hypo-echoic and is depicted as a rather homogeneous greyish-black background

on which hyperechoic parenchyma stands out in white granular patches of variable size (Figure 12.5). For these characteristics, the sensitivity of sonography is not affected, as is mammography, by the presence of parenchyma, which, on the contrary, offers the ideal hyper-echoic background for hypo-echoic circumscribed lesions, either benign or malignant (Figure 12.6). On the other hand, the postmenopausal breast, made essentially of fat and fibrous septa, offers the worst contrast on sonography, and some intermediate hypo-echoic lesions (mostly benign fibroadenomas) may be difficult to differentiate from fat lobules (Figure 12.7).

Benign breast disease

The appearance of benign lesions of the breast is often typical, but in some cases the differential diagnosis with breast cancer is not easy, as they may share the same mammographic/sonographic features. Clinical evidence or patient's age and history may help, but in some cases fine-needle aspiration cytology (FNAC) or even surgical biopsy are necessary to define the exact nature of the lesion.

The most common benign lesions and the diagnostic problems that may arise for each of them are discussed below.

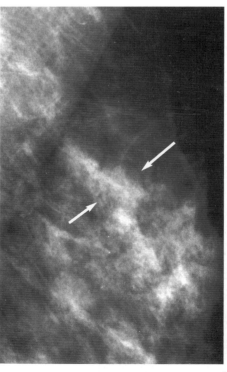

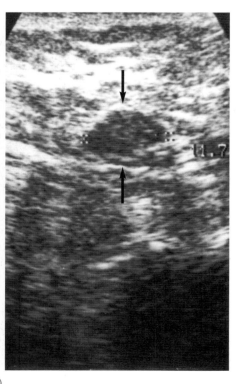

Figure 12.6 Premenopausal breast: on mammography (a), a small fibroadenoma (arrows) is masked in the radiologically dense parenchyma, which, on the contrary, offers the best hyperechoic contrast on sonography (b) (arrows).

(a)   (b)

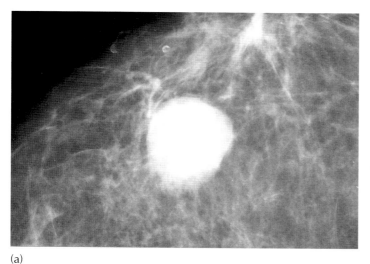

(a)

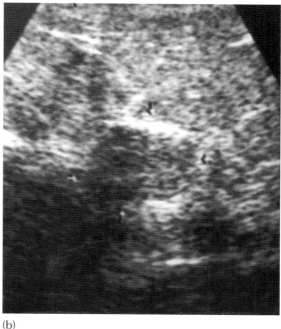

(b)

Figure 12.7 Postmenopausal breast: on mammography (a), a fibroadenoma stands out as a sharp opacity on the radiolucent fat background, whereas it is much less evident on sonography (b), being almost iso-echoic to fat.

Cysts

Cysts are very common, especially among women in their 30s and 40s. When not masked by surrounding parenchymal opacities, a cyst is depicted on mammography as a sharp-bordered round opacity (Figure 12.8) though incompletely filled cysts may be oval. Calcifications of the cyst wall have a typical appearance (Figure 12.9) but are infrequent. It is almost impossible to differentiate a cyst from other sharp-bordered non-calcified opacities (e.g. fibroadenoma and medullary carcinoma), although suspicion of cancer should arise only for isolated opacities in older women.

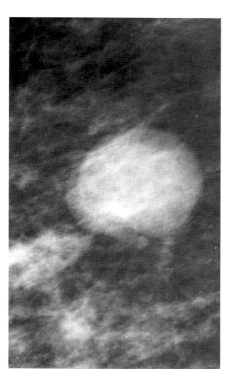

Figure 12.8 Cyst: typical appearance on mammography.

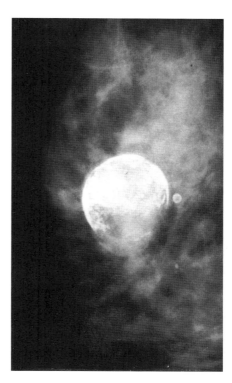

Figure 12.9 Cyst: typical calcification of cystic walls.

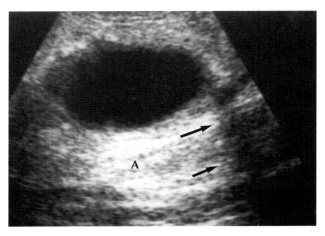

Figure 12.10 Cyst: typical appearance on sonography – an anechoic lesion, with posterior acoustic enhancement (A) and lateral acoustic shadowing (arrows).

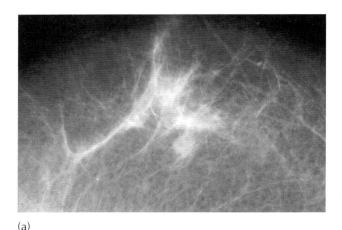

(a)

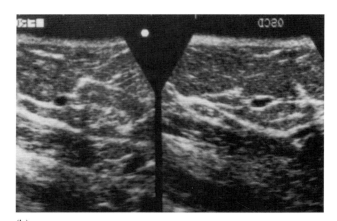

(b)

Figure 12.11 Circumscribed opacity on mammography (a) may suggest medullary carcinoma in an elderly woman, but sonography (b) demonstrates a cyst, and no other assessment is necessary.

Sonography is the ideal instrumental method to diagnose a cyst, as the anechoic appearance (usually with posterior acoustic enhancement and lateral acoustic shadowing) is typical of this lesion (Figure 12.10). Sonography may be particularly useful in diagnosing small cysts in elderly women, which may be suspected to be circumscribed carcinomas on mammography (Figure 12.11). Aspiration is the simplest, cheapest and fastest method of diagnosing a cyst, and is therapeutic at the same time, as the majority of cysts will not refill after complete aspiration.[4]

In the presence of an isolated palpable mass, aspiration can be useful. If the mass is a cyst then diagnosis and treatment will be achieved at the same time. If the mass is solid then aspiration will provide material for cytological examination, which will help the differential diagnosis between cancer and solid benign lesions.

Some clinicians, especially radiologists, oppose the extensive use of aspiration, and prefer to confirm the presence of a cyst by sonography. In our experience, a woman will not be fully satisfied with a diagnosis of a benign cyst if she has a breast lump. Aspiration of the cyst will by far compensate for the minimal discomfort of skin puncture, and the woman's anxiety will be relieved.

Aspiration allows evaluation of the characteristics of the cyst fluid. A non-blood-stained cyst content is associated with a negligible risk of an intracystic growth. Even when the cyst fluid is blood-stained, no intracystic lesion is found in the majority of cases, and the few cases of intracystic lesions are usually benign papillomas (Table 12.2). Intracystic cancer (i.e. an otherwise unapparent cancer growing

Table 12.2	**Probability of intracystic growth according to the appearance of cyst fluid on aspiration**[a]		
Intracystic lesion	**Total no. of aspirated cysts**	**Cyst fluid appearance**	
		Blood-stained	**Non-blood-stained**
Cancer[b]	1	1	—
Papilloma	5	5	—
None	6776	119	6657

[a]Modified from Ciatto et al.[5]
[b]Accidental finding of in situ lobular carcinoma adjacent to the cyst.

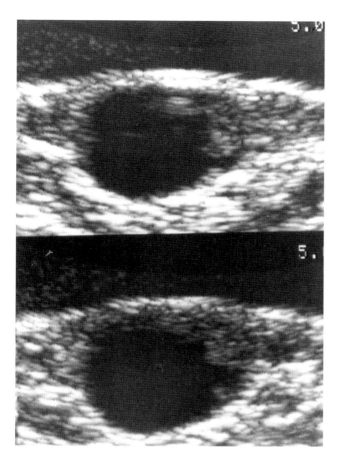

Figure 12.12 Intracystic papilloma: evidence of intracystic growth on sonography.

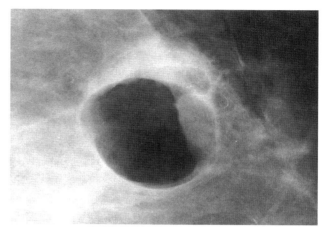

Figure 12.13 Intracystic papilloma: evidence of intracystic growth on pneumocystography.

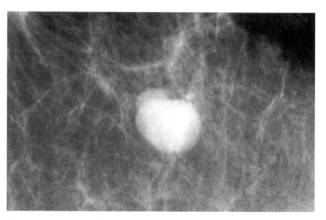

Figure 12.14 Fibroadenoma: typical appearance on mammography.

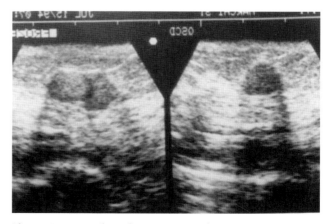

Figure 12.15 Fibroadenoma: typical appearance on sonography.

from the inner face of the cystic wall) is an infrequent event. Most reports of intracystic cancer have dealt with clinically or radiologically evident carcinomas, associated with haemorrhagic pseudocysts, that have been described erroneously as intracystic.

When the cyst fluid is blood-stained, evaluation of the cyst wall is important in order to assess the presence of intracystic growth. Sonography (Figure 12.12) is far simpler than pneumocystography (Figure 12.13), which is no longer used. Cytological examination of the cyst fluid may reveal cells from papilloma or cancer but its sensitivity is low and it should be performed only on blood-stained aspirates (Table 12.2). Surgery is justified only when an intracystic growth is suspected.

Fibroadenomas

Fibroadenomas are also very common. They are typical breast lumps in the teenage years, but they may also occur in older age groups. On mammography, fibroadenomas appear as homogeneous intense opacities with sharp margins, virtually indistinguishable from cysts except for their oval rather than rounded shape (Figure 12.14). On sonography, fibroadenomas are homogeneously hypo-echoic. In young women, sonography is much

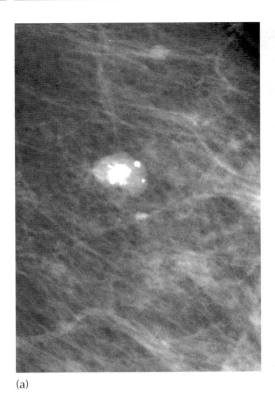

(a)

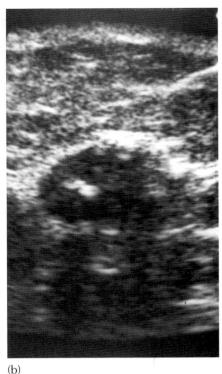

(b)

Figure 12.16
Fibroadenoma: typical calcifications evidenced on mammography (a) or sonography (b).

more reliable, as it shows the whole margin of the lesion (Figure 12.15), being unaffected by the opacity of surrounding parenchyma, whereas in postmenopausal women, fibroadenomas may be difficult to appreciate as they are often iso-echoic to the surrounding fat. After the menopause, typical coarse 'wax drop' macrocalcifications may be evident within the fibroadenoma, and may be easily shown either on mammography or on sonography (Figure 12.16). Unfortunately, it is not possible to reliably differentiate diagnosis between small non-

calcified fibroadenomas and small carcinomas with regular borders on either mammography or sonography (Figure 12.17). Age and history may be helpful, but aspiration cytology is a useful approach, which avoids an excess of excision biopsies, which are unnecessary as fibroadenoma is a benign lesion carrying no risk of progression to cancer. Doubts about the nature of the lesion may arise when palpation and imaging suggest a benign fibroadenoma (solid, hard, mobile, with sharp borders and an oval shape) and cytology is abnor-

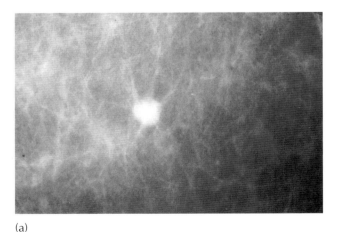

(a)

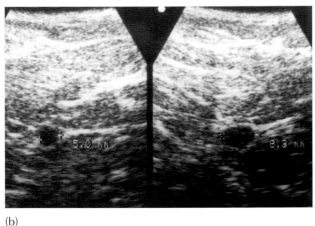

(b)

Figure 12.17   Medullary carcinoma: the lesion has sharp margins on mammography (a), and on sonography (b). A false-benign report is common in these cases.

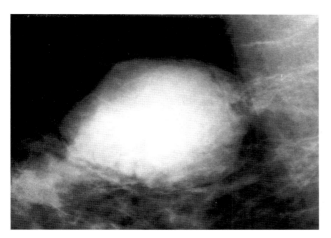

Figure 12.18   Benign phyllodes tumour: the appearance on mammography is the same as that of a fibroadenoma.

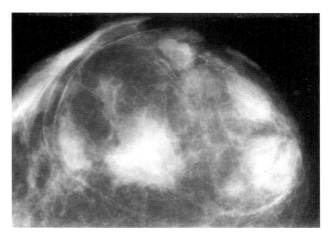

Figure 12.19   Lipoma: typical radiolucent appearance on mammography.

mal with cellular atypia of varying degree. In the majority of such cases, the lesion is a fibroadenoma with cellularity of the epithelial component, and does not necessarily need excision. A core biopsy confirming the benign nature of the lesion may spare unnecessary surgery.

Benign phyllodes tumours

When the lesion has not reached a very large size, the benign variety of phyllodes tumour is indistinguishable from a fibroadenoma, as both mammography and sonography will depict it as a hypo-echoic lesion with regular margins (Figure 12.18).

A history of rapid growth might suggest the diagnosis of a phyllodes tumour, but surgical biopsy will always be necessary to confirm its benign or malignant nature.

Core biopsy may provide histological evidence of phyllodes tumor, but usually surgical excision is necessary because of the risk that the needle may have missed scattered areas of degeneration. Phyllodes tumours should be excised with a narrow margin of normal breast tissue.

Lipomas

The mammographic diagnosis is straightfroward, as lipomas are radiolucent (Figure 12.19). It may be difficult to differentiate a lipoma from the surrounding fat either on mammography or on sonography, but this has almost no clinical relevance as the diagnosis of lipoma is generally already evident on physical examination, and no further diagnostic procedure is necessary.

Nipple discharge and papilloma

Nipple discharge is a frequent cause of referral to a breast clinic for consultation. Although in most cases it has no sinister significance, in a few cases nipple discharge may be the only sign of cancer. The likelihood of cancer is associated with the type of discharge, being minimal for milky or coloured discharges, and high for blood-stained discharges and for clear discharge in elderly women (Table 12.3).

For practical purposes, isolated milky or coloured discharge and even clear discharge in premenopausal women does not warrant further assessment, which should be limited to blood-stained

Table 12.3	**Prevalence (%) of otherwise unapparent breast cancer associated with nipple discharge, according to the type of discharge (5035 consecutive cases)[a]**

Type of discharge	Age			Total
	<40	40–59	>59	
Clear	0.00	0.16	2.70	0.16
Milky	0.09	0.18	0.00	0.13
Purulent	0.00	0.44	28.60[b]	0.83
Blood-stained	2.61	2.89	8.82	3.96

[a]Modified from Ciatto et al.[6]
[b]2 of 7 cases.

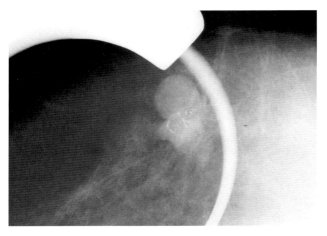

Figure 12.20 Subareolar gross intraductal papilloma identifiable by the presence of coarse calcifications.

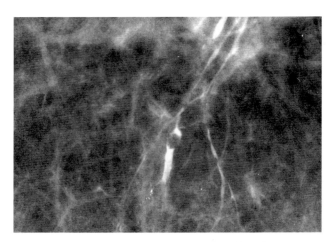

Figure 12.21 Galactography: a filling defect due to an isolated papilloma is evident in the injected duct.

discharge or clear discharge in postmenopausal women. Multiductal and bilateral discharge is also associated with minimal risk, as cancer is usually associated with uniductal and unilateral discharges confined to a single duct.

Mammography and sonography have limited use in diagnosis of papilloma, except for larger lesions, which are usually subareolar, and may contain coarse calcifications (Figure 12.20). Thus assessment should be based on cytological examination and galactography. Cytology may reveal cancer and papilloma cells in the discharge, but although the

test is highly specific, it is not very sensitive (Table 12.4). A negative or inadequate cytological report is not completely reliable in excluding malignancy.

On galactography, papillomas are usually depicted as small spherical masses (Figure 12.21) but more than one filling defect may be due to multiple papillomas as well as intraductal carcinomas (Figure 12.22). The majority of blood-stained discharges are not associated with papilloma or cancer, and routine resection of major subareolar ducts represents overtreatment in most cases, and may miss peripherally located lesions.

Table 12.4	**Frequency of suspicious findings at different diagnostic procedures in 18 cancer cases associated with nipple discharge[a]**		
Procedure	Intraductal carcinoma	Invasive carcinoma	Total no. of cancers
Palpation	3/8	6/10	9/18
Mammography	1/8	5/10	6/18
Discharge cytology	2/8	5/10	7/18
Galactography	2/8	5/10	7/18
All above	5/8[b]	8/10[c]	13/18

[a]Modified from Ciatto et al.[7]
[b]3 cases of intraductal carcinoma underwent surgery with a galactographic diagnosis of multiple papilloma.
[c]2 cases of invasive carcinoma underwent surgery for persistent blood-stained discharge with no other evidence.

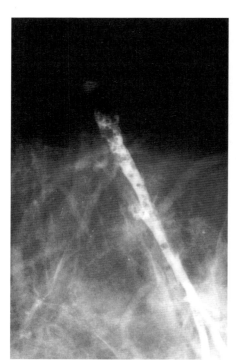

Figure 12.22 Galactography: multiple filling defects due to papillomas are evident in the injected duct.

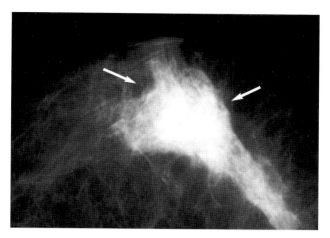

Figure 12.23   Acute mastitis: an abscess is visualised on mammography as a pseudonodular area of increased density (arrows).

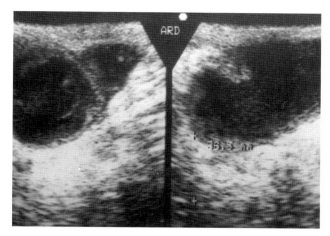

Figure 12.24   Acute mastitis: an abscess is visualised on sonography as an irregular mass with a predominant anechoic component and scattered hyperechoic foci and septa.

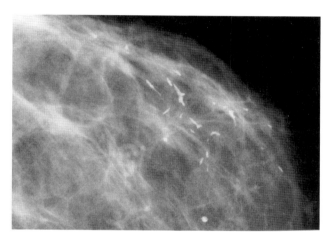

Figure 12.25   Chronic mastitis: typical periductal linear calcifications.

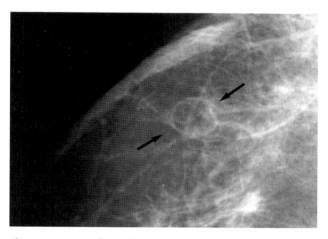

Figure 12.26   Effect of previous surgery: radiolucent circumscribed area due to fat necrosis (oil cyst: arrows).

Galactography is fundamental in assessing the presence and the site of an intraductal growth, and allows guided limited resection. When no lesion is shown on galactography and malignant cells are evident on cytological examination, the whole injected ductal tree should be resected.

Mastitis

Acute mastitis can occur in non-pregnant non-lactating women. Mammography and sonography will confirm the presence of skin and breast oedema, but they do not allow any reliable distinction from inflammatory carcinoma. The latter is currently based on the typical signs of acute mastitis (sudden onset, pain, circumscribed skin reddening and fever) and on aspiration cytology.[8]

When an abscess is present, it may be revealed on mammography as a circumscribed opacity with irregular, poorly defined margins (Figure 12.23), which may suggest the presence of carcinoma. On sonography, differential diagnosis may also be difficult, but the central part of the abscess is often anechoic with scattered hyperechoic foci due to necrotic fragments (Figure 12.24). Aspiration is the simplest and fastest method to achieve a definitive diagnosis when purulent material is aspirated.

Chronic mastitis may be associated with breast lumps and skin dimpling, which can mimic cancer. On mammography, the diagnosis of chronic mastitis may be confidently made if typical linear periductal calcifications, usually bilateral, are evident (Figure 12.25).

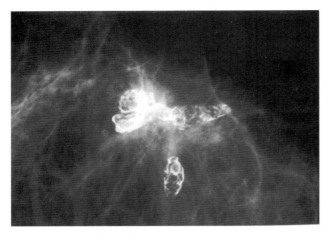

Figure 12.27 Effect of previous surgery: typical gross calcifications within the surgical scar.

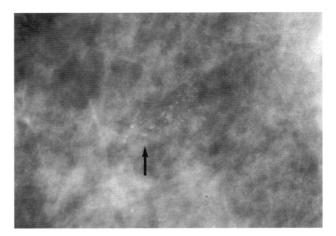

Figure 12.28 Tea-cup-like benign microcalcifications (arrow).

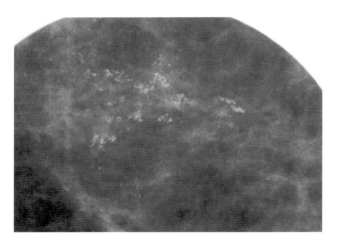

Figure 12.29 Punctate benign microcalcifications.

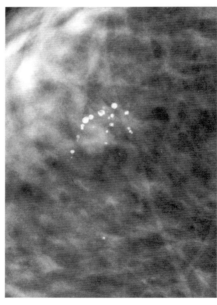

Figure 12.30 Anular/circular benign micro-calcifications.

Effects of previous surgery

Previous surgery can lead to diagnostic problems on subsequent breast imaging, due to the presence of the scar causing star-like opacities or parenchymal distortion. The presence of circumscribed areas of liponecrosis (oil cysts) (Figure 12.26) or of gross coarse calcifications (Figure 12.27) is typical of previous surgery, but when these features are absent, the differential diagnosis from cancer may be difficult and tissue acquisition may be necessary. This is one of the reasons for reducing the frequency of unnecessary surgical biopsies as much as possible. Cytology is often inadequate in these cases, due to the fibrous nature of the lesion, and only core biopsy may provide reliable microscopic evidence, if needed.

Benign microcalcifications

Microcalcifications are often present in the normal breast. For some of them, there is no diagnostic uncertainty when they are diffuse and bilateral with a typical benign morphology: tea-cup (Figure 12.28), punctate (Figure 12.29) or anular/circular (Figure 12.30).

In some other cases, benign microcalcifications may be unilateral and clustered and have a crystalline granular morphology (Figure 12.31). In these cases, differential diagnosis may be very difficult on mammography, prompting a large number of unnecessary biopsies.[9]

Sonography is of no help in these cases,[10] and stereotaxic cytology may be employed to reduce the

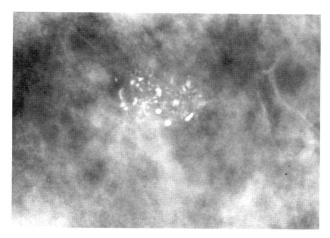

Figure 12.31   A cluster of benign crystalline granular microcalcifications, which may be misinterpreted as malignant and thus lead to an unnecessary surgical biopsy.

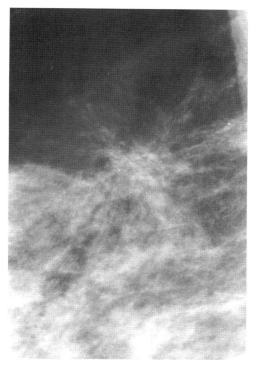

Figure 12.32   Sclerosing adenosis: an irregular opacity with infiltrating-like margins simulating cancer.

number of unnecessary biopsies.[11] Core biopsy allows radiological confirmation of the presence of calcifications in the core (which is anecdotal on the cytological smear), and is much more reliant than cytology in the event of a negative report.

Cancer-like lesions

Some benign lesions that are neither precancerous nor associated with increased risk of cancer may simulate breast cancer on mammography. This occurs with sclerosing adenosis (Figure 12.32) or radial scar (Figure 12.33), which have a star-like distorted appearance that may often justify a false-positive mammographic report. Although some characteristics (radiolucent central area, absence of palpable mass and visualisation on single view only) may be diagnostic, they are not sufficiently specific,[12] and most cases undergo surgical biopsy due to the high predictive value associated with this mammographic pattern.[9] Even on microscopic examination, these lesions may create problems of differential diagnosis with scirrhous or tubular carcinoma. This diagnostic difficulty might account for reports of an association between radial scar and cancer.[13]

Reporting benign lesions in clinical or screening practice

The criteria for reporting of benign lesions may differ between clinical and screening practice. In clinical practice, radiologists are usually requested to comment on a suspicious palpable lesion, and they

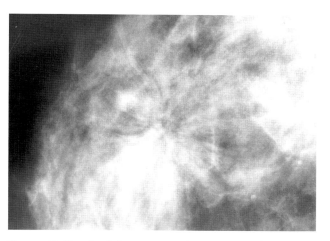

Figure 12.33   Radial scar: typical mammographic appearance with gross distortion, radiating spicules and radiolucent central core.

should report typical benign signs (e.g. innocent calcifications, cysts or periductal mastitis on mammography, and cystic features on sonography). This will support a benign diagnosis, reassure the clinician and avoid unnecessary surgical biopsy. In screening practice, the situation is quite different: healthy asymptomatic women are invited for screening without a clinical examination. The aim of screening is to detect early cancer and not to report on the presence of benign abnormalities that carry no increased risk of cancer. Reporting a benign lesion might generate anxiety and unnecessary further assessment or even biopsy. Thus it is a common policy for screening radiologists not to comment on benign lesion(s) detected on routine screening, the report being limited to a 'negative' or to an 'absence of suspicious findings' formula. This policy should also be extended to benign lesions detected on clinical mammography in areas of the breast other than the site of the palpable or symptomatic lesion for which the woman is referred.

What can be asked of imaging?

Some clinicians expect that breast imaging should classify women according to their relative risk of developing breast cancer, either by applying some classification based on mammographic pattern, such as Wolfe's, or simply by identifying the presence of 'dysplasia', or 'fibrocystic change' – often assumed to be consistent with 'dense breast tissue'.

It should be clear that breast imaging has no such capability. Mammographic parenchymal patterns cannot be scored in a consistent manner, as originally described Wolfe. In the literature, the average relative risk associated with high-risk patterns (P2-DY) is around 2:1, a figure that does not justify any special surveillance. Breast imaging does not recognise the presence of 'dysplasia', atypical ductal or lobular hyperplasia has no mammographic or sonographic correlate, and the presence of radiologically dense breasts is not a synonym for fibrocystic change, which may be diagnosed only when cysts are visible on sonography. Moreover, in the presence of hyperplasia fibrocystic change is associated with a negligible increase in the risk of developing breast cancer, and justifies no special action or surveillance. The presence of a radiologically dense breast tissue should only warn the clinician about the reliability of a negative mammographic report. Thus breast imaging allows no accurate and consistent prediction of breast cancer risk in current practice, and should not be used as an excuse to justify excessively frequent surveillance of selected patients.

References

1. Wolfe JN. Breast patterns as an index of risk for developing breast cancer. AJR Am J Roentgenol 1976; 126: 1130–9.
2. Rosselli Del Turco M, Ciatto S, Mezzalira LP et al. The role of mammographic patterns in the selection of women for periodical mass screening. Int J Breast Mammary Pathol Senol 1983; 2: 75–8.
3. Egan RL, Mosteller RC. Breast cancer mammographic patterns. Cancer 1977; 40: 2087–90.
4. Ciatto S, Rosselli Del Turco M, Cariaggi P. Diagnostic and therapeutic role of breast pneumocystography. Int J Breast Mammary Pathol Senol 1983; 2: 27–9.
5. Ciatto S, Cariaggi P, Bulgaresi P. The value of routine cystologic examination of breast cyst fluids. Acta Cytol 1987; 31: 301–4.
6. Ciatto S, Bravetti P, Cariaggi P. Significance of nipple discharge clinical patterns in the selection of cases for cytological examination. Acta Cytol 1986; 30: 17–20.
7. Ciatto S, Bravetti P, Berni D et al. The role of galactography in the detection of breast cancer. Tumori 1988; 74: 177–81.
8. Cardona G, Ciatto S. Criteria of clinical and radiological diagnosis in nonpuerperal acute phlogistic-like processes of the breast: considerations on 97 consecutive cases. Tumori 1981; 67: 31–4.
9. Ciatto S, Cataliotti L, Distante V. Nonpalpable lesions detected with mammography: review of 512 consecutive cases. Radiology 1987; 165: 99–102.
10. Ciatto S, Catarzi S, Morrone D, Rosselli Del Turco M. Fine needle aspiration cytology of nonpalpable breast lesions: US V8 stereotaxic guidance. Radiology 1993; 188: 195–8.
11. Ciatto S, Rosselli Del Turco M, Bravetti P. Nonpalpable breast lesions: stereotaxic fine needle aspiration cytology. Radiology 1989; 173: 57–9.
12. Ciatto S, Morrone D, Catarzi S et al. Radial scars of the breast: review of 38 consecutive mammographic diagnoses. Radiology 1993; 187: 757–60.
13. Fisher ER, Palekar AS, Kotwal N. A non-encapsulated sclerosing lesion of the breast. Am J Clin Pathol 1979; 71: 240–6.

13 The radial scar

Nick Perry, Lia Bartella, Iain Morrison

Introduction

The radial scar/complex sclerosing lesion is a proliferative and benign condition demonstrating architectural distortion as its major radiological feature. There may be an associated soft tissue element, but whether or not there is a central tumour nidus, the predominant feature is that of deformity of the breast architecture with variable retraction of the surrounding soft tissues (Figure 13.1).

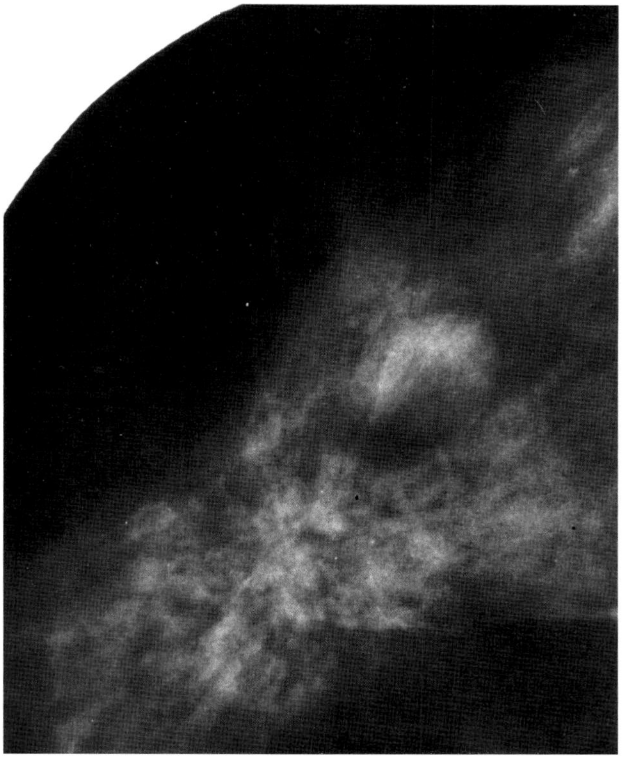

These so-called stellate lesions may be easy to detect mammographically, but if small they can be extremely difficult to identify within a dense fibroglandular breast. Providing there has been no trauma or previous surgical intervention to the area, the important differential diagnosis lies between the radial scar/complex sclerosing lesion and invasive malignancy. The two of course may coexist; likewise, a radial scar may be associated with in situ malignancy.

Pathological features

The radial scar[1,2] is a benign pathological entity characterised by central fibro-elastosis, surrounded by radiating parenchymal and epithelial structures (Figure 13.2). Previous and alternative terms include sclerosing adenosis with pseudo-infiltration,[3] infiltrating epitheliolosis,[4] non-encapsulated sclerosing lesion[5] and indurative mastopathy.[6] Andersen and

Figure 13.1 Typical appearance of a radial scar with quite marked architectural distortion but little in the way of a central mass. The size of this may be judged in comparison with a 7 mm cyst that was incidentally present just anteriorly.

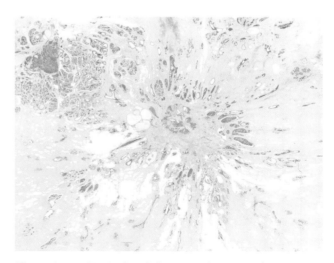

Figure 13.2 Typical radial scar with surrounding epithelial hyperplasia.

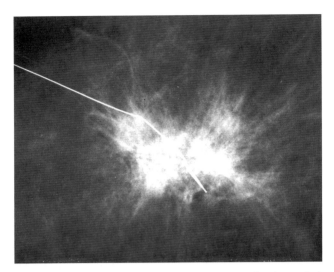

Figure 13.3   A complex sclerosing lesion. Like the radial scar, this is also more complex in its radiological appearance. It is larger and denser than a typical radial scar, although there is not so much a central mass as central thickening, and the predominant feature is once again that of distortion. The guidewire illustrates the fact that, despite its size and appearance, this lesion was impalpable.

Gram[7] reported a high incidence of associated papillomatosis, epithelial hyperplasia and microcalculus formation.

The UK Royal College of Pathologists Working Group[8] has set down guidelines that a radial scar be defined as a lesion 10 mm or less in maximum diameter with a dense and poorly cellular fibroelastotic centre with radiating epithelial structures in a stellate formation. A complex sclerosing lesion (Figure 13.3) has similar features but measures more than 10 mm in maximum diameter and generally has more complex and extensive benign changes peripherally, such as sclerosing adenosis.

Risk of malignancy

Studies suggest an increased incidence of malignancy in association with radial scar.[9,10] The widespread use of population-based mammographic breast screening programmes has drawn attention in recent years to the presence and significance of stellate lesions. The National Health Service Breast Screening Programme (NHSBSP) in the UK screens over one million women a year, and as image quality continues to improve, a breast assessment centre may expect to deal with a substantial number of these lesions. Tabar and Dean[11] have reported a screening incidence of 0.9 per 1000 women screened. The increasing use of full-field digital

systems and computer-aided detection may increase this number further.

The radiological appearance of a stellate lesion carries a significant risk of malignancy of approximately 40–50%.[12] Differentiation, however, needs to be made between this radiological appearance and the spiculate mass, where there is a central mass with spiculate margination. The positive predictive value for malignancy here is much higher – in the region of 90–95%.

There has in the past been much controversy over whether a radial scar is a completely benign entity or whether it carries a premalignant association. Notable proponents of a totally benign character include Fenoglio,[13] Tremblay,[14] Azzopardi[4] and Rickert.[6] Eminent supporters of the premalignant theory include Fisher,[5] Linell[2] and Sloane and Mayers.[9]

The Breast Unit at St Bartholomew's Hospital, London recorded cases of radial scar since computerised records were commenced in 1989 up until 1995, due to the observed frequent incidence of atypical hyperplasia or carcinoma in association with radial scars. They analysed 45 patients with radial scar, 40 of whom were screen-detected: 16 (35%) had associated malignancy and a further 8 cases (18%) showed atypical hyperplasia (Table 13.1). A later separate analysis of 32 cases between 1994 and 1998 from the same unit showed an associated incidence of 18% invasive malignancy and 12% ductal carcinoma in situ (DCIS) with radial scars.[15]

On the basis of these figures, in conjunction with other published data, this unit would support the premalignant theory. Many major breast units now believe that there is at least sufficient circumstantial evidence to admit the possibility that radial scars/complex sclerosing lesions may be associated with the development of malignancy and that this should be taken into account when considering their management. Tubular carcinoma is the malignancy

Table 13.1	Analysis of associated pathology in 45 radial scars
	Number
Uncomplicated radial scar	21 (47%)
Associated atypical hyperplasia	8 (18%)
Associated invasive malignancy	7 (16%)
Associated in situ malignancy	9 (20%)

most commonly associated with a radial scar; it is frequently discovered in a young population and has a favourable prognosis.

Most cases will be found through screening, as a radial scar presenting through the symptomatic service will in most cases have been discovered as a chance finding rather than a palpable mass. The decision to biopsy here is usually standard. In screening, however, the importance lies with what investigation and management the radiologist and multidisciplinary team should pursue. Is it a reasonable policy to leave these abnormalities on the basis that the typical appearance of a radial scar is most likely to be benign, or should they all be referred for surgery? Indeed, can radiological appearances reliably predict the presence of a radial scar without significant associated pathology?

Imaging characteristics

Classical radial scar features are those of architectural distortion with typical lack of a central tumour nidus. Different radiologists refer to 'black stars' or 'white stars', which in many cases probably reflects no more than their personal visual subjective biases. The 'black star' theory holds that the multiple lucent linear markings are due to elastosis causing distortion of fat. A 'wheatsheaf' or clumping appearance of spicule branching may be seen (Figure 13.4). This correlates with the common finding that the appearance of a radial scar varies according to the radiographic projection. It is quite typical to be able to visualise this lesion mammographically with ease in one projection but to have extreme difficulty visualising it in the orthogonal projection. This may lead to difficulty during wire localisation. Microcalcification is often associated with radial scars, and is usually of a non-specific scattered punctate and scanty appearance. There may be some distribution in association with the strand-like elements.

Sonographically, there is often an irregular hypo-echoic area with dense acoustic shadowing and some distortion of the surrounding structures. However, these features are not reliable and cannot with certainty be differentiated from malignancy or previous surgical scarring, fat necrosis, etc. The use of sonography can be very helpful in the clinical setting, as it can allow ultrasonically guided intervention. Sonography has also proven valuable in assessing multicentricity and multifocality of disease in the setting of malignancy.

Unfortunately, both the mammographic and sonographic features of radial scars are insufficiently specific to differentiate a benign lesion from a carci-

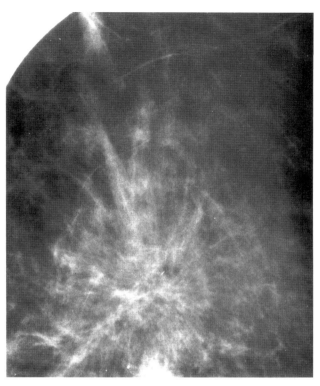

Figure 13.4   Another classical radial scar appearance, demonstrating spicule bunching.

noma,[16–18] thus producing a need for more specific imaging modalities in order to reduce the benign core biopsy rate for radial scars.

Magnetic resonance imaging (MRI) has to date proven to be of some limited but promising value. Several studies have demonstrated a 100% negative predictive value (NPV) for the presence of carcinoma in a non-enhancing radial scar on MRI.[19–21] This means that, on current evidence, we can reliably exclude the presence of malignancy in a radial scar, usually seen as a spiculate lesion on MRI, when this does not demonstrate any enhancement. Unfortunately, the use of MRI is not so helpful when the spiculate lesion shows evidence of enhancement, as both benign and malignant lesions can enhance, and there is insufficient evidence regarding the enhancement characteristics to allow confident differentiation between the two. A multicentre study is underway in the UK that will hopefully provide more useful evidence using larger patient numbers.[22]

Prediction of malignancy

A widely held view is that, if palpable, this mammographic lesion is most likely to represent malignancy. However, most aspirators will bear testament to the toughness of a radial scar on fine-needle aspiration. Some have experienced the bending of a needle while attempting to aspirate such pathology. The literature to date strongly suggests that by far the majority of carcinomas associated with radial scars are impalpable. Another classically described feature is that the spicules of a radial scar will not traverse the subcutaneous tissue and tether the skin, whereas malignancy may do this. Change in the shape or size of a lesion over time is not a reliable predictive factor for malignancy or benignity. Both radial scars and many grade 1 invasive tumours with a high desmoplastic reaction, as well as tubular malignancies, may remain relatively static over many years. In a series of 126 radial scar/complex sclerosing lesions, Sloane and Mayers[9] found a relationship between the size of the lesion and the presence of malignancy. Of 50 lesions that were 7 mm or more in size, 38 had associated malignancy or atypical hyperplasia, as opposed to only 6 out of 76 that were 6 mm or smaller. These same authors also report an association with age: 37 out of 66 lesions studied where the woman was aged over 50 had associated malignancy or atypical hyperplasia, as opposed to only 7 out of 56 in women up to the age of 50.

The presence of microcalcification in our series was found to be of some help in predicting associated pathology, although it was not entirely reliable. Retrospective analysis of the 21 screen-detected cases where distortion was the predominant mammographic feature showed microcalcification associated with 8 out of 11 cases where there was associated significant pathology, as opposed to 3 out of 10 uncomplicated radial scars (Table 13.2). We further analysed 14 screening cases that had typical appearances mammographically of a radial scar, and of these, 6 out of 6 cases where there was associated pathology showed microcalcification, as opposed to 1 out of 8 uncomplicated radial scars (Table 13.3)

Jacobs et al[23] concluded that radial scars are an independent histological risk factor for breast cancer. They studied 1396 women who underwent benign breast biopsies, including 255 women who went on to develop breast cancer. Women with radial scars had a relative risk factor of 1.8 of developing breast cancer compared with those without radial scars. Where atypical hyperplasia was present in breast biopsies, those with radial scars showed a relative risk of 5.8, compared to 3.8 without radial scars.

Cytology is unreliable for determining the presence of malignancy, and can only be regarded as useful when malignant cells are demonstrated. Although Kirwan et al[24] have suggested that core biopsy can confidently exclude the presence of malignancy in stellate lesions, many clinicians would not feel satis-

Table 13.2 Analysis with regard to microcalcification content of 21 radial scars where distortion was the predominant feature mammographically

	Number	Micro-calcification
Uncomplicated radial scar	10	3 (30%)
Associated atypical hyperplasia	6	4 (67%)
Associated carcinoma	5	4 (80%)

Table 13.3 Analysis of the importance of microcalcification in 14 cases having typical radiological features of a radial scar

	Number	Micro-calcification
Uncomplicated radial scar	8	1 (13%)
Associated atypical hyperplasia	3	3 (100%)
Associated carcinoma	3	3 (100%)

fied without proceeding to surgical excision of the lesion. Jackman et al[25] had a 40% cancer underestimation rate in radial scars from a 14G core biopsy. If a stellate lesion is due to a cancer then there would appear to be a very high chance of core biopsy demonstrating this. If, however, the stellate lesion is due to a radial scar with an associated focus of malignancy, a sampling error with core biopsy must be considered. A large series reported by Brenner et al[26] concluded that it was safe to leave radial scars diagnosed by core biopsy if at least 12 cores had been obtained and there was no associated atypical hyperplasia.

No study has to date been published specifically looking at cancer underestimation rates in radial scars using an 11G vacuum-assisted biopsy device, but Philpotts et al[27] reported a low (1.6%) carcinoma underestimation in masses, with a higher percentage (16.3%) for mammographic calcifications. Interestingly, however, this same paper reports a zero cancer underestimation rate for mammographic lesions that were excised completely. This is also supported by Liberman et al[28] in a study where all mammographic evidence of a lesion was removed by this technique. Unfortunately, a 73% residual carcinoma rate was shown in this series, demonstrating the need for definitive surgical treatment in these cases.

Sufficient evidence exists to support the use of an 11G mammotome device over a 14G core biopsy when deciding which percutaneous biopsy technique to use for sampling of a radial scar lesion. Although evidence to date suggests that complete excision of the mammographic lesion is highly likely to demonstrate any evidence of coexisting carcinoma, a larger trial is needed before the need for surgery can be eliminated in the presence of a radial scar.

Tabar[29] has proposed a policy of opting for immediate surgical excision without further interventional diagnostic workup, on the grounds that, due to the high associated risk of atypical ductal hyperplasia, atypical lobular hyperplasia, low-grade DCIS and tubular carcinoma, surgical excision is the safest option to eliminate under- or overdiagnosis. Many would support this viewpoint as a cost-effective and timely way of making a definitive diagnosis.

Conclusion

The collective experience of many units now indicates a high incidence of hyperplasia and carcinoma in association with radial scars, lending support to the premalignant theory. Lesions that are radiologically classical for radial scars are frequently associated with significant pathology. Microcalcification, when present, was a good predictor of associated pathology in our own series.

Is it safe to leave such a lesion, when in retrospect, it is possible to identify it on a previous mammographic study? This would not seem advisable – certainly not without the woman's informed consent. There are several recorded cases of malignant 'radial scars' where there had been no radiological change over several years, and the decision to biopsy was prompted by a change of policy to excision of all such lesions. The removal of a suspected radial scar is still advocated by many workers even in the presence of a negative core biopsy. However, the use of vacuum-assisted percutaneous biopsy techniques may prove to be diagnostically definitive.

References

1. Hamperl H. [Radial scars (scarring) and obliterating mastopathy]. Virchows Arch A Pathol Anat Histol 1975; 369: 55–68.
2. Linell F, Ljungberg O, Andersson I. Breast carcinoma. Aspects of early stages, progression and related problems. Acta Pathol Microbiol Scand Suppl 1980; 272: 1–233.
3. McDivitt R, Stewart F, Berg J. Tumors of the Breast. Atlas of tumor pathology. Washington, DC: Armed Forces Institute of Pathology, 1968.
4. Azzopardi JG, Ahmed A, Millis RR. Problems in breast pathology. Major Probl Pathol 1979; 11: 1–466.
5. Fisher ER, Palekar AS, Kotwal N, Lipana N. A nonencapsulated sclerosing lesion of the breast. Am J Clin Pathol 1979; 71: 240–6.
6. Rickert RR, Kalisher L, Hutter RV. Indurative mastopathy: a benign sclerosing lesion of breast with elastosis which may simulate carcinoma. Cancer 1981; 47: 561–71.
7. Andersen JA, Gram JB. Radial scar in the female breast. A long-term follow-up study of 32 cases. Cancer 1984; 53: 2557–60.
8. Royal College of Pathologists. Pathology Reporting in Breast Cancer Screening, 2nd edn. Sheffield: NHS Breast Screening Programme, 1995.
9. Sloane JP, Mayers MM. Carcinoma and atypical hyperplasia in radial scars and complex sclerosing lesions: importance of lesion size and patient age. Histopathology 1993; 23: 225–31.
10. Frouge C, Tristant H, Guinebretiere JM et al. Mammographic lesions suggestive of radial scars: microscopic findings in 40 cases. Radiology 1995; 195: 623–5.
11. Tabar L, Dean P. Teaching Atlas of Mammography, 2nd edn. Stuttgart: Georg Thieme Verlag, 1985.
12. Ciatto S, Morrone D, Catarzi S et al. Radial scars of the breast: review of 38 consecutive mammographic diagnoses. Radiology 1993; 187: 757–60.
13. Fenoglio C, Lattes R. Sclerosing papillary proliferations in the female breast. A benign lesion often mistaken for carcinoma. Cancer 1974; 33: 691–700.
14. Tremblay G, Buell RH, Seemayer TA. Elastosis in benign sclerosing ductal proliferation of the female breast. Am J Surg Pathol 1977; 1: 155–66.
15. Mokbel K, Price R, Mostafa N et al. Radial scar and carcinoma of the breast: Microscopic findings in 32 cases. Breast 1999; 8: 339–342.
16. Vega A, Garijo F. Radial scar and tubular carcinoma. Mammographic and sonographic findings. Acta Radiol 1993; 34: 43–7.
17. Cohen MA, Sferlazza SJ. Role of sonography in evaluation of radial scars of the breast. AJR Am J Roentgenol 2000; 174: 1075–8.
18. Sheppard DG, Whitman GJ, Huynh PT et al. Tubular carcinoma of the breast: mammographic and sonographic features. AJR Am J Roentgenol 2000; 174: 253–7.
19. Baum F, Fischer U, Fuzesi L et al. [The radial scar in contrast media-enhanced MR mammography]. Rofo Fortschr Geb Rontgenstr Neuen Bildgeb Verfahr 2000; 172: 817–23.
20. Nunes LW, Schnall MD, Orel SG et al. Correlation of lesion appearance and histologic findings for the nodes of a breast MR imaging interpretation model. Radiographics 1999; 19: 79–92.

21. Nunes LW, Schnall MD, Orel SG. Update of breast MR imaging architectural interpretation model. Radiology 2001; 219: 484–94.

22. Manton D, Turnbull L. Magnetic resonance mammography of radial scars: potential for reduction in benign biopsy rates. In: RCR Breast Group Annual Scientific Meeting Abstracts, 2000.

23. Jacobs TW, Byrne C, Colditz G et al. Radial scars in benign breast-biopsy specimens and the risk of breast cancer. N Engl J Med 1999; 340: 430–6.

24. Kirwan SE, Denton ER, Nash RM et al. Multiple 14G stereotactic core biopsies in the diagnosis of mammographically detected stellate lesions of the breast. Clin Radiol 2000; 55: 763–6.

25. Jackman RJ, Nowels KW, Rodriguez-Soto J et al. Stereotactic, automated, large-core needle biopsy of nonpalpable breast lesions: false-negative and histologic underestimation rates after long-term follow-up. Radiology 1999; 210: 799–805.

26. Brenner RJ, Jackman RJ, Parker SH et al. Percutaneous core biopsy of radial scars of the breast: when is excision necessary. AJR Am J Roentgenol 2002; 179: 1179–1184.

27. Philpotts LE, Lee CH, Horvath LJ et al. Underestimation of breast cancer with II-gauge vacuum suction biopsy. AJR Am J Roentgenol 2000; 175: 1047–50.

28. Liberman L, Dershaw DD, Rosen PP et al. Percutaneous removal of malignant mammographic lesions at stereotactic vacuum-assisted biopsy. Radiology 1998; 206: 711–15.

29. Tabar L. Teaching Course in Diagnostic Breast Imaging. Mammography Education, 2001.

14 Circumscribed breast masses

A Robin M Wilson

Introduction

A circumscribed mass demonstrated on mammography can be defined as a localised rounded lesion of predominantly homogeneous density with convex margins, in contrast to an asymmetric density, which is made up of tissue of mixed density and has predominantly concave margins, and a spiculate mass, which is associated with surrounding radial architectural distortion.[1]

Circumscribed masses in the breast demonstrated on mammography account for between 15% and 20% of breast carcinomas detected at screening. Review of interval screening breast cancers has shown that up to 25% of false-negative cases are represented on previous screening mammograms as circumscribed masses, many of these occurring in the 'review areas' (the retro-areolar area and behind, inferior and medial to the breast disc).[2,3]

Screening radiologists should pay particular attention to these areas. Similarly, a review of incident screen-detected cancers has shown that a significant proportion are demonstrated on the previous screening mammograms as subtle small circumscribed masses. However, the vast majority of circumscribed masses seen on mammography are benign.[4,5] Distinguishing benign from malignant circumscribed masses on the basis of their mammographic features alone is not usually a problem, but these lesions require careful evaluation at the time of screen reading.

Further assessment of those that do not fulfil the radiological criteria of benignity should include imaging (with mammography and ultrasound) clinical examination, and needle biopsy (fine-needle aspiration (FNA) for cytology and/or core needle biopsy) where indicated (triple assessment).[6-9] Only by doing so can unnecessary open surgical procedures be avoided for what prove to be benign abnormalities. This approach to assessment also has the advantage of providing a definitive preoperative diagnosis of malignancy, allowing the breast team to plan treatment and the patient to make informed decisions about treatment options supported by a breast care nurse.

Detecting and distinguishing significant circumscribed masses demonstrated on mammography

A large number of both normal and abnormal processes can appear as circumscribed masses on mammography; a comprehensive list of causes is shown in Table 14.1. Features that are helpful in differentiating benign from malignant masses include:

- number
- size
- density
- composition
- position
- character of margin
- contour
- any associated features
- patient age

Each of these is described separately below, but it should be stressed that all these features need to be considered together when weighing up the probabilities of a mass representing malignancy and no single characteristic should be regarded as diagnostic.

Single or multiple masses

The differential diagnoses of single and multiple circumscribed masses are shown in Table 14.1; malignancy is more likely with a solitary lesion than with multiple lesions. However, before dismissing

Table 14.1 **Round masses on mammography**

Multiple round masses
- Cysts
- Fibroadenomas
- Papillomas
- Multifocal carcinoma
- Galactocoele
- Metastases:
  — Carcinoma
  — Melanoma
- Lymphoma

Solitary round masses
- Normal structures:
  — Nipple
  — Normal breast lobule
  — Intramammary lymph node
  — Vascular structures
  — Skin lesion (mole, sebaceous cyst, naevus)
- Common causes:
  — Cyst
  — Fibroadenoma
  — Carcinoma
  — Abscess
  — Haematoma
  — Galactocoele
  — Papilloma
- Uncommon causes:
  — Phyllodes tumour
  — Hamartoma
  — Metastasis (contralateral breast, melanoma, lung, ovary)
  — Adenoma
- Rare causes:
  — Sarcoma
  — Fibromatosis
  — Tuberculosis
  — Sarcoid
  — Haemangioma
  — Neurofibroma
  — Leiomyoma
  — Granular cell tumour

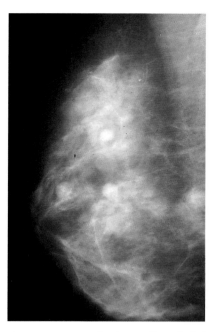

Figure 14.1   Multiple small well-defined masses demonstrated on mammography. Simple cysts are the most likely diagnosis – confirmed on ultrasound.

identified at any stage in their development.[5] However, as a general rule, a well-circumscribed mass that is less than 1 cm in diameter is unlikely to be malignant, while any circumscribed mass over 2 cm in diameter warrants further assessment (Figure 14.2). An ill-defined mass of any size requires additional investigation.

multiple masses as benign, they must all be seen to have similar features and a careful search made for a mass with significantly different characteristics that may warrant further assessment. Figure 14.1 shows the typical mammographic features of multiple benign circumscribed masses.

Size

On its own, the size of an abnormality is not of particular importance, as malignant tumours may be

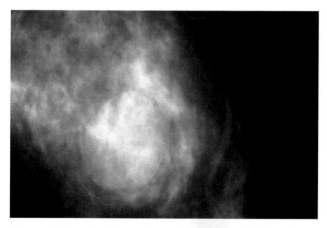

Figure 14.2   A solitary 2.5 cm diameter well-defined mass as shown on mammography. A surrounding halo is clearly demonstrated. This appearance is strongly in favour of a benign lesion; a cyst is the mostly likely diagnosis.

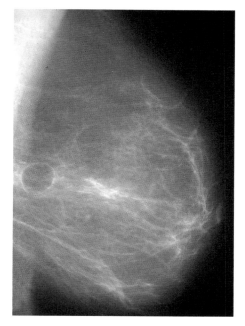

Figure 14.3 A well-defined reduced-density mass demonstrated on mammography – the typical appearances of an oil cyst.

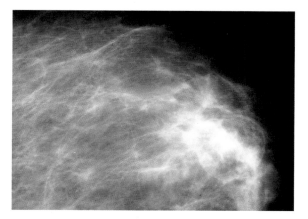

Figure 14.4 A mammogram demonstrating a mixed-density mass behind the nipple.

Density and composition

Density and composition are important in assessing the nature of a mass found on mammography.[10] Masses of reduced density compared with normal adjacent tissue (radiolucent) are very likely to be benign (Figure 14.3). The commonest causes of radiolucent masses are oil cysts, lipomas and galac-

tocoeles; these rarely cause much diagnostic difficulty.

Masses of mixed density containing tissue of fat density are also highly likely to be benign (Figure 14.4). The differential diagnosis includes normal lymph nodes (Figure 14.5), fibroadenoma (Figure 14.6), galactocoele and haematoma.

Masses showing increased density deserve careful evaluation, as most malignant circumscribed lesions are radio-opaque (Figure 14.7).

However, increased density is a non-specific feature, with many benign lesions (e.g. cysts and fibroadenomas) often showing significantly increased

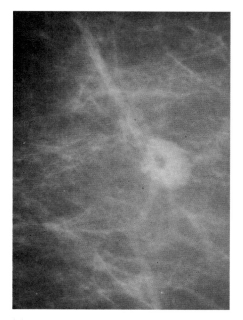

(a)

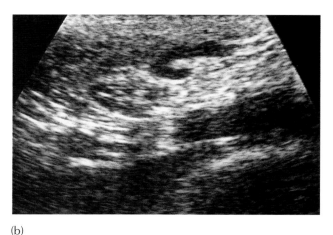

(b)

Figure 14.5 The mammographic (a) and ultrasound (b) appearances of a normal intramammary lymph node. (a) The lucent central area represents fat in the lymph node hilum. (b) The morphology correlates with that shown on mammography.

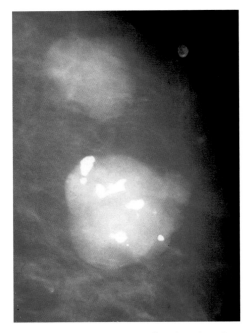

Figure 14.6 Mammography showing the typical appearances of two fibroadenomas, one shown as a simple lobulated mass and the other containing characteristic coarse 'popcorn' calcification.

density when compared with the adjacent normal breast tissue.[11]

Position

A circumscribed mass can occur in any part of the breast. However, masses demonstrated in certain

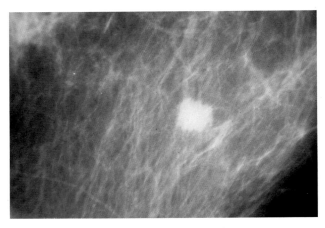

Figure 14.7 A small circumscribed malignant mass on mammography showing markedly increased density compared with the adjacent normal breast tissue and ill-defined margins (cf. Figure 14.6).

areas deserve special attention. These areas are often referred to as the 'review areas', and include the retro-areolar area, the retroglandular space on the mediolateral oblique projection (Figure 14.8), the medial aspect of the breast and the inframammary angle (Figures 14.9 and 14.10). The majority of circumscribed masses in the axillary tail of the breast are normal lymph glands, but all such masses should be carefully reviewed and further assessment arranged if there is any doubt about their nature.

Margin

The nature of the margin of a circumscribed mass is probably the most important single feature in decid-

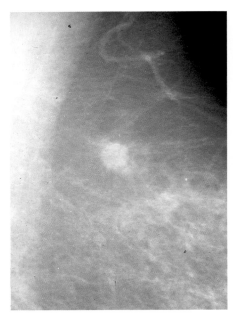

(a)

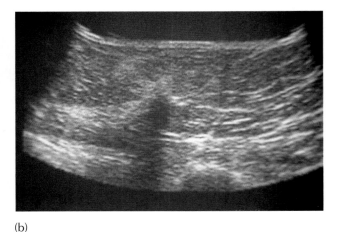

(b)

Figure 14.8 (a) A small invasive carcinoma represented by the ill-defined mass lying behind the breast disc on a mediolateral oblique mammogram. (b) Ultrasound of the same lesion, showing an ill-defined hypoechoic mass with distal acoustic shadowing.

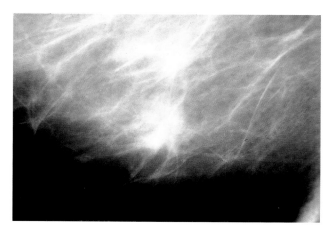

Figure 14.9 A small circumscribed carcinoma lying in the inframammary angle as shown on a mediolateral oblique mammogram.

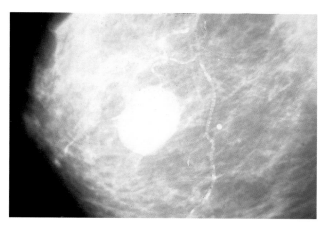

Figure 14.11 Mammography showing the typical well-circumscribed margins, with a clearly visible surrounding 'halo', of a benign mass.

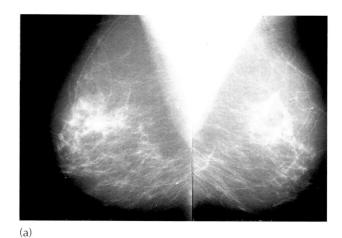

(a)

ing the need for further assessment. A well-defined mass with clearly circumscribed margins, where there is a sharp differentiation between tumour edge and normal breast tissue is unlikely to represent malignant disease (Figure 14.11); the risk of malignancy in a solitary well-defined mass is reported to be between 0.5% and 2%. Benign circumscribed masses often show a surrounding halo which is either partial or complete (Figures 14.2 and 14.11) – a feature that is rarely seen in malignant lesions.

However, if the margins of the circumscribed lesion are ill defined, such that there is no clear distinction between the margin of the mass and adjacent normal breast tissue (Figure 14.12), then the risk of malignancy is significant; all poorly defined circumscribed

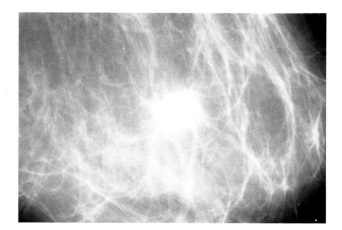

(b)

Figure 14.10 A small circumscribed carcinoma with associated disturbance of architecture is clearly demonstrated medially in the breast on a craniocaudal mammogram (a); the lesion is very difficult to identify on the mediolateral projection (b).

Figure 14.12 An example of a poorly defined mass demonstrated on mammography. On comparing this with Figure 14.11, the distinction between probably benign and probably malignant masses on the basis of their margins is clearly demonstrated.

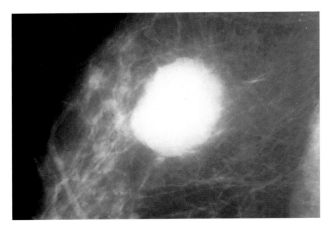

Figure 14.13 A circumscribed mass with a clearly defined anterior border but a poorly defined posterior border.

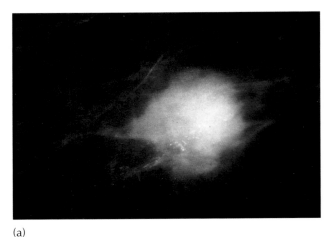

(a)

(b)

Figure 14.14 (a) Mammogram showing a mass with a lobulated contour with associated pleomorphic microcalcification representing ductal carcinoma in situ both within the mass and in the surrounding tissues. (b) Ultrasound of the same malignant mass clearly demonstrating the lobulated irregular contour.

masses require further assessment. Virtually all circumscribed masses that represent invasive carcinoma will have ill-defined margins; only a few benign lesions will show this feature. Circumscribed masses with margins that are mostly well-defined but with a portion that is ill-defined (Figure 14.13) should be managed in the same way as other ill-defined masses. Most of these will prove to be benign, the ill-defined portion of their margin being caused by overlying normal breast parenchyma, but the risk of malignancy is such that at least further imaging is required.

Contour

Benign circumscribed masses are almost always circular or oval and often show lobulation (Figure 14.6). The exceptions are haematoma and infection (abscess), but the history usually points to the diagnosis in these cases.

Most malignant lesions show some degree of irregularity to their contour; some circumscribed malignancies also show lobulation, particularly papillary and medullary carcinomas (Figure 14.14).

Palpability

Another feature, of less importance, is whether or not the abnormality is palpable. A circumscribed lesion that is palpable at small size on imaging (approximately 1 cm or less in diameter) is more likely to be malignant than one that is not. This is true because the desmoplastic reaction induced in the surrounding breast tissue is often palpable around the tumour mass, exaggerating the true size of the lesion.

However, this is not a reliable means of differentiation between benign and malignant lesions – small benign inflammatory lesions may be easily palpable while small invasive carcinomas very often are not.

Associated features

The presence of calcification in and around a circumscribed breast lesion is often a helpful feature in deciding its nature. Macrocalcification within a mass can be characteristic of fibroadenoma that has undergone partial hyaline degeneration (Figure 14.6). This appearance is diagnostic and needle biopsy is unnecessary; malignant change within a fibroadenoma is extremely rare.

On the other hand, pleomorphic calcifications in or around a circumscribed lesion are of much more significance and should suggest a diagnosis of ductal carcinoma in situ (DCIS; Figure 14.14a); the soft tissue mass in these circumstances does not necessarily indicate the presence of invasive malignant disease, as, not infrequently, the mass represents a localised non-malignant inflammatory response to the in situ disease.

Patient age

The differential diagnosis of circumscribed masses is influenced by the age of the patient. Those presenting in women aged under 35 are very likely to be benign, fibroadenoma being the most likely diagnosis. Between ages 35 and 45, cysts are common, but after age 35, all circumscribed masses should be assessed fully if they show equivocal benign features on imaging.[4,5]

Histological correlation

Circumscribed breast carcinomas without evidence of adjacent desmoplastic reaction to produce architectural distortion are considered more likely to be of high histological grade as the tumour grows rapidly without stimulation of a response from the adjacent breast tissue. The most likely diagnosis of a poorly defined circumscribed mass in the breast that is malignant is invasive ductal carcinoma of no specific type. However, any type of breast cancer can give this appearance, including lobular carcinoma. Mucinous and medullary carcinoma typically produce a circumscribed mass in the breast as opposed to a stellate lesion or a spiculate mass.

Assessment of circumscribed breast lesions

If there is any doubt in the mind of the mammogram film reader about the nature of the circumscribed lesion then further imaging and clinical assessment are mandatory. The assessment process for circumscribed masses is straightforward. The single most useful complementary imaging tool is ultrasound, which, using frequencies of at least 7.5 MHz, should be the routine initial imaging investigation for circumscribed masses detected on routine mammography. It will demonstrate the majority of masses and facilitate image-guided biopsy should this be indicated. Ultrasound will readily differentiate solid from cystic lesions (Figures 14.15 and 14.16); where there is doubt, needle aspiration should be

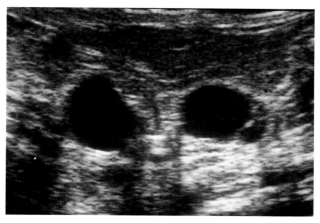

Figure 14.15 Ultrasound showing the characteristic features of a simple cyst – an anechoic mass with crisp well-defined margins, posterior wall bright-up and distal acoustic enhancement.

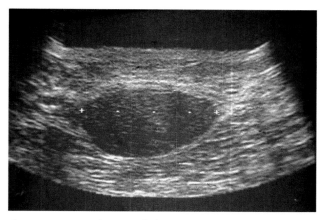

Figure 14.16 Ultrasound showing the typical features of a well-defined solid lesion (cf. Figure 14.15) – all solid circumscribed lesions identified at assessment require FNA or core biopsy regardless of their imaging features.

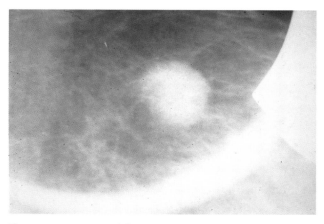

Figure 14.17 A paddle compression mammogram clearly showing the ill-defined nature of the contour of a circumscribed malignant mass.

attempted. All solid lesions deemed worthy of further assessment should undergo FNA for cytology and/or core needle biopsy.

If a circumscribed lesion is not visible on ultrasound then further mammography is indicated. It should not be assumed that a mass that is not seen on ultrasound either does not exist as a true mass or is benign. Paddle compression is particularly useful in confirming the presence of a circumscribed mass, and will often give more information about the contour and margins (Figure 14.17).[12,13] X-ray-guided FNA or core biopsy should be performed if the mass is not clearly benign.

Summary

Circumscribed masses are common findings on screening mammography, and the majority are benign. Differentiation of definitively benign from possibly malignant circumscribed masses is usually straightforward, with mass margin and density being the most important mammographic features. Ultrasound is the most useful imaging tool for further assessment of circumscribed masses.

References

1. Kopans DB, Swann CA, White GW et al. Asymmetric breast tissue. Radiology 1989; 171: 639–43.
2. Bird R, Wallace T, Yankaskas B. Analysis of cancers missed at screening mammography. Radiology 1992; 184: 613–17.
3. Burrell H, Sibbering D, Wilson ARM et al. The mammographic features of interval cancers and prognosis compared with screen detected symptomatic breast cancers. Radiology 1996; 199: 811–17.
4. Stomper P, Leibowich S, Meyer J. The prevalence and distribution of well circumscribed nodules on screening mammography: analysis of 1500 mammograms. Breast Dis 1991; 4: 197–203.
5. Sickles E. Nonpalpable, circumscribed, noncalcified, solid breast masses: likelihood of malignancy based on lesion size and age of patient. Radiology 1994; 192: 439–42.
6. Feig S. Breast masses: mammographic and sonographic evaluation. Radiol Clin North Am 1992; 30: 67–92.
7. Ellis I, Galea M, Locker A et al. Early experience in breast cancer screening: emphasis on development of protocols for triple assessment. Breast 1993; 2: 148–53.
8. Sickles E, Parker S. Appropriate role of core breast biopsy in the management of probably benign lesions. Radiology 1993; 188: 315.
9. Sickles E, Parker S. Appropriate role of core biopsy in the management of probably benign lesions. Radiology 1993; 188: 315.
10. Tabar L, Dean P. Teaching Atlas of Mammography. Stuttgart: Georg Thieme Verlag, 1985.
11. Jackson V, Dines K, Bassett L et al. Diagnostic importance of the radiographic density of noncalcified breast masses: analysis of 91 lesions. AJR Am J Roentgenol 1991; 157: 25–8.
12. Berkowitz JE, Gatewood OMB, Gayler BW. Equivocal mammographic findings: evaluation with spot compression. Radiology 1989; 171: 369–71
13. Sickles EA. Breast masses: mammographic evaluation. Radiology 1989; 173: 297–303.

15 Microcalcifications

Rosalind Given-Wilson

Introduction

Microcalcifications of the breast are common. They are seen in approximately one-third of all mammograms. The great majority are benign, but a small percentage are markers of malignancy.

In a typical mammographic screening population, malignancy will be detected in 0.5–0.8% of women. Twenty percent of this is due to ductal carcinoma in situ (DCIS). This is usually detected by the presence of calcification.[1] In the remaining 80% of malignancies, half will have microcalcification accompanied by other signs such as a mass or distortion.

Thus, although malignant microcalcification is seen in up to 0.5% of all mammograms, it accounts for only 1/60 of all cases of microcalcifications visualised. Over 98% of microcalcifications are due to benign processes. It is therefore essential to be able to distinguish benign from malignant microcalcifications, both to detect malignancy and to reduce unnecessary biopsies.

Some microcalcifications are characteristically benign and do not warrant further evaluation. Others need further assessment, which may include special views, ultrasound and guided needle biopsy. Stratification of the radiological level of suspicion for malignancy (Table 15.1)[2] contributes to decisions on further management, particularly the need for surgical excision.

It is important to have an understanding of the pathological processes producing calcifications and the anatomical structures within which they arise. These determine their shape, density and distribution, the features that allow differential diagnosis. Malignant calcifications are typically pleomorphic (variable in shape and size), clustered (>5 calcifications/cm²), linear and branching.

Calcifications occur in many structures in the breast. Of importance to the radiologist are those arising in ducts and lobules, which commonly represent or simulate malignancy. Knowledge of the natural history of conditions associated with calcifications facilitates the determination of a management strategy.

Calcifications classified by structure of origin

Calcifications outside ducts and lobules

These are benign and rarely cause diagnostic difficulty. They are characteristically ringed, tubular or curvilinear. All are benign shapes.

Vascular calcification

This is very common and is usually associated with medial calcific sclerosis, which is calcium deposition in the media of small to medium-sized muscular arteries. This produces curvilinear and tubular calcifications and may be widespread throughout the breast. It may rarely cause diagnostic difficulties if

Table 15.1	**Grading of imaging reports of microcalcifications according to risk of malignancy**	
Grade	**Degree of suspicion**	**Mammographic appearance**
1	Normal	No abnormality seen
2	Consistent with a benign lesion	Popcorn, ring, micro cystic or diffuse bilateral calcification
3	Atypical or indeterminate but probably benign	Localised cluster of round, fine or punctate calcification
4	Suspicious of malignancy	Localised cluster of granular calcification
5	Consistent with malignancy	Comedo calcification

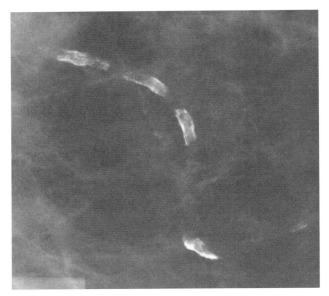

Figure 15.1 Vascular calcification. Calcium within the wall of a small artery produces parallel linear densities outlining the vessel's course.

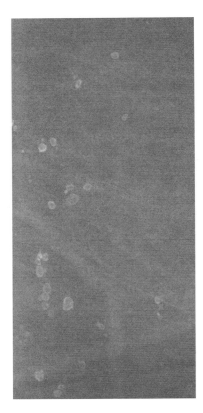

Figure 15.2 Intradermal calcification. This consists of small clusters of benign-appearing lucent-centred rings of calcium, commonly seen within calcified sebaceous glands. These are most frequent in the areolar skin inframammary folds and axillae, but can be present over the skin of the whole breast. On tangential views, their intradermal location can be confirmed.

there is only a small area and typical parallel lines and curves cannot be seen. It is commoner in patients with diabetes, renal failure, coronary artery disease and those undergoing dialysis (Figure 15.1).[3,4]

Sebaceous gland calcification

This is distinguished by its intradermal location and can be clearly demonstrated by tangential views if necessary. It consists of small clusters of 2–6 calcifications, individually measuring about 1 mm in diameter, within sebaceous glands. These tend to be concentrated in the inframammary fold, the areola and the axilla, but may occasionally be scattered over the breasts. They are likely to be due to inflammation such as chronic folliculitis (Figure 15.2). Epidermal inclusion cysts may also be associated with heterogeneous microcalcifications. These are associated with a high-density well-circumscribed mass on mammography and a superficial cystic lesion on ultrasound, allowing easy diagnosis.[5] Skin calcification and ossification can also be seen in Albright's hereditary osteodystrophy and osteoma cutis and Klippel–Trenaunay syndrome.[6,7]

Fat necrosis

Liponecrosis microcystica calcificans is well-defined ring calcification, 1–4 mm in diameter, that occurs around small areas of fat necrosis. These are more common in association with trauma such as surgery or with plasma cell mastitis, but are often scattered in the breast with no obvious underlying cause (Figure 15.3). Larger areas of fat necrosis up to several centimetres across can follow trauma

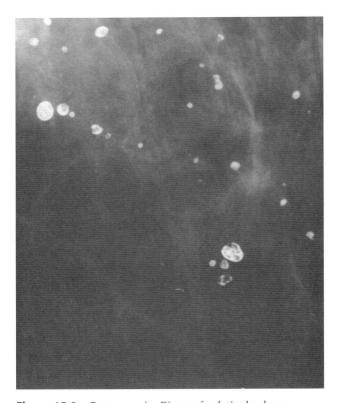

Figure 15.3 Fat necrosis. Rings of relatively dense calcium with lucent centres are scattered throughout the breast in this asymptomatic patient, corresponding to small areas of fat necrosis, otherwise known as liponecrosis microcystica calcificans.

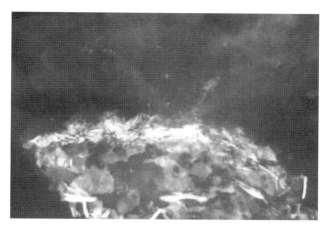

Figure 15.4 Coarse fat necrosis. In this woman with a history of previous surgical implant removal, amorphous sheets of fat necrosis are seen around the region of the previous implant.

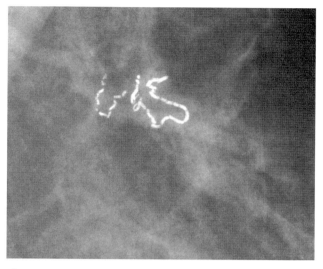

Figure 15.6 Calcified parasitic worms. On this screening mammogram in a woman of sub-Saharan African origin, several small calcified worms lie in a cluster.

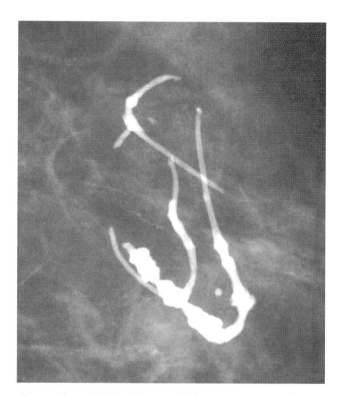

Figure 15.5 Calcified suture. This woman gave a history of previous wide local excision and radiotherapy for an invasive cancer. Ten years later, calcified suture material is visible at the site of previous surgery. A small amount of vascular calcification can also be seen both superior and inferior to this. Calcification of sutures is unusual unless radiotherapy has been given.

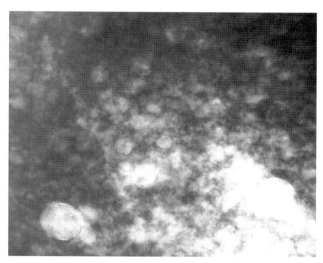

Figure 15.7 Calcified foreign material. This woman had undergone direct silicone injections into the breasts for augmentation over 20 years prior to this screening mammogram. Multiple globules of high-density silicone can be seen within the breast, and show rim calcification.

Occasionally, in the early stages of development, rim calcification around fat necrosis or sheet calcification may simulate malignant calcification, as may irregular calcification in diffuse, saponified fat. In addition, fat necrosis can cause stellate distortion, leading to confusion.[8]

Foreign bodies

Calcification can occur in reaction to any foreign body. Its shape will depend on that of the structure

(including cyst aspiration, biopsy, lumpectomy, radiation therapy, reduction mammoplasty, breast reconstruction, implant removal and anticoagulant therapy), and may have a striking appearance with a dense rim or sheets of calcification (Figure 15.4).

to which it is responding. Surgical sutures lead to curvilinear and tubular calcification around a scar, similar to vascular calcification shapes. Calcification of suture material commonly occurs following irradiation, but is rarely seen in the non-irradiated breast (Figure 15.5).[9] Parasitic worms, not surprisingly, cause small worm-shaped calcifications. They are rare, but are commoner in women of African origin (Figure 15.6). Schistosomiasis is also rare, but has been reported to cause breast calcifications indistinguishable from malignancy,[10–12] and *Trichinella* can cause pectoral muscle calcification. Implants may cause sheets of fat necrosis-type calcification around them. Direct injection into the breast has been practised for augmentation. Silicone injection has been carried out in North America and paraffin has been used in a similar fashion in the Far East. This results in subsequent granulomas and calcification (Figure 15.7). Lipiodol ultra fluid has in the past been used for galactography. It may persist in breast ducts or cysts for some years, mimicking intraductal calcifications.[13]

Stromal calcifications

Occasionally, calcifications of unknown aetiology occur in fibrous breast stroma. These may be variable and quite bizarre in shape, with punctate well-defined calcifications mixed with large linear and sheet-like shapes. These can occasionally simulate malignancy, but are usually more extensive and bilateral. Heterotopic metaplastic ossification can rarely occur in the stroma of the breast, producing pleomorphic calcification suggestive of malignancy. This has been described as an incidental finding in a patient with no known breast pathology, but also occurs in relation to breast tumours of mesenchymal origin (such as sarcomas and mesenchymomas) primary localised amyloid of the breast and occasionally with other benign conditions.[14,15]

Artefacts simulating calcification

These can arise from a variety of sources. Talcum powder, deodorants and creams in the axilla or inframammary fold may become aggregated into small rods and balls. These can simulate malignant calcification, but their distribution should allow distinction (Figure 15.8). Intradermal densities can be caused by tattoos and warts. A careful record by the radiographer of any visible skin lesions should avoid confusion. Also, the patient's scalp hair should be pulled well back during mammography to avoid it being projected on the film, where it can cause blurred curvilinear densities, usually seen on the back of the craniocaudal view (Figure 15.9).

Careful inspection of the films should distinguish by their brightness the small white artefacts that arise

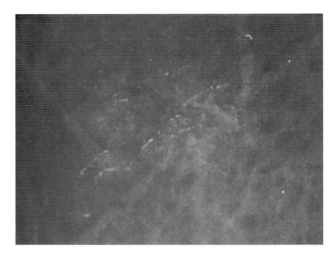

Figure 15.8 Artefact – talcum powder. On this craniocaudal view, talcum powder in the inframammary fold has rolled into small balls and rods, coating the lower aspect of the breast. This produces tiny punctate and linear artefacts mimicking malignant calcification.

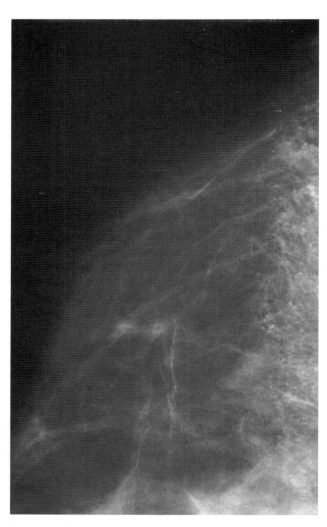

Figure 15.9 Hair artefact. Overlying hair projected at the back of the craniocaudal view simulates calcifications.

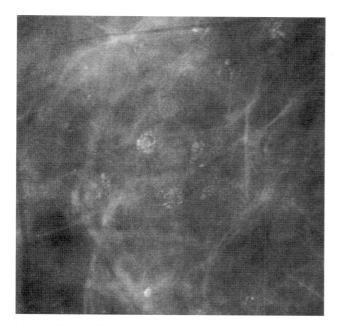

Figure 15.10 Benign breast change. This is a woman with stable screening mammograms and extensive fine punctate calcifications in both breasts contained within rounded clusters, consistent with benign breast change such as adenosis/epitheliosis.

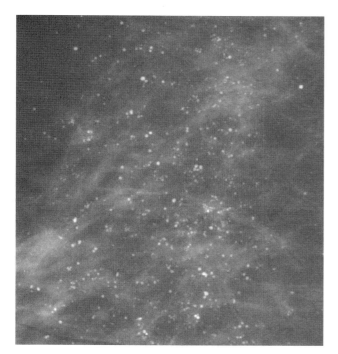

Figure 15.11 Benign breast change – adenosis. Extensive small rounded pearl-like calcifications are seen, some lying singularly and some in small round clusters in this woman, whose screening mammograms were unchanged on two subsequent screening rounds. The appearances are consistent with a lobular distribution and benign breast change such as adenosis/epitheliosis.

due to dirt on the screens, film scratches or pick-off produced during processing from calcification. Fingerprints on the films should be recognisable by their whorled patterns.

The Chinese herbal treatment Go-yak has been used for the treatment of breast abscess and results in residual lead deposits in the region of the previous abscess, which may mimic microcalcification. They can be distinguished by the unusually high density of deposits and a relevant history.[16] In addition, lead deposits in the breast simulating microcalcification have been described following a rifle shot to the breast.[17]

Calcification in the lobule

Lobules are the commonest site of breast calcifications. The majority are markers of benign breast disease (fibrocystic changes). Those that are malignant represent lobular carcinoma in situ (LCIS – see below) and cannot be distinguished from benign lobular calcifications radiologically. Adenosis, sclerosing adenosis and microcystic disease are variants of fibrocystic benign breast disease.

Adenosis
Overgrowth of the epithelium lining the terminal duct lobular unit can lead to calcium deposits within distended lobules. These concretions are rounded pearl-like calcifications, of uniform density and size and arranged in tiny round clusters (likened to 'little raspberries' or 'dog's paw prints') or in ones or twos (like diplococci) (Figure 15.10). They are often scattered throughout both breasts wherever there is glandular tissue and are frequently associated with a spectrum of benign breast disease. When localised, they may cause diagnostic difficulties. Following fatty involution, scattered lobular calcifications may remain within adipose tissue with no visible surrounding glandular tissue (Figure 15.11).

Sclerosing adenosis
In this variant, there is a greater degree of stromal fibrosis associated with epithelial hyperplasia within the lobules. This results in distortion of normal lobular architecture and can produce calcifications, which show variations in density, shape and size.

There may also be architectural distortion of breast stroma visible on a mammogram. These appearances simulate malignancy. Alternatively, amorphous, powdery calcifications within tiny cysts may produce softer, less dense, lobular calcifications

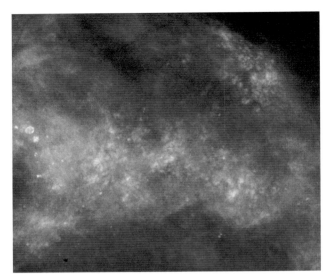

Figure 15.12 Sclerosing adenosis. This woman's mammograms showed extensive benign-type calcification, unchanged over three yearly subsequent screening mammograms. The calcifications show a lobular distribution with extensive fine cumulus cloud-type calcification that is associated with a spectrum of benign breast changes such as sclerosing adenosis.

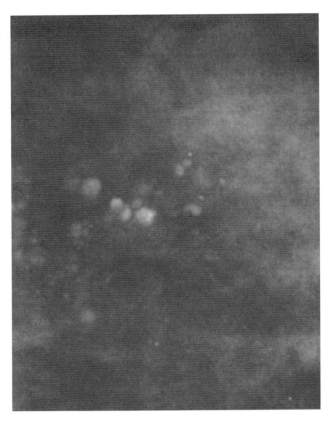

Figure 5.13 Microcystic disease: craniocaudal view. The calcifications appear as lower-density and rounded.

giving a cumulus cloud effect on mammography (Figure 15.12).

Microcystic disease

Again as part of the spectrum of benign breast disease – and often seen in association with the conditions above, and with macrocystic disease – the calcifications may be scattered or clustered. The lobules enlarge to form tiny cysts 1–5 mm in diameter. The epithelium secretes fluid containing calcium salts, which precipitate within the cysts, producing a layer of sludge at the bottom. This appearance has been likened to 'tea leaves in a tea cup'.

These have a characteristic mammographic appearance. When viewed from the side on a true lateral horizontal X-ray film, crescents of calcium are seen lying horizontally. When viewed from above on a craniocaudal film, the calcifications are seen as rounded lower-density pearls. It is worthwhile searching for this appearance with a true lateral and craniocaudal magnification view, as it represents a definite benign disease process (Figures 15.13–15.15).

Lobular carcinoma in situ (LCIS)

LCIS is not a direct precursor of malignancy, but is a marker of increased risk. Thus some authors prefer

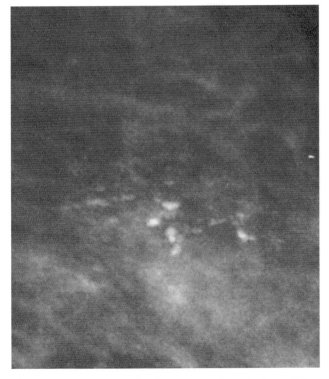

Figure 5.14 Microcystic disease: true lateral view of the same cluster of calcification as in Figure 15.13. A higher-density crescent shape is seen, indicating the presence of benign microcystic disease.

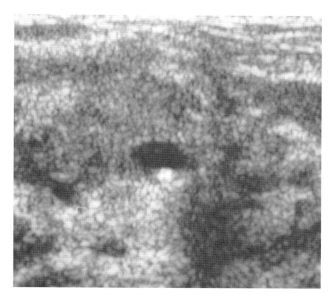

Figure 15.15 Ultrasound appearances of microcystic disease. This highly magnified ultrasound image in a woman with microcystic calcification visible on her mammogram shows a tiny cyst with calcium layering posteriorly within it.

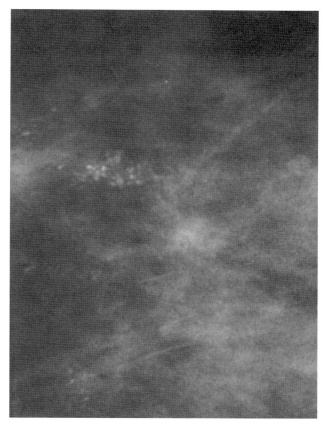

Figure 15.16 Lobular carcinoma in situ (LCIS). Small rounded clusters of punctate slightly variable calcifications cannot be distinguished radiologically from other causes of indeterminate calcifications, such as benign breast change and low-grade ductal carcinoma in situ (DCIS).

the term 'lobular neoplasia'. It is commonly multi-centric (60–90%) and bilateral (35–59%).[18] It indicates a risk of 1% per year of developing invasive cancer, of either ductal or lobular type, in either breast (a sevenfold-increased risk above the general population). Neoplastic cells replace the normal epithelium of acini and intralobular ductules. The abnormal cells cause expansion of individual acini, as well as enlargement of the entire lobule. On rare occasions, it leads to the formation of calcifications, which are indistinguishable from the lobular calcifications that are seen in adenosis or sclerosing adenosis. These conditions are much commoner than LCIS. For all practical purposes therefore, LCIS is not a diagnosis that is made mammographically. It is usually an incidental finding in breast biopsies and its management is as yet uncertain. Commonly, an expectant surveillance policy is adopted (Figure 15.16).

Calcification in ducts

The majority of breast cancers arise from ductal epithelium and a proportion start as DCIS. DCIS appears to be a direct precursor of invasive tumours, evolving into invasive cancer in up to 50% of cases.[19] It is a diagnosis most commonly made on mammography, accounting for up to 20% of screen-detected malignancy and about 5% of symptomatic cancers. Benign ductal calcifications also occur in plasma cell mastitis (PCM) and atypical ductal hyperplasia (ADH). PCM should be easily distin-guishable from DCIS radiologically. ADH is more difficult to identify.

Large non-calcified ducts are frequently seen in the subareolar region. Individual ducts may be several millimetres in width, but when subareolar or symmetrical they are not of clinical significance. Dilated ducts that are in other areas of the breast, that change and become more prominent over time and that are associated with linear calcifications are associated with malignancy.[20]

Plasma cell mastitis (PCM)

In this benign condition, also known as mammary duct ectasia, enlarged ectatic ducts are filled with inspissated eosinophilic material, lipid-containing histiocytes and desquamated duct epithelium. Sometimes ovoid crystalline bodies and cholesterol crystals are present. These may calcify within the ducts, giving rods or needles or dense well-circum-scribed round-ended calcium of up to a centimetre long and 1–3 mm thick. They are frequently

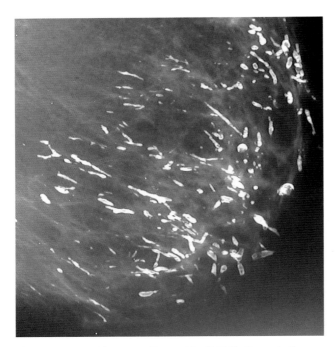

Figure 15.17 Plasma cell mastitis (PCM). Smooth linear calcifications in needle shapes mixed with lucent-centred ovals outline the ducts in this asymptomatic woman with PCM/mammary duct ectasia on mammography.

distributed throughout both breasts in a ductal pattern converging on the nipple, although they may occupy a single segment. They are most common in the subareolar area. Duct inflammation is invariably present. Rupture may also occur and lead to oval, lucent-centred, ductally distributed calcifications interspersed with the rods. Rings of fat necrosis may also be associated. PCM calcification tends to be widely spaced within the breast. This and the smooth well-defined borders of individual calcifications usually allow differentiation from DCIS (Figure 15.17).

In a fatty breast, enlarged ducts in this condition may be visible. There is often long-standing slit-like nipple inversion. Although women may present with pain or nipple discharge, the majority are asymptomatic. Diffuse bilateral benign intraductal microcalcification has also been described following recent lactation, and may be related to milk stasis or apoptosis associated with lactation.[21]

Ductal carcinoma in situ (DCIS)

In DCIS, malignant cells are confined within the basement membrane of the ducts. DCIS can be extensive within a duct system and may involve adjacent lobules (cancerisation of the lobules). Tiny foci of invasion (up to 1 mm diameter) may also be present and are defined as micro-invasion. Areas of invasive carcinoma larger than 1 mm in diameter are classed as invasive cancers rather than micro-invasion. DCIS can be multifocal (more than one lesion, single quadrant) or multicentric (more than one quadrant involved) and in these cases breast-conserving surgery may be inappropriate (recently, the difficult distinction between multifocal and multicentric disease has been abandoned by histopathologists, with all forms regarded as multi-focal).

In the past, DCIS has been classified according to the architecture of the growth pattern into comedo and non-comedo groups, with categories within the non-comedo group including cribriform, micropapillary, solid and papillary. It was found, however, that this classification did not give useful prognostic information, and the classification of DCIS is now based on cytonuclear morphology rather than growth pattern. There is further subdivision on the basis of the presence or absence of necrosis within affected ducts.[22] In the UK, there are national guidelines for grading of DCIS into low, intermediate and high grades.[23] With this classification, DCIS is divided into low-grade (small cells with infrequent mitoses and commonly a cribriform or micropapillary growth pattern), intermediate-grade (moderate variation in size and shape of cells and variable architecture) and high-grade (marked variability in nuclear size and shape, with large cells, often a comedo growth pattern and frequently associated necrosis). A single area of DCIS will often contain a mixture of areas of cytological grades and architectural growth patterns, and should be graded according to the worst area within the lesion.

The majority of high-grade lesions show a comedo growth pattern, which produces radiologically visible calcification in 94% of cases.[24] It accounts for the majority of screen-detected DCIS. Large malignant cells fill and expand the involved ducts. They undergo central necrosis and the necrotic tissue calcifies, producing casts of the ducts with linear and irregularly shaped calcifications.[25] These are very variable in shape and size, but may be up to several millimetres long. Although these are the hallmark of comedo DCIS, there is often, in addition, extensive granular and punctate calcification. Presumably, this represents calcification in necrotic debris that has not yet coalesced to form casts. Fourteen percent have granular calcification alone. Casting calcifications may branch and form X or Y shapes. There is marked variation in density, both within and between calcifications, and they have very irregular borders. They follow a ductal distribution, and thus cluster shapes are typically linear or triangular with convergence on the nipple (Figure 15.18).

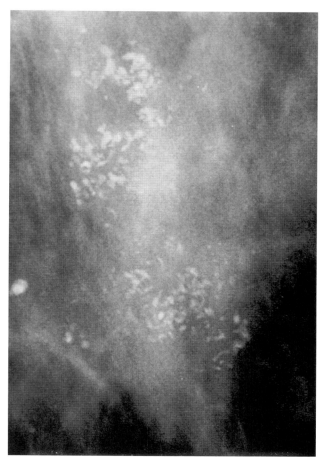

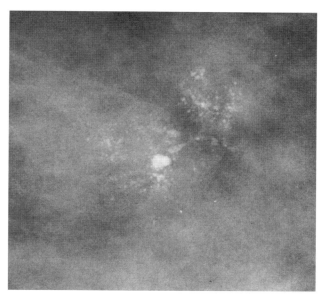

Figure 15.19 Low-grade DCIS. A small cluster of fine punctate calcification was present in the woman with a single associated coarse calcification. The appearance was classified as indeterminate, and biopsy confirmed the presence of low-grade DCIS with a cribriform growth pattern. There was no invasion.

Figure 15.18 High-grade ductal carcinoma in situ (DCIS) with invasive cancer. In this 39-year-old woman with a palpable lump, mammography shows an area of increased density with casting comedo calcification. Note the irregular linear and Y-shaped forms of calcium and the marked variability in size, shape and density between the individual calcifications. This was proven to represent high-grade DCIS associated with grade 3 invasive carcinoma.

The calcifications that are visible in comedo DCIS are likely to be representative of the extent of disease. In cases of pure comedo DCIS, 88% show less than 20 mm discrepancy between mammographic and histological measurements of the extent of disease. Comedo DCIS, however, has a relatively high recurrence rate following local treatment.

Intermediate- and low-grade DCIS tend to show cribriform or micropapillary architecture. In these cases, the involved ducts are expanded by malignant cells, but these grow in a regular fashion, with sieve-like spaces between arches of malignant cells, or small papillary projections with intervening clefts. Crystalline calcifications are produced from active secretion into these spaces. Necrosis is not a major feature.

It appears that only about half of cribriform/micropapillary DCIS (53%) produce radiologically visible calcification. This type is more likely to be mammographically occult than comedo-type DCIS and may present symptomatically.[24] When calcification is visible, it is likely that the disease extends well beyond the area of calcification. Mammography therefore underestimates the histological extent of disease by more than 20 mm in 44% of cases of pure micropapillary/cribriform-type DCIS. The calcifications in this condition tend to be small (<0.5 mm diameter) and granular, leading to confusion with benign lobular calcifications. However, they show greater variability in density, shape and size than in benign conditions, and their distribution is ductal, linear and segmental. These features should give rise to suspicion. In addition, there is overlap with 22% of calcified small cell DCIS showing linear calcification similar to that of comedo DCIS (Figure 15.19).[25]

Other forms of DCIS – clinging and solid – may also produce calcifications of variable, but often punctate shape, and a high index of suspicion is needed to make the diagnosis. These patterns are associated with low-grade DCIS.

When diagnosing DCIS by mammography, the presence of linear branching calcifications is highly predictive of high-grade comedo DCIS. In one study, 100% of cases of linear branching calcifications represented comedo DCIS, as did 80% of cases of linear non-branching calcifications. These features were more important than the number of calcifications, the density, or the size of the cluster. Granular and punctate calcifications occur both in low- and intermediate-grade non-comedo DCIS and in benign disease. Whereas suspicious linear calcifications may be classified as M5, granular calcifications tend to be categorised as M3 or M4, depending on the degree of variability that they show – indeterminate to suspicious.[26,27]

It is possible, to some extent, to predict the likelihood of finding invasion within mammographically detected DCIS. When core biopsy has shown high-grade DCIS and there are more than 40 microcalcifications present, 48% of cases of DCIS show areas of invasion at surgical histology. However, only 15% of areas of high-grade DCIS, with less than 40 calcifications present, contained invasive disease.[28] In this series of 116 cases, those with non-high-grade DCIS on core biopsy did not show any foci of invasive disease at surgical excision. Features not shown to be predictive of the presence of invasion were the clinical presentation, the morphology of the calcifications and the cluster size.

Factors influencing the recurrence rate after local excision of DCIS are the size of the lesion (>2.5 cm is associated with a high recurrence rate), the margin of excision and a high pathological grading.[1] High-grade (large cell) DCIS has a higher recurrence rate than low-grade (small cell) type.

Although screen-detected DCIS is usually diagnosed on the basis of microcalcifications it can have a variety of less common manifestations, without calcifications. For instance, it may produce a stellate lesion, duct thickening, asymmetry, or a circumscribed or ill-defined mass.[29]

Atypical ductal hyperplasia (ADH)
In this condition, there is an intraductal epithelial proliferation with cells that show architectural and/or cytological atypia. However, the degree of atypia is insufficient quantitatively or qualitatively to allow a diagnosis of DCIS. ADH is a risk marker for malignancy and carries a four- to fivefold-increased risk of subsequently developing invasive malignancy.[30] This risk is doubled if there is a family history of breast cancer in a first-degree relative, giving an absolute risk of breast cancer of 20% at 15 years. ADH is commonly found on biopsy, in combination with a spectrum of benign breast disease.

ADH is present in up to 31% of biopsies undertaken for benign microcalcifications.[31] The calcifications that it produces are usually in secretions in the lumen of affected ducts, with irregular punctate and linear forms. Because of its ductal origin, the calci-

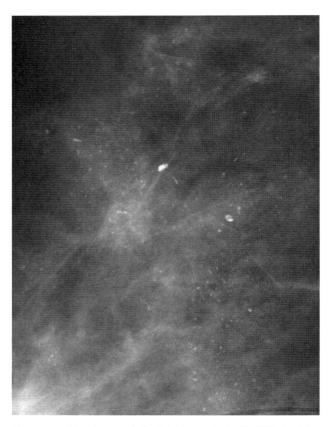

Figure 15.20 Atypical ductal hyperplasia (ADH). In this woman, indeterminate calcification was distributed over a quadrant of the breast containing some linear and many punctate forms, with variability in size and shape of calcifications. Biopsy confirmed the presence of ADH, a risk marker for malignancy. Excision showed only ADH and no evidence of malignancy.

fications tend to show a segmental linear distribution and may simulate DCIS or benign breast disease such as sclerosing adenosis (Figure 15.20).

With the increasing use of core biopsy, it is becoming more common to diagnose ADH on diagnostic wide-bore needle biopsy. In this instance, it is advisable to go on to surgical excision of the area, as ADH on core biopsy is associated with a final diagnosis of carcinoma in between 25% and 75% of cases in reported series.[32,33]

Calcifications associated with masses

Most types of breast masses can have associated calcifications. The form of these may aid diagnosis of the mass. They may be benign or malignant.

Carcinoma
Many invasive cancers show DCIS-type calcification, either within the mass or surrounding it. This

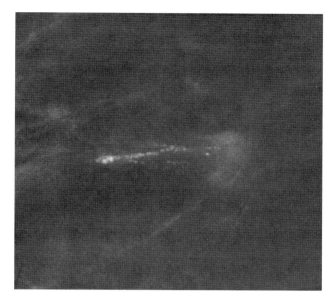

Figure 15.21 Comedo DCIS with a small invasive tumour. Linear, irregular comedo-type calcification in this high-grade DCIS is associated with a small 5 mm invasive ductal carcinoma.

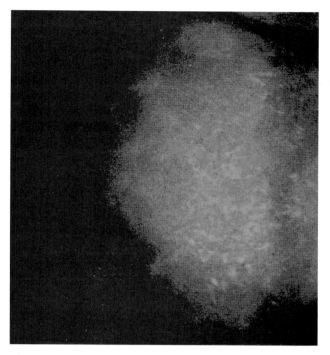

Figure 15.22 Calcifications seen within a lymph node metastasis. Metastases to lymph nodes can occasionally produce casting DCIS-type calcification.

may indicate the extent of associated DCIS and aid in planning surgery. Invasive carcinoma also often shows coarser dystrophic calcifications, usually within areas of necrotic tumour. When extensive DCIS is seen in association with invasive tumour, there is an increased risk of recurrence after local treatment. Data from the Swedish Two-County Trial suggest that the presence of casting-type calcification in association with small invasive cancers up to 14 mm in diameter indicates a subgroup of women with a poorer prognosis. Women with tumours smaller than 10 mm where casting-type calcification was present had a 7.51-fold relative risk of dying of breast cancer compared with women with circumscribed masses without calcification (Figure 15.21).[34]

Very rarely (two reported cases), invasive mucinous breast carcinoma presents mammographically as clustered pleomorphic calcifications without any evidence of an associated mass.[35,36]

Inflammatory breast cancer may produce only nonspecific signs of inflammation (skin thickening, increased breast density and trabecular thickening). In 47% of cases, however, malignant-type microcalcification is present. In association with inflammatory signs, it allows the diagnosis of locally advanced carcinoma to be made on mammography.[37]

Lymph nodes

Rarely, nodes containing metastases from breast carcinoma will calcify.[38] This can be typical DCIS-type calcification within ductal structures formed by

a well-differentiated tumour. Alternatively, as in primary tumours, more amorphous calcifications will occur in necrotic areas and can be up to several millimetres across. More commonly, however, nodes show calcification of benign aetiology, usually inflammatory. Popcorn-type calcification is common

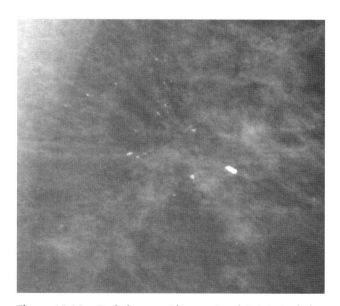

Figure 15.23 Radial scar with associated DCIS. Radial scars often contain calcification – usually within benign breast change associated with the radial lesion. There may also be associated DCIS producing linear and punctate calcification around the scar, as in this case.

following tuberculosis. Also, punctate nodal calcification can occur following gold therapy for rheumatoid arthritis (Figure 15.22).

Radial scars

These often show calcifications. They are highly proliferative epithelial lesions and the majority of calcifications represent a spectrum of benign breast disease within and around the main lesion.[39] In up to 39% of screen-detected radial scars, however, there is associated malignancy. Typical DCIS-type calcifications associated with the radial scar may suggest this (Figure 15.23).[40]

Fibroadenomas and papillomas

These are common in the screening population. Their nature is usually obvious, particularly if a benign-appearing mass is accompanied by typical, dense clumps of popcorn-type calcification within its fibrous stroma or eggshell-like rim calcification. Often the original fibroadenoma has become hyalinised and only the calcification remains visible. Again this should cause no diagnostic difficulty. Calcifications in fibroadenomas, however, are also common within the epithelium-lined clefts, which curve within the tumour. This calcification is then linear and branching. It is generally well defined and often the branches have characteristic clubbed ends formed by the blunt ends of the cleft. It should form a rounded or oval cluster, and the circumscribed border of the soft tissue mass may be visible around it. These features, when present, will allow differentiation from malignant causes of calcification, but this is not always possible (Figure 15.24).

Calcifications within a papilloma may be very similar. These masses tend to be near the nipple and aligned within the ducts. Single papillomas are normally benign, but multiple papillomatosis is a risk marker for malignancy, indicating a four- to fivefold-increased risk.

Fibroadenomatoid hyperplasia

This unusual benign breast lesion shows composite features histologically between those of a fibroadenoma and fibrocystic change. It may present on mammography as a soft tissue mass with ill-defined borders. It commonly shows granular microcalcifications in an irregularly shaped cluster, which may or may not be associated with a mass. In 64% of cases, in one series, rod-shaped calcifications were also seen. The microcalcifications may appear indeterminate or suspicious on mammography (Figure 15.25).[41]

Fibroadenolipomas

These have such a characteristic radiological appearance that they should not cause confusion. However, they contain elements of normal breast tissue and these can contain benign breast disease.

PCM has been seen producing linear calcification within a fibroadenolipoma. Malignancy within a fibroadenolipoma has not been described.

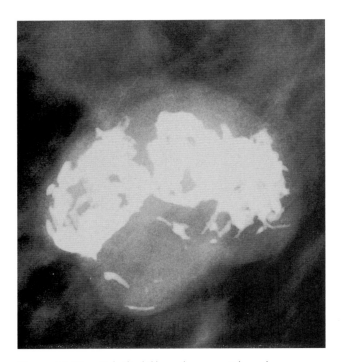

Figure 15.24 Calcified fibroadenoma. Fibroadenomas may hyalinise and calcify over time, showing dense popcorn-like calcification. Calcium may also be seen in linear coarse forms, showing clubbed ends, where calcium lies within the epithelial cleft of fibroadenomas. Similar calcifications can be seen within papillomas.

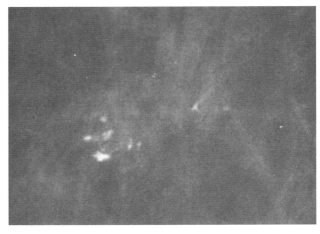

Figure 15.25 Fibroadenomatoid hyperplasia. Note the presence of calcification of variable size and shape with linear forms in this case proven to represent fibroadenomatoid hyperplasia. In this condition, the calcification often simulates malignant appearances.

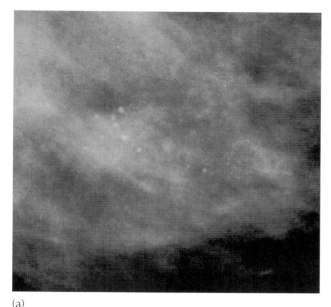

(a)

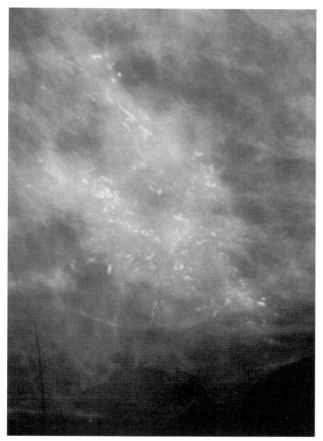

(b)

Figure 15.26 Increasing calcification. In this woman a small cluster of punctate calcification indeterminate on the initial mammogram (a) has increased markedly on a subsequent screening mammogram 3 years later (b). It now shows clearly malignant, casting and comedo calcifications with an associated soft tissue mass. Surgery at this time confirmed the presence of a 10 mm grade 2 invasive ductal carcinoma with associated high-grade DCIS.

Galactocoeles

These can contain clumpy thick calcification, but will rarely be seen in the screening population.

Haemangiomas

These may contain thick, clumpy or variable bizarre-shaped calcification.

Warts

These may also show irregular calcifications, but should be clinically obvious.

Changing calcification

Calcifications of benign aetiology obviously start at some point in time and must change and develop after this. However, change is a feature of malignancy, and therefore any change in breast calcification should be regarded with suspicion. The commonest change in malignant calcification is an increase in the number and extent of particles with time (Figure 15.26). In one series of screening patients, 30% of new microcalcifications seen after a 3-year screening interval yielded malignancy. In this series, all cases of malignancy contained calcifications classified as pleomorphic or linear, and none had new punctate calcifications.[42] The amount of time taken for a visible change, indicating malignancy to happen is variable, but if no change has occurred in 3 years, malignancy is unlikely. Alternatively, calcification may decrease and resolve with time; this can also be a marker of malignancy as it indicates an active disease process. In a series of 37 cases of spontaneously resolving microcalcification, 36% of a group with initially indeterminate calcification subsequently developed malignancy at the site of the disappearing calcification. In these cases, the usual sequence of events is for a soft tissue mass to appear subsequently in the same area. The presence of spontaneously disappearing indeterminate calcification in association with a new soft tissue mass should be regarded as highly suspicious of malignancy. There may be difficulties with management, as disappearing calcifications become more difficult to biopsy (Figure 15.27).[43]

Management

When reading mammograms, to be certain to identify the finest microcalcifications, a thorough examination should include the use of a magnifying glass. The identification of abnormalities, including microcalcifications, is improved when films are double-read. Computer-aided detection (CAD) systems are now available that can provide evaluation of a digitised mammographic image and place prompts on areas of possible microcalcifications or

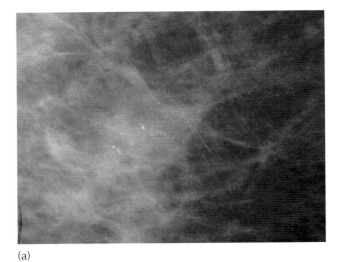
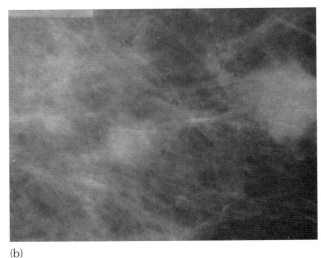

(a)   (b)

Figure 15.27   Disappearing calcification. Indeterminate calcification initially visualised (a) has spontaneously resolved 1 year later (b), but two small irregular soft tissue masses have appeared in the same area. Histology confirmed a 5 and 10 mm grade 2 invasive ductal carcinoma with associated DCIS.

masses, to assist radiological detection of abnormalities. CAD systems are more accurate in detecting microcalcification than masses. In one series, 98% of malignant microcalcifications and 80% of benign microcalcifications were marked by the CAD system. In this study, however, there was no statistically significant increase in sensitivity for the detection of malignant microcalcification by experienced mammographers using the CAD system.[44]

The majority of calcifications seen on screening or symptomatic mammograms will appear clearly benign. These will include cases with widespread diffuse, punctate, lobular-type calcifications, microcystic calcifications and calcifications outside the duct lobular system, such as those in calcified fibroadenomas or vessels. For these kinds of cases, no recall or further investigation is necessary (Figure 15.28).

When clustered calcifications are present (>5/cm²) and are isolated in one area, or appear dominant or different on a background of diffuse calcification, further investigation is warranted. In the first instance, it is helpful to obtain any previous mammograms. If the calcifications have a benign appearance and have been present and unchanged for over 3 years then the likelihood of a benign aetiology is very strong and no further investigation is necessary.

Women with suspicious or new clustered microcalcifications should undergo further assessment. This will include a history and clinical examination as well as magnification views of the area of the calcification in the true lateral and craniocaudal projections. The use of two magnification views taken from

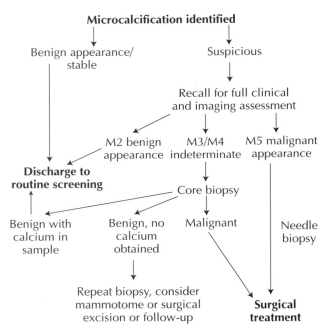

Figure 15.28   Management of microcalcifications: final outcome should be definitive diagnosis of benign aetiology with discharge or malignancy.

these different projections allows the assessment of any alteration in the shape of the calcification between the two views, which may allow a diagnosis of microcystic disease to be made. (See Table 15.2 for diagnostic features of calcifications seen on standard and magnification mammographic views.) When calcifications show a definitive benign appearance, such as microcystic disease or vascular calcification, on magnified views, the woman can be reassured and discharged without further investigation.

Feature	Benign	Malignant
Distribution	Single or diffuse	Clustered (>5 in a small area)
Cluster shapes	Round	Linear, triangular, rhomboid
Form	Round, popcorn rings, needles, parallel lines	Casting, (linear and branching) granular, pleomorphic
Size	Uniform	Variable
Density	Uniform	Variable – within and between calcification

Table 15.2 Diagnostic features of calcifications

The presence of typical benign calcifications does not exclude co-existent malignancy and each area of calcification within a breast should be judged separately (Figure 31a–d).

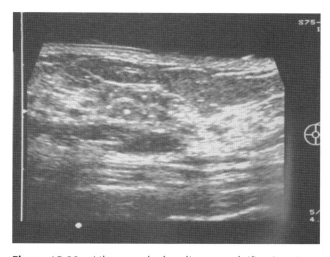

Figure 15.29 Ultrasound of malignant calcification. In this 38-year-old with high-grade DCIS, ultrasound shows an ill-defined hypoechoic area with hyperechoic flecks of calcium in the centre of the image.

High-frequency breast ultrasound is now routinely used in breast assessment clinics. It is worthwhile examining with ultrasound the area of calcification identified on the mammogram. High rates of sensitivity (75–100%) have been reported in depicting breast masses associated with malignant microcalcifications.[45,46] The ultrasound appearance of microcalcifications has been described as that of twinkling stars (bright dots in different planes) in a dark sky (contrasted against ill-defined hypoechoic patches), corresponding on histopathology to groups of expanded ducts with increased cell density with or without necrosis (Figure 15.29).[47] It has also been

reported that when there is distortion of the soft tissues on ultrasound in association with microcalcifications, this corresponds to comedo-type DCIS. By contrast, a pattern of prominent ducts visible on ultrasound is suggestive of non-comedo DCIS.[48] Ultrasound is much more likely to demonstrate an associated soft tissue mass when microcalcifications are of malignant, rather than benign, aetiology (100% versus 59% sensitivity in one series).[46] Power Doppler can also be used to assess areas of soft tissue abnormality seen on ultrasound in association with microcalcifications. Abnormal increased vascularity may be seen on power Doppler in both benign and malignant areas of calcification and is not helpful in distinguishing aetiology. It can, however, help to guide needle biopsy, including identifying the area of an invasive focus within a region of DCIS.[49]

Magnetic resonance imaging (MRI) can be used to assess areas of calcification. Areas of DCIS may enhance in either a linear or a segmental fashion during the early phase of contrast-enhanced dynamic MRI. The sensitivity of dynamic imaging for detecting DCIS is lower than that for invasive cancer. In one study, the sensitivity was reported as 45% with a specificity of 72% and an overall accuracy of 56% in differentiating benign from malignant microcalcifications. In no case was surgical management altered by MRI findings in this study.[50] Other authors have reported higher sensitivity for the detection of DCIS: up to 93%.[48]

When full clinical and imaging assessment is complete, the radiologist should be able on the basis of magnification mammography and ultrasound to classify the clustered calcifications according to the level of suspicion (M1–M5)[2] or the BIRADS system (Table 15.1). Calcifications falling in the category M3–M5 (indeterminate to suspicious) should be further assessed with needle biopsy. This may be either fine-needle aspiration cytology (FNAC) or wide-bore needle biopsy (core needle biopsy), according to local preference. Wide-bore needle biopsy is preferable. It allows histological information to be obtained and differentiation to be made between in situ and invasive malignancy, as well as being more accurate in achieving a diagnosis.[51] Larger bore biopsy devices, such as vacuum assisted mammotomy (11g), will further increase diagnostic accuracy.

Before guided needle biopsy is undertaken, the woman should be given a full explanation of the probable cause and level of suspicion attached to her calcifications. Her consent should be obtained for the procedure and a management plan discussed with her. When the calcifications are classed as M5 (highly suspicious of malignancy), surgical excision will be needed even if the needle biopsy result proves inadequate or benign. In this instance, excision will be for diagnostic rather than therapeutic reasons. It is, however, extremely desirable to obtain a malignant diagnosis on needle biopsy prior to surgery when malignancy is present. This will allow preoperative counselling of the patient and for therapeutic surgery to be planned. This might include an axillary procedure when invasive malignancy is present, thus potentially avoiding the need for more than one operation.

Needle biopsy for calcifications may be undertaken under either ultrasound or stereotactic guidance, depending on preference and the ease of visualisation of the area with each technique.

In many cases, the conclusion from imaging assessment is that calcification is indeterminate (M3 or M4). The majority of women with indeterminate calcification will have benign disease and surgical excision biopsy should be avoided for them. If guided needle biopsy indicates atypical or malignant change, including ADH, referral for surgical excision is indicated. When, however, the calcification is classified as indeterminate and the cytology or histology obtained at needle biopsy is benign, further management will depend on the type of biopsy undertaken. When benign histology from core biopsy has been obtained and X-ray of the core biopsy specimens has confirmed the presence of representative calcification within the sample, the woman can be reassured and discharged without further follow-up. When guided core biopsy of an area of calcification has been undertaken and no radiological calcification is identified in the specimens, consideration should be given to repeating the biopsy or to diagnostic excision to obtain representative calcification. The alternative strategy is to adopt a surveillance policy, and this may also be undertaken when FNAC has been used and has yielded a benign result. It is reasonable to repeat the clinical and imaging assessment at 1 year. Assuming that these show no change, a screening mammogram can then be performed at 2 years, giving a total of 3 years' follow-up.[52]

Any change with either an increase or a decrease in the number of calcifications during the period of follow-up should prompt a reassessment with repeat needle biopsy and careful consideration again of the need for excision biopsy. Management will always be tempered by consideration of the woman's wishes. Most women, having received a full explanation, will tolerate a policy of follow-up well, but a few cannot sustain any uncertainty and will prefer to have excision biopsy. Following benign core needle biopsy, the delayed false-negative rate is low (<2%),[53] but occasionally delayed change in the mammographic appearance indicates malignancy despite a previous benign core biopsy. For this reason, some centres advocate repeat screening mammography at 1 year after biopsy for follow-up, even in cases with a clear benign diagnosis.

It is more difficult to obtain adequate cytological samples from microcalcifications than other breast lesions. Lofgren et al[54] found a 29% inadequate sample rate from calcifications versus 26% overall for impalpable lesions on FNAC. On those occasions when the cytology is insufficiently cellular for diagnosis, it should ideally be repeated after an interval or core biopsy added. Diagnostic cytology results are more likely to be obtained if a cytopathologist or cytotechnologist is present at the time of aspiration so that adequacy can be assessed immediately. Further passes can then be made if the sample is insufficient.

Postoperative changes

Benign histology

In a proportion of cases, when surgical biopsy has been recommended by the radiologist because of suspicious mammographic findings, benign histology will be found. When the calcifications have been completely excised, no further follow-up is necessary. In some of these, however, usually – when the calcifications are extensive – only an incisional biopsy will have been performed and there will be residual calcifications. Assuming that the specimen contains representative calcification, it appears safe to follow a policy of mammographic surveillance rather than repeat excision. In 39 such cases followed for an average of 32 months, Homer[55] found no cases of malignancy developing.

Malignancy

When malignancy is found on surgical biopsies performed for microcalcification, in up to 40% of cases, incomplete excision may be suspected because the tumour was close to the margins of the surgical specimen (within 5 mm). This may happen when the original biopsy was diagnostic rather than therapeutic, or because of the difficulty of identifying the extent of calcifications intraoperatively. Postoperative mammography can be used to help guide re-excision if breast-conserving surgery is planned. It should be delayed at least 1 month after surgery to allow wound healing. When more than five residual calcifications are seen in women with DCIS, the mammogram is a good predictor of residual disease.[56]

Some centres are routinely undertaking postlumpectomy mammograms in patients who have presented with suspicious microcalcification and have been treated with breast conservation. Even when the mammographic lesion is thought to be entirely removed on postexcision specimen radiographs, and the surgical margin of excision was thought to be adequate, a significant number of patients (17% in one series) had residual microcalcifications. Of those undergoing re-excision, 67% were found to have residual malignancy, representing 9% of the whole group.[57,58] In view of this, a number of centres have now adopted routine follow-up mammography, post breast-conserving surgery for calcifications. This is especially helpful in those with DCIS.

Following breast-conserving surgery for malignant microcalcification, continuing mammographic surveillance is advisable to allow early detection of recurrence. It should initially be carried out annually, and then on a tapering protocol.

Recurrent calcification

Non-excised residual calcifications may or may not disappear post radiation therapy. If they persist, this does not necessarily indicate viable tumour, but careful follow-up is necessary to ensure stability. New calcifications in a treated breast following breast-conserving surgery may be due to recurrent malignancy or benign postoperative changes. When microcalcifications appear at the site of surgery within 3 years and when their appearance is benign, the risk of malignancy is low. Benign appearances following surgery include thick calcified sheets and elongated dystrophic calcifications commonly seen with scarring. When calcifications have a malignant appearance or develop more than 3 years following surgery, they should be regarded with a high degree of suspicion and biopsy should be undertaken.[59–61]

Forty-three percent of recurrences detected by mammography manifest as calcifications.[62] The distribution and appearance of these calcifications are similar to those of malignant calcifications in the pretreated breast. Recurrence after breast conservation treatment is commonest at the site of previous surgery (70%), but may occur elsewhere in the breast. Cases originally treated for DCIS usually manifest recurrent malignancy as microcalcifications and recurrent DCIS. When the original cancer has been invasive, the appearance of local recurrence is more variable.[63] However, 20–25% of irradiated breasts develop benign calcifications within fat necrosis, sutures or duct ectasia. It is important to recognise these and avoid unnecessary biopsy.[64]

Composition of microcalcifications

Microcalcifications detected by radiology may not be easily visualised by the pathologist. Larger calcifications may be fragmented and lost during the preparation and cutting of slices for histological examination. Finer calcifications fall into two main categories.

Type I

Calcium oxalate dihydrate (wedellite)
This forms small polyhedral shapes, which may be difficult to see on mammograms. It is usually associated with benign or borderline lesions. The crystals are birefringent and may also be difficult to visualise on microscopy except with the use of polarised light. The frequency of polyhedral microcalcifications on screening mammograms is 3%.[65]

Type II

Amorphous calcium phosphate or hydroxyapatite
This is non-crystalline. It is associated with both benign and malignant conditions. It stains readily with haematoxylin and is more readily visualised on microscopy.[66]

Hydroxyapatite is a bone-specific mineral. The mechanism of formation of this crystal within breast cancer is not fully understood. It has, however, been shown that breast cancer cells express several bone matrix proteins, including bone sialoprotein, which is involved in the initiation of hydroxapatite crystallisation. Specific staining of tissue sections containing hydroxyapatite crystals has shown that the calcifications contain cells and may represent the fossils of cancer cells.[67]

It has also been found that there are elevated levels of certain elements, including aluminium, calcium, chloride, iron and zinc, in tumour tissues. It is possible that these raised elemental concentrations may be related to the formation of microcalcification.[68]

The pathologist examining breast lesions needs to be aware that microcalcifications were present on the mammogram, so that a specific search can be carried out to confirm their presence in the histological specimen. Otherwise, they may be missed (Table 15.I).

Further reading

Lanyi M. Diagnosis and Differential Diagnosis of Breast Calcifications. New York: Springer-Verlag, 1988.

Tabar L, Dean PB. Teaching Atlas of Mammography. 3rd edn. Stuttgart: Georg Thieme Verlag, 2001.

References

1. Bassett LW. Mammographic analysis of calcifications. Radiol Clin North Am 1992; 30: 93–105.

2. Roche NA, Given-Wilson RM, Thomas VA, Sacks NPS. Assessment of a screening system for breast imaging. Br J Surg 1998; 85: 669–72.

3. Evans AJ, Cohen MEL, Cohen GF. Patterns of breast calcification in patients on renal dialysis. Clin Radiol 1992; 45: 343–4.

4. Kagel PJ, Aquino MO, Fiorella R, Chapman J. Clinical radiographic, and pathologic features on medial calcific sclerosis in the breast. South Med J 1997; 90: 518–21.

5. Denison CM, Ward VL, Lester SC et al. Epidermal inclusion cysts of the breast: three lesions with calcifications. Radiology 1997; 204: 493–6.

6. Kopans DB, Meyer JE, Homer MJ, Grabbe J. Dermal deposits mistaken for breast calcifications. Radiology 1983; 149: 592–4.

7. Apesteguia L, Pina L, Inchusta M et al. Klippel–Trenaunay syndrome: a very infrequent cause of microcalcifications in mammography. Eur Radiol 1997; 7: 123–5.

8. Hogge JP, Robinson RE, Magnant CM, Zuurbier RA. The mammographic spectrum of fat necrosis of the breast. Radiographics 1995; 15: 1347–56.

9. Stacey-Clear A, McCarthy KA, Hall DA et al. Calcified suture material in the breast after radiation therapy. Radiology 1992; 183: 201–8.

10. Gorman JD, Champaign JL, Sumida FK, Canavan L. Schistosomiasis involving the breast. Radiology 1992; 185: 423–4.

11. Sloan BS, Rickman LS, Blau EM, Davis CE. Schistosomiasis masquerading as carcinoma of the breast. South Med J 1996; 89: 345–7.

12. Peyromaure M, Antoine M, Gadonneix P, Villet R. Schistosomiasis: an unusual cause of breast microcalcifications. J Gynecologie 2000; 29: 790–2.

13. Frouge C, Cazenave A, Pham E et al. Mammographic pattern due to residual Lipiodol after galactography. Eur Radiol 1997; 7: 204–7.

14. Keyoung JA, Zuurbier RA, Tsangaris TN, Azumi N. Idiopathic metaplastic ossification of the breast. Clin Radiol 2001; 56: 775–7.

15. Bisceglia M, Carosi I, Murgo R et al. Primary amyloid tumor of the breast. Case report and review of the literature. Acta Pathol 1995; 87: 162–7.

16. Moon WK, Park JM, Im JG et al. Metallic punctate densities in the breast after Chinese herbal treatment: mammographic findings. Radiology 2000; 214: 890–4.

17. Bertrand AF, Dubois-Toussaint S, Lorimier G et al. Breast micro-opacities of lead origin mimicking microcalcifications. J Radiologie 1995; 76: 213–5.

18. Meloni GB, Becchere MP, Soro D et al. Lobular carcinoma in situ: the mammographic aspects and the therapeutic problems. Radiol Med 1996; 91: 360–3.

19. Rosen PP, Braun DW Jr, Kinne DW. The clinical significance of pre-invasive breast carcinoma. Cancer 1980; 46: 919–25.

20. Huynh PT, Parellada JA, de Paredes ES et al. Dilated duct pattern at mammography. Radiology 1997; 204: 137–41.

21. Stucker DT, Ikeda DM, Hartman AR et al. New bilateral microcalcifications at mammography in a postlactational woman: case report. Radiology 2000; 217: 247–50.

22. Holland R, Pertese JL, Millis RR et al: Ductal carcinoma in situ – a proposal for a new classification. Semin Diagn Pathol 1994; 11: 167–80.

23. National Co-ordinating Group for Breast Screening Pathology. Pathology Reporting in Breast Cancer Screening. NHSBSP Publication 31. Sheffield: NHS Breast Screening Programme, 1995.

24. Holland R, Hendriks JHCL, Verbeek ALM et al. Extent, distribution, and mammographic/histological correlations of breast ductal carcinoma in situ. Lancet 1990; 335: 519–22.

25. Stomper PC, Connolly JL. Ductal carcinoma in situ of the breast: correlation between mammographic calcification and tumour subtype. AJR Am J Roentgenol 1992; 159: 483–5.

26. Dinkel HP, Gassel AM, Tschammler A. Is the appearance of microcalcifications on mammography useful in predicting histological grade of malignancy in ductal carcinoma in situ? Br J Radiol 2000; 73: 938–44.

27. Hermann G, Keller RJ, Drossman S et al. Mammographic pattern of microcalcifications in the preoperative diagnosis of comedo ductal carcinoma in situ: histopathologic correlation. Can Assoc Radiol J 1999; 50: 235–40.

28. Bagnall MJC, Evans AJ, Robin A et al. Predicting invasion in mammographically detected microcalcification. Clin Radiol 2001; 56: 828–32.

29. Ikeda DM, Anderson I. Ductal carcinoma in situ: atypical mammographic appearances. Radiology 1989; 172: 661–6.

30. Dupont WD, Page DL. Risk factors for breast cancer in women with proliferative breast disease. N Engl J Med 1985; 312: 146–51.

31. Stomper PC, Cholewinski SP, Penetrante RB et al. Atypical hyperplasia: frequency mammographic and pathologic relationships in excisional biopsies guided with mammography and clinical examination. Radiology 1993; 189: 667–71.

32. Brem RF, Behrndt VS, Sanow L, Gatewood OM. Atypical ductal hyperplasia: histologic underestimation of carcinoma in tissue harvested from impalpable breast lesions using 11-gauge stereotactically guided directional vacuum-assisted biopsy. AJR Am J Roentgenol 1999; 172: 1405–7.

33. Bazzocchi M, Facecchia I, Zuiani C et al. Atypical ductal hyperplasia of the breast. Its diagnostic imaging and the role of percutaneous needle biopsy with a 14-gauge needle. Radiol Med 1999; 98: 133–7.

34. Tabar L, Chen H-H, Duffy SW et al. A novel method for predication of long-term outcome of women with T1a, T1b, and 10–14 mm invasive breast cancers: a prospective study. Lancet 2000; 355: 429–33.

35. Pina Insausti LJ, Sogo Garcia E. Mucinous breast carcinoma showing as a cluster of suspicious

microcalcifications on mammography. Eur Radiol 1998; 8: 1666–8.

36. Goodman DN, Boutross-Tadross O, Jong RA. Mammographic features of pure mucinous carcinoma of the breast with pathological correlation. Can Assoc Radiol J 1995; 46: 296–301.

37. Tardivon AA, Viala J, Corvellec Rudelli A et al. Mammographic patterns of inflammatory breast carcinoma: a retrospective study of 92 cases. Eur J Radiol 1997; 24: 124–30.

38. Helvie MA, Rebner M, Sickles EA, Oberman HA. Calcifications in metastatic breast carcinoma in axillary lymph nodes. AJR Am J Roentgenol 1988; 151: 921–2.

39. Greenstein Orel S, Evers K, I-Tien Yeh, Troupin RH. Radial scar with microcalcifications: Radiologic, pathologic correlation. Radiology 1992; 183: 479–82.

40. Sloane JP, Mayers MM. Carcinoma and atypical hyperplasia in radial scars and complex sclerosing lesions: importance of lesion size and patient age. Histopathology 1993; 23: 225–31.

41. Kamal M, Evans AJ, Denley H et al. Fibroadenomatoid hyperplasia: a cause of suspicious microcalcification on mammographic screening. AJR Am J Roentgenol 1998; 171: 1331–4.

42. Hussain HK, Ng YY, Wells CA et al. The significance of new densities and microcalcification in the second round of breast screening. Clin Radiol 1999; 54: 243–7.

43. Seymour HR, Cooke J, Given-Wilson RM. The significance of spontaneous resolution of breast calcification. Br J Radiol1999; 72: 3–8.

44. Brem RF, Schoonjans JM. Radiologist detection of microcalcifications with and without computer-aided detection: a comparative study. Clin Radiol 2001; 56: 150–4.

45. Moon WK, Im JG, Koh YH et al. US of mammographically detected clustered microcalcifications. Radiology 2000; 217: 849–54.

46. Gufler H, Buitrago-Tellez CH, Madjar H et al. Ultrasound demonstration of mammographically detected microcalcifications. Acta Radiol 2000; 41: 217–21.

47. Huang CS, Wu CY, Chu JS et al. Microcalcifications of non-palpable breast lesions detected by ultrasonography: correlation with mammography and histopathology. Ultrasound Obstet Gynaecol 1999; 13: 431–6.

48. Satake H, Shimamoto K, Sawaki A et al. Role of ultrasonography in the detection of intraductal spread of breast cancer: correlation with pathologic findings. Eur Radiol 2000; 10: 1726–32.

49. Teh WL, Wilson AR, Evans AJ et al. Ultrasound guided core biopsy of suspicious mammographic calcifications using high frequency and power Doppler ultrasound. Clin Radiol 2000; 55: 390–4.

50. Westerhof JP, Fischer U, Moritz JD, Oestmann JW. MR imaging of mammographically detected clustered microcalcifications: is there any value? Radiology 1998; 207: 675–81.

51. Britton PD, McCann J. Needle biopsy in the NHS Breast Screening Programme: How much and how accurate? Breast 1999; 8: 5–11.

52. Sickles EA. Breast calcifications: mammographic evaluation. Radiology 1986; 160: 280–93.

53. Lee CH, Philpotts LE, Horvath LJ, Tocino I. Follow-up of breast lesions diagnosed as benign with stereotactic core-needle biopsy: frequency of mammographic change and false-negative rate. Radiology 1999; 212: 189–94.

54. Lofgren M, Andersson I, Lindholm K. Stereotactic needle aspiration for cytologic diagnosis of non palpable breast lesions. AJR Am J Roentgenol 1990; 154: 1191–5.

55. Homer MJ. Nonpalpable breast microcalcifications: frequency, management and results of incisional biopsy. Radiology 1992; 185: 411–13.

56. Gluck BS, Dershaw DD, Liberman L, Deutch BM. Microcalcifications on postoperative mammograms as an indicator of adequacy of tumor excision. Radiology 1993; 188: 469–72.

57. Aref A, Youssef E, Washington T et al. The value of post lumpectomy mammogram in the management of breast cancer patients presenting with suspicious microcalcifications. Cancer J Sci Am 2000; 6: 25–7.

58. Waddell BE, Stomper PC, DeFazio JL et al. Postexcision mammography is indicated after resection of ductal carcinoma in situ of the breast. Ann Surg Oncol 2000; 7: 665–8.

59. Vora SA, Wazer DE, Homer MJ. Management of microcalcifications that develop at the lumpectomy site after breast-conserving therapy. Radiology 1997; 203: 667–71.

60. Krishnamurthy R, Whitman GJ, Stelling CB, Kushwaha AC. Mammographic findings after breast conservation therapy. Radiographics 1999; 19 (Spec No):S53–62; quiz S262–3.

61. Greenstein Orel S, Troupin RH, Patterson EA, Fowble BL. Breast cancer recurrence after lumpectomy and irradiation: role of mammography in detection. Radiology 1992; 183: 201–6.

62. Stomper PC, Recht A, Berenberg AL et al. Mammo-graphic detection of recurrent cancer in the irradiated breast. AJR Am J Roentgenol 1987; 148: 39–43.

63. Giess CS, Keating DM, Osborne MP, Rosenblatt R. Local tumor recurrence following breast-conservation therapy: correlation of histopathologic findings with detection method and mammographic findings. Radiology 1999; 212: 829–35.

64. Mendelson EB. Radiation changes in the breast. Semin Roentgenol 1993; 28: 344–62.

65. Frouge C, Guinebretiere JM, Juras J et al. Polyhedral micro-calcifications on mammograms: prevalence and morpho-metric analysis. AJR Am J Roentgenol 1996; 167: 621–4.

66. Frouge C, Meunier M, Guinebretiere J-M et al. Polyhedral microcalcifications at mammography: histologic correlation with calcium oxalate. Radiology 1993; 186: 681–4.

67. Castronovo V, Bellahcene A. Evidence that breast cancer associated microcalcifications are mineralized malignant cells. Int J Oncol 1998; 12: 305–8.

68. Ng KH, Bradley DA, Looi LM. Elevated trace element concentrations in malignant breast tissues. Br J Radiol 1997; 70: 375–82.

16 Asymmetry of breast tissue and distortion of architecture

Caroline M Kissin

Introduction

Distortion of the breast parenchyma is a very worrying mammographic finding and, if previous trauma and surgery can be excluded, there is a high likelihood that it is due to malignancy. Even the benign radial scar has been found to contain foci of malignant or premalignant change in up to 19% of cases,[1] and the overlap between the mammographic features of benign and malignant radial lesions is so great that carcinoma cannot be excluded without surgery. However, if the breast is known to be, or is likely to be, scarred from previous injury, accurate assessment of mammographic and ultrasound features can be very difficult.

In contrast, some degree of asymmetry of the breast tissue is a common mammographic finding[2] and statistically is usually benign. However, such asymmetry may hide an underlying mass lesion or may contain parenchymal distortion or microcalcification that is not initially evident. The presence of any of these features would greatly increase the risk of malignancy. An area of asymmetrical breast tissue therefore warrants full and thorough assessment, although the rate of detection of malignancy may be relatively low.

Assessment

All mammograms showing definite or possible parenchymal distortion need full assessment unless there is a clear history of significant injury or surgery to the breast. Focal compression views will confirm or refute the presence of distortion (Figure 16.1). Where distortion is confirmed to be present, the cause must be pursued thoroughly, even if relative mammographic stability has been documented, and needle biopsy will be necessary.

Similarly, most areas of asymmetry, whether large or more focal, that are present in two views (or in one view if only one projection is available) need to be recalled for assessment and further evaluation. However, if the mammographic appearances of this asymmetry have been stable over a period of time, malignancy is much less likely and recall may not be necessary.

At assessment, clinical evaluation is vital, and ultrasound may be very helpful in identifying a focal lesion or architectural disturbance in the relevant quadrant of the breast. Specialist mammographic views over the area of asymmetry, using focal compression and magnification, will provide considerable additional diagnostic information. Such 'paddle views' can increase the internal pressures within the breast by up to 60% compared with those pressures experienced during routine mammography,[3] and this may confirm or reveal parenchymal distortion or identify a mass lesion or

Table 16.1	**The value of focal compression and magnification views in the mammographic assessment of architectural distortion and of asymmetry.**

In asymmetry	In suspected distortion
To reveal underlying distortion	To confirm presence of distortion (Figure 16.1)
To identify underlying mass lesion (Figure 16.8)	To assess presence and density of tumour core (Figure 16.11)
To identify microcalcification (Figure 16.10)	To identify microcalcification
To assess skin changes	To assess length and lucency of spicules (Figure 16.11)

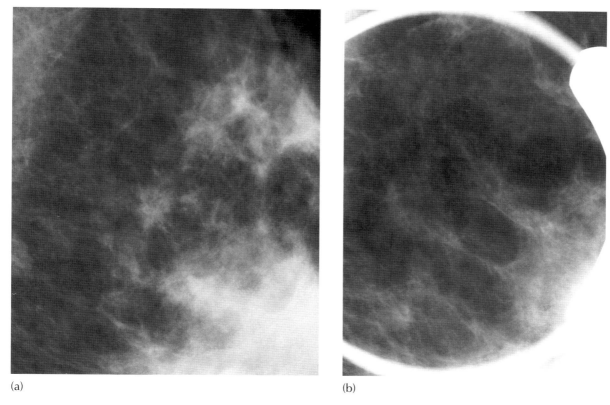

(a)   (b)

Figure 16.1   An unmagnified focal compression view (b) reveals that the suspected distortion (a) is merely a positional shadow.

calcification. The presence of any of these features will help to indicate the underlying pathology, and will also increase the risk of associated malignancy (Table 16.1).

These assessment techniques will usually be supplemented with needle sampling in order to provide accurate triple assessment.

Mammographic assessment of an area of asymmetry may therefore reveal asymmetry alone (either generalised or localised), asymmetry with an underlying mass lesion, asymmetry with underlying microcalcification or asymmetry with underlying distortion. These appearances will help to indicate the underlying pathology.

Asymmetry only

Generalised

Radiotherapy
The irradiated breast typically shows a generalised diffuse increase in density, marked trabecular prominence and skin thickening. The diffuse density is due to oedema of the breast tissue, which occurs maximally 6 months after starting radiotherapy and then starts to resolve in the subsequent 3–6 months.[4] The associated phenomenon of collagen bundle oedema causes the distinctive trabecular thickening and prominent reticular pattern (Figure 16.2), which resolves more slowly than the diffuse density, possibly due to the development of associated fibrosis. Generalised skin thickening is usually obvious at 6 months after radiotherapy and contributes to the increased density of the treated breast. In 35% of cases, this has resolved by 3 years,[5] but local or periareolar thickening may persist for long periods due to induced fibrosis and surgical interference with normal lymph drainage. Coarse, rounded, benign-type calcifications can be seen in approximately 25% of irradiated breasts and are believed to be a direct result of the radiation. These may develop up to 6 years after radiotherapy.[5]

Inflammatory carcinoma
Inflammatory carcinoma of the breast is characterised by erythema, warmth and induration of the skin over all or part of the breast, with accentuation of the depressions around the hair follicles causing a 'peau d'orange' appearance.[6,7] This is due to tumour infiltration of the subdermal lymphatics causing oedema of the skin and also often to meta-

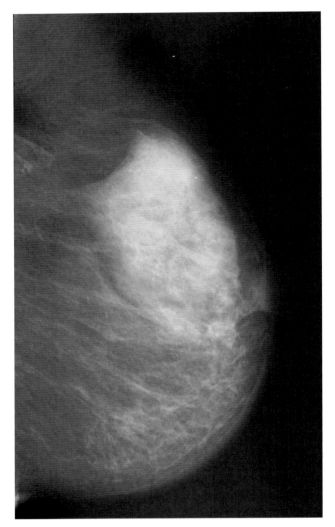

Figure 16.2 A prominent reticular pattern is clearly seen in the lower half of the left breast 1 year after radiotherapy.

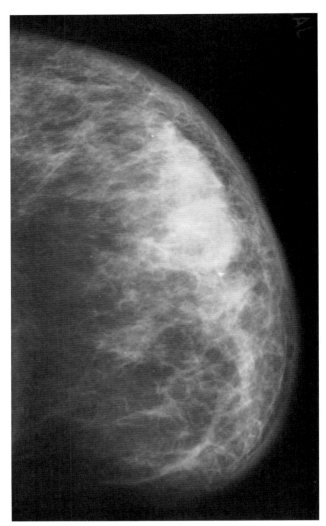

Figure 16.3 Skin thickening, diffuse increased density and a prominent reticular pattern are seen in this craniocaudal view of an inflammatory carcinoma.

stases to the axillary lymph nodes. This leads to an appearance very similar to that seen after radiotherapy, with diffuse density, prominent reticular pattern, skin thickening and distention of the lymphatics in the subcutaneous tissues (Figure 16.3). Within this, it may not be possible to identify the underlying malignancy, but in some cases focal asymmetrical density, architectural distortion, malignant microcalcification or a mass lesion may be present.[8,9] Enlarged axillary lymph nodes are also a common finding.

Other causes

Oedema of the breast causing the typical picture of skin thickening, diffuse increased density, trabecular thickening and a prominent reticular pattern can also be seen in acute mastitis and where there is obstruction to the lymphatic or venous drainage of the breast. It has also been described unilaterally or bilaterally in patients on renal dialysis.[10]

Hypoplasia of the opposite breast

It is usually clinically apparent when there is an underdevelopment of the breast parenchyma on the one side rather than a generalised increased density on the other. Such unilateral hypoplasia of breast tissue may be an isolated finding or it may be associated with absence of the pectoralis major muscle on that side (Poland's syndrome[11]).

Localised

Accessory breast tissue

Accessory breast tissue is a localised area of normal breast tissue lying slightly separate from the

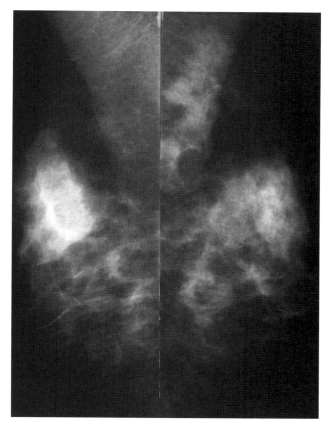

Figure 16.4 Accessory breast tissue is clearly visible in the upper part of the left breast.

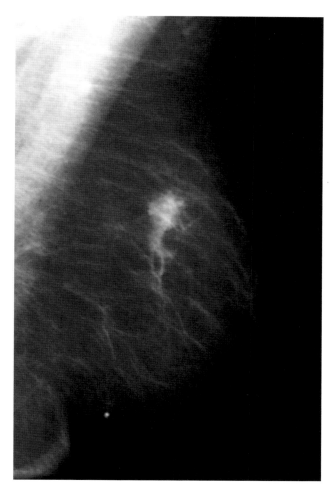

Figure 16.5 Core biopsy of a new area of focal asymmetry in the right breast revealed histological changes consistent with HRT use only.

remainder of the breast. This is most commonly seen in the axillary tail of the breast (Figure 16.4) but may lie anywhere along the milk line, which extends from the axilla to the groin. The accessory tissue may drain into the duct system of the main breast or may have its own nipple. There is no detectable ultrasound abnormality and no evidence of distortion on paddle views.

Patchy involution

Uneven involution of breast parenchyma after the menopause may temporarily leave a residual island of otherwise normal breast tissue that can create diagnostic confusion. Again there is no evidence of mammographic distortion in association, no microcalcification and no associated ultrasound abnormality. Needle biopsy will reveal normal breast tissue only and the diagnosis is therefore largely made by exclusion.

Hormone replacement therapy

The use of hormone replacement therapy (HRT) causes demonstrable mammographic changes in a significant proportion of women within a short time.[12] Increased breast density has been described in 17–73% of women, particularly with the continuous use of combined preparations of oestrogen and progesterone.[13,14] In some women, this is a bilateral generalised diffuse increase in density (58%), but in others, there are more focal or patchy changes (Figure 16.5), including the development of unifocal or multifocal asymmetrical parenchymal densities (17%), the development or increase in size of cysts (25%), and increase in size of fibroadenomas.[12,15]

Carcinoma

While an ill-defined asymmetrical density is a well-described appearance of invasive lobular carcinoma (ILC), this can also be seen with invasive ductal carcinoma (IDC) and ductal carcinoma in situ (DCIS). ILC is seen as an asymmetrical density only, with no evidence of a central tumour nidus, in 7–27% of cases, and up to 85% are of a density no greater than that of the surrounding normal breast tissue.[16,17] This can therefore make the mammographic manifestations subtle and detection can be

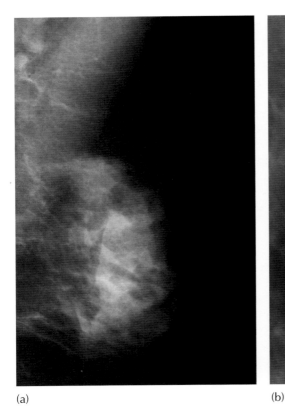

(a)

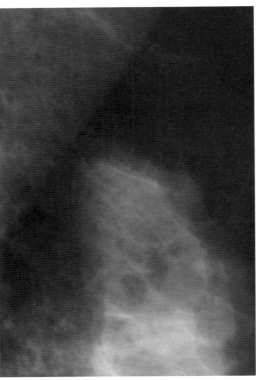

(b)

Figure 16.6 (a) A 20 mm diameter grade 3 invasive ductal carcinoma presenting as a localised asymmetrical opacity in the oblique projection. (b) Paddle magnification shows no distortion or spiculation, indicating rapid growth.

difficult, leading to a reported false-negative rate of up to 19%.[18] Up to 4% of IDCs present as an asymmetrical mammographic opacity only, with no evidence of spiculation or parenchymal distortion.[16] These are largely found to be aggressive grade 3 tumours that are growing fast and have not excited a significant connective tissue response within the surrounding breast tissue (Figure 16.6). DCIS is most commonly seen as suspicious clustered microcalcifications (62%), but up to 15% may be identified only as a nodular or more diffuse mammographic density with or without architectural distortion.[19]

Minor trauma

Injury to the breast, as a result of accidental trauma, fine-needle aspiration biopsy (FNAB) or core biopsy, can cause local oedema and haemorrhage, resulting in an ill-defined focal parenchymal density and possibly some thickening of the overlying skin.

These parenchymal mammographic changes associated with needle biopsies are common but short-lived. The small haematomas produced by FNABs of solid lesions can cause misleading and worrying X-ray changes in up to 36% of cases if imaged within 7 days of the needle test. However, these appearances have invariably resolved by 2 weeks.[20] Stereotactic core biopsies (CBs) of the breast cause mammographically detectable haematomas in 51%

of cases imaged immediately after the procedure,[21] but there are no long-term mammographic changes at 6–8 months, even when as many as 13 14-gauge automated needle specimens or 25 14-gauge vacuum-assisted specimens have been taken from a single lesion.[22] Significantly greater injury to the breast can, however, cause an initial haematoma and then lead on to long-standing mammographic changes of fat necrosis (parenchymal density, architectural distortion and calcified oil cysts).

Inflammation

Inflammation of the breast is usually clinically obvious, but mammographically there may be no more than an ill-defined area of increased parenchymal density, due to inflammatory infiltrate and oedema, with overlying skin thickening. Ultrasound will show skin thickening and a diffuse increase in the subcutaneous fat echoes, with some irregular areas of hypoechogenicity and posterior attenuation within the parenchyma (Figure 16.7).

Previous surgery on the opposite breast

The excision of breast tissue from one breast can give an impression of localised asymmetrical increase in density on the opposite side. Evidence of parenchymal scarring and skin thickening or deformity may be seen on the treated side.

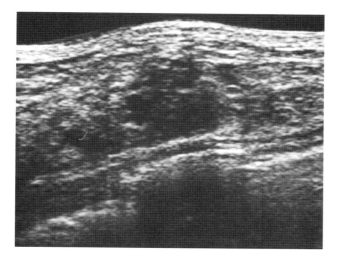

Figure 16.7 A 41-year-old woman presented with sudden onset of pain in the right breast. A palpable lump and reddening of the overlying skin quickly developed. Ultrasound examination revealed an ill-defined irregular hypoechoic lesion consistent with infection.

Asymmetry with an underlying mass lesion

Well-defined mass

Focal compression views may reveal a well-defined mass within an area of asymmetry. The differential diagnosis of this includes a simple cyst, an intra-mammary lymph node, a long-standing fibroadenoma and a phyllodes tumour. If the lesion is found to be solid, it requires needle sampling in order to clarify the diagnosis.

Simple breast cysts are commonly seen both in perimenopausal women and in those taking HRT. The typical smooth, sharp, rounded mammographic margins may be obscured by the generalised or patchy increased density in both breasts, which often also accompanies HRT,[14] but the true nature of the lesion should be readily identifiable with ultrasound.

Irregular mass

An irregular or spiculate mass within an area of asymmetry is likely to be a carcinoma (Figure 16.8), but this appearance can be seen with fat necrosis. Thickening of the overlying skin, adjacent distortion and calcifications may be seen in both conditions.

Asymmetry with microcalcification

Magnification views of an area of parenchymal asymmetry may reveal underlying microcalcifica-

(a)

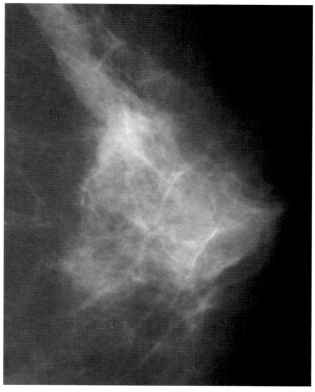

(b)

Figure 16.8 (a, b) A paddle view over an area of asymmetry laterally in the left breast reveals an underlying irregular mass lesion. Histology showed a 12 mm grade 1 invasive ductal carcinoma.

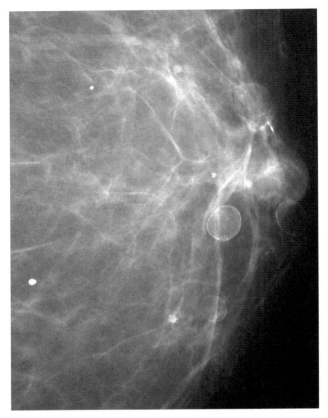

Figure 16.9   Severe bruising to the left breast had occurred after seat belt injury. Four months later, calcified oil cysts are seen, confirming fat necrosis.

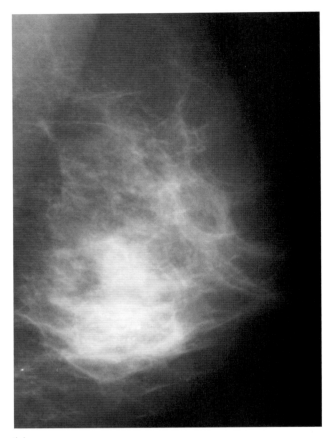

(a)

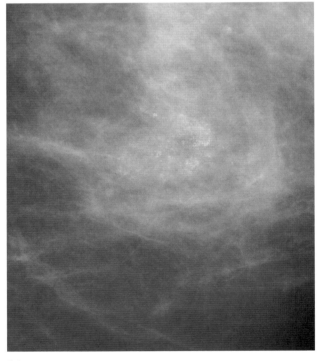

(b)

tion. The morphology of the particles may help in establishing their pathological cause.

Benign

The commonest types of benign breast change to cause microcalcification are adenosis (simple, sclerosing or blunt duct), microcystic involution and fibrocystic change.[23] Accumulation of secretions within the acini may calcify, producing multifocal powdery calcifications or characteristic sedimentary shapes (known as 'teacupping'). Without these typical benign features, needle biopsy will be necessary to exclude malignancy.

Alternatively, magnification views may reveal characteristic mural calcification in a simple cyst or an oil cyst (Figure 16.9).

Malignant

Both IDCs and ILCs may present as asymmetrical densities with suspicious calcifications within (Figure 16.10). The presence of a soft tissue density

Figure 16.10   A relatively large area of localised asymmetry is seen in the lower part of the left breast (a). A magnified view over this (b) shows extensive microcalcification within the asymmetry. Histology revealed a 14 mm grade 2 invasive ductal carcinoma.

associated with pleomorphic microcalcification usually indicates that the malignancy is invasive, but occasionally DCIS alone may produce an asymmetrical density or even a mass lesion.[19]

Asymmetry with distortion

Benign

Fat necrosis

Fat necrosis of the breast is often confused with carcinoma, both clinically and radiologically.[24,25] In a significant number of patients, there is no definite history of trauma (38–48%),[26,27] but in some, there has been recent injury, such as from a seat belt or surgery (often followed by radiotherapy). There is a wide spectrum of mammographic appearances, ranging from radiolucent oil cysts (27%) (with or without curvilinear mural calcifications) (Figure 16.9), through ill-defined asymmetrical densities (15.8%), round opacities (12.6%) or suspicious spiculate masses (3.9%), to dystrophic calcifications (26.9%) and clustered pleomorphic microcalcifications (3.9%).[24,26] The presence of oil cysts is characteristic of the condition, but the other features are non-specific. Ultrasound[27] and core biopsy[25] will help to distinguish between fat necrosis and malignancy.

Radial scar

Focal compression over an area of asymmetry may reveal underlying radial distortion. Certain features may suggest that this is due to a radial scar, but overall the appearances are very similar to those of malignancy. Radial scars, and their larger counterparts, complex sclerosing lesions (CSLs), are benign pseudo-infiltrative lesions characterised by a central zone of fibroelastosis from which epithelial structures radiate out. Their diagnostic significance lies in their close mammographic resemblance to low-grade invasive carcinoma and in the fact that a significant number contain or develop foci of malignant or premalignant change.[1]

The radial scar is classically seen to have long slender spicules, paralleled by linear radiolucencies, and the absence of a solid central tumour commensurate in size to the length of the spicules (Figure 16.11).[28] Microcalcification is relatively uncommon (8–29%) as is the presence of an associated clinically palpable lesion (25–31%).[29,30] However, more than 50% are visible on ultrasound and have features identical to those of a carcinoma.[29,31] In addition, up to 19% of histological radial scars have been shown to have a focus of atypical hyperplasia or carcinoma associated (IDC, ILC, DCIS, LCIS,

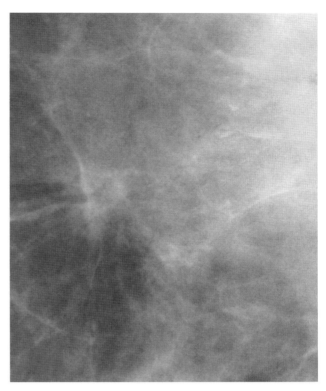

Figure 16.11 Paddle magnification view revealing the typical features of a radial scar.

atypical ductal hyperplasia (ADH) or atypical lobular hyperplasia (ALH)). This is usually located around the periphery of the lesion and is found more commonly in lesions greater than 7 mm in diameter and in women over the age of 50.[1] Clearly, therefore, even if benign tissue is obtained by needle sampling, all radial distortions within the breast should be excised.

Malignant

Invasive lobular carcinoma

Both IDC and DCIS can be seen mammographically as a diffuse area of asymmetry with subtle architectural distortion (13.5% and 15%, respectively),[16,19] but more often these features suggest the diagnosis of ILC.

ILC often presents problems in mammographic detection.[32] It constitutes approximately 10% of all breast malignancies yet accounts for up to 33% of mammographically occult cancers[33] and up to 16% of interval cancers.[17] It may present as a spiculate mass lesion, but 27–57% are seen as a diffuse ill-defined area of parenchymal asymmetry with subtle architectural distortion or distortion only visible on focal compression (Figure 16.12).[16,34] It characteristically spreads by diffuse infiltration as single rows (or 'Indian files') of cancer cells into the surrounding parenchyma in a manner that does not destroy the glandular anatomy or generate substantial connective tissue reaction. This contributes to the frequent absence of a well-defined tumour nidus and to the relatively low radiographic density of the lesion (52–85% are of a density less than or equal to that of the surrounding parenchyma, compared with only 17% of IDCs).[16,17] Radiographic definition can vary markedly with projection (up to 32% being seen in one projection only),[16] and the rarity of microcalcifications within ILCs (0–28%)[16,32,34] further contributes to the difficulty in diagnosis.

In addition, ultrasound has been found to have relatively low sensitivity in the detection of ILC, especially where it presents with subtle or nonspecific mammographic findings. The reported

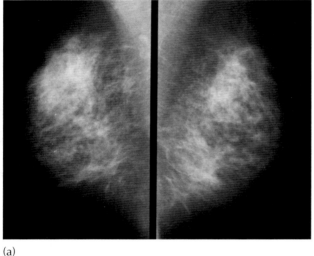

(a)

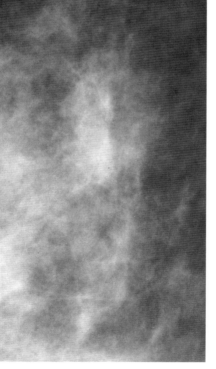

(b)

Figure 16.12 (a) A diffuse area of increased density is present in the upper half of the right breast. (b) Paddle magnification view shows underlying architectural distortion, and histology revealed a 40 mm invasive lobular carcinoma.

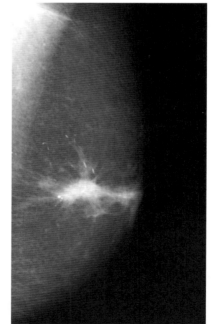

(a)

(b)

Figure 16.13
This 69-year-old woman had undergone wide local excision of a left-sided invasive ductal carcinoma 7 years previously. The surgical scarring is far more obvious in the oblique view (b) than in the craniocaudal view (a).

sensitivity of ultrasound ranges from 95% for stellate or circumscribed masses to only 30% for those ILCs presenting as an asymmetrical density only.[35–38]

Thus the absence of a sonographic lesion cannot be regarded as a completely reassuring finding when investigating asymmetry. In these circumstances, a core biopsy is more likely to give a definitive diagnosis than cytological sampling (up to 48% of FNABs for ILC may be negative for malignancy or yield an inadequate sample).[39]

Tumour recurrence

Breast-conserving surgery, particularly where there has been haematoma or seroma formation, can cause marked cicatrisation of the parenchyma. The resultant stellate distortion is characteristically planar rather than volumetric (i.e. much more obvious in one view than two) (Figure 16.13) and, radiographically, fat may be seen centrally within the scar.[40] Ring calcification may be evident in the walls of lipid cysts due to fat necrosis and coarse, rounded, benign-type calcifications can develop up to 6 years after radiotherapy.[41] However, in a patient who has had previous surgery for malignancy, comparison with old films is invaluable to assess whether the degree of distortion or asymmetry is increasing, or if a new mass or, morphologically suspicious, microcalcification is developing in association.

These features, possibly with an associated clinical abnormality, would suggest the development of local recurrence (Figure 16.14).

Conclusion

Some degree of asymmetry of breast tissue is a common mammographic finding and is usually benign. The asymmetry may, however, be hiding an underlying mass lesion, microcalcification or distortion, any of which make malignancy more likely. Thorough assessment is therefore needed, although the likelihood of detection of cancer may be low.

In contrast, distortion of breast parenchyma is a very worrying mammographic finding. If previous injury can be excluded, there is a high probability that it is due to malignancy. Aggressive evaluation with needle biopsy is thus needed and surgical excision is often necessary.

References

1. Sloane JP, Mayers MM. Carcinoma and atypical hyperplasia in radial scars and complex sclerosing lesions: importance of lesion size and patient age. Histopathology 1993; 23: 225–31.

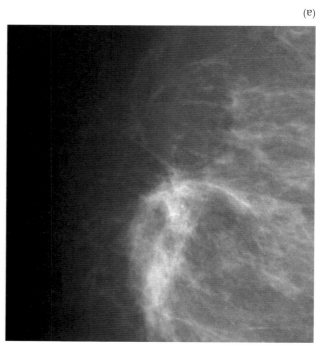
(a)

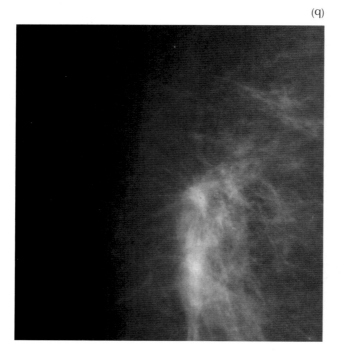
(b)

Figure 16.14 (a,b) Microcalcification and increasing distortion are noted, developing over 5 years at the site of a previous microdochectomy (performed 10 years previously). Histology revealed a 15 mm invasive ductal carcinoma.

2. Kopans DB, Swann CA, White G et al. Asymmetric breast tissue. Radiology 1989; 171: 639–43.

3. Russell DG, Ziewacz JT. Pressures in a simulated breast subjected to compression forces comparable to those of mammography. Radiology 1995; 194: 383–7.

4. Buckley JH, Roebuck EJ. Mammographic changes following radiotherapy. Br J Radiol 1986; 59: 337–44.

5. Dershaw DD, Shank B, Reisinger S. Mammographic findings after breast cancer treatment with local excision and definitive irradiation. Radiology 1987; 164: 455–61.

6. Kopans DB. Breast Imaging, 2nd edn. Philadelphia: Lippincott-Raven, 1998: 591.

7. Harris, JR. Breast Diseases. Philadelphia: Lippincott-Raven, 1987: 571–7.

8. Kushwaha AC, Whitman GJ, Stelling CB et al. Primary inflammatory carcinoma of the breast. AJR Am J Roentgenol 2000; 174: 535–8.

9. Dershaw DD, Moore MP, Liberman L, Deutch BM. Inflammatory breast carcinoma: mammographic findings. Radiology 1994; 190: 831–4.

10. Kuerer HM, Wilson MW, Bowersox JC. Innominate vein stenosis mimicking locally advanced breast cancer in a dialysis patient. Breast J 2001; 7: 128.

11. Samuels TH, Haider MA, Kirkbride P. Poland's syndrome: a mammographic presentation. AJR Am J Roentgenol 1996; 166: 347–8.

12. Stomper PC, Van Voorhis BJ, Ravnikar VA, Meyer JE. Mammographic changes associated with postmenopausal hormone replacement therapy: a longitudinal study. Radiology 1990; 174: 487–90.

13. Dixon JM. Hormone replacement therapy and the breast. BMJ 2001; 323: 1381–2.

14. Persson I, Thurfjell E, Holber L. Effect of estrogen and estrogen-progestin replacement regimes on mammographic breast parenchyma density. J Clin Oncol 1997; 15: 3201–7.

15. Cyrlak D, Wong CH. Mammographic changes in postmenopausal women undergoing HRT. AJR Am J Roentgenol 1993; 161: 1177–83.

16. Newstead GM, Baute PB, Toth HK. Invasive lobular and ductal carcinoma: mammographic findings and stage at diagnosis. Radiology 1992; 184: 623–7.

17. Hilleren DJ, Andersson IT, Lindholm K, Linnell FS. Invasive lobular carcinoma: mammographic findings in a 10 year experience. Radiology 1991; 178: 149–54.

18. Krecke K, Gisvold J. Invasive lobular carcinoma of the breast: Mammographic findings and extent of disease. AJR Am J Roentgenol 1993; 161: 957–60.

19. Ikeda DM, Andersson I. Ductal carcinoma in situ: atypical mammographic appearances. Radiology 1989; 172: 661–6.

20. Sickles EA, Klein DL, Goodson WH, Hunt TK. Mammography after needle aspiration of palpable breast masses. Am J Surg 1983; 145: 395–7.

21. Hann LE, Liberman L, Dershaw DD et al. Mammography immediately after stereotaxic breast biopsy: is it necessary? AJR Am J Roentgenol 1995; 165: 59–62.

22. Burbank F. Mammographic findings after 14-gauge automated needle and 14-gauge directional, vacuum assisted stereotactic breast biopsies. Radiology 1997; 104: 153–6.

23. In Tot T, Tabar L, Dean P. Practical Breast Pathology. Stuttgart: Thieme Verlag, 2002.

24. Bilgen IG, Ustun EE, Memis A. Fat necrosis of the breast: clinical, mammographic and sonographic features. Eur J Radiol 2001; 39: 92–9.

25. Harrison RL, Britton P, Warren R, Bobrow L. Can we be sure about a radiological diagnosis of fat necrosis of the breast? Clin Radiol 2000; 55: 119–23.

26. Bassett LW, Gold RH, Cove HC. Mammographic spectrum of traumatic fat necrosis. AJR Am J Roentgenol 1978; 130: 119–22.

27. Soo MS, Kornguth PJ, Hertzberg BS. Fat necrosis in the breast: sonographic features. Radiology 1998; 206: 261–9.

28. Tabar L, Dean PB. Teaching Atlas of Mammography. Stuttgart: Thieme Verlag, 1985: 88–90.

29. Wallis MG, Devakumar R, Hosie KB et al. Complex sclerosing lesions (radial scars) of the breast can be palpable. Clin Radiol 1993; 48: 319–20.

30. Ung OA, Lee WB, Greenberg ML, Bilous M. Complex sclerosing lesion: the lesion is complex, the management is straightforward. Aust NZ J Surg 2001; 71: 35–40.

31. Cohen MA, Sferlazza SJ. Role of sonography in evaluation of radial scars of the breast. AJR Am J Roentgenol 2000; 174: 1075–8.

32. Sickles EA. The subtle and atypical mammographic features of invasive lobular carcinoma. Radiology 1991; 178: 25–6.

33. Holland R, Hendriks JH, Mravunac M. Mammographically occult breast cancer. Cancer 1983; 52: 1810–19.

34. Cornford EJ, Wilson AR, Athanassiou E et al. Mammographic features of invasive lobular and invasive ductal carcinoma of the breast: a comparative analysis. Br J Radiol 1995; 68: 450–3.

35. Rissanen T, Tikkakoski T, Autio AL, Apaja-Sarkkinen M. Ultrasound of invasive lobular breast carcinoma. Acta Radiol 1998; 39: 285–91.

36. Paramagul CP, Helvie MA, Adler DD. Invasive lobular carcinoma: Sonographic appearance and role of sonography in improving diagnostic sensitivity. Radiology 1995; 195: 231–4.

37. Cole-Beuglet C, Soriano RZ, Kurtz AB, Goldberg BB. Ultrasound analysis of 104 primary breast carcinomas classified according to histopathology type. Radiology 1983; 147: 191–6.

38. Evans N, Lyon K. The use of ultrasound in the diagnosis of invasive lobular carcinoma of the breast less than 10 mm in size. Clin Radiol 2000; 55: 251–3.

39. Sadler GP, McGee S, Dollimore NS et al. Role of fine-needle aspiration cytology and needle-core biopsy in the diagnosis of lobular carcinoma of the breast. Br J Surg 1994; 81: 1315–17.

40. Dershaw DD. Mammography in patients with breast cancer treated by breast conservation (lumpectomy with or without radiation). AJR Am J Roentgenol 1995; 164: 309–16.

41. Libshitz HL, Montague ED, Paulus DD. Calcifications and the therapeutically irradiated breast. AJR Am J Roentgenol 1977; 128: 1021–5.

17 Ultrasound in the diagnosis of small breast carcinomas

Eleanor Moskovic

Introduction

While mammography is the primary diagnostic tool for breast screening in the general population, high-resolution breast ultrasound has become an invaluable adjunct for assessment, and is now used widely in breast diagnostic units, surgical outpatient clinics and general radiology departments. The advantages of ultrasound are its safety, speed, cost-effectiveness and role in diagnostic biopsy/aspiration.[1] It is used increasingly to solve problems in younger women in whom mammography is either not indicated or not interpretable due to breast density. Used in conjunction with mammography, ultrasound has been shown to increase diagnostic accuracy.[2] Most breast radiologists and indeed many surgeons now rely on breast ultrasound as an integral part of the imaging process in 'triple assessment' for breast screening, and it is now the first port of call for the diagnosis and biopsy of small solid masses.

Ultrasound technology and equipment

Sound whose frequency is higher than the upper limit of audibility (>20 KHz) is defined as 'ultrasound'. Because the spatial resolution in an ultrasound image is proportional to the frequency used, as high a frequency as possible is preferred for imaging. However, attenuation (absorption) of the ultrasound beam by the tissues through which it passes increases in proportion to frequency, so for optimal imaging a balance has to be reached between frequency and penetration. In practice, with new ultrasound technology, frequencies between 12 and 15 MHz are now used for breast examination, with the ability to reduce frequency down to 8 MHz for large breasts or particularly dense breast tissue (Figure 17.1). Following the

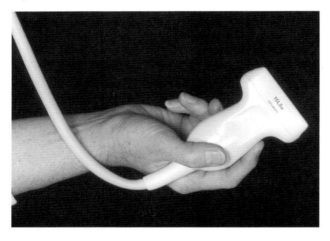

Figure 17.1 A 15 MHz transducer for breast and small parts scanning (Acuson, Mountainview, CA).

application of acoustic coupling gel on the breast to reduce impedance created by intervening air, a hand-held transducer that emits high-frequency sound waves is placed continuously on the skin surface. These sound waves pass through the breast and bounce off the various layers of soft tissue within it. Reflected sound waves are received back again by the transducer at varying frequencies according to the reflectivity or echogenicity of the tissues through which they pass. A computer assigns a visual greyscale to the frequencies obtained and constructs a 'real-time' picture, providing a moving image on the ultrasound screen as the transducer is moved over the skin. As described, for breast work, probe frequencies of 8–15 MHz are now used, allowing good tissue penetration of approximately 7–10 cm from the skin surface (which is adequate for most breast and small part work) while providing excellent spatial resolution in the near field.[3] By exploitation of the Doppler shift effect, velocity of blood flow in small vessels within the soft tissues

can be detected using ultrasound and the vascularity of breast masses can be assessed (Figure 17.2).

Ultrasound in breast diagnosis: cystic and solid lesions

The chief roles of ultrasound in the diagnosis of breast disease are for the differentiation of cystic from solid masses and for intervention to obtain tissue. If a mass is detected on mammography, certain features may suggest a simple cyst (smooth circular contour, multiplicity), but X-ray mammography cannot be definitive since, for example, a low-grade carcinoma may also be well defined and circular in shape. Because of the rapid transmission (low impedance) of sound waves through fluid, cysts are easily recognised on ultrasound as well-marginated echo-free, rounded or oval lesions with a characteristic band of posterior echo enhancement. Typically, a cyst will appear as a 'black hole' on the ultrasound image (Figures 17.3 and 17.4). Sometimes, a cyst contains internal debris, which is seen as internal echoes within it; this can occasionally cause confusion with a solid lesion although circular contour, and through-transmission of sound can often resolve this. A solid, non-cystic mass attenuates sound waves and therefore will produce an image containing echoes, the appearance of which will vary according to the nature of the mass. For example, a common benign solid lesion is the fibroadenoma, which on ultrasound appears as a smooth, usually oval or lobulated, mass that has uniform internal echoes and is of low vascularity

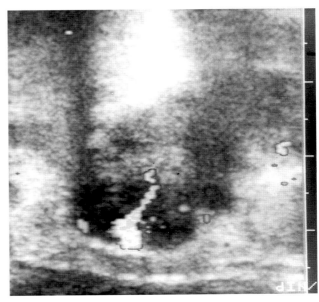

Figure 17.2 Doppler signal in breast carcinoma, showing a solid mass with abnormal vascularity.

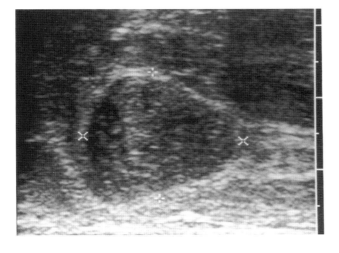

Figure 17.3 A simple breast cyst, showing through-transmission of sound (bright-up).

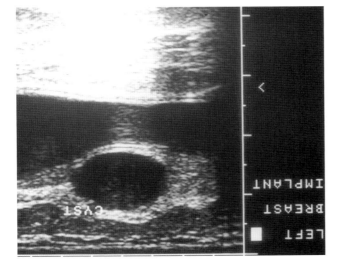

Figure 17.5 A fibroadenoma – a solid, well-circumscribed mass with homogeneous internal echotexture.

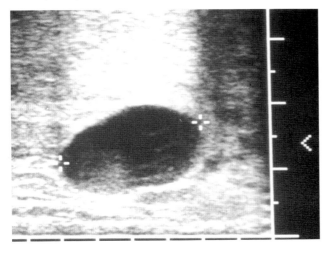

Figure 17.4 A simple cyst overlying a breast implant; the implant is also sonolucent and appears cystic.

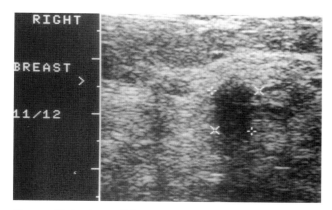

Figure 17.6 A small breast carcinoma measuring less than 1 cm with posterior acoustic shadowing.

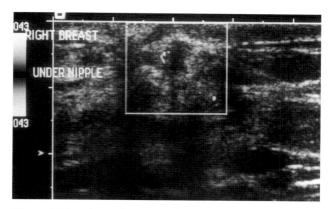

Figure 17.7 A small retroareolar carcinoma – irregular solid mass with abnormal vascularity on Doppler.

(Figure 17.5). Features of breast carcinoma on ultrasound include an irregular margin, strong attenuation of sound waves causing shadowing behind the lesion, disruption of surrounding tissue planes, and an increase in vascularity on Doppler (Figures 17.6 and 17.7). Inhomogeneity of internal echotexture in malignant masses is due to the presence of fibrosis, necrosis and calcification.

All of the features of benign and malignant breast masses described above are more obvious when the mass is large. A small breast carcinoma (<1 cm) may mimic a fibroadenoma, especially if it is well differentiated (i.e. low-grade), and similarly a benign solid lesion can have sonographically suspicious features.[4]

The advantage of ultrasound in these circumstances is that, unlike mammography, it lends itself easily to guided fine-needle aspiration cytology (FNAC) or core biopsy, which can be performed rapidly in most centres.

Ultrasound and breast screening

The main limitation of ultrasound in relation to early breast cancer diagnosis is that it is relatively poor at detecting fine calcification, since the density of calcium provides an interface that is 'opaque' to sound waves at this frequency. Thus calcified or ductal tumours such as ductal carcinoma in situ (DCIS) that have no soft tissue or invasive component are better shown by mammography, and ultrasound is not used as a primary screening technique. Nevertheless, if a mammographically screen-detected calcified tumour is carefully sought using ultrasound, it can normally be found, however small it is, particularly with the advent of higher-frequency transducers.[5]

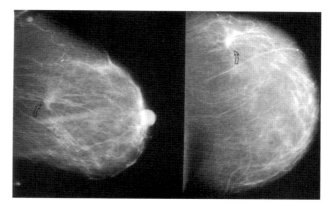

Figure 17.8 A screening mammogram showing a small early breast carcinoma (arrowed).

As described, mammography is used as the primary diagnostic test in the screening population (aged over 50), and ultrasound in this cohort is used mainly to characterise masses seen on the screening mammogram and, when appropriate, to guide biopsy or FNAC (Figures 17.8 and 17.9). The benefits of obtaining accurate cytology and especially histology from a non-palpable screen-detected lesion without resorting to formal biopsy are undisputed. In the case of a carcinoma, knowing accurate histology with data about lymphovascular invasion prior to surgery allows planning of the appropriate operation and may dictate whether axillary dissection should be considered. Information about tumour markers such as oestrogen receptor status can also be obtained from the biopsy specimen. In the case of a small X-ray-detected breast carcinoma, ultrasound can be used both to confirm the diagnosis cytologically or histologically and for subsequent wire localisation.[6–8] Sensitivity and specificity are extremely high for ultrasound-guided procedures, and in experienced hands, ultrasound-guided aspiration, biopsy and localisation are at least as accurate and generally faster than

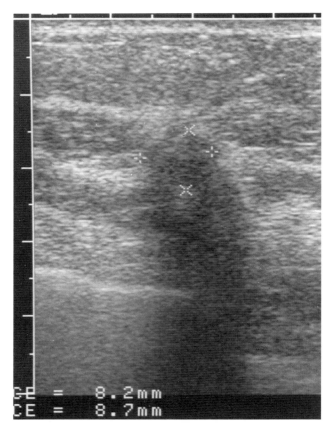

Figure 17.9 Ultrasound of the case shown in Figure 17.8, confirming a small carcinoma with posterior acoustic shadowing.

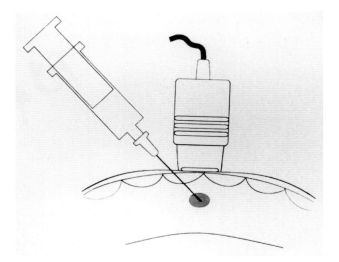

Figure 17.10 Diagram of ultrasound-guided fine-needle aspiration cytology (FNAC).

mammographically guided techniques. If required, confirmation of the position of the wire tip after ultrasound-guided localisation can always be undertaken using mammography.[9]

Technique of ultrasound-guided aspiration and biopsy

Ultrasound is a highly effective method of guiding successful FNAC and core-cut biopsy in small breast cancers (i.e. masses well <1 cm).[1,9,10]

Individual practices vary, and each operator develops a technique with which they are most comfortable.

Fine-needle aspiration cytology (FNAC)

Our practice is to have one person assisting the procedure by scanning and locating the lesion, with the operator being free to use both hands to manoevre the needle and apply suction to the

syringe. Many centres prefer to add a connecting tube to the needle to allow the assistant to provide suction while the operator directs the needle. We have not found it necessary to use commercially available needle guides attached to the ultrasound transducer. The consent of the patient is obtained following explanation, and the lesion to be aspirated is located using ultrasound, with the patient positioned so that the distance between the skin surface and the mass is minimised. This often requires the patient to lie in the lateral decubitus or oblique position if the lesion lies laterally within the breast. The transducer is sterilised with an appropriate cleaning solution, and sterile acoustic coupling gel is also used. The surface marking of the underlying lesion is inked on the skin and 2 ml of 2% lidocaine is infiltrated subcutaneously into that area. The use of local anaesthetic is preferable, since it improves patient confidence and permits repeated needle passage if necessary without pain. It also allows the use of a wide-bore 19-gauge needle for aspiration, thereby improving the chances of a more cellular smear. For almost all aspirates, our choice of fine needle is a simple 1.5 inch 19-gauge hypodermic needle, which is universally available and inexpensive. It can be visualised easily with ultrasound due to the sharp reflecting needle bevel, air within the lumen and movement of the needle itself. For aspiration of a small solid lesion, a 10 ml syringe is required to obtain good suction; larger syringes can be cumbersome and do not enhance the outcome. To facilitate expulsion of the contents of the syringe after aspiration, it helps in advance to withdraw the syringe plunger by about 1 ml prior to attaching the needle and inserting it. The transducer is placed on the skin surface, with the lesion to be aspirated lying in the midline of the scan so that the

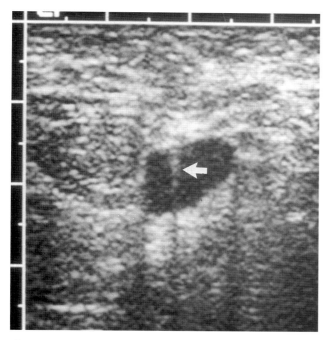

Figure 17.11 Ultrasound-guided FNAC. The needle is seen transfixing a small solid mass (arrowed).

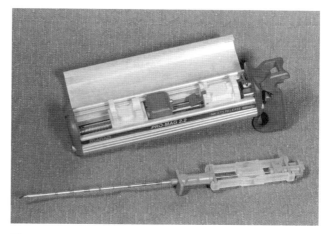

Figure 17.12 An example of a spring-loaded automatic biopsy device (Pro-Mag 2.2, Medical Device Technologies Inc.) with core-cut biopsy needle prior to loading.

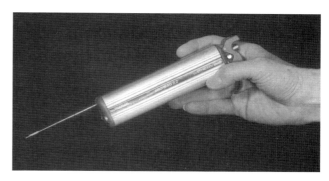

Figure 17.13 The device loaded with a needle and ready for biopsy.

operator can insert the needle along the path of the beam under direct vision (Figure 17.10). Once the needle tip is seen within the mass, the operator simultaneously applies maximum suction to the plunger while moving the needle to and fro and angling it in a fanlike fashion throughout the mass, observing the screen all the while so that the needle tip does not exit from the region of interest (Figure 17.11). Suction on the syringe is terminated before the needle is withdrawn from the mass, so that the contents of the needle lumen and syringe are not contaminated by normal overlying tissue or blood. The contents of the syringe and needle are discharged onto a series of dry microscope slides and smeared so that their adequacy can be assessed. Some centres prefer to have a cytopathologist to hand to assess the adequacy of the smear; in our experience, the usual reason for failure is inadequate suction on the syringe while moving the needle in a controlled manner. Lesions that are technically hard to aspirate successfully include fibroadenomas, scarred or irradiated tissue, and lesions near vital structures such as the chest wall or a breast prosthesis. However, with practice, all of these can be sampled satisfactorily. Simple pressure followed by a small plaster applied to the aspiration site is all that is needed after the procedure, which is tolerated well in all circumstances. Intercurrent medication with anticoagulants is not a contraindication to FNAC; a 20- or 21-gauge needle may be preferred in this circumstance, and pressure on the skin for a full 5 minutes after the procedure is advisable.

Ultrasound-guided core-cut biopsy

Large-core needle biopsy can also be guided with ultrasound using spring-loaded automatic biopsy devices (Figures 17.12 and 17.13); this method of biopsy is rapidly becoming the preferred diagnostic technique as a core provides diagnostic information that may direct surgery (see the section on ultrasound and breast screening above) and cytology cannot differentiate between DCIS and invasive carcinoma.[11] Consent must again be obtained for this procedure, which is more uncomfortable than an FNAC and may cause bruising. Essentially, the same technique is used as with FNAC, taking care to fully anaesthetise the lesion of interest and surrounding tissues, as the core biopsy needle is larger (14- to 16-gauge). Again the transducer is positioned over the lesion and the needle in the biopsy device is manoevred into place on one side of the mass in a plane oblique to the chest wall. The spring-loaded device is fired through the mass and a core of tissue

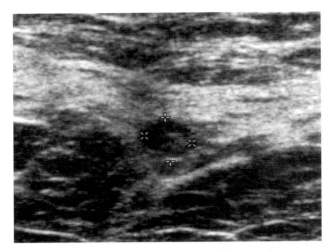

Figure 17.14 A small solid mass on ultrasound.

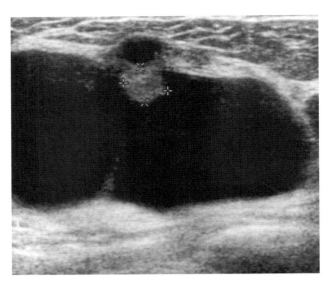

Figure 17.16 A small solid mass within the wall of a cyst.

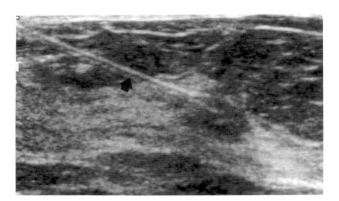

Figure 17.15 The core-cut biopsy needle positioned for sampling the lesion in Figure 17.14; note the alignment of the needle parallel to the chest wall (arrowed).

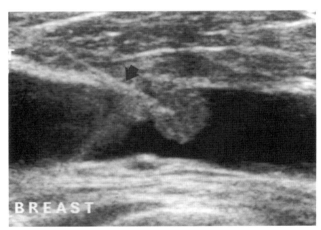

Figure 17.17 The core-cut biopsy needle sited in the mass in Figure 17.14 (arrowed).

obtained. Care must be taken to ensure that the chest wall is not breached, by aligning the needle track parallel to the skin (Figures 17.14–17.17). Usually 2–4 cores are obtained at one sampling.

Ultrasound assessment of regional nodes

No diagnostic imaging modality including ultrasound has yet been able to identify tumour micrometastases in normal-sized axillary nodes with accuracy, but the axilla is always interrogated as part of an ultrasound scan of the breast, whether for suspected benign or malignant breast disease. Despite the advent of sentinel lymph node biopsy, ultrasound with guided FNAC of lymph nodes can be important in making management decisions in exceptional circumstances if the need for an axillary dissection is in doubt.[12] In early breast cancer, nodes are usually normal, with less than 20% of Stage I

tumours under 2 cm having axillary metastasis. If the axilla is clinically normal, ultrasound will always identify small lymph nodes, but their pathological status if normal in size, shape and vascularity on ultrasound criteria cannot be ascertained, since the presence of microscopic metastatic disease is beyond the resolution of the scan.

However, much recent research has centred on ultrasound nodal morphology and especially vascularity. Various studies have shown that incorporating colour Doppler scanning of axillary nodes improves the detection rate of metastatic disease, with sensitivities of 70–75% for involvement and specificities of 98–100%, yielding a positive predictive value of 96–100%.[13–15] As a general rule, certain sonographic features of nodes may be considered normal and abnormal. A normal axillary node is oval in shape,

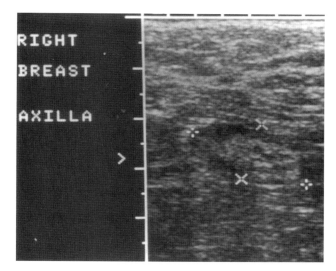

Figure 17.18 Ultrasound of a normal axillary node, showing an oval shape, central sinus echogenicity and little peripheral lymphoid tissue.

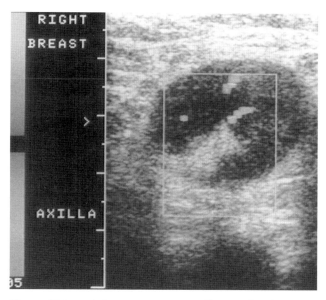

Figure 17.20 A large metastatic axillary node, showing a circular contour and abnormal vascularity on Doppler.

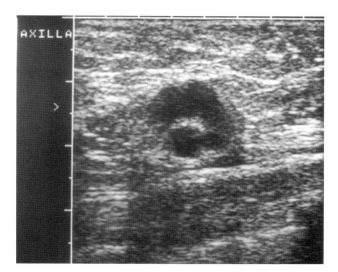

Figure 17.19 Ultrasound of an abnormal axillary node in metastatic breast cancer, showing an irregular shape, low attenuation, and loss of most of the central sinus echoes.

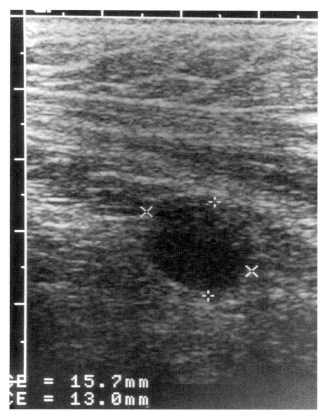

Figure 17.21 An abnormal infraclavicular lymph node lying below the insertion of the pectoral muscle. Although oval in shape, the node is diffusely hypoechogenic and has lost central sinus echoes due to tumour replacement.

contains echogenic hilar fat and has a rim of more sonolucent lymphoid tissue (Figure 17.18). Pathological nodes are always visible on ultrasound if palpable, and have certain characteristic features. They are often multiple, are round rather than oval (altered long/short ratio), are echo-poor, and have little or no hilar fat, the lymphoid tissue and fat having been destroyed by tumour (Figure 17.19). The distribution of neovascularity in metastatic nodes tends to be peripheral, i.e. subcapsular on Doppler, which is an important finding (Figure 17.20).[16,17] Other areas of nodal involvement, such as the infra- and supraclavicular regions, can easily be

examined and needled using ultrasound if appropriate; however, metastases to these sites are very uncommon in early breast cancer (Figure 17.21). The

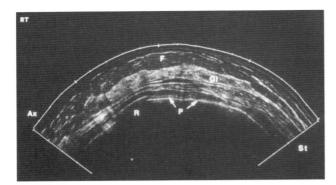

Figure 17.22 Extended field of view (EFOV) scan through the breast from axilla to sternum. Ax, Axilla; R, rib; Gl, gland; F, fat; P, pectoral muscle; St, sternum.

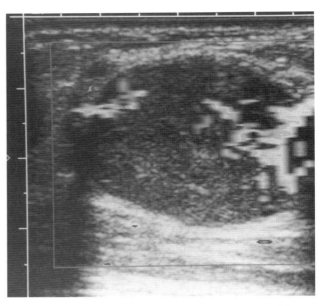

Figure 17.23 Ultrasound of a breast carcinoma with profuse vascularity on colour Doppler flow.

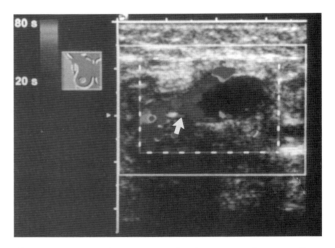

Figure 17.24 Enhancement of a breast carcinoma using microbubble contrast; the image shows the arrival of contrast bolus (arrowed).

other important main route of lymphatic spread, namely the internal mammary chain is less accessible to ultrasound, although careful scanning of the intercostal parasternal spaces may sometimes reveal an enlarged node.

Recent advances in breast ultrasound

Rapid progress in ultrasound technology over recent years has produced refinement of existing applications as well as novel approaches to increased resolution and diagnostic accuracy.[18,19] A brief outline of new developments in breast ultrasound is given below.

Improvement of the signal-to-noise ratio, which is critical in high-frequency scanning, is evolving by the addition of digital scanners and composite transducers, which allow depiction of breast ducts with diameters smaller than 5 mm.[20]

B-Flow (GE Medical Systems), or so-called 'greyscale Doppler', provides direct visualisation of blood flow with greyscale so that flowing blood can be visualised without contrast agents. In comparison with conventional colour Doppler ultrasound, it has wide-band resolution and a higher frame rate. This is especially useful for simultaneous imaging of tissue and blood flow similar to an angiogram and is easy to use, with no complex control parameters.[18]

Ultrasound computed tomography (CT) or extended field of view (EFOV), which is currently available on some ultrasound scanners, facilitates comparison of textures across the whole breast and is useful for follow-up studies (Figure 17.22). Three-dimensional (3D) datasets can be obtained and are easily reproducible for monitoring lesions.[18,21]

Neovascularity (angiogenesis) is a feature of carcinomas, and the presence of increased Doppler signals within or around a breast mass makes the diagnosis of malignancy more likely (Figure 17.23).[22,23] The recent development of ultrasound contrast agents has allowed the amplification of normal and especially abnormal vascularity, which can help differentiate benign from malignant masses. The introduction of ultrasound contrast agents in the form of microbubbles injected intravenously during scanning has improved the display of small vessels down to 100 μm and also makes 3D Doppler studies more informative (Figure 17.24).[24,25] Several studies have shown that more complete display of malignant neovascularity improves

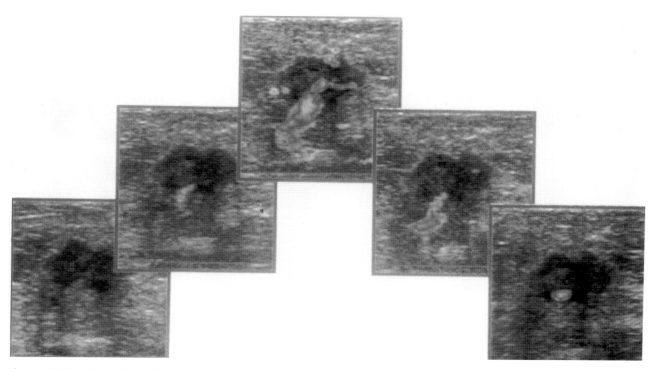

Figure 17.25 Wash-in/wash-out images of a bolus of intravenous contrast in a breast carcinoma.

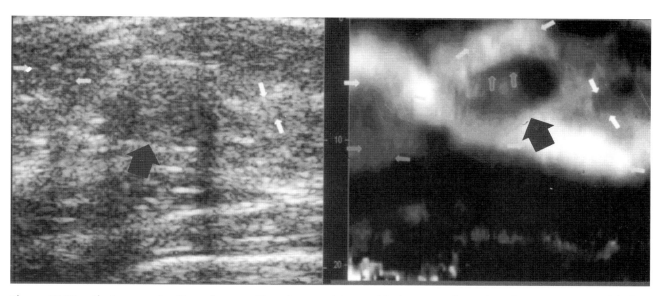

Figure 17.26 Elastogram of a fibroadenoma. The ultrasound image (a) shows an almost isoechoic breast mass (black arrow). (b) The resultant elastogram showing the lesion as an area of stiffness centrally (black arrow).

diagnostic accuracy. Microbubbles also allow the performance of functional studies by timing the wash-in and wash-out following a bolus intravenous injection (Figure 17.25).[26]

A fascinating new technique is elasticity imaging, which depicts the distortion or strain of the breast as it responds to a stress applied via the transducer. Because the stiffness or Young's modulus of tissue tends to increase with disease (i.e. tumour formation), the elasticity of abnormal tissue can be measured when pressure is applied to the breast as a whole and a stiffer area can be imaged with greater contrast (Figure 17.26).[27,28]

References

1. Liberman L. Percutaneous image-guided core breast biopsy. Radiol Clin North Am 2002; 40: 483–500.
2. Zonderland HM, Coerkamp EG, Hermans J et al.

Diagnosis of breast cancer: contribution of US as an adjunct to mammography. Radiology 1999; 213: 413–22.

3. Tohno E, Cosgrove DO, Sloane JP. Ultrasound Diagnosis of Breast Diseases. Edinburgh: Churchill Livingston, 1994.

4. Skaane P, Engedal K. Analysis of sonographic features in the diferentiation of fibroadenoma and invasive ductal carcinoma. AJR Am J Roentgenol 1998; 170: 109–14.

5. Cheung YC, Wan YL, Chen SC et al. Sonographic evaluation of mammographically detected microcalcifications without a mass prior to stereotactic core needle biopsy. J Clin Ultrasound 2002; 30: 323–31.

6. Fornage BD, Coan JD, David CL. Ultrasound-guided needle biopsy of the breast and other interventional procedures. Radiol Clin North Am 1992; 30: 167–85.

7. Sneige N, Fornage BD, Saleh G. Ultrasound-guided fine needle aspiration of non-palpable breast lesions: cytologic and histologic findings. Am J Clin Pathol 1994; 102: 98–101.

8. Rissanen TJ, Makarainen HP, Mattila SI et al. Wire localized biopsy of breast lesions: a review of 425 cases found in screening or clinical mammmography. Clin Radiol 1993; 47: 14–22.

9. Fornage BD, Sneige N, Edeiken BS. Interventional breast sonography. Eur J Radiol 2002; 42: 17–31.

10. Schiller VL, Gurfinkel F, Wolke J, Kushwaha D. Ultra-sound diagnosis of mammographically occult minimal carcinoma of the breast. J Diagn Med Sonogr 1995; 11.

11. Litherland JC. Should fine needle aspiration cytology in breast assessment be abandoned? Clin Radiol 2002; 57: 81–4.

12. Lernevall A. Imaging axillary lymph nodes. Acta Oncol 2000; 39: 277–81.

13. Dixon JM, Walsh J, Paterson D, Chetty U. Colour Doppler studies of benign and malignant breast lesions. Br J Surg 1992; 79: 259–60.

14. Walsh JS, Dixon JM, Chetty U, Patterson D. Colour Doppler studies of axillary node metastases in breast carcinoma. Clin Radiol 1994; 49: 189–91.

15. Yang WT, Ahuja A, Tang A et al. Ultrasonographic demonstration of normal axillary lymph nodes; a learning curve. J Ultrasound Med 1995; 14: 823–7.

16. Steinkamp HJ, Mueffelman M, Bock, JC. Differential diagnosis of lymph node lesions: a semiquantitative approach with colour Doppler ultrasound. Br J Radiol 1998; 71: 828–33.

17. Ahuja A, Ying M, Yuen YH, Metreweli C. Power Doppler sonography of cervical lymphadenopathy. Clin Radiol 2001; 56: 965–9.

18. Harvey CJ, Pilcher JM, Eckersley RJ et al. Advances in ultrasound: Review article. Clin Radiol 2002; 57: 157–77.

19. Samuels TH. Breast imaging. A look at current and future technologies. Postgrad Med 1998; 104: 91–101.

20. Cosgrove DO, Eckersley RJ. Breast. Ultrasound Med Biol 2000; 26 (Suppl 1): S110–15.

21. Kruker J, Meyer C, LeCarpentier G et al. Volume registration for 3-D compounding of ultrasound images. Radiology 1999; 213: 101.

22. Cosgrove DO, Kedar RP, Bamber JC et al. Breast diseases: color Doppler US in differential diagnosis. Radiology 1993; 189: 99–104.

23. Holcombe C, Pugh N, Lyons K et al. Blood flow in breast cancer and fibroadenoma estimated by colour Doppler ultrasonography. Br J Surg 1995; 82: 787–8.

24. Cosgrove DO. Ultrasound contrast agents. In: Dawson P, Cosgrove DO, Grainger RG, eds. Textbook of Contrast Media. Oxford: ISIS Medical Media, 1999: 451–587.

25. Huber S, Helbich T, Kettenbach J et al. Effects of a microbubble contrast agent on breast tumours: computer assisted quantitative assessment with colour Doppler US – early experience. Radiology 1998; 208: 485–9.

26. Albrecht T, Patel N, Cosgrove DO et al. Enhancement of Power Doppler signals from breast lesions with the ultrasound contrast agent EchoGen emulsion: subjective and quantitative assessment. Acad Radiol 1998; 5 (Suppl 1): S195–8.

27. Fuechsel, FG, Bush NL, Bamber JC et al. An interactive display of freehand elasticity imaging (FEI) on breast masses in combination with ultrasound for improved understanding of breast pathology and better differential diagnosis. Radiology 2000; 217: 706.

28. Bamber JC. Ultrasound elasticity imaging: definition and technology. Eur Radiol 1999; 9 (Suppl 3): S327–30.

18 New radiological techniques: digital mammography, MRI, scintimammography, PET and some more for 'Tomorrow's World'

Ruth Warren

with contributions from Charlotte Fowler, Will Teh, Tarik Massoud and Vincent Wallace

Introduction

Over the last few years, alternative techniques have increasingly come into use for the imaging of breast cancer. Diagnosis so far has largely used an integrated combination of clinical examination, mammography, high-frequency ultrasound and a variety of targeted methods of obtaining cellular material for definitive diagnosis. Given the availability of this well-researched array of techniques, one may speculate on why anything more is needed. Many radiologists and clinicians caring for breast cancer patients do not seek any further diagnostic tests.

It should be noted that mammography is one of the best-researched radiological examinations of all – probably second only to the chest X-ray. Because of its use in mammography screening over the last three decades, mammography has been tested in randomised controlled trials on whole populations of healthy women, so its sensitivity and specificity are known on standardised case material with longitudinal follow-up and in the investigation of a single disease. This is a more focused research scenario than anything else in radiology, including the chest X-ray.[1] The motivation for this scrupulous research is the controversy that has surrounded breast screening of the healthy population by mammography at its inception and since. Further debate has taken place on its use in women aged under 50 and in those with a family history of breast cancer. The risk

of cancer induction in the breast by ionising radiation has been a factor driving the controversy. From all this research the limitations of mammography are well known. Other techniques have been used to cover these limitations, and in standard practice, ultrasound and biopsy techniques give most of the answers.

There are many newer, and perhaps more exciting techniques for diagnosis that use different methods of imaging. In some instances these harness functional features. Enthusiasts for each of these techniques wish to prove that their new 'toy' is better than all previous ones, and propose it as an imaging technique for breast cancer. Certain well-known deficiencies of mammography could helpfully be surpassed by the perfect newer technique, and each new technique claims to have the answer. Breast cancer experts must find a way of keeping an open mind to innovation, while protecting their patients from ever more studies of techniques with unknown sensitivity and specificity, and lacking biopsy methods for confirmation.

The mammographic limitations, which may be addressed are as follows:

- Mammography uses ionising radiation, which may cause cancer of the breast, particularly in young individuals, those with genetic defects or with repeated use.

- The sensitivity of mammography in the dense breast is poor
- Even in a breast of mixed density, there is a definite false-negative rate
- Women do not like to have the breast compressed for examination.

The features that are favoured to support the use of newer modalities are the absence of radiation dose (or the use of lower dose than in mammography), high sensitivity in dense breast tissue and acceptability to women. Mammography is a cheap investigation, and so price is seldom a favourable factor with new techniques. Specificity with some of the newer techniques is poor, which may cause confusing results and additional tests. The remainder of this chapter is divided into two parts: realistic alternatives to present techniques and others which claim to hold promise as future applications.

Newer imaging modalities that are recommended for exploration

It is not anticipated that breast clinicians will wish to use all of these, but the following are in a state of development that may justify further scrutiny:

- digital mammography
- computerised interpretation
- Doppler ultrasound
- contrast-enhanced magnetic resonance imaging (MRI)
- scintimammography
- sentinel node biopsy
- lymphoscintigraphy
- positron emissions tomography (PET)

Digital mammography

The digital revolution in radiology has touched all forms of plain-film radiographic imaging with mammography being one of the last to be so affected. The reasons for this are the high level of detail that has been attained with film/screen mammography. This level of detail is required for the detection of small cancers and accurate interpretation of radiographic features. The need for images with large numbers of pixels of small size and giving a high level of resolution has challenged developers. Large volumes of data storage are required. Monitors are needed that allow review of the entire area of the breast, comparison with previous studies and the review of small areas with zoom

facilities. Systems are coming into clinical use, but the cost is high. At present, we do not know whether they can achieve the same level of diagnostic accuracy as film/screen mammography. Even if this were to be the case, the cost may be difficult to justify, in the absence of additional benefit. Such benefits might be improved sensitivity and specificity, the use of computer-aided diagnosis to further increase diagnostic accuracy; and the ability to store and retrieve the archive more efficiently. The present methods of archiving and display are dependent upon meticulous technician labour, which is both costly and boring and risks diagnostic failure through loss or human error.

The features of mammography that might potentially be improved are:

- better latitude in the context of high contrast
- the trade-off between detail and dose
- the need for compression to offset the problem of overlapping dense tissue

The improvements that might be achieved by digital mammography are:

- the potential for computer-aided image processing, allowing the contrast and brightness to be optimised
- a wider dynamic range
- a linear response curve to radiation rather than a sigmoid one, as in the case of film/screen mammography

Three approaches have been used in the design of systems for full-field mammography:

- a scanning slot device with caesium iodide (CsI) phosphor
- large area detectors with caesium oxide (thallium) (CsI(Tl)) phosphor coated onto photodiodes
- an array of multiple modules containing a fibre-optic taper and charge-coupled device.

The technical aspects have been well reviewed by Williams et al[2] and Feig and Yaffe.[3] The first technology in this field was computed mammography. Cowen et al reviewed the comparison between this and full-field digital mammography.[4] This is still a technology in development and is far from full clinical evaluation.[5,6] Comparisons of this technology with film/screen mammography are becoming available.[7–9] One may expect that in the next decade, full-field digital mammography will supplant film/screen mammography unless the costs cannot be reduced to an affordable level. There will be pressures for this to happen as hospitals and departments of radiology become fully digital. Such facilities will not wish to retain a film archive for mammography alone.

Figure 18.1 shows an area of calcification on a digital film demonstrating the ability of the computer method to maximise definition.

Computerised interpretation

See Chapter 11

Doppler ultrasound

See Chapter 17 and later section in this chapter

Contrast enhanced MRI

MRI has transformed many aspects of oncological radiology because of the entirely new physical parameters used to obtain the tomographic images. Whereas X-ray computed tomography (CT) has little to offer the breast imager, the capacity of MRI to obtain soft tissue detail is of real value in imaging the breast. This could not be exploited until gadolinium contrast was employed. This innovation of the mid-1980s has become a powerful tool in breast imaging. Gadolinium is taken up in tumours, and the characteristics of enhancement of carcinomas generally differ from those of benign lesions for which they may be mistaken. The features that are of particular value are the high sensitivity of the technique for invasive cancer and the capacity to demonstrate tumours in breasts that are mammographically dense. Moreover, the tomographic images provide a level of detail that cannot be obtained with mammography. The computer data are amenable to various forms of digital manipulation that further enhance the information about the breast lesion. MRI has the following features that make it a useful technique:

- It has a high sensitivity for invasive tumour.
- It does not use ionising radiation.
- The breast does not need to be compressed to obtain the images.
- Subtraction and three-dimensional (3D) reconstruction techniques give an attractive map for surgeons.

These advantages are offset by some adverse features:

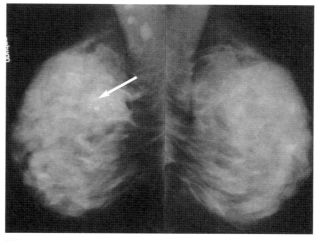

(a)

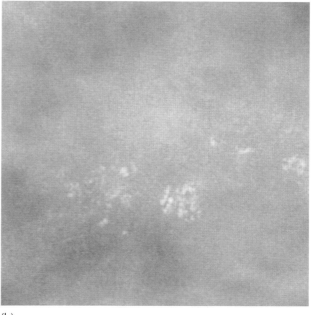

(b)

Figure 18.1 (a) An area of calcification on a digital film demonstrating the ability of the computer method to maximise definition. (b) Magnification view. The patient was aged 40 and had a mass in the right breast. The digital image shows the malignant calcification well in the dense glandular tissue. Such images can be manipulated and subjected to computerised image analysis methods. (See also Chapter 11.)

- The technique is time-consuming for patient and radiologist.
- It is expensive, exceeding by a factor of ten times the cost of a mammographic study.
- Its specificity is rather poor and depends on the quality of the interpretation.

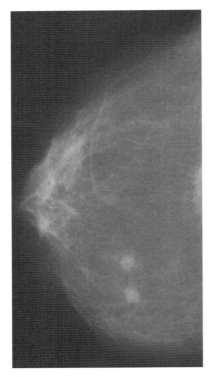

(a)

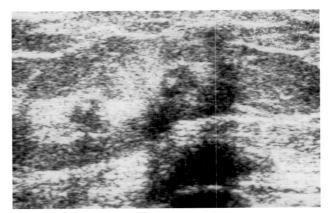

(b)

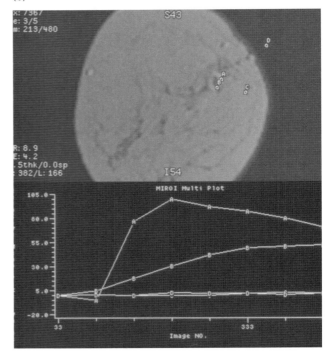

(c)

Figure 18.2 This shows the case of a woman aged 59, who 6 years earlier had a wide local excision for a grade 3 invasive, node-positive ductal carcinoma that was treated postoperatively with chemotherapy and radiotherapy followed by tamoxifen. At her last surveillance mammogram, two small nodules were seen (a). MRI (c,d) shows contrast uptake in the small masses, and locates these areas of tumour recurrence in the line of the surgical resection scar. Biopsy confirmed a further grade 3 oestrogen receptor/progesterone receptor/c-*erb*B-2-negative tumour. (a) shows the mammographic findings. (b) shows the ultrasound appearances. (c), from the 3D dynamic contrast-enhanced series, shows the enhancing lesions in the scar with their malignant time–intensity curve. (d) is a fat-saturated high-detail image taken 10 minutes after the contrast injection. It shows tumour masses in the scar line from previous surgery.

- There are no well-established biopsy techniques for lesions found on MRI only, which, with the previous point, poses a management problem for clinicians.
- A contrast injection is required for most applications, and so this is an invasive technique.

Breast MRI has now been in widespread use for more than a decade and there is an extensive literature, evaluating it, and indicating how the technique may assist the occasional user. A number of review articles are available[10–14] as is a recent book.[15] Breast MRI may be clinically useful in a number of situations.

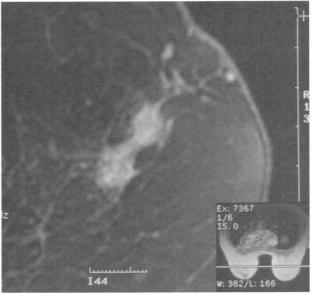

(d)

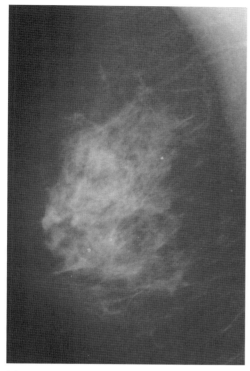

(a)

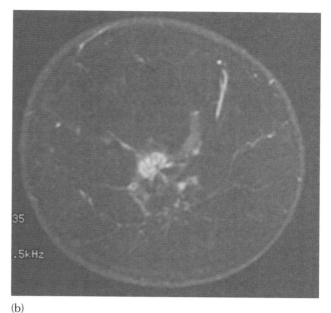

(b)

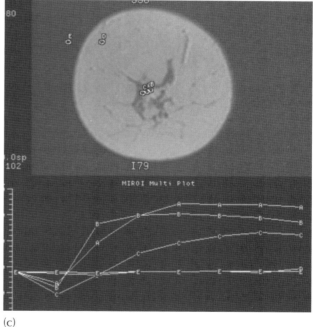

(c)

Figure 18.3 This shows the case of a woman aged 65 who had a breast cancer 10 years before. The dense mammogram was reported normal. MRI undertaken because of a clinical query on the side of the surgery confirmed no recurrence, but showed a small tumour on the opposite (right) side. It could not be seen on review of the mammogram, but ultrasound was used to obtain a biopsy specimen. (a) Right mammogram, MLO view. (b) A fat-saturated high-definition image after contrast shows the small enhancing lesion with morphology suspicious of malignancy. (c) The suspicious curve on 3D dynamic contrast-enhanced MRI. (d) The small tumour has now been shown on ultrasound prior to successful biopsy. Reproduced with permission from Warren R, Coulthard A (eds). Breast MRI in Practice. London: Martin Dunitz, 2002.

Breast MRI for the detection of tumour recurrence (Figure 18.2)

The high sensitivity of contrast-enhanced breast MRI for invasive tumours makes it an ideal test to exclude recurrence of tumour in a conserved breast where the patient has had wide local excision and postoperative radiotherapy followed by tamoxifen or ovarian ablation. In this situation, some of the possible causes of confusing benign lesions are absent:

- There is no cyclical uptake of contrast, as these patients are postmenopausal (natural or treatment-induced).

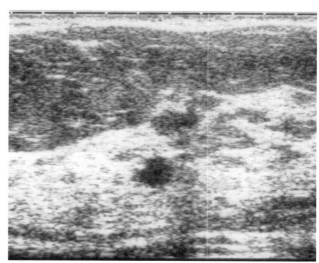

(d)

- The fibrosis of surgery and subsequent radio-therapy reduce the probability that there will be contrast uptake in the breast parenchyma.
- Most recurrences are invasive tumours, and even when the primary lesion has been ductal carcinoma in situ (DCIS) recurrence is in many cases an invasive tumour.

It should be noted that the sensitivity for DCIS is less than for invasive tumour.[12] A number of recent studies have confirmed the usefulness of MRI in the diagnosis of recurrence after conservation surgery.[16–19]

Breast MRI for the demonstration of tumour in dense glandular tissue (Figure 18.3)

This enables more complete preoperative staging. The basis of breast MRI is the detection of gadolinium contrast uptake in tumour tissue after injection. Both morphological and dynamic features are analysed. These features can be clearly seen even in breasts that may be completely dense on mammography. A dense mammographic pattern is found more frequently in younger women, those taking hormone replacement therapy (HRT) and in those at elevated risk by reason of family history.[20] It is also associated with the more aggressive grade 3 tumours.[21,22]

Breast MRI for the demonstration of multifocality (Figure 18.4)

One of the most useful aspects of breast MRI in staging primary cancer is the demonstration of multifocality. This can lead to more extensive surgery, for example conservation surgery may be planned but MRI demonstrates the need for mastectomy or even contralateral surgery.[23–25]

Breast MRI for monitoring tumour response in neoadjuvant chemotherapy (Figure 18.5)

There is no consensus in the literature on the best way to estimate response to neoadjuvant chemotherapy. Clinical measurements sometimes give a good estimate of the response, but are not always reliable, and give under- or overestimates. Repeat mammography may be unhelpful in dense breasts. Ultrasound gives quite a good image, but measurements can be difficult in multifocal or irregular tumours. MRI provides 3D information in tumours of the sort commonly treated with neoadjuvant chemotherapy. These are often large, grade 3, multifocal tumours in dense breasts and may be permeative in nature. MRI data can also be manipulated to show the change in the dynamic curve and volume reduction in the mass in relation to the size of the whole breast. The ability of MRI to determine accurately whether there is residual tumour is not yet established. Contrast uptake may be seen when no further active tumour cells survive, and there may be residual viable cells when the contrast uptake has been eradicated by the treatment. Newer methods of data manipulation have been undertaken that attempt to determine after the first cycle of chemotherapy whether response is occurring.[26] This would be useful if it enables a change in the treatment regime to be instituted, and expensive and unpleasant cycles of chemotherapy stopped when ineffective.[26–29]

Breast MRI to diagnose axillary lymphadenopathy with unknown primary tumour (Figure 18.6)

This clinical situation arises from time to time. There are occasions when breast examination is normal but the histology of the lymph node suggests breast origin, or when the breast is too dense for reliable assessment. With its high sensitivity, MRI can help in this situation. The assumption that any enhancing lesion in the breast is the primary tumour may be tempting, but the diagnostic criteria for cancer must be present, and it is wise to confirm this by biopsy.[30–32]

Breast MRI for the diagnosis of the problem mammogram (Figure 18.7)

There are occasional cases where MRI helps elucidate a mammographic query in an exceptionally useful way. These cases must be selected carefully, and if this selection is correct, then the technique can be extraordinarily useful in locating a lesion or establishing a diagnosis.[33]

Breast MRI for screening women at high risk of breast cancer (Figure 18.8)

Breast MRI, with its high sensitivity, absence of ionising radiation and ability to make a diagnosis in dense breasts, may be ideally suited for a screening test in women at high risk by reason of family history. Trials are underway of its use in this situation, and early results suggest that such screening is possible and does not necessarily have adverse effects. The poor specificity, the problem of hormonal contrast enhancement in young women and the lack of effective biopsy techniques are the potential problems in this clinical scenario. The expense of breast MRI will need to be evaluated in formal cost-effectiveness analysis.[34–40]

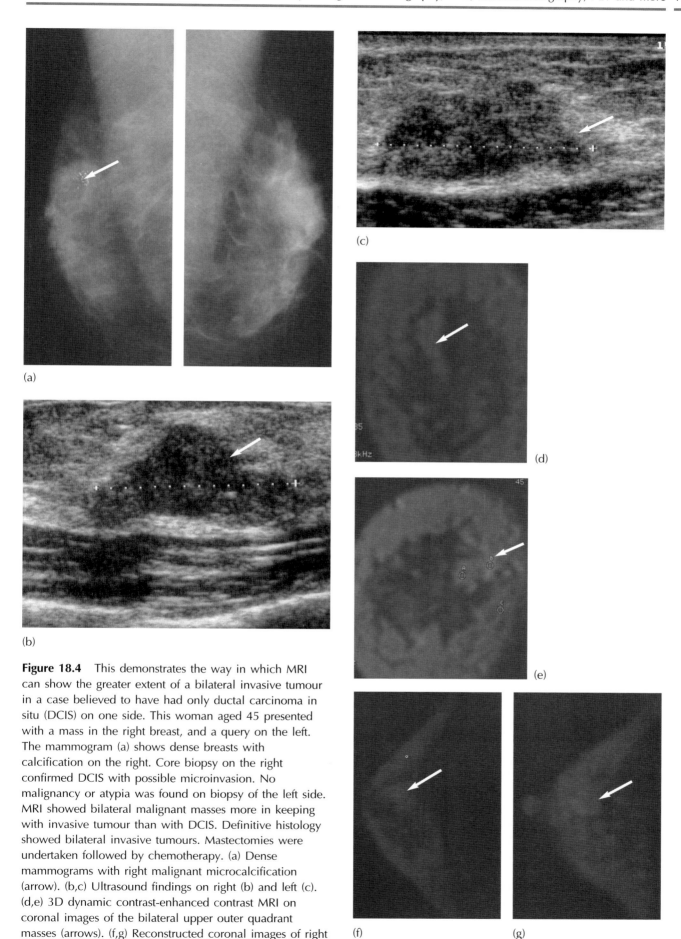

Figure 18.4 This demonstrates the way in which MRI can show the greater extent of a bilateral invasive tumour in a case believed to have had only ductal carcinoma in situ (DCIS) on one side. This woman aged 45 presented with a mass in the right breast, and a query on the left. The mammogram (a) shows dense breasts with calcification on the right. Core biopsy on the right confirmed DCIS with possible microinvasion. No malignancy or atypia was found on biopsy of the left side. MRI showed bilateral malignant masses more in keeping with invasive tumour than with DCIS. Definitive histology showed bilateral invasive tumours. Mastectomies were undertaken followed by chemotherapy. (a) Dense mammograms with right malignant microcalcification (arrow). (b,c) Ultrasound findings on right (b) and left (c). (d,e) 3D dynamic contrast-enhanced contrast MRI on coronal images of the bilateral upper outer quadrant masses (arrows). (f,g) Reconstructed coronal images of right and left breasts, with contrast uptake in the masses.

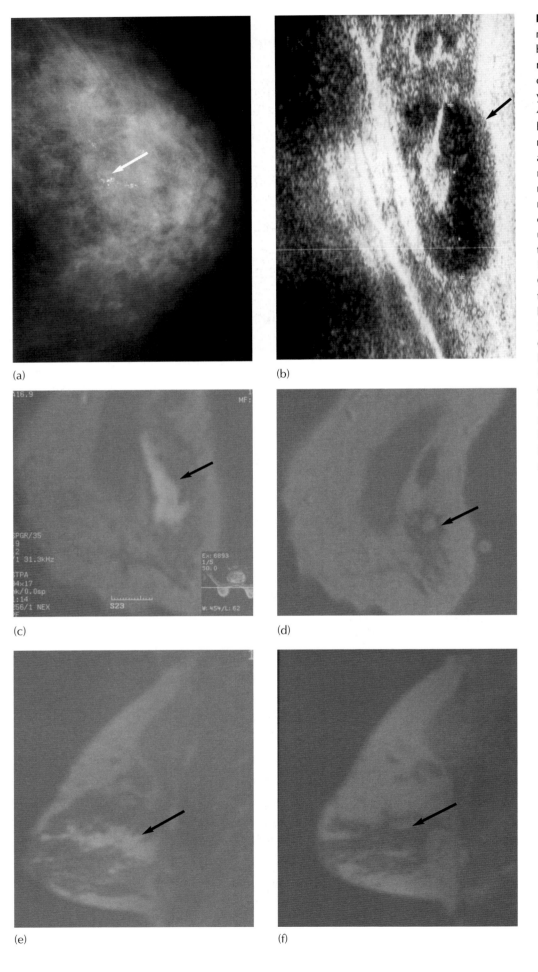

(a)

(b)

(c)

(d)

(e)

(f)

Figure 18.5 A large multifocal tumour before and after neoadjuvant chemotherapy in a young patient. This 49-year-old woman had a large multifocal tumour and enlarged axillary nodes. (a) The dense mammogram with malignant calcification. (b) An ultrasound image of the large axillary lymph nodes. (c,d) Coronal images of the same area of breast in a dynamic 3D contrast-enhanced series before (c) and after (d) neoadjuvant chemotherapy. (e,f) Coronal reconstructed images before (e) and after (f) taxane chemotherapy.

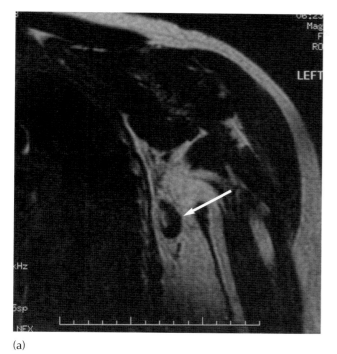

(a)

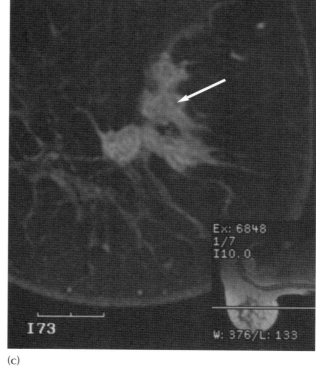

(c)

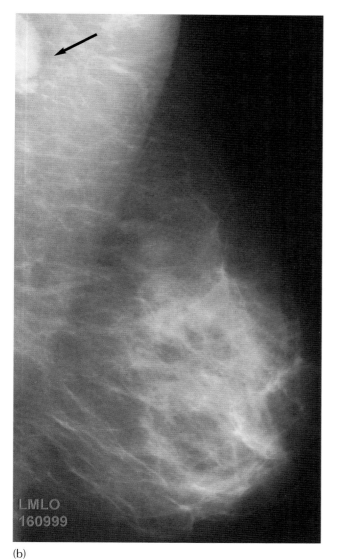

(b)

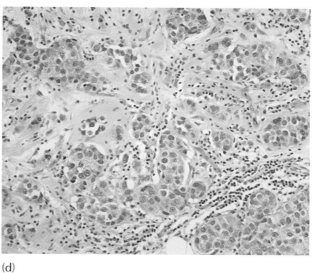

(d)

Figure 18.6 This shows the case of a woman aged 63 who had an enlarged lymph node at the left axilla. She had a right mastectomy for carcinoma 19 years before. Axillary node biopsy showed recurrent carcinoma, and MRI was undertaken to check the breast, which was dense on mammography. The mass was shown and confirmed by ultrasound biopsy, but was undetected by mammography. (a) Axillary node (arrow) on coronal T1-weighted MRI. (b) Dense mammogram with large lymph node (arrow). (c) Fat-saturated high-detail MRI sequence, showing the irregular tumour in the glandular tissue of the breast plate. (d) Tumour on histology. Reproduced with permission from Warren R, Coulthard A (eds). Breast MRI in Practice. London: Martin Dunitz, 2002.

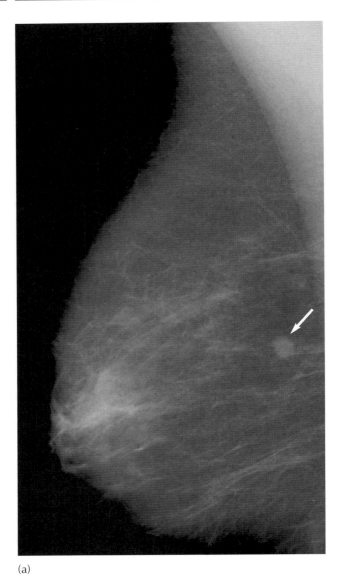

(a)

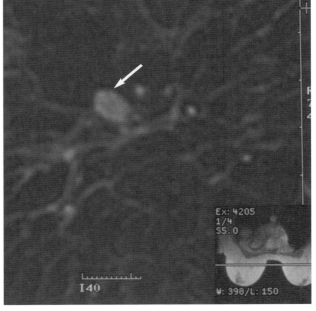

(b)

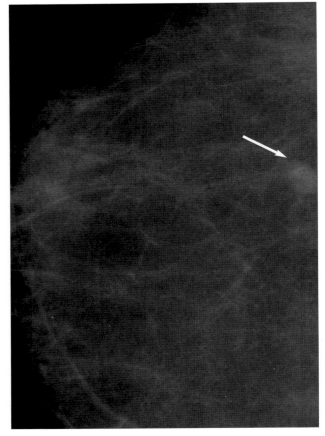

(c)

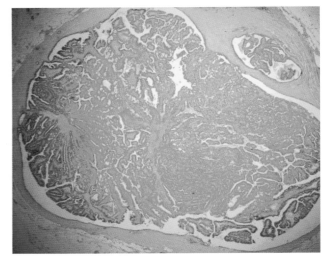

(d)

Figure 18.7 (a) Screening mammogram of a woman aged 51 with a small lesion (arrow). This could not be located on the craniocaudal (CC) view, but the position is resolved by MRI. (b) Fat-saturated high-detail sequence showing the small oval mass. The CC view now shows the position and allows diagnostic removal of a small papilloma. (d) Histology (courtesy of Dr Lynda Bobrow, University of Cambridge.) Reproduced with permission from Warren R, Coulthard A (eds). Breast MRI in Practice. London: Martin Dunitz, 2002.

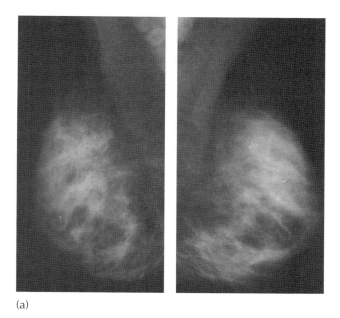

(a)

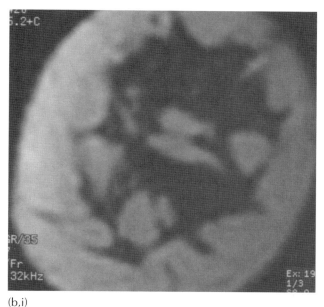

(b,i)

Figure 18.8 A screen-detected cancer in a high-risk woman aged 37 with dense mammographic pattern demonstrated by MRI. (a) Dense mammograms without any evidence of a lesion. (b) Images taken from the 3D dynamic contrast-enhanced series, showing an area of dense glandular tissue with contrast enhancement. (c) The time–intensity curve is of malignant character, confirmed by the finding of an invasive ductal carcinoma. Case kindly provided by Dr Graham Crothers of Belfast.

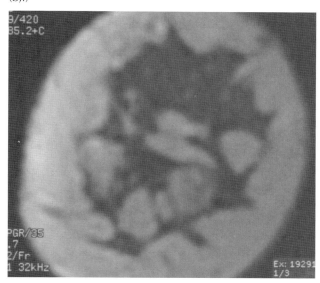

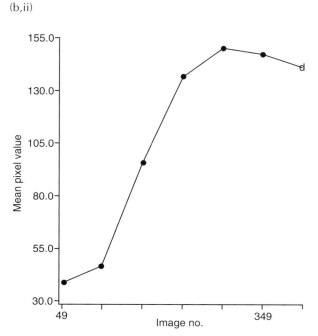

(b,ii)

Implant integrity and the diagnosis of cancer in the presence of implants

Breast MRI is widely recognised as the best technique for both these scenarios. Many of the standard techniques used for cancer diagnosis have limitations, which make them ineffective. Therefore, breast clinicians who have access to MRI will often use it in this situation. The diagnosis of implant rupture is characterised by some typical radiological signs, one of which is the linguine sign shown in Figure 18.9. A good relationship and co-operation between the referring surgeon and the radiologist helps avoid errors that arise from inadequate knowledge of implant details.

Breast MRI – in conclusion

Breast MRI has the potential to resolve some of the outstanding problems that remain when mammography, high-frequency ultrasound and tissue biopsy techniques are used to their limits. It is extensively researched, and appears to have a role that will be

(c)

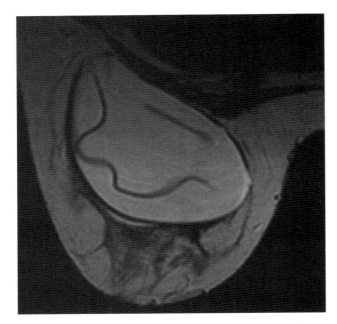

Figure 18.9 The linguine sign of implant rupture. This axial image shows the silicone implant. Within its contour, the inner layer of the skin shows a wavy appearance reminiscent of pasta. This sign is said to be pathognomonic of internal implant rupture.

acknowledged in due course.[1] It is an expert technique, but open to errors of interpretation, and therefore should be carried out by radiologists who have sufficient workload to become highly competent.

Advanced MR techniques

MR spectroscopy

There are newer and adjunctive experimental techniques used with MRI for more accurate diagnosis. Recently MR localised proton (hydrogen 1) magnetic resonance spectroscopy has been used in the characterisation of contrast material-enhanced breast lesions on the basis of choline detection. Several in vitro studies of breast cancer and benign breast tissues showed that choline metabolism was altered in breast cancer and that the detection of choline in tissues might be the means for improving tissue characterisation in vivo.[41,42] This has been applied in several observational studies in patients with breast cancer and benign breast disease.[43,44] In a study by Yeung,[45] the detection of choline by MR spectroscopy in 30 women (mean age 50 years (range 20–80)) gave a sensitivity of 92%, specificity of 83% and accuracy of 90%. Whether these methods become incorporated into regular clinical breast practice awaits further research.

Diffusion weighting, magnetisation transfer, elastography (MRI techniques)

Current breast MRI is constructed upon a single foundation; that of lesion vascular supply, reflected by the time signal response to an intravenous bolus of extracellularly distributed contrast media. Improvements in technology may be used to exploit further the established intrinsic contrast mechanisms of MRI. Diffusion weighting and magnetisation transfer contrast are examples that may be used, as well as intriguing techniques, such as tissue stiffness contrast using MR elastography.[46]

Scintimammography (Figures 18.10–18.12)

'Scintimammography' describes the technique in which images of the breast are obtained using a gamma camera, following intravenous injection of a radiopharmaceutical that accumulates in breast tumours. In common with other nuclear medicine studies, scintimammography reveals a functional image. This provides information, which is complementary to the anatomical information provided by mammography and ultrasound. Scintimammography, which is performed with a standard gamma camera using readily available radiopharmaceuticals, has recently been shown to be as effective as FDG-PET[47,48] and MRI[49] in the diagnosis of primary breast tumours.

If the consistently encouraging results of scintimammography in comparative studies are confirmed, it should become established as a useful complementary diagnostic method. It has yet to find a precise role within the armamentarium of diagnostic methods used in breast cancer management, and covers some common ground with breast MRI.

Tracers used in scintimammography

Technetium 99m (Tc99) MIBI (methoxyisobutylisonitrile) is the tracer most commonly used for scintimammography. It is the only agent which has received FDA approval for this purpose and is the tracer used in the vast majority of published studies. It is taken up by many types of tumours, with in vitro studies showing that Tc99-MIBI concentrates to four times the normal level in malignant tissue.[50] In heart tissue, 90% of the MIBI is sequestered within the mitochondria.[51] A similar mechanism is likely in malignant tissue. Tc99-MIBI's concentration in neoplasia probably depends also on angioneogenesis, metabolic rate, mitotic rate, and mitochondrial density. MIBI is a substrate of P-glycoprotein 170, and is therefore extruded from

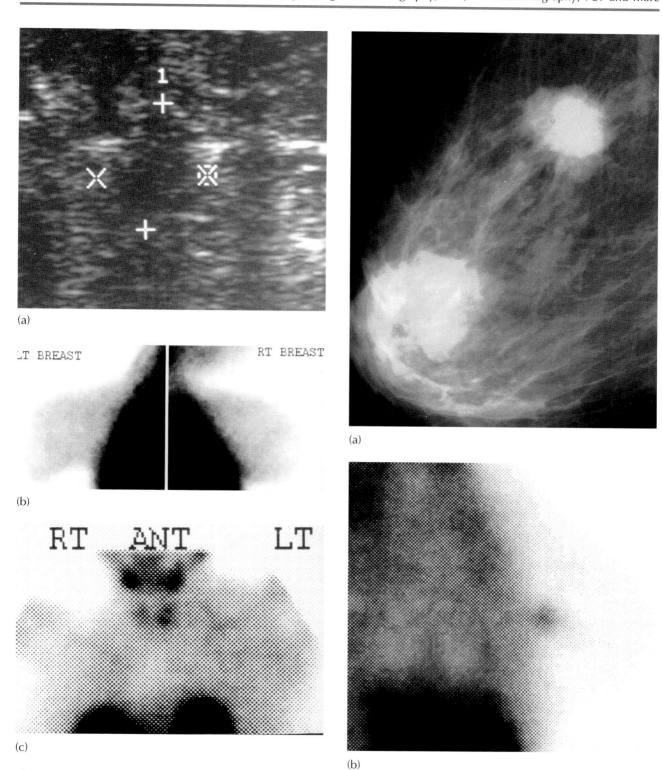

(a)

(b)

(c)

(a)

(b)

Figure 18.10 A true-negative case by scintimammography. A woman aged 80 had had breast carcinoma 22 years previously. Mammography showed post-treatment changes but no focal abnormality. A mass was found on examination, and on ultrasound had features highly suspicious of malignancy (a). (b,c) Cytology was suspicious for malignancy (C4). Scintimammography was normal. The patient has remained well during 3 years of follow-up. This case was kindly supplied by Dr TF El Sayed, Watford General Hospital, UK.

Figure 18.11 A true-positive case by scintimammography. (a) A woman aged 85, with a palpable mass, was found on mammography to have two focal regions of abnormality on the right, raising the possibility of multifocal breast carcinoma. Biopsy was contraindicated due to a blood dyscrasia. (b) Scintimammography demonstrated a single focus of uptake, which was confirmed as invasive carcinoma on subsequent excision. This case was kindly supplied by Dr TF El Sayed, Watford General Hospital, UK.

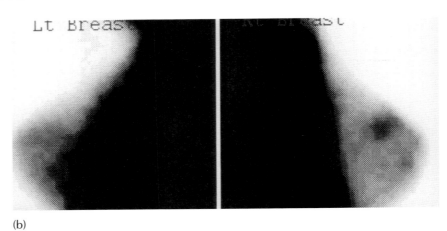

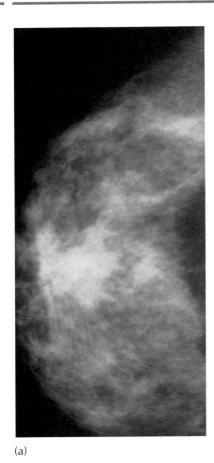

(a)

(b)

Figure 18.12   A false-positive by scintimammography. A woman aged 52 had undergone excision of a benign breast abnormality 2 years previously. She was found to have a focal highly suspicious abnormality in the retroareolar region on mammography (a), which also had features of neoplasia on ultrasound. A true-cut biopsy showed granulomatous change only, with no features of malignancy. (b) Scintimammography performed a fortnight later showed an intense but poorly defined focus of activity. An excision biopsy was found to contain fibrocystic and inflammatory changes, with no evidence of malignancy. The false-positive scintimammography was due to inadequate delay for healing following the core biopsy. Note the poor delineation of the lesion when compared with Figure 18.11(b). This case was kindly supplied by Dr TF El Sayed, Watford General Hospital, UK.

cells which over-express the multidrug resistant (MDR1) gene.[52] This explains the occasional false negative study when imaging is delayed, and the developing role of MIBI imaging in the prediction of chemotherapy response.[53]

MIBI is not the only radiopharmaceutical available for scintimammography. Nuclear imaging of breast cancer started in 1946 with ^{32}P-phosphorous.[54] Since then a wide range of radiopharmaceuticals have been used in research, ranging from highly targeted immunoscintigraphy,[55] to non-specific tracers such as standard bone (MDP) and renal imaging agents (DMSA, DTPA) amongst many others. The majority of non-specific tracers are likely to rely on the abnormal vasculature of breast tumours for focal tracer uptake and lack the specific accumulation in tumour cells seen with MIBI. MDP is an interesting exception. Research in one large centre has shown that MDP may have a particular role in DCIS, perhaps because of uptake into regions of microcalcification.[56]

Technique and technical pitfalls

Dose: The standard dose of 500–700 MBq of Tc-MIBI provides a whole body dose of 5mSV. Only a very small percentage of tracer accumulates in the breast,

with the heart, liver and biliary tract receiving the majority of the dose.

Timing: In addition to uptake in tumours, MIBI accumulates in regions of inflammation. It is therefore recommended that to avoid iatrogenic false positives scintimammography with MIBI is performed either before intervention or after an appropriate time to allow healing: 10 days after fine needle aspiration cytology (FNA), 4–6 weeks after core biopsy (CB), or 2–3 months from surgery or radiotherapy.

Increased breast uptake has been reported during the luteal phase of the menstrual cycle. In premenopausal patients, it is recommended that scintimammography be performed during the first 10 days of the cycle.

Injection site: When upper limb injection is used, extravasated tracer may be taken up by draining lymph nodes. This may simulate axillary nodes involved by tumour. The injection should therefore preferably be made in the foot. However, many centres find the contralateral upper limb acceptable.

Positioning and acquisitions: The prone lateral position has been shown to be the most successful for imaging. The relaxation of pectoral muscles and dependent breast allow good separation of the breast from the heart, liver and chest wall. Mattresses with cut-outs for the breast are commercially available . These allow the breast being imaged to hang free while the other breast is either compressed or shielded to prevent shine-through. Images are acquired starting 5 minutes after the injection, with 10-minute acquisitions. The standard protocol includes prone lateral acquisitions of both breasts, and a supine anterior acquisition with the arms fully abducted, the field of view including both breasts and axillae. Images obtained after a delay have not been found to improve results, nor has SPECT.[57]

Diagnosis of breast lesions

MIBI is taken up not only by breast tumours, but also by benign entities such as fibroadenomas, epithelioid hyperplasia and acute inflammation. The differentiation between benign and malignant lesions by scintimammography depends on the focality of the lesion, with malignant lesions being better delineated from background than benign entities.[58]. Unfortunately, there is substantial overlap of target to background ratios for malignant and benign breast lesions,[59] so quantitative analysis alone is unreliable. Experienced practitioners advocate the use of monitors rather than hard copies when analysing scintimammography to allow image manipulation, which maximises sensitivity and specificity of interpretation. Managing clinicians may therefore have difficulty if they only have access to hard copies.

Results

There have been many large studies comparing MIBI scintimammography with histological analysis. A meta-analysis of MIBI scintimammography across 21 studies, including two prospective multicentre trials, involving over 2000 patients, reveals 85% sensitivity, 89% specificity, PPV of 89% and NPV of 84%.[60] Compared to mammography, the overall sensitivity of scintimammography is equivalent, and specificity much higher.

Unfortunately, the sensitivity of the method falls with size of the lesion, with values ranging from 98%, for lesions between 16 and 25mm, to 55% for invasive carcinoma under 11mm in size.[61] This is because, for lesions under 10mm in size, the inherently poor resolution of currently available gamma cameras is inadequate to delineate the tumour. This is reflected in the much higher sensitivity of the method for palpable lesions (95%), than non palpable (72%).[62] The implication of this poor sensitivity for small lesions (which account for approximately 25% of breast cancers detected on screening

mammography) is that there is no role for scintimammography in screening, nor in the investigation of known lesions under 10 mm.

However, unlike mammography in which sensitivity drops off from the usual 80–90% in fatty breasts of older women, to 60–70% in dense breast tissue (premenopausal women or those on HRT), or when there is architectural distortion following breast surgery or radiotherapy,[63] there is no such change in scintimammography sensitivity. A recent study found a significant reduction in false negative mammography with increasing age, but no corresponding significant change in scintimammography sensitivity.[64]

With the increased use of HRT and the improved survival of treated breast cancer patients, the proportion of difficult breasts being evaluated on mammography has risen in some centres from 25% to 35–40%,[65] and scintimammography is anticipated to establish a role for itself in this setting. Certainly, mammography and scintimammography appear to have complementary roles, with areas under ROC curves revealing a combination of mammography and scintimammography to have significantly more accuracy than the individual tests performed alone.[66]

The role of scintimammography

How scintimammography should fit into established breast imaging protocols is a subject of debate. The triple diagnostic test of clinical examination, radiology and core cytology/biopsy is the standard, well-established, cost-effective method for diagnosis of breast disease. Some maintain that the primary role for scintimammography should be as a complementary method in cases where there is discordance between the results of these three components. This frequently occurs in patients with dense breasts and a recent study has shown that a combination of the triple test and scintimammography showed significant improvement in detecting cancer in dense breasts with a sensitivity of 100%.[67] Others anticipate that the use of the method may be more intrusive with its high negative predictive value being used to avoid unnecessary biopsies in certain groups.[68] Others argue instead that its role will be in aiding in the planning of the extent of surgery for non-palpable lesions.[69]

Advocates of the method advise scintimammography use in the following clinical scenarios for lesions over 10 mm:

- When there is discordance between the components of the triple diagnostic test.

- When mammography is difficult to interpret (e.g. in dense breasts or breasts with architectural distortion due to surgery, chemo or radiotherapy and breast implants).
- For patients intolerant of compression required for mammography.
- When biopsy is not possible due to a medical contraindication.
- In the identification of an occult breast primary.
- In the prediction of response to neoadjuvant chemotherapy.

It should be noted that these indications are exactly those identified earlier in the chapter for breast MRI. A comparative study between MRI and scintimammography found that the two had similar sensitivity for palpable lesions, but that scintimammography had significantly higher specificity for breast carcinoma than MRI.[48]

Axillary staging is a potential benefit of scintimammography, with sensitivity for involved nodes of 85%; however, this is not as sensitive as sentinel lymphoscintigraphy with probe directed biopsy, and axillary staging is not an indication for scintimammography at present.

New developments

The two main limitations of scintimammography in the management of patients are currently being addressed. First, the poor inherent resolution of gamma cameras is being tackled by the development of new dedicated small field of view cameras which, with breast compression, offer improved sensitivity for lesions less than 10 mm from 50 to 80%, with lesions as small as 3 mm being successfully identified.[70] Second, scintimammographic directed needle biopsy using stereotactic techniques has been shown to be feasible.[71] If these developments are continued, the shortcomings of the technique may be successfully resolved such that scintimammography assumes a more central position in the imaging and management of breast patients.

The place of FDG-PET in imaging, staging and therapy of breast cancer

FDG-PET scanning uses 18 fluorodeoxyglucose (FDG) which is taken up by cells metabolising glucose. Breast malignancy, acute inflammation and some benign breast lesions such as fibroadenomas show increased FDG uptake. Due to its cost, the availability of PET scanning has not been sufficiently widespread to allow it to be considered a current technique for breast imaging, and there have been no prospective multicentre trials conducted to evaluate its use in the diagnosis of primary breast cancer. Its place in the imaging of breast cancer is not yet fully mapped out. A recent review[72] summarises in a commendably critical manner, the potential of this promising method. One limitation, which it has in common with scintimammography using sestaMIBI, is poor sensitivity for lesions less than 1 cm in size. The positive predictive value of FDG PET for cancer is over 96% and so the finding of an FDG-avid lesion merits biopsy. FDG PET is likely to be of use in detecting mammary chain and mediastinal involvement by breast cancer,[73] and can be helpful in assessing axillary recurrence. There appear to be limitations to its use in primary axillary staging.[72,74] It will be valuable in the detection of bony metastases[75] and is likely that FDG PET imaging may have potential for monitoring response to chemotherapy.[72] Comparative studies have been undertaken comparing the role of FDG PET with that of MRI.[76]

Sentinel node

See Chapter 37.

Lymphoscintigraphy

See Chapters 36 and 37.

Advanced ultrasound techniques

Doppler ultrasound in breast disease (see also Chapter 17)
Dr WL Teh

Doppler ultrasound examination in the breast relies on the ability to detect vascularity. Malignant tumours are associated with angiogenesis; the production of angiogenesis factors enables malignant tumours to recruit new blood vessels allowing rapid cellular proliferation to take place.[77] Associations between neoangiogenesis and adverse prognostic factors,[78,79] such as shorter relapse-free survival, nodal disease, and the presence of distant micrometastases, have been described. The earliest studies using Doppler shift analysis showed that malignant breast tumours exhibit strong signals with higher maximum systolic frequencies and lower minimum diastolic frequencies. Colour Doppler enabled the visualisation of blood flow within a sample volume, allowing qualitative measurements and the number of blood vessels to be counted. In general, malignant lesions displayed

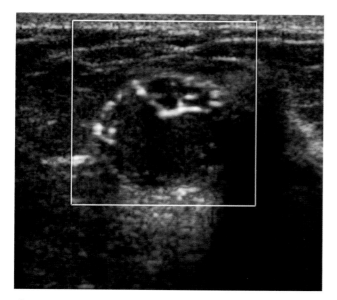

Figure 18.13 Power Doppler ultrasound image of a grade 3 malignant ductal carcinoma. There are multiple peripheral vessels and some penetrating branching vessels.

more vessels compared to benign lesions but there is a degree of overlap so a definitive numerical cut-off value for benign-malignant differentiation cannot be applied. Quantitative measurements of blood flow velocity[80–85] generally demonstrate malignant vasculature to have higher maximum peak systolic velocities ranging from 5 to 34 cm/sec with the majority demonstrating a peak systolic velocity exceeding 15 cm/sec. Other malignant characteristics include higher resistance (usually exceeding 0.7) and pulsatility indices with sinusoidal or bi-directional flow; this is attributed to arterio-vascular shunts. The morphological features of vascularity also showed malignant lesions to have penetrating and abnormally branching vessels.[86] In particular, there is an association between histological grade and the degree of power Doppler vascularity, and abnormal branching, central or penetrating vessels (Figure 18.13). Increased vascularity not only occurs with infiltrative breast tumours but may also arise in areas of in-situ carcinoma.[87–89] This can be successfully exploited to detect areas of both high-grade DCIS as well as invasive disease, allowing ultrasound guided core biopsy to be performed.[90]

The visualisation of vascularity can be utilised in other ways. Colour Doppler examination has also been described as useful in breast reconstructive surgery.[91, 92] Preoperative mapping of the perforating arteries supplying the transverse rectus abdominis myocutaneous (TRAM) flap enables the surgeon to have detailed information of the flap vasculature, i.e.

the location, size and quality of blood flow. Other investigators have also studied Doppler imaging as a method of measuring response to chemotherapy in patients with advanced breast cancer.[93]

Microbubble contrast agents

The use of microbubbles as ultrasound contrast agents significantly improves visualisation of tumour vascularity, thus aiding the specificity of the sonographic examination.[94–96] A rapid uptake of contrast is seen in high-grade malignancies.[97] Other potential applications include the differentiation between scar and recurrent tumour. Studies comparing colour Doppler with ultrasound contrast enhancement have shown ultrasound contrast agent to increase accuracy of differentiation between scar tissue and recurrent disease[98–100] much in the same way as MRI shows enhancement in recurrent disease. Though colour Doppler alone does not increase the accuracy of benign–malignant differentiation of nodal involvement, use of microbubble contrast agents shows a greater number of peripheral vessels with increased enhancement duration to be associated with nodal involvement.[96]

Resistance index (ultrasound)

Colour-coded Doppler sonography can be used to calculate resistance index, from the spectral Doppler tracings. This has been used as a means of offsetting the poor specificity of ultrasound. As might be expected, results have shown an overlap between benign and malignant lesions such that biopsy is often necessary.[84]

Techniques for tomorrow's world

- Light scan
- Impedance imaging, TransScan, Electropotential measurements
- Microwave radiometric imaging
- Synchrotron radiation
- Terahertz imaging
- Molecular imaging

Light scan – a new look

In the mid 1980s, equipment was developed that transilluminated the breast with light. This equipment was claimed to have the potential to image breast cancer without the use of the ionising radiation of mammography. This technology fell out of use after the field trials showed that its sensitivity and specificity were not satisfactory for diagnosis.[101] Mammography had been improved, dose reductions had been achieved and ultrasound had shown advances. The concept of light being the imaging source has, however, not been lost. New equipment is now being subjected to trials in Illinois, which uses light but with much more sophisticated detectors, that can image with minute amounts of light energy, and which present the information digitally.[102] A group in Germany have now developed the use of a contrast agent that has been tested in rat models, designed to improve sensitivity and specificity.[103] The technique is undergoing clinical trials,[104] and may show greater usefulness than its precursor.

Impedance imaging (TransScan), electropotential measurements (Biofield)

In recent years equipment has been designed that detects electrical currents at the breast's surface. Electrical impedance imaging is the name given to this technology, currently produced by TransScan Medical Ltd (Migdal Ha'Emek, Israel)[105] in association with clinical teams in Germany and elsewhere.[106] This technique shows quite high sensitivity in the range of 90%, but poorer specificity, particularly in premenopausal women, where it may relate to cyclical hormonal changes in the breast.[107] This technology is undergoing further field trials, and has been promoted to improve sensitivity of diagnosis by existing methods, the operators having found surveillance methods to overcome the false positives. This does not appear to be an improvement on existing methods using mammography, ultrasound and core biopsy/fine needle aspiration cytology.

A related technology developed by Biofield has used electropotential measurements in the breast to detect malignant and premalignant lesion,[108] which has been assessed by a high quality multicentre study with sophisticated statistical analysis and full pathology review by an expert. It showed sensitivity of 90% and a specificity of 55% and recommended the use in symptomatic clinics to avoid other diagnostic tests in women expected to have benign breast change. This study examined the technique's potential for detecting and correctly assigning borderline breast pathologies.

Synchrotron radiation

Over recent years, experimental work has been undertaken to see whether diagnostic benefit can be obtained by imaging the breast with synchrotron radiation. This use of X-rays detects phase-perturbation effects in tissue, which are higher than absorption effects for soft tissue in the energy range of 15–25 keV. Detection of phase-perturbation effects is possible because of the high degree of coherence of synchrotron radiation sources. Images have been obtained of mammography phantoms and of ex-vivo breast tissue specimens, and yield images of high quality at an acceptable delivered dose. A further use of the capabilities of synchrotron radiation described by Pisano[109] uses diffraction-enhanced imaging on specimens and showed improved conspicuity of lesions. The technology, by which this would be applied to diagnosis in vivo, has not been developed, and whether this technique can find a useful place in the diagnostic armamentarium cannot be predicted. There is some literature on this topic, which describes experimental use to date, together with application in other fields of medicine.[110,111]

Microwave radiometric imaging

This is a technology that lays claim to useful potential in soft tissues, and therefore has particular relevance to the breast. It has yet to make any impact in the field of breast imaging, but claims to have clinical potential.[112]

Terahertz imaging
Vincent Wallace

Over the last decade, advances in laser and semiconductor technology have allowed us to investigate the terahertz region of the electromagnetic spectrum as a possible tool for medical imaging.[113] The terahertz frequency range covers the far infrared wavelengths and is sensitive to librational and vibrational modes of molecules. Terahertz radiation is non-ionizing and does not undergo as much scattering as wavelengths in the near infrared.[114]

Terahertz pulse imaging has already demonstrated it effectiveness by differentiating between benign and malignant tissue in vitro, in particular basal cell carcinoma.[115] Terahertz radiation is heavily attenuated by water but it is hoped that, due to the increased lipid content in breast tissue, we should potentially be able to image through thicknesses of several centimetres. Figure 18.14 shows the technique used in basal cell carcinoma of skin compared with adjacent normal tissue.

Molecular imaging
Tarik F Massoud

Improved and more specific diagnostic techniques are necessary to enhance the contribution of the imaging sciences to the understanding of breast

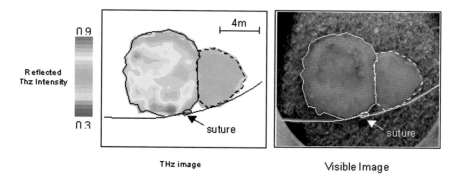

Figure 18.14 Terahertz (THz) imaging. Fifteen basal cell carcinoma samples were imaged. The study was performed blind and the results were compared with histology. The figure shows a control of healthy tissue alongside the diseased tissue, from the same patient. This work was done in collaboration with Dr Richard Pye, Addenbrooke's Hospital, Cambridge, UK.

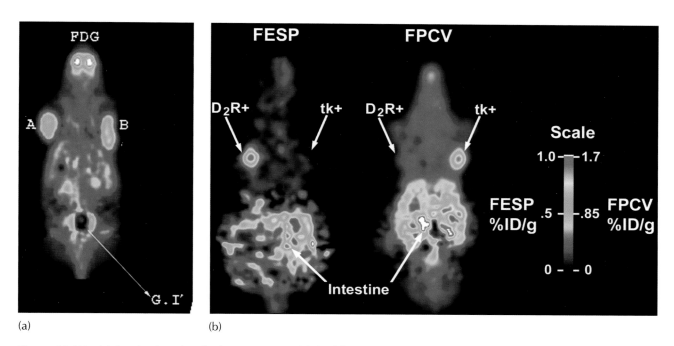

Figure 18.15 Molecular imaging for breast cancer. (a) [^{18}F]fluorodeoxyglucose (FDG) picture of a mouse imaged in a microPET (1 hour after injection of FDG via tail vein). The cells are from an MCF-7 breast cancer cell line. One million cells were injected subcutaneously in each shoulder region. G.I' is gut uptake (nonspecific). Reproduced with kind permission of Dr SS Gambhir of the Crump Institute for Molecular Imaging, UCLA School of Medicine, USA. (b) Imaging of D$_2$R and HSV1-tk PET reporter genes in the same animal. The mouse carrying a C6-stb-tk+ tumour (right) and a D$_2$R tumour (left) was imaged by microPET for HSV1-tk reporter gene expression (using FPCV) and D2R reporter gene expression (using FESP). Both images are displayed using the same global maximum to allow direct comparison. A quantitative scale is shown on the right. The images shown were reconstructed with the MAP reconstruction algorithm. Highly specific localization of FPCV and FESP was found in tumours expressing the HSV1-tk and D2R genes respectively. (Reproduced with permission from Iyer et al 2001.[126])

cancer biology and to the clinical management of women with this disease. Although still mostly confined to the laboratory setting, the recent rapid emergence of in vivo molecular imaging strategies has become possible by advances in molecular cell biology techniques, the availability of transgenic animal models, highly specific imaging drugs that are activated by target interaction, new methods of combinatorial drug design, and the emergence of novel imaging techniques. These molecular imaging strategies include receptor mapping; imaging of apoptosis/hypoxia, peptide uptake, anti/angiogenesis, invasion/metastasis, cell-cycle progression, and tumour antigens; imaging of gene delivery and gene expression, and imaging cell trafficking in vivo. Molecular imaging arises from a need to create a new paradigm that links established in vitro experimental assays to in vivo imaging studies. Thus, molecular imaging would allow: (i) the study of pathogenesis in intact microenvironments in vivo; (ii) the provision of three-dimensional information quickly, noninvasively, and with less labour; and (iii) the assessment of therapeutic effectiveness at a molecular level, long before phenotypic change.[116]

Folate receptors are overexpressed on many neoplastic cells, including those of breast cancer. These receptors could be a potential target for tumour imaging, providing a rational way of selecting patients for treatment with antifolates such as methotrexate. Attempts at this have been made using ^{67}Ga deferoxamine-folate[117] and ^{111}In-DTPA-folate,[118] and in breast tumour-bearing rats using ^{99m}Tc-ethylenedicysteine-folate.[119]

The assessment of tumour hypoxia before radiotherapy could provide rational means of selecting patients for treatment with radiosensitizers or bioreductive drugs such as mitomycin C. The differentiation of hypoxic radioresistance from well-oxygenated active tumour may be possible by labelling misonidazole with different radioisotopes for PET and SPECT imaging. Recent experimental studies in breast tumour-bearing rats have also demonstrated the usefulness of ^{99m}Tc-ethylenedicysteine-nitroimidazole for targeting tumour hypoxia.[119]

Annexin V binds to phosphotidylserin, which is overexpressed by tumour apoptotic cells. Imaging assessment of neoplastic cell apoptosis, which occurs following chemotherapy and radiotherapy, has been shown in breast tumour-bearing rats using ^{99m}Tc-ethylenedicysteine-annexin V.[119]

High uptake of amino acids is observed in viable tumour cells. Labelling glutamic acid peptide may be useful in differentiating the degree of malignancy of tumours. The use of peptide imaging in breast tumour-bearing rats has been shown with ^{99m}Tc-ethylenedicysteine-glutamic acid pentapeptide.[119]

Angiogenesis is the formation of new blood vessels. These vessels provide a direct route for neoplastic cells to exit the primary tumour site and enter the circulation to form metastases. One strategy for imaging angiogenesis entails the use of ^{99m}Tc-MIBI (sestamibi),[120–122] initially developed for myocardial perfusion imaging. It has been shown that this agent may be used to predict tumour angiogenesis and that its uptake correlates well with tumour microvessel density. Antiangiogenesis is a strategy for starving tumours by interrupting their blood supply. Promising antiangiogenic drugs such as TNP 470 (AGM-1470), fumagillin, heparin-steroid conjugates, ovalicin, paclitaxel, taxotere, and epithilone are small organic molecules that can be labelled with various isotopes for PET and SPECT imaging.[119] Higher uptake in tumours could be a prognostic indicator of a higher incidence of tumour metastasis due to an underlying high tumour vascular density. The usefulness of ^{99m}Tc-ethylenedicysteine-colchicine for imaging tumour angiogenesis has been shown in breast tumour-bearing rats.[119]

Some of the more exciting recent developments in targeted molecular imaging of cancer have been in reporter gene and transgene expression imaging using microPET or in vivo optical charge-coupled devices (CCD).[123] 'PET reporter genes (PRG)' are genes whose protein products are either (i) receptors for positron-labelled 'PET reporter ligand probes' or (ii) enzymes that metabolise positron-labelled 'PET reporter substrate probes' to sequestered intracellular products. Using tomographic imaging, it is possible to repeatedly quantify in living animal tissue localisation and levels of expression of PRG driven by specific promoters. Alternatively, cells stably expressing the PRG can also be tracked over time. Gambhir et al.[124] have developed a PET based imaging assay for determining the location(s), magnitude, and persistence of Herpes Simplex Type 1 thymidine kinase (HSV1-tk) reporter gene expression or the Dopamine-2 receptor (D2R) reporter gene expression. An adenoviral-directed delivery mechanism has been used, in which a replication-deficient adenovirus carrying the PRG, driven by the cytomegalovirus promoter, is used to deliver the PRG primarily to the murine liver when injected intravenously, or to cell lines in vitro (Figure 18.15). Alternatively, the PRG can be knocked-in the genetic construct of transgenic models. Similar strategies apply to use of the optical reporter gene firefly luciferase; this provides a simple low-cost approach for CCD imaging of low levels of light from living animals. For a comprehensive review of the rapidly evolving field of imaging endogenous or transferred gene expression and its applications to breast cancer the reader is directed to the recent work of Berger and Gambhir.[125]

Conclusion

By the time that the next edition of this text is published, the topics discussed here will have evolved, and the space needed for the various modalities may have changed reflecting the shifting importance of all these different emerging techniques. The author's prediction is reflected in the space allocated: that digital mammography will in due course take over from film/screen mammography, but the overall dominance of X-ray mammography will remain as the baseline imaging and screening tool in women over 40 years of age for many years to come. MRI will show further development and will become part of the presurgical assessment of tumours in women with premenopausal breast cancer, and in those with dense breasts. MRI will lilely have a part in the surveillance of treated breast cancer. Nuclear medicine tests will remain optional, considered useful by some and ignored by others, until FDG PET is freely available. However, this will be partnered or even overtaken by the functional potential of molecular imaging. Whether other newer technical modalities of litescan, impedance imaging, synchrotron radiation or terahertz imaging ever take a hold will be an unfolding story, but some will certainly pass unnoticed into history. There are exciting years ahead, and these predictions may be wholly wrong. If this conclusion had been written in 1950, 1970 or even 1990, would the current front-runners have been recognised? – maybe not and woe betide the referee who would have turned down the grant application from the physicist who had the germ of an idea for ultrasound or MRI in 1950!

Acknowledgements

Figures contributed kindly by:
Geoff Parkin, University of Leeds, UK
William Teh, Northwick Park, Harrow UK
Vincent Wallace, Cambridge UK
TF El Sayed, Watford General Hospital, UK
Lynda Bobrow, Department of Histopathology, Cambridge, UK
Graham Crothers, Royal Victoria Hospital, Belfast
SS Gambhir of the Crump Institute for Molecular Imaging, UCLA School of Medicine, USA.

References

1. Warren R. Is breast MRI mature enough to be recommended for general use? Lancet 2001; 358: 1745–46.
2. Williams M, Pisano E, Schnall M, Fajardo L. Future directions in imaging of breast diseases. Radiology 1998; 206: 297–300.
3. Feig SA, Yaffe MJ. Digital mammography. Radiographics 1998; 18: 893–901.
4. Cowen AR, Parkin GJ, Hawkridge P. Direct digital mammography image acquisition. Eur Radiol 1997; 7: 918–30.
5. Chan HP, Helvie MA, Petrick N et al. Digital mammography: observer performance study of the effects of pixel size on the characterization of malignant and benign microcalcifications. Acad Radiol 2001; 8: 454–66.
6. Kimme-Smith C. New digital mammography systems may require different X-ray spectra and, therefore, more general normalized glandular dose values. Radiology 1999; 213: 7–10.
7. Pisano ED, Cole EB, Major S et al. Radiologists' preferences for digital mammographic display. The International Digital Mammography Development Group. Radiology 2000; 216: 820–30.
8. Pisano ED, Yaffe MJ, Hemminger BM et al. Current status of full-field digital mammography. Acad Radiol 2000; 7: 266–80.
9. Venta LA, Hendrick RE, Adler YT et al. Rates and causes of disagreement in interpretation of full-field digital mammography and film-screen mammography in a diagnostic setting. AJR Am J Roentgenol 2001; 176: 1241–8.
10. Kuhl CK. MRI of breast tumors. Eur Radiol 2000; 10: 46–58.
11. Harms SE. Breast magnetic resonance imaging. Semin Ultrasound CT MR 1998; 19: 104–20.
12. Kinkel K, Hylton NM. Challenges to interpretation of breast MRI. J Magn Reson Imaging 2001; 13: 821–9.
13. Kumar NA, Schnall MD. MR imaging: its current and potential utility in the diagnosis and management of breast cancer. Magn Reson Imaging Clin N Am 2000; 8: 715–28.
14. Orel SG. MR imaging of the breast. Radiol Clin North Am 2000; 38: 899–913.
15. Warren R, Coulthard A. Breast MRI in Practice. London: Martin Dunitz; 2002.
16. Kramer S, Schulz-Wendtland R, Hagedorn K et al. Magnetic resonance imaging in the diagnosis of local recurrences in breast cancer. Anticancer Res 1998; 18: 2159–61.
17. Drew PJ, Kerin MJ, Turnbull LW et al. Routine screening for local recurrence following breast-conserving therapy for cancer with dynamic contrast-enhanced magnetic resonance imaging of the breast. Ann Surg Oncol 1998; 5: 265–70.
18. Mumtaz H, Davidson T, Hall-Craggs MA et al. Comparison of magnetic resonance imaging and conventional triple assessment in locally recurrent breast cancer. Br J Surg 1997; 84: 1147–51.
19. Viehweg P, Heinig A, Lampe D et al. Retrospective analysis for evaluation of the value of contrast-enhanced MRI in patients treated with breast conservative therapy. Magma 1998; 7: 141–52.
20. Kerlikowske K, Grady D, Barclay J et al. Effect of age, breast density, and family history on the sensitivity of first screening mammography [see comments]. JAMA 1996; 276: 33–8.
21. Sala E, Solomon L, Warren R et al. Size, node status, and grade of breast tumours: association with mammographic parenchymal patterns. European Radiology 2000; 10: 157–61.
22. Sala E, Warren R, McCann J et al. Mammographic parenchymal patterns and mode of detection: implications for the breast screening programme. J Med Screen 1998; 5: 207–12.
23. Malur S, Wurdinger S, Moritz A et al. Comparison of written reports of mammography, sonography and magnetic resonance mammography for preoperative evaluation of breast lesions, with special emphasis on magnetic resonance mammography. Breast Cancer Res 2001; 3: 55–60.
24. Fischer U, Kopka L, Grabbe E. Breast carcinoma: effect

of preoperative contrast-enhanced MR imaging on the therapeutic approach. Radiology 1999; 213: 881–8.

25. Mumtaz H, Hall-Craggs MA, Davidson T et al. Staging of symptomatic primary breast cancer with MR imaging. AJR Am J Roentgenol 1997; 169: 417–24.

26. Padhani AR, Husband JE. Commentary. Are current tumour response criteria relevant for the 21st century? Br J Radiol 2000; 73: 1031–3.

27. Harms SE. Integration of breast magnetic resonance imaging with breast cancer treatment. Top Magn Reson Imaging 1998; 9: 79–91.

28. Trecate G, Ceglia E, Stabile F et al. Locally advanced breast cancer treated with primary chemotherapy: comparison between magnetic resonance imaging and pathologic evaluation of residual disease. Tumori 1999; 85: 220–8.

29. Abraham DC, Jones RC, Jones SE et al. Evaluation of neoadjuvant chemotherapeutic response of locally advanced breast cancer by magnetic resonance imaging. Cancer 1996; 78: 91–100.

30. Stomper PC, Waddell BE, Edge SB, Klippenstein DL. Breast MRI in the evaluation of patients with occult primary breast carcinoma. Breast J 1999; 5: 230–4.

31. Orel SG, Weinstein SP, Schnall MD et al. Breast MR imaging in patients with axillary node metastases and unknown primary malignancy. Radiology 1999; 212: 543–9.

32. Tilanus-Linthorst MM, Obdeijn AI, Bontenbal M, Oudkerk M. MRI in patients with axillary metastases of occult breast carcinoma. Breast Cancer Res Treat 1997; 44: 179–82.

33. Lee CH, Smith RC, Levine JA et al. Clinical usefulness of MR imaging of the breast in the evaluation of the problematic mammogram. AJR Am J Roentgenol 1999; 173: 1323–9.

34. Plevritis SK. A framework for evaluating the cost-effectiveness of MRI screening for breast cancer. Eur Radiol 2000; 10(Suppl 3): S430–2.

35. Tilanus-Linthorst MM, Obdeijn IM, Bartels KC et al. First experiences in screening women at high risk for breast cancer with MR imaging. Breast Cancer Res Treat 2000; 63: 53–60.

36. Kuhl CK, Schmutzler RK, Leutner CC et al. Breast MR imaging screening in 192 women proved or suspected to be carriers of a breast cancer susceptibility gene: preliminary results. Radiology 2000; 215(1): 267–79.

37. Brown J, Buckley D, Coulthard A et al. Magnetic resonance imaging screening in women at genetic risk of breast cancer: imaging and analysis protocol for the UK multicentre study. Magn Reson Imaging 2000; 18: 765–76.

38. The UK MRI Breast Screening Study (MARIBS) Brown J, Coulthard A, Dixon A, Dixon J et al. Protocol for a national multi-centre study of magnetic resonance imaging screening in women at genetic risk of breast cancer. The Breast 2000; 9: 78–82.

39. The UK MRI Breast Screening Study (MARIBS), Brown J, Coulthard A, Dixon A, et al. Rationale for a national multi-centre study of magnetic resonance imaging screening in women at genetic risk of breast cancer. The Breast 2000; 9: 72–7.

40. Schnall MD. Application of magnetic resonance imaging to early detection of breast cancer. Breast Cancer Res 2001; 3: 17–21.

41. Mackinnon WB, Barry PA, Malycha PL et al. Fine-needle biopsy specimens of benign breast lesions distinguished from invasive cancer ex vivo with proton MR spectroscopy. Radiology 1997; 204: 661–6.

42. Cheng LL, Chang IW, Smith BL, Gonzalez RG. Evaluating human breast ductal carcinomas with high-resolution magic-angle spinning proton magnetic resonance spectroscopy. J Magn Reson 1998; 135: 194–202.

43. Roebuck JR, Cecil KM, Schnall MD, Lenkinski RE. Human breast lesions: characterization with proton MR spectroscopy. Radiology 1998; 209: 269–75.

44. Kvistad KA, Bakken IJ, Gribbestad IS et al. Characterization of neoplastic and normal human breast tissues with in vivo (1)H MR spectroscopy. J Magn Reson Imaging 1999; 10: 159–64.

45. Yeung DK, Cheung HS, Tse GM. Human breast lesions: characterization with contrast-enhanced in vivo proton MR spectroscopy—initial results. Radiology 2001; 220: 40–6.

46. Lawrence AJ, Rossman PJ, Mahowald JL et al. Assessment of breast cancer by magnetic resonance elastography. In: 7th Annual Meeting of the International Society for Magnetic Resonance in Medicine, Philadelphia. 1999. p. 525.

47. Yutani K, Shiba E, Kusuoka H et al. Comparison of FDG-PET with MIBI-SPECT in the detection of breast cancer and axillary lymph node metastasis. J Comput Assist Tomogr 2000; 24: 274–80.

48. Palmedo H, Bender H, Grunwald F et al. Comparison of fluorine-18 fluorodeoxyglucose positron emission tomography and technetium-99m methoxyisobutylisonitrile scintimammography in the detection of breast tumours. Eur J Nucl Med 1997; 24: 1138–45.

49. Imbriaco M, Del Vecchio S, Riccardi A et al. Scintimammography with 99mTc-MIBI versus dynamic MRI for non-invasive characterization of breast masses. Eur J Nucl Med 2001; 28: 56–63.

50. Maublant JC, Zhang Z, Rapp M et al. In vitro uptake of technetium-99m-teboroxime in carcinoma cell lines and normal cells: comparison with technetium-99m-sestamibi and thallium-201. J Nucl Med 1993; 34: 1949–52.

51. Carvalho PA, Chiu ML, Kronauge JF et al. Subcellular distribution and analysis of technetium-99m-MIBI in isolated perfused rat hearts. J Nucl Med 1992; 33: 1516–22.

52. Piwnica-Worms D, Chiu ML, Budding M et al. Functional imaging of multidrug-resistant P-glycoprotein with an organotechnetium complex. Cancer Res 1993; 53: 977–84.

53. Ciarmiello A, Del Vecchio S, Silvestro P et al. Tumor clearance of technetium 99m-sestamibi as a predictor of response to neoadjuvant chemotherapy for locally advanced breast cancer. J Clin Oncol 1998; 16: 1677–83.

54. Berg GR, Kalisher L, Osmond JD et al. 99mTc-diphosphonate concentration in primary breast carcinoma. Radiology 1973; 109: 393–4.

55. Baum RP, Brummendorf TH. Radioimmunolocalization of primary and metastatic breast cancer. Q J Nucl Med 1998; 42: 33–42.

56. Lastoria S, Piccolo S, Muto P. Breast imaging with 99mTc Methylene Diphosphonate. In: Taillefer R, Khalkhali I, Waxman A, eds. Radionuclide imaging of the breast. New York: Marcell Dekker 1998. p. 299.

57. Danielsson R, Bone B, Agren B et al. Comparison of planar and SPECT scintimammography with 99mTc-sestamibi in the diagnosis of breast carcinoma. Acta Radiol 1999; 40: 176–80.

58. Khalkhali I, Vargas HI. The role of nuclear medicine in breast cancer detection: functional breast imaging. Radiol Clin North Am 2001; 39: 1053–68.

59. Arslan N, Ozturk E, Ilgan S et al. 99Tcm-MIBI scintimammography in the evaluation of breast lesions and axillary involvement: a comparison with mammography and histopathological diagnosis. Nucl Med Commun 1999; 20: 317–25.

60. Taillefer R. The role of 99mTc-sestamibi and other conventional radiopharmaceuticals in breast cancer diagnosis. Semin Nucl Med 1999; 29: 16–40.

61. Howarth D, Sillar R, Clark D, Lan L. Technetium-99m sestamibi scintimammography: the influence of histopathological characteristics, lesion size and the presence of carcinoma in situ in the detection of breast carcinoma. Eur J Nucl Med 1999; 26: 1475–81.

62. Waxman AD. The role of (99m)Tc methoxyisobutylisonitrile in imaging breast cancer. Semin Nucl Med 1997; 27: 40–54.

63. Meyer JE, Eberlein TJ, Stomper PC, Sonnenfeld MR. Biopsy of occult breast lesions. Analysis of 1261 abnormalities. JAMA 1990; 263: 2341–3.

64. Lumachi F, Ferretti G, Povolato M et al. Usefulness of 99m-Tc-sestamibi scintimammography in suspected breast cancer and in axillary lymph node metastases detection. Eur J Surg Oncol 2001; 27: 256–9.

65. Jackson V, Hendrick R, Feig S, Kopans D. Imaging of the radiographically dense breast. Radiology 1993; 188: 297–301.

66. Buscombe JR, Cwikla JB, Holloway B, Hilson AJ. Prediction of the usefulness of combined mammography and scintimammography in suspected primary breast cancer using ROC curves. J Nucl Med 2001; 42: 3–8.

67. Danielsson R, Reihner E, Grabowska A, Bone B. The role of scintimammography with 99mTc-sestamibi as a complementary diagnostic technique in the detection of breast cancer. Acta Radiol 2000; 41: 441–5.

68. Mirzaei S, Zajicek SM, Knoll P et al. Scintimammography enhances negative predictive value of non-invasive pre-operative assessment of breast lesions. Eur J Surg Oncol 2000; 26: 738–41.

69. Aguilar J, Andres B, Nicolas F et al. Value of 99mTc-MIBI scintimammography in women with impalpable breast lesions seen on mammography. Eur J Surg 2001; 167: 344–6.

70. Scopinaro F, Pani R, De Vincentis G et al. High-resolution scintimammography improves the accuracy of technetium-99m methoxyisobutylisonitrile scintimammography: use of a new dedicated gamma camera. Eur J Nucl Med 1999; 26: 1279–88.

71. Khalkhali I, Mishkin FS, Diggles LE, Klein SR. Radionuclide-guided stereotactic prebiopsy localization of nonpalpable breast lesions with normal mammograms. J Nucl Med 1997; 38: 1019–22.

72. Wahl RL. Current status of PET in breast cancer imaging, staging, and therapy. Semin Roentgenol 2001; 36: 250–60.

73. Eubank WB, Mankoff DA, Takasugi J et al. 18fluorodeoxyglucose positron emission tomography to detect mediastinal or internal mammary metastases in breast cancer. J Clin Oncol 2001; 19: 3516–23.

74. Greco M, Crippa F, Agresti R et al. Axillary lymph node staging in breast cancer by 2-fluoro-2-deoxy-D-glucose-positron emission tomography: clinical evaluation and alternative management. J Natl Cancer Inst 2001; 93: 630–5.

75. Kim TS, Moon WK, Lee DS et al. Fluorodeoxyglucose positron emission tomography for detection of recurrent or metastatic breast cancer. World J Surg 2001; 25: 829–34.

76. Brix G, Henze M, Knopp MV et al. Comparison of pharmacokinetic MRI and [18F] fluorodeoxyglucose PET in the diagnosis of breast cancer: initial experience. Eur Radiol 2001; 11: 2058–70.

77. Harris AL, Horak E. Growth factors and angiogenesis in breast cancer. Recent Results Cancer Res 1993; 127: 35–41.

78. Gasparini G, Harris AL. Clinical importance of the determination of tumor angiogenesis in breast carcinoma: much more than a new prognostic tool. J Clin Oncol 1995; 13: 765–82.

79. Horak ER, Harris AL, Stuart N, Bicknell R. Angiogenesis in breast cancer. Regulation, prognostic aspects, and implications for novel treatment strategies. Ann N Y Acad Sci 1993; 698: 71–84.

80. McNicholas MM, Mercer PM, Miller JC et al. Color Doppler sonography in the evaluation of palpable breast masses. AJR Am J Roentgenol 1993; 16: 765–71.

81. Huber S, Delorme S, Knopp MV et al. Breast tumors: computer-assisted quantitative assessment with color Doppler US. Radiology 1994; 192: 797–801.

82. Peters-Engl C, Medl M, Leodolter S. The use of colour-coded and spectral Doppler ultrasound in the differentiation of benign and malignant breast lesions. Br J Cancer 1995; 71: 137–9.

83. Madjar H, Prompeler HJ, Sauerbrei W et al. Differential diagnosis of breast lesions by color Doppler. Ultrasound Obstet Gynecol 1995; 6: 199–204.

84. Youssefzadeh S, Eibenberger K, Helbich T et al. Use of resistance index for the diagnosis of breast tumours. Clin Radiol 1996; 51: 418–20.

85. Hollerweger A, Rettenbacher T, Macheiner P, Gritzmann N. New signs of breast cancer: high resistance flow and variations in resistive indices evaluation by color Doppler sonography. Ultrasound Med Biol 1997; 23: 851–6.

86. Raza S, Baum JK. Solid breast lesions: evaluation with power Doppler US. Radiology 1997; 203: 164–8.

87. Lee AH, Happerfield LC, Bobrow LG, Millis RR. Angiogenesis and inflammation in ductal carcinoma in situ of the breast. J Pathol 1997; 181: 200–6.

88. Guidi AJ, Schnitt SJ, Fischer L et al. Vascular permeability factor (vascular endothelial growth factor) expression and angiogenesis in patients with ductal carcinoma in situ of the breast. Cancer 1997; 80: 1945–53.

89. Engels K, Fox SB, Whitehouse RM et al. Distinct angiogenic patterns are associated with high-grade in situ ductal carcinomas of the breast. J Pathol 1997; 181: 207–12.

90. Teh WL, Wilson AR, Evans AJ et al. Ultrasound guided core biopsy of suspicious mammographic calcifications using high frequency and power Doppler ultrasound. Clin Radiol 2000; 55: 390–4.

91. Berg WA, Chang BW, DeJong MR, Hamper UM. Color Doppler flow mapping of abdominal wall perforating arteries for transverse rectus abdominis myocutaneous flap in breast reconstruction: method and preliminary results. Radiology 1994; 192: 447–50.

92. Pacifici A, Cirocchi R, Flamini FO et al. [Pre- and postoperative color Doppler ultrasonography of myocutaneous flaps in reconstructive surgery of the breast]. Minerva Chir 1997; 52: 247–50.

93. Seymour MT, Moskovic EC, Walsh G et al. Ultrasound assessment of residual abnormalities following primary chemotherapy for breast cancer. Br J Cancer 1997; 76: 371–6.

94. Schroeder RJ, Maeurer J, Vogl TJ et al. D-galactose-based signal-enhanced color Doppler sonography of breast tumors and tumorlike lesions. Invest Radiol 1999; 34: 109–15.

95. Moon WK, Im JG, Noh DY, Han MC. Nonpalpable breast lesions: evaluation with power Doppler US and a microbubble contrast agent-initial experience. Radiology 2000; 217: 240–6.

96. Yang WT, Metreweli C, Lam PK, Chang J. Benign and malignant breast masses and axillary nodes: evaluation with echo-enhanced color power Doppler US. Radiology 2001; 220: 795–802.

97. Teh WL, Shah B, Shah K. Dynamic contrast enhanced ultrasound examination of malignant breast tumours: comparison against dynamic breast MRI and histological features. Radioogy 2001; 221: 606.

98. Baz E, Madjar H, Reuss C et al. The role of enhanced Doppler ultrasound in differentiation of benign vs. malignant scar lesion after breast surgery for malignancy. Ultrasound Obstet Gynecol 2000; 15: 377–82.

99. Stuhrmann M, Aronius R, Schietzel M. Tumor vascularity of breast lesions: potentials and limits of contrast- enhanced Doppler sonography Am J Roentgenol 2000; 175: 1585–9.

100. Bonifacino A, Ranieri E, Tella S, Vecchione A. Ultrasonography of local recurrent breast cancer. J d'Echographie et de Medecine par Ultrasons 1998; 19: 81–5.

101. Alveryd A, Andersson I, Aspegren K et al. Lightscanning versus mammography for the detection of breast cancer in screening and clinical practice. A Swedish multicenter study. Cancer 1990; 65: 1671–7.

102. Franceschini MA, Moesta KT, Fantini S et al. Frequency-domain techniques enhance optical mammography: initial clinical results. Proc Natl Acad Sci USA 1997; 94: 6468–73.

103. Ebert B, Sukowski U, Grosenick D et al. Near-infrared fluorescent dyes for enhanced contrast in optical mammography: phantom experiments. J Biomed Opt 2001; 6: 134–40.

104. Cerussi AE, Berger AJ, Bevilacqua F et al. Sources of absorption and scattering contrast for near-infrared optical mammography. Acad Radiol 2001; 8: 211–18.

105. Assenheimer M, Laver-Moskovitz O, Malonek D et al. The T-SCAN technology: electrical impedance as a diagnostic tool for breast cancer detection. Physiol Meas 2001; 22: 1–8.

106. Malich A, Fritsch T, Anderson R et al. Electrical impedance scanning for classifying suspicious breast lesions: first results. Eur Radiol 2000; 10: 1555–61.

107. Perlet C, Kessler M, Lenington S et al. Electrical impedance measurement of the breast: effect of hormonal changes associated with the menstrual cycle. Eur Radiol 2000; 10: 1550–4.

108. Cuzick J, Holland R, Barth V et al. Electropotential measurements as a new diagnostic modality for breast cancer. Lancet 1998; 352: 359–63.

109. Pisano ED, Johnston RE, Chapman D et al. Human breast cancer specimens: diffraction-enhanced imaging with histologic correlation—improved conspicuity of lesion detail compared with digital radiography. Radiology 2000; 214: 895–901.

110. Arfelli F, Bonvicini V, Bravin A et al. Mammography with synchrotron radiation: phase-detection techniques. Radiology 2000; 215: 286–93.

111. Thomlinson W, Berkvens P, Berruyer G et al. Research at the European Synchrotron Radiation Facility medical beamline. Cell Mol Biol (Noisy-le-grand) 2000; 46: 1053–63.

112. Leroy Y, Bocquet B, Mamouni A. Non-invasive microwave radiometry thermometry. Physiol Meas 1998; 19: 127–48.

113. Mittleman D, Jacobson R, Nuss M. T-ray imaging. J Sel. Top Quantum Electron 1992; 2: 679–92.

114. Arnone D, Ciesla C, Corchia A et al. Applications of Terahertz (THz) Technology to Medical Imaging. In: Terahertz Spectroscopy and Applications – II. SPIE Proceedings. pp. 209–19.

115. Woodward R et al. Terahertz Pulse Imaging of in vitro basal cell carcinoma samples. In: OSA Trends in Optics and Photonics (TOPS); 2001; Washington DC; pp. 329–30.

116. Weissleder R, Mahmood U. Molecular imaging. Radiology 2001; 219: 316–33.

117. Mathias CJ, Wang S, Lee RJ et al. Tumor-selective radiopharmaceutical targeting via receptor-mediated endocytosis of gallium-67-deferoxamine-folate. J Nucl Med 1996; 37: 1003–8.

118. Wang S, Luo J, Lantrip D et al. Design and synthesis of 111In-DTPA-folate for use as a tumor-targeted radio-pharmaceutical. Bioconjugate Chem 1997; 8: 673–9.

119. Yang D, Inoue T, Kim E. Radiopharmaceuticals for tumor-targeted imaging: Overview. In: Kim E, Yang D, eds. Targeted Molecular Imaging in Oncology. New York: Springer; 2001. pp. 62–82.

120. Scopinaro F, Schillaci O, Scarpini M et al. Technetium-99m sestamibi: an indicator of breast cancer invasiveness. Eur J Nucl Med 1994; 21: 984–7.

121. Yoon JH, Bom HS, Song HC et al. Double-phase Tc-99m sestamibi scintimammography to assess angiogenesis and P-glycoprotein expression in patients with untreated breast cancer. Clin Nucl Med 1999; 24: 314–18.

122. Omar WS, Eissa S, Moustafa H et al. Role of thallium-201 chloride and Tc-99m methoxy-isobutyl-isonitrite (sestaMIBI) in evaluation of breast masses: correlation with the immunohistochemical characteristic parameters (Ki-67, PCNA, Bcl, and angiogenesis) in malignant lesions. Anticancer Res 1997; 17: 1639–44.

123. Lok C. Picture perfect. Nature 2001; 412: 372–4.

124. Gambhir SS, Herschman HR, Cherry SR et al. Imaging transgene expression with radionuclide imaging technologies. Neoplasia 2000; 2: 118–38.

125. Berger F, Gambhir SS. Recent advances in imaging endogenous or transferred gene expression utilizing radionuclide technologies in living subjects: applications to breast cancer. Breast Cancer Res 2001; 3: 28–35.

126 Iyer M, Barrio JR, Namavari M, Bauer E, Satyamurthy N, Nguyen K et al. 8-[18F]Fluoropenciclovir: an improved reporter probe for imaging HSV1– tk reporter gene expression in vivo using PET. J Nucl Med 2001; 42: 96–105.

19 Fine-needle aspiration cytology

Jolanta G McKenzie, Jean Dalrymple

Introduction

The use of fine-needle aspiration cytology (FNAC) in the diagnosis of palpable breast lesions is well established and has superseded diagnostic biopsy with frozen section in most cases. The relative merits of the two techniques were described by Trott and Randall[1] in 1979 and are shown in Table 19.1. Following the Forrest report,[2] which recommended the use of FNAC in the triple approach for the assessment of screen-detected lesions, its use has become widespread in assessment centres where experienced cytopathologists are in post.

In our unit, following 10 years of experience of FNAC work on palpable lesions, this technique has been used in a screening programme that started in 1987, and it continues to be the primary diagnostic technique. FNAC has been accepted as a valuable diagnostic aid that is cost-effective and that has enabled the planning of surgical treatment in advance, with appropriate counselling of the patient. However, for certain mammographic abnormalities (e.g. microcalcification), image-guided core biopsy is now accepted as being more appropriate, Microcalcification can be confirmed to be present within core biopsies by X-raying the cores once they have been taken. An X-ray of the tissue block can also be performed to confirm the presence of microcalcification if required.

There is continuing debate about who should undertake the aspiration – surgeon, radiologist or pathologist – but in the final analysis, the quality of the aspirate is all-important and obviously reflects the expertise of the aspirator. The cytopathologist can only report on the material present on the slide. It is important to remember that a positive result is of significance, whereas a negative one may not be so. The reasons for this will be discussed later in this chapter.

Table 19.1	Relative merits of surgical biopsy and fine-needle aspiration cytology (FNAC)	
	Surgical biopsy	**FNAC**
Diagnosis	Histopathological	Cytopathological
Diagnostic facility	Narrow	Broad
Anaesthetic needed?	Yes	No
Length of procedure	>5 min	<5 min
Wait for report	Long (1–2 days)	Short (30 min if necessary; reduces patient anxiety)
False-positives	None	Rare
False-negatives	Few	Some
Cost	High	Low
Specimen obtained	In operating theatre	As outpatient anywhere
Trauma?	Yes	Little, if any

For cytology to be of benefit in a breast screening programme, the inadequacy rate and benign biopsy rate must be as low as possible. Inadequate aspirates usually need to be repeated or a core biopsy considered if repeated inadequate cytology is obtained. This, however, adds to the cost and causes unnecessary patient anxiety. Benign biopsies add to the surgical cost, cause anxiety and trauma to the patient, and may affect the appearance of future mammograms.

It is imperative that the cytological opinion and any core biopsy findings be considered as part of the triple approach in the assessment of screen-detected lesions, and weekly multidisciplinary meetings should be held at which the relevant findings can be reviewed and discussed.

Preparation of material and staining

The aspirate is either directly smeared on slides or put in saline and cytospin preparations made. The latter are not used in our unit, as the cytospin preparation appears to alter the 'architecture' of the aspirate, which may be helpful in the interpretation of the smear. In addition, they are expensive in technical time and support.

We prefer to take two direct smears from each case: one air-dried and one fixed specimen. It is essential that fixation be immediate and air drying be facilitated by gently waving the slide in the air, thus preserving cellular material and minimising artefact. All slides are labelled with the patient's name and number and are carefully matched with the request form. The fixed slide is stained with haematoxylin and eosin (H&E) and the air-dried slide with May–Grunwald–Giemsa using automatic staining machines. Other centres use the Papanicolau stain rather than an H&E stain, and it is a matter of personal preference which stains are employed. We feel that as the majority of breast carcinomas are of glandular origin, an H&E stain is preferable and cytological appearances are easily compared with subsequent histology. The use of the Giemsa and H&E stains is helpful and the appearances are complementary. The air-drying process results in enlargement of cells, but cellular detail and in particular nuclear detail are preserved, which is critical in the evaluation of whether an aspirate is malignant. Wet fixation results in a reduction in cell size but minimises artefact, and cellular preservation is good. Some centres offer instant reporting in the assessment clinic. Our unit is a busy district hospital pathology department, and it has not been possible to offer this facility on a regular basis due to restricted technical and medical time, although a quick technical and medical result in approximately half an hour can be given if requested by the clinician in a specific case. Slides are double-screened by two pathologists and reported without prior knowledge of the radiological appearances to avoid bias. While obviously positive or negative reports are straightforward, a significant proportion of aspirates from impalpable lesions need careful, quiet consideration and discussion. In our opinion, the additional pressure for instant results makes the reporting of these latter cases particularly difficult, and will increase the number of unhelpful and possibly incorrect reports.

A one-stop diagnostic facility is, however, offered in the one-stop symptomatic clinic for palpable lumps. The pathologist attends the clinic, providing an instant diagnosis on the air-dried slide using a rapid staining technique. The wet fixed slide is then stained routinely in the laboratory after the clinic. Infrequently, a diagnosis is deferred until the fixed slide has been examined.

Technical staff who undertake the staining of the aspirates are encouraged to look at cases, after reporting, and there are several in our department who are able to offer a valuable opinion. This is important in maintaining the level of interest in the service.

General diagnostic patterns

The criteria used for distinguishing between a benign and malignant aspirate are given in Table 19.2. A wide range of histological appearances are seen in the breast, and this is reflected in the cytological appearances. Some of the more difficult diagnostic categories and their cytological appearances are described in more detail later.

Reporting categories

The Marsden grading is used in our unit:

- C1: inadequate
- C2: benign
- C3: suspicious probably benign
- C4: suspicious probably malignant
- C5: malignant

The C1, C2 and C5 categories are relatively straightforward diagnostic groups; however, the C3 and C4 categories are difficult for the cytopathologist to interpret. These categories in particular require careful discussion at the multidisciplinary meetings

Table 19.2   General diagnostic criteria for the recognition of benign and malignant conditions[3]

Criterion	Benign	Malignant
Cellularity	Usually poor or moderate	Usually high
Cell-to-cell cohesion	Good, with large well-defined clusters of cells	Poor, with cell separation resulting in dissociated cells with cytoplasm or small groups of intact cells
Cell arrangement	Even, usually in flat sheets (monolayers)	Irregular with overlapping and 3-dimensional arrangement
Cell types	Mixtures of epithelial, myoepithelial and other cells with fragments of stroma	Usually uniform cell population
Bipolar (elliptical) bare nuclei	Present, often in high numbers	Not conspicuous
Background	Generally clean, except in inflammatory conditions	Occasionally necrotic debris and sometimes inflammatory cells, including macrophages
Nuclear characteristics:		
Size (in relation to red blood cell diameter)	Small	Variable, often large (depending on tumour type)
Pleomorphism	Rare	Common
Nuclear membranes (Pap stain)	Smooth	Irregular with identations
Nucleoli (Pap stain)	Indistinct or small and single	Variable, but may be prominent, large and multiple
Chromatic (Pap stain)	Smooth or fine	Clumped and may be irregular
Additional features	Apocrine metaplasia, foamy macrophages	Mucin, intracytoplasmic lumina

where the radiological, cytological and clinical appearances are considered together and appropriate action taken. The C3 category is a particularly difficult grade, and we would prefer the description 'atypical probably benign'.

Aspirates obtained from palpable lesions are usually representative of that lesion, with a relatively uniform cell population. Aspirates from impalpable lesions may include cells through which the needle has passed, and therefore a dual population of both benign and malignant cells in a single aspirate is not uncommon. This makes reporting more difficult.

Many mammographic abnormalities show microcalcification of both benign and malignant types. The absence of microcalcification in the aspirate from such a site may be significant and may indicate that the needle is not in the lesion. Our aim is to provide a useful result, wherever possible giving a definitive diagnosis of malignancy or benignity with the object of minimising the benign biopsy rate.

C1: inadequate

An aspirate may be inadequate for a variety of reasons:

- poor cellularity with less than five epithelial cell clusters
- artefacts making interpretation difficult – these include heavily bloodstained smears, thick or unevenly spread smears, air-drying artefact, and artefact due to vigorous spreading

The reason for inadequacy must always be stated in the report.

C2: benign (Figures 19.1–19.5)

The components of a benign aspirate include:

- bare nuclei (bipolar cells or myoepithelial cells)
- stromal fragments

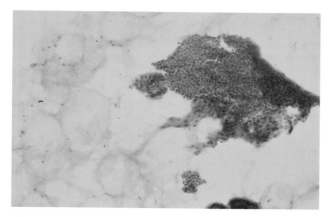

Figure 19.1 Monolayered sheet of cohesive, uniform benign epithelial cells, including apocrine cells; there are background bare nuclei. (H&E, ×20.)

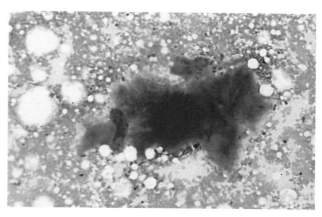

Figure 19.4 Fibroadenoma: myxoid stroma. (Giemsa, ×40.)

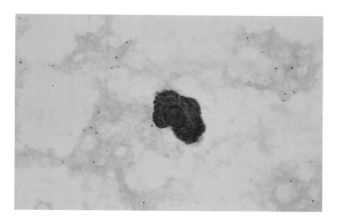

Figure 19.2 Cluster of benign epithelial cells with microcalcification; there are background bare nuclei. (H&E, ×20.)

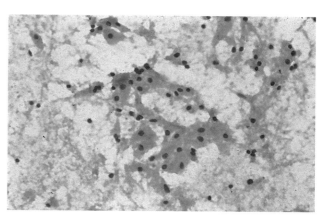

Figure 19.5 Granular cell tumour: groups and single epithelial cells with eosinophilic granular cytoplasm and indistinct cell borders. (H&E, ×20.)

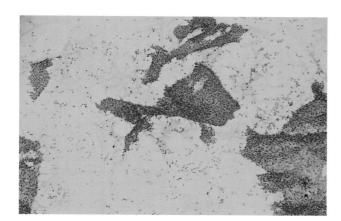

Figure 19.3 Fibroadenoma: papillary monolayered fragment and abundant background bare nuclei. (H&E, ×20.)

- cohesive clusters of uniform epithelial cells with benign cytological features

If the aspirate is from an area of breast tissue showing benign fibrocystic change then the aspirate may also show:

- some background debris with foamy macrophages
- apocrine cells, which may show cytological atypia with variably sized nuclei and prominent central nucleoli with some cell dispersion – the recognition of cytoplasmic granularity and staining characteristics (slate blue on Giemsa and red on H&E) should identify the cell type
- microcalcification

Other features may also be seen in the aspirate if it is from a discrete entity such as a fibroadenoma.

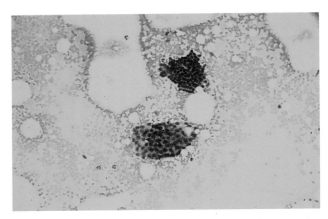

Figure 19.6 C3: the upper cluster shows nuclear enlargement but a normal chromatin pattern; there are scanty background bare nuclei. (Giemsa, ×20.)

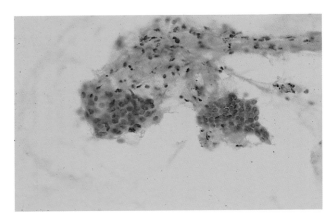

Figure 19.7 C3: there are two epithelial groups, with one cluster showing nuclear enlargement but a normal chromatin pattern. (H&E, ×20.)

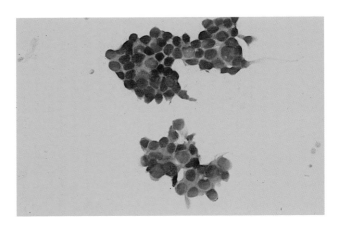

Figure 19.8 C3: clusters show variations in nuclear size and shape but a normal chromatin pattern. (Giemsa, ×40.)

C3: atypical probably benign (Figures 19.6–19.8)

This is perhaps the least helpful category for the radiologist/surgeon, but it is nevertheless occasionally necessary to report smears as such, and it is our aim to keep this category to a minimum. The aspirate will show benign features, but in addition may also show the following:

- increased cellularity
- nuclear cytological atypia with nuclear irregularity, overlapping and nuclear enlargement
- some loss of cohesion with dispersion
- only scanty 'bare' bipolar nuclei
- changes due to treatment or hormonal effect (e.g. hormone replacement therapy, irradiation or even pregnancy)

It appears that aspirates from breast tissue showing epithelial hyperplasia often show the above features, and it has to be accepted that this is a grey area for the pathologist and that the limitations of cytology in this area have become apparent. It may be that, with time and experience, we may learn to recognise particular cytological appearances for this diagnostic group.

C4: suspicious of malignancy (Figures 19.9–19.11)

The aspirate, although suspicious, is not diagnostic of malignancy. This may be for a variety of reasons:

- a scanty specimen showing malignant features
- artefactual changes due to poor preservation or preparation, making a definite opinion difficult
- an aspirate with a predominantly benign pattern but very occasional malignant cells

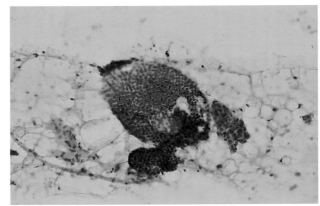

Figure 19.9 C4: dual population with a predominance of benign epithelial cells. There is a small cluster of larger epithelial cells with suspicious nuclear characteristics and a dirty background with scanty bare nuclei. (H&E, ×20.)

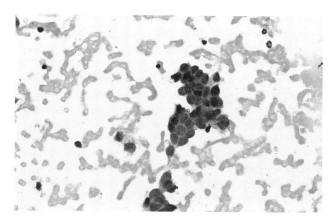

Figure 19.10 C4: large epithelial cells with some dissociation. There is nuclear atypia, but the cells are not clearly malignant. (Giemsa, ×40.)

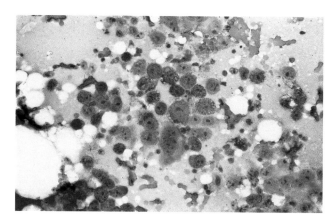

Figure 19.12 C5: large dissociated malignant cells with prominent nuclear cytological atypia, nucleoli and mitotic figures. (Giemsa, ×40.)

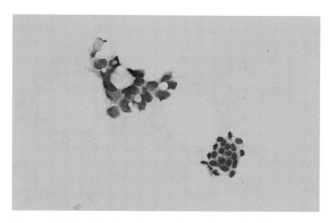

Figure 19.11 C4: the larger cluster shows highly suspicious features but poor preservation. (Giemsa, ×40.)

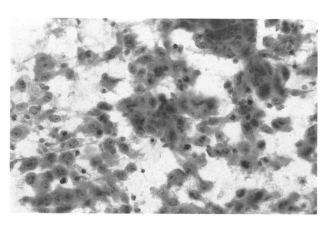

Figure 19.13 C5: large dissociated malignant cells with prominent nuclear cytological atypia, nucleoli and mitotic figures. This is small cell carcinoma. (H&E, ×40.)

- aspirates from well-differentiated carcinomas (e.g. tubular and lobular) where the epithelial cells are small and relatively uniform and cytological atypia is not marked

C5: malignant (Figures 19.12–19.18)

The aspirate shows the cytological features of malignancy (see Table 19.2). Malignant cells should be present in significant numbers. It is important to appreciate that in our experience it is not possible to distinguish between in situ and invasive lesions. Some pathologists have reported that malignant cells seen in stromal fragments indicate invasion. In our opinion, this is not reliable. In many aspirates from malignant tumours of the breast, stroma is scanty and sometimes even absent.

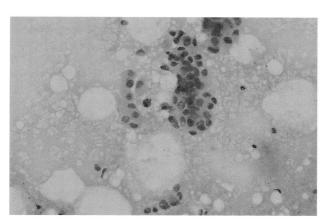

Figure 19.14 Epithelial cells show dispersion with Indian file formation. (H&E, ×40.)

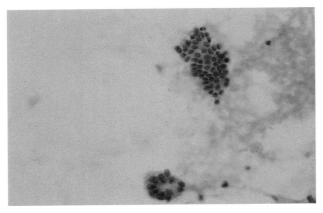

Figure 19.15 Tubule formation. (H&E, ×20.)

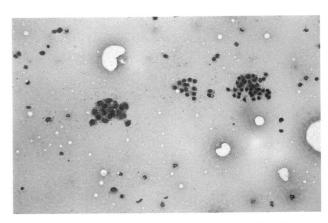

Figure 19.18 Dissociated small epithelial cells with intracytoplasmic vacuoles. This is a lobular carcinoma. (Giemsa, ×20.)

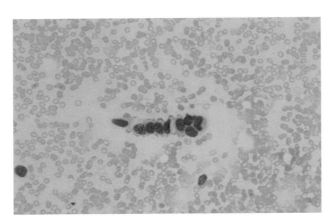

Figure 19.16 Indian file with moulding of cells. (Giemsa, ×40.)

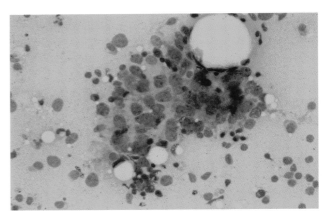

Figure 19.19 Large malignant epithelial cells with associated lymphocytes. This is a medullary carcinoma. (H&E, ×40.)

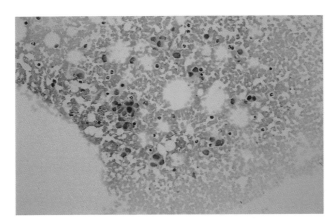

Figure 19.17 Dissociated small epithelial cells. (Giemsa, ×20.)

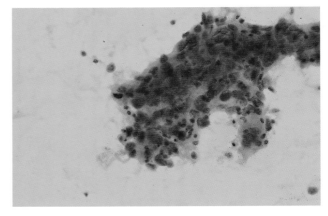

Figure 19.20 Large malignant epithelial cells with associated lymphocytes. This is a medullary carcinoma. (Giemsa, ×40.)

With regard to the reporting of malignant aspirates, some helpful suggestions can be made concerning the particular type of cancer. However, it is important to remember that the aspirate may not be representative of the entire lesion, and mixed tumours do occur:

- An assessment of cell size may indicate whether the tumour is of large cell or small cell type.
- The arrangement of cells in tubular or 'Indian file' profiles suggests tubular or lobular differentiation.
- The presence of abundant mucin is suggestive of colloid carcinoma.
- Abundant lymphocytes associated with large pleomorphic epithelial tumour cells suggests a medullary carcinoma (Figures 19.19 and 19.20). Lymphocytes may also be seen in association with other tumour types.

At present, we do not apply formal grading systems to cytological samples; however, we do comment upon well differentiated and poorly differentiated features.

Immunocytochemical techniques are not routinely performed, but are at present used as a research tool.

Diagnostic difficulties leading to a potentially false-positive result

There are a number of conditions that make the reporting of aspirates difficult and must always be remembered when reporting.

'Hyperplasia'

In our experience, one of the most difficult areas is the interpretation of aspirates from hyperplastic lesions. The aspirates invariably are responsible for the C3 category and occasionally C4. False-positive diagnoses can be avoided if strict diagnostic criteria are adhered to. It is particularly important to discuss these cases carefully with the surgeon and radiologist. These lesions are among the major causes of benign diagnostic surgical biopsies.

Fibroadenoma

The interpretation of aspirates from fibroadenomas can be difficult. They are usually extremely cellular with some cell dispersion and cytological atypia, but the presence of abundant bare bipolar nuclei and myxoid stroma should avoid a false-positive diagnosis.

Papillary tumours

Aspirates from intraductal papillomas can be very cellular with papillary aggregates, and can be difficult to distinguish from in situ and invasive papillary carcinomas. The presence of bare nuclei strongly suggests benign papilloma, while nuclear pleomorphism, necrosis, the absence of bare nuclei and apocrine cells favour diagnosis of malignancy.

Apocrine cells

These can show a variable appearance, particularly in hyperplastic lesions and complex sclerosing lesions/radial scars. It may not always be obvious that the cells are of apocrine origin.

Granular cell tumours

These lesions are composed of cells with indistinct cell membranes and prominent granular cytoplasm that is eosinophilic on the H&E preparation. The nuclei can be variable in size and show some nuclear atypia. Positivity with an S100 immunohistochemical stain and periodic acid–Schiff (PAS) positivity confirm the diagnosis.

Adenomyoepithelial lesions (Figure 19.21)

These lesions are uncommon and as yet incompletely understood. Aspirates from these lesions can show suspicious features with high cellularity and a tendency to dispersion of rather pleomorphic cells, which are actually myoepithelial. Obvious benign epithelial cell clusters and normal bare bipolar nuclei are also present.

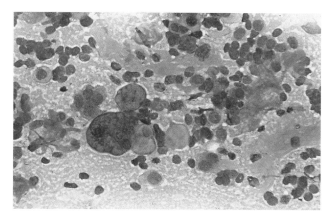

Figure 19.21   Globules of basement membrane material with dissociated myoepithelial cells and epithelial cells. (Giemsa, ×40.)

Radiotherapy

Aspirates from breast tissue that has been irradiated are usually of low cellularity and can show prominent irradiation fibroblasts, which can be mistaken for malignant cells. In addition, epithelial cell changes occur, and marked nuclear pleomorphism and dissociation can be present. Caution should always be taken when reporting such aspirates.

Diagnostic difficulties leading to a potentially false-negative result

The commonest cause of a false-negative result is when the needle is not in the lesion, resulting in an aspiration miss. If the mammographic abnormality is microcalcification and this is not seen in the aspirate, it suggests that the needle may not be in the lesion and the aspirate may therefore not be representative of the abnormality. There are particular tumours that may produce a false-negative result.

Well-differentiated carcinomas (Figures 19.14–19.18)

Tubular carcinomas, cribriform carcinomas and lobular carcinomas will by definition yield aspirates that, on initial inspection, show much in common with benign aspirates. Important features to look for include:

- an absence of bare nuclei
- individual cells and small groups with cytoplasm
- tubular profiles and 'Indian files'
- intracytoplasmic lumina (lobular carcinomas)
- mild cytological atypia.

Such tumours may also result in a C3 or C4 diagnosis.

Sclerotic carcinomas

These tumours, by definition, have abundant fibrous stroma and therefore may yield either an acellular aspirate or stromal fragments only.

Other lesions

Lymph nodes

It is always important to remember that intramammary lymph nodes are present within the breast and that they can be benign or malignant. The recognition of a lymphoid origin is important. It is also important to remember that some in situ and invasive carcinomas are associated with a lymphoid response, without this necessarily being typical of a medullary carcinoma.

Metastatic carcinoma in lymph nodes may be the presenting feature of breast cancer when the primary tumour may be small and undetected. Lymph nodes can be almost entirely replaced by metastatic tumour and an aspirate may not show an obvious lymph node origin.

Primary lymphoma of the breast does occur, as does lymphomatous involvement. Clinical information is all important, and immunocytochemistry will be helpful in such cases.

Metastatic tumours

Metastatic small cell carcinoma ('oat cell' carcinoma) of the lung has been seen rarely in breast aspirates. Metastatic melanoma has also been reported, and careful attention must be paid to the cytological appearance and pattern, especially if melanin pigment is absent.

Other metastatic tumours have been reported, including ovarian and renal carcinomas.

Stromal lesions

Fibromatosis can occur in the breast, and typical fibroblasts, spindle-shaped with regular nuclei, are present in the aspirate. Malignant stromal tumours occur, but are rare.

Metaplastic carcinomas are more common, and should be considered first in any aspirate showing sarcomatous features.

Phyllodes tumours

The benign variants will show cytological appearances similar to that of a fibroadenoma; however, a clue to the diagnosis is an excess of bare bipolar nuclei, and cellular stromal fragments with myxoid material.

Malignant variants will show benign epithelial cells with malignant characteristics in spindle-shaped cells.

Results

FNAC has been used in our unit since November 1987. Table 19.3 shows an analysis of the cytology results for the prevalence round (1987–90) and an incidence round (1991–93). The suggested minimum values shown are taken from the NHSBSP Publication.[3] It is reassuring to note that in comparing the prevalence and incidence rounds, the inadequacy and false-negative rates have improved and that sensitivity and specificity rates are well above the recommended minimum values.

Table 19.4 shows the biopsy results since 1987. The malignant-to-benign ratio illustrates the learning curve in the early years and emphasises the small number of benign biopsies since 1991.

Conclusion

The use of FNAC has been shown to decrease the benign biopsy rate, to assist in the early diagnosis of breast cancer and to allow planned cost-effective treatment in the breast screening unit. In addition, for the patient, it reduces the number of operations and allows pretreatment discussion and counselling.

References

1. Trott PA. Fine needle aspiration cytology. Lancet 1979; ii: 253.
2. The Forrest Report, 1986.
3. Cytology Sub-Group of the National Coordinating Committee for Breast Screening Pathology. Guidelines for Cytology Procedures and Reporting in Breast Cancer Screening. NHSBSP Publication 22. Sheffield: NHS Breast Cancer Screening Programme, 1992.

Table 19.3 Cytology results in prevalence and incidence rounds

	Prevalence round	Incidence round	Suggested minimal value
Absolute sensitivity (%)	71.8	69.6	>60
Complete sensitivity (%)	87.2	88.8	>80
Specificity (full) (%)	74.7	78.3	>60
Positive predictive value (C5) (%)	100.0	99.1	>95
False-negative rate (%)	6.2	3.1	<5
False positive rate (%)	0.00	0.6	<1
Inadequacy rate (%)	12.6	8.0	<25

Table 19.4 Biopsy results 1987–94

Year	Benign	Malignant	Total	Malignant/ benign
1987/8	24	50	74	2.0
1989	28	100	128	3.5
1990	21	106	127	5.0
1991	13	82	95	6.3
1992	13	60	73	4.6
1993	16	45	61	2.8
1994	5	42	47	8.4

20 Core and diagnostic biopsies

Peter Britton, Michael WE Morgan

Introduction

Tissue diagnosis of the breast can be carried out by one of four available techniques:

- fine needle-aspiration cytology (FNAC)
- core biopsy (CB)
- incisional biopsy
- excisional biopsy.

High-quality needle biopsy, whether FNAC or CB, is essential for accurate patient diagnosis. A high level of preoperative cancer diagnosis will enable suitable patient counselling prior to definitive cancer surgery. High needle biopsy specificity will reduce the number of patients requiring unnecessary surgery or follow-up. Clearly, no diagnostic test is 100% accurate and there will be instances when patients require a surgical excision to reach a definitive diagnosis. Such patient management decision-making should be taken in a multidisciplinary team setting where clinical, imaging and needle biopsy findings can all be taken into consideration.

Core biopsy

FNAC has been the mainstay of breast needle biopsy since the introduction of the UK National Health Service Breast Screening Programme (NHSBSP) in the late 1980s. More recently, however, there has been an increasing use of wide-bore needle CB in breast diagnosis.[1] Solid cores of breast tissue are removed, sufficient for paraffin-embedded histological examination allowing assessment of both breast architecture and cellular morphology. This has several advantages over FNAC. Although skilled interpretation is required, the services of a highly specialised breast cytopathologist are not needed. Diagnosis of definite malignancy or benignity can frequently be reached with fewer equivocal biopsy results. Invasive versus in situ malignancy, tumour grade and hormone receptor status can also be evaluated. More recently, vacuum-assisted biopsy (VAB) devices have been developed. These deliver larger amounts of tissue and promise a higher degree of diagnostic accuracy, but at increased expense.[2]

Clearly, no percutaneous biopsy technique will be foolproof. Interpretation of all biopsy results should be undertaken in a multidisciplinary team setting where clinical and imaging information is also available. Where diagnostic uncertainty or concern regarding malignancy persists, diagnostic surgical biopsy is required.

Technique

CB should be performed using an automated gun, as these yield larger samples than disposable devices. The original Biopty device has made way for lighter more flexible devices. Best results are obtained using larger gauge (14G) needles with longer throw (23 mm).[3] The procedure is performed under local anaesthetic and a 2–3 mm skin nick is required to introduce the needle. Although breast lumps can be biopsied using manual palpation, image guidance does allow more accurate needle placement. For impalpable sonographically visible lesions, the method of choice is to perform CB using ultrasound guidance (Figure 20.1). Two needle passes are usually sufficient to achieve a reliable diagnosis. For sonographically invisible lesions, which include the majority of microcalcifications, stereotactic mammographic guidance is necessary. The majority of such units consist of 'add-on' devices attached to standard upright mammography units, using either analogue or digital technology to produce an image (Figure 20.2). Dedicated prone stereotactic biopsy units are available, and have the advantage of increased comfort with consequently less patient movement and syncope. The disadvantages of such units are their great expense and their limitation to biopsy only. When microcalcification is biopsied, 5–10 or even more passes are required to achieve

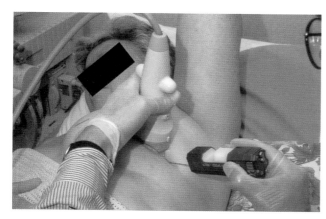

Figure 20.1 A patient undergoing ultrasound-guided breast biopsy using a spring-loaded biopsy device (Bard Magnum).

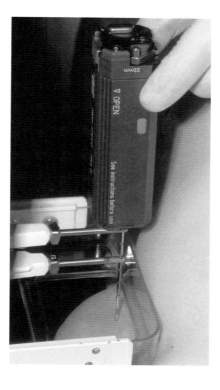

Figure 20.2 A patient undergoing a stereotactically guided breast biopsy using an 'add-on' unit and a 14-gauge biopsy needle.

reliable diagnostic accuracy,[4] and it is mandatory to perform specimen radiography to confirm that representative calcification has been retrieved.[5]

Complications

Ecchymosis of varying degree is almost universal, but the incidence of serious complications is remarkably low. The rate of surgical haematoma formation (with or without infection) requiring surgical drainage is of the order of 0.2%.[6] Tumour epithelial seeding along the biopsy track has been reported, but its precise incidence and, more importantly, its significance remain unclear.[7]

Table 20.1 Core biopsy reporting categories used in the UK NHS Breast Screening Programme[8]

Reporting category	Tissue type	Notes
B1	Normal tissue	Pathology includes: • Lipomas or hamartomas Note that this category may also indicate that a lesion has not been sampled
B2	Benign lesion	Pathology includes: • A wide variety of benign changes • Epithelial hyperplasia of usual type (HUT)
B3	Lesion of uncertain malignant potential	Pathology includes: • ADH with moderate degrees of atypia • Lobular neoplasia (ALH and LCIS) • Papillary lesions • Phyllodes tumour
B4	Suspicious of malignancy	Pathology includes: • Probable carcinoma cells but where the sample is too small, crushed or poorly preserved for diagnostic certainty • ADH with a high degree of atypia
B5	Malignant	This should state whether invasive or in situ malignancy is demonstrated Estimation of tumour grade and hormone receptor status can also be made

ADH, atypical ductal hyperplasia; ALH, atypical lobular hyperplasia; LCIS, lobular carcinoma in situ.

Table 20.2   Performance results comparing FNAC with CB under stereotactic and ultrasound guidance using published data on over 17,000 needle biopsies[9]

	Stereotactic biopsy		Ultrasound biopsy	
	FNAC (%)	CB (%)	FNAC (%)	CB (%)
Absolute sensitivity	62.4	90.5	83.1	96.7
Complete sensitivity	83.1	94.6	95.1	98.5
Specificity	86.9	98.3	84.0	98.7
Positive predictive value malignant (B5) biopsy	99.3	99.5	98.3	100
False-positive rate	0.5	0.4	1.4	0
Inadequate rate	6.4	1.0	12.8	0.05
Inadequate rate in cancers	5.0	1.5	2.1	0

Table 20.3   Performance results comparing FNAC with CB in the NHS Breast Screening Programme in 1996–97[10] and 1996–2000[8]

	1996–97		1996–2000	
	FNAC median (%)	CB median (%)	FNAC median (%)	CB median (%)
Absolute sensitivity	53.6	75	57.1	76.4
Complete sensitivity	81.8	76.6	81.5	84.5
Specificity	57.8	84.2	58.4	81.2
Positive predictive value malignant (B5) biopsy	100	100	99.6	100
False-positive rate	0	0	0.2	0
False-negative rate	6.3	13.0	6.3	15.1[a]
Inadequate rate	23.2	10.6	23.4	NA
Inadequate rate in cancers	10.6	7.4	9.8	NA

NA, not available.
[a]Miss rate (B1 + B2) from cancer.

Reporting categories

In the NHSBSP, CB results are classified into five groups (B1 to B5).[8] This classification is described in Table 20.1.

Performance results: CB versus FNAC

A review of the literature comparing CB with FNAC performance in over 17 000 biopsies is shown in Table 20.2.[9] CB has both higher sensitivity and increased specificity when compared with FNAC. Studies of the results using FNAC and CB in the NHSBSP also show overall better results for CB (Table 20.3) with one important exception: the false-negative rate (a benign needle biopsy result in the presence of a cancer) is significantly higher for CB than for FNAC.[8,10]

Although overall results are better for CB, it is clear that some units have extremely good results using FNAC.[10] FNAC also has the advantages of being cheaper and capable of same-session reporting so that truly 'one-stop' clinics can be undertaken. Whatever biopsy technique is performed, it is vital that both unit and individual clinician performance be openly monitored.

Problem areas for CB (Table 20.4)

False-negative CB
Examination of the NHSBSP (Table 20.3) shows that operators using CB are more likely to have obtained

Table 20.4   **Problem areas for core biopsy**
• False-negative core biopsy
• Ductal carcinoma in situ versus invasive disease
• Atypical ductal hyperplasia
• Lobular neoplasia (lobular carcinoma in situ and atypical lobular hyperplasia)
• Radial scar

an erroneous benign biopsy result in the presence of a cancer.[8] This is likely to represent poor targeting and sampling of lesions rather than pathological misinterpretation and underlines the importance of adherence to meticulous technique.[10] It also illustrates the importance of interpreting all biopsy results in a multidisciplinary team setting. If suspicion regarding potential malignancy persists following a benign biopsy result then the biopsy should either be repeated or diagnostic surgical biopsy undertaken.

Ductal cancer in situ versus invasive malignancy

CB may underestimate the presence of invasive disease. Twenty percent of CBs that reveal ductal cancer in situ (DCIS) only will be found to have invasive disease at subsequent surgery.[7,11] Patients with a preoperative CB diagnosis of DCIS should therefore be warned that subsequent surgery may reveal invasive disease, which would usually necessitate surgical staging of the axilla.

Atypical ductal hyperplasia

CB may also underestimate the presence of DCIS. In 40–50% of cases where the CB reveals atypical ductal hyperplasia (ADH), subsequent surgical histology will reveal DCIS.[7,12] Any patient whose CB produces a diagnosis of ADH should therefore undergo diagnostic surgical excision.

Lobular neoplasia

Lobular carcinoma in situ (LCIS) and atypical lobular hyperplasia (ALH) are pathological entities that are occasionally diagnosed on CB and are collectively referred to as 'lobular neoplasia'. They are encountered as incidental findings or may occasionally account for a mammographic abnormality, usually a cluster of microcalcification.[13] The reported incidence of ALH varies from 0.05% to 0.5% of needle biopsies. In those patients subsequently undergoing surgical excision, carcinoma can be found in up to 20%.[7,14,15] The reported incidence

of LCIS also varies widely, from 0.02% to 2% of needle biopsies, and must reflect different histopathological reporting patterns. However, in those patients undergoing surgical excision, up to 30% can be found to have carcinomas.[7,14,15] The exact incidence and significance of lobular neoplasia is still emerging. It is, however, associated with increased breast cancer risk in general, as well as adjacent to the needle biopsy site. We would therefore advocate that when LCIS or ALH is diagnosed on needle biopsy, subsequent surgical excision be undertaken.[13]

Radial scar

Radial scars are benign lesions usually detected by screening mammography as areas of parenchymal distortion or spiculation often mimicking a carcinoma. Although CB can frequently suggest a diagnosis of radial scar, it will frequently not diagnose the associated areas of malignancy that can occur in these lesions.[7] In addition, there may be overlap in the histopathological appearances of radial scars and tubular carcinomas, and care is required to prevent a false-positive CB result.[10]

Vacuum-assisted biopsy

More recently, VAB probes (Mammotome, Ethicon Endosurgery and Minimally Invasive Breast Biopsy, US Surgical) have been developed. Probe sizes vary from 8G to 14G and although most frequently used with stereotactic guidance, they may now also be introduced using ultrasound control. The advantage of such devices is that substantially larger specimens can be obtained than with conventional CB without an increase in the complication rate. VAB is more successful than CB in retrieving microcalcification.[12] Small clusters of calcification are not infrequently removed by the VAB device. In such instances, a small metallic clip can be inserted to mark the biopsy site if subsequent surgery is required. Underestimation of disease is also lower with VAB than with conventional CB. When ADH is diagnosed on VAB, subsequent surgical histology reveals DCIS in only approximately 15% (compared with 40–50% for conventional core biopsy).[12] Where VAB reveals a diagnosis of DCIS only, invasive carcinoma is found at subsequent surgery in approximately 10% of patients (compared with 20% with conventional CB).[16] The main disadvantage of VAB is the expense of the probe, which is 15–20 times more expensive than conventional CB. However, this should be offset against reduced surgical costs.

CB and VAB are able to diagnose benign and malignant breast conditions with a high degree of accuracy. However, no technique is perfect and interpretation of a biopsy should take place in a multidisciplinary team setting. If concern regarding malignancy persists even in the presence of a benign needle biopsy result then surgical diagnostic biopsy should be undertaken. Surgical excision should also be performed on all patients with 'borderline' pathology such as ADH, ALH and LCIS.

Surgical biopsy

Incisional biopsy

During this procedure, a portion of the mass is excised – usually under general anaesthesia, although local anaesthetia may be used for smaller masses. It is usually performed when there is an index of suspicion either mammographically or cytologically that cannot be confirmed by either modality. Common situations in which this would arise are:

- widespread mixed calcification
- spiculated masses with benign cytology
- areas of increased density with atypical cytology
- where the CB or FNAC does not correlate with the mammographic abnormality.

Excisional biopsy

This approach is frequently used for small localised lesions and again it can be carried out under local anaesthesia for superficial lesions or general anaesthetia for those lesions that are more deeply placed. It is recommended in a number of situations:

- *Patient desire* – despite counselling and reassurance, a number of patients will not rest until a mammographic lesion has been removed.
- *Lesion increasing in size* despite benign FNAC or CB (e.g. fibroadenoma).
- *Radial scars* – although a histological diagnosis, mammographically these frequently mimic small invasive tumours.
- *Small expanding lesions* in which the needle biopsy result may not be representative in view of their small size.
- *Lesions radiologically and needle biopsy suspicious without definite evidence of malignancy* – these lesions would include 'borderline' pathology such as ADH, ALH and LCIS on CB.

Operation

Prior to the operation – indeed ideally at the assessment visit – the patient will have been counselled to allay fear and to explain the operative procedure and reassured that nothing more than the procedure for which she has consented will be carried out. On the day of the operation, the patient must be examined by the operating surgeon and palpable lesions marked accurately. Impalpable lesions will have been localised with a guidewire either by stereotaxis or ultrasound or by measurement marking using the true lateral and craniocaudal view, allowing the surgeon to place the needle at the point of surgical incision.

Occasionally, two guidewires are used to mark the distal limits of more extensive lesions, thus allowing, after X-ray confirmation of the specimen, more adequate total excision of the abnormality. The current mammogram must be available and mounted on a viewing box in the operating theatre at the time of operation. This allows review of the mammogram during the operative procedure and, when excision of the mammographic abnormality is carried out with X-ray confirmation of the specimen, comparison with a specimen X-ray mammogram as a check for adequacy of excision.

When excising benign lesions within 5 cm of the areola, a periareolar incision not encompassing more than half the circumference of the areola will allow good access, and the lesion is easily removed either with skin retraction or by tunnelling through the subcutaneous breast tissue. This usually results in an excellent scar.

When operating on any breast mass with a suspicion of malignancy, one must always place the incision such that it would not compromise the incisions for a mastectomy that may be advised following the result of the diagnostic biopsy.

For lesions more than 5 cm from the areola or lesions with a suspicion of malignancy, a curvilinear incision over the mass and parallel to the areola will allow good access and heal well. More peripheral lesions in the medial and lateral sixths are best approached via a radial incision for the reasons mentioned above. Of particular difficulty are lesions inferior to the nipple close to the periphery of the breast. For these, better cosmetic results are sometimes obtained via a radial incision. The acceptable incisions are indicated in Figure 20.3.

Biopsy excision technique

Excision of palpable lesion

The mass will have been marked preoperatively. It is necessary to re-examine the breast on the unprepared patient in the operating theatre to reorientate oneself with the clinical picture. It is remarkable

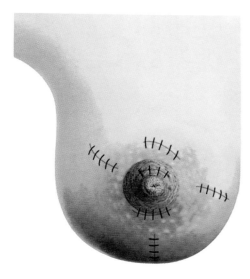

Figure 20.3 Acceptable incisions for breast biopsies.

how difficult it can be to palpate the lump intraoperatively. With lumps that are difficult to feel, it is sometimes helpful to insert a 21G hypodermic needle through the skin into the mass, thereby fixing it, and using this needle as an intraoperative guide.

The skin and subcutaneous tissue are incised and all bleeding points secured. The mass is palpated, the extent assessed and the mass excised. Depending on the size of the residual cavity, the breast tissue may be opposed with absorbable sutures and, unless the cavity is very small, all wounds are best drained for 24 hours.

Excision of impalpable lesion
The lesion will have been marked pre-operatively with a guidewire. An incision is made close to the guidewire, the subcutaneous tissue dissected and the guidewire delivered into the wound. A small self-retaining retractor is placed into the wound and the incision with a knife carried down into the breast tissue adjacent to the guidewire until the lesion is reached. If there is a high degree of suspicion, the lesion is excised together with a 1 cm clearance of normal breast tissue around the lesion. If the index of suspicion is low, simple excision alone is sufficient.

One should avoid using cutting diathermy, as this frequently scars the margins and makes histological interpretation difficult. In addition, if the diathermy touches the guidewire, the latter will either melt or vaporise. Similarly, scissors should be avoided, as these can frequently cut through the guidewire. The size of the residual cavity will dictate whether the breast tissue should be closed and whether the wound should be drained. The specimen removed

from the patient is marked. Many methods have been described, but the simplest is to place a nylon suture at the nipple end of the specimen and a silk suture at the skin surface of the specimen, which is then sent for immediate X-ray to confirm that the mammographic abnormality has been removed. The specimen is then sent fresh without fixative to the pathology department with sutures as described and a pathology request form showing the site of the lesion in the breast to orientate the specimen.

Antibiotics

Antibiotics are rarely indicated for diagnostic biopsies, although there may be clinical situations in which they are recommended, such as patients with diabetes or who are immunocompromised, HIV-infected or on steroids.

Day surgery

It is not good policy to admit patients to day surgery units. This removes them from the team support that is so essential, and it is unlikely that specimen X-rays will be available on day surgery units. However, the operation may be performed as a day case within the breast unit environment.

Conclusions

In a breast care programme, it is imperative to keep the number of benign diagnostic open biopsies performed to a minimum. 'Triple' assessment involving clinical examination, imaging (mammography and ultrasound) and needle biopsy enables a high degree of diagnostic accuracy in the majority of cases. Interpretation of diagnostic information should take place in a multidisciplinary team setting. Teamwork and regular monitoring of working practices will result in high quality and safe patient care and will reduce the number of unnecessary diagnostic surgical operations to a minimum.

References

1. Britton PD, Flower CDR, Freeman, AH et al. Changing to core biopsy in an NHS breast screening unit. Clin Radiol 1997; 52: 764–7.
2. Burbank F, Parker SH, Fobarty TH. Stereotactic breast biopsy: Improved tissue harvesting with the mammotome. Am Surg 1996; 9: 738–43.
3. Nath ME, Robinson TM, Tobson H et al. Automated large-core needle biopsy of surgically removed breast

lesions: Comparison of samples obtained with 14-, 16-, and 18-gauge needles. Radiology 1995; 197: 739–42.

4. Liberman L, Dershaw DD, Rosen PP et al. Stereotaxic 14-gauge breast biopsy: how many core biopsy specimens are needed? Radiology 1994; 192: 793–5.

5. Bagnall MJC, Evans AJ, Wilson ARM et al. When have mammographic calcifications been adequately sampled at needle core biopsy? Clin Radiol 2000; 55: 548–53.

6. Parker SH, Burbank F, Jackman RJ et al. Percutaneous large-core breast biopsy: a multi-institutional study. Radiology 1994; 193: 359–64.

7. Liberman L. Clinical management issues in percutaneous core breast biopsy. Radiol Clin North Am 2000; 38: 791–807.

8. Ellis IO, Humphreys S, Michell M et al. Guidelines for Non-operative Diagnostic Procedures and Reporting in Breast Cancer Screening. NHSBSP Publication 50. Sheffield: NHS Breast Screening Programme, 2001.

9. Britton PD. Fine needle aspiration or core biopsy. Breast 1999; 8: 1–4.

10. Britton PD, McCann J. Needle biopsy in the NHS Breast Screening Programme 96/97: How much and how accurate? Breast 1999; 8: 5–11.

11. Jackman RJ, Burbank F, Parker SH et al. Stereotactic breast biopsy of nonpalpable lesions: determinants of ductal carcinoma in situ underestimation rates. Radiology 2001; 218: 497–502.

12. Jackman RJ, Burbank F, Parker SH et al. Atypical ductal hyperplasia diagnosed at stereotactic breast biopsy: improved reliability with 14-gauge, directional, vacuum-assisted biopsy. Radiology 1997; 204: 485–8.

13. O 'Driscoll D, Britton PD, Bobrow L et al. Lobular carcinoma in situ on core biopsy – what is the clinical significance? Clin Radiol 2001; 56: 216–20.

14. Reynolds HE. Core needle biopsy of challenging benign breast conditions: a comprehensive literature review. AJR Am J Roentgenol 2000; 174: 1245–50.

15. Berg WA, Mrose HE, Ioffe OB. Atypical lobular hyperplasia or lobular carcinoma in situ at core-needle breast biopsy. Radiology 2001; 218: 503–9.

16. Jackman RJ, Nowels KW, Rodriguez-Soto J et al. Stereotactic, automated, large-core needle biopsy of nonpalpable breast lesions: false-negative and histologic underestimation rates after long-term follow-up. Radiology 1999; 210: 799–805.

21 Preoperative localisation of impalpable breast abnormalities

Guidubaldo Querci della Rovere, Ashraf Patel, Nicola Roche, Gina Brown, Lorenzo Orzalesi, John R Benson

Introduction

The detection and excision of impalpable breast lesions is an increasingly common event due to the number of abnormalities identified with mammographic screening. Preoperative localisation of impalpable breast lesions permits accurate surgical excision and minimises cosmetic deformity. A successful outcome depends upon the following criteria being met:

- The impalpable lesion is accurately localised (usually with a guidewire).
- The surgical incision is appropriately placed.
- An adequate volume of breast tissue is excised compatible with complete surgical excision of the tumour and good cosmesis.

The techniques for excising impalpable lesions constitute a relatively new surgical challenge, and the precise methods employed for both radiological localisation and surgical approach vary between centres.

Historical perspective

Dodd et al[1] first described the technique for localisation of impalpable breast lesions in 1966. Several different techniques for preoperative localisation have subsequently been described, involving either positioning of some form of needle[2–5] or hook wire[6–8] or alternatively injection of dye/isotope.[9–12] Whichever form of localisation is used, accurate placement is undertaken with stereotactic devices,[13,14] perforated grids[15,16] or combined radiological/clinical measurements.[17]

Needle and/or hookwire

In 1976, Frank et al[6] first proposed the use of a needle and hookwire for localisation, and this is currently the most commonly employed method. Following infiltration with local anaesthetic, the hookwire and needle are introduced through a small skin incision. Once in the correct position, the hookwire is advanced slightly and the outer needle withdrawn, thus leaving the inner hookwire in situ. The simplest method for guiding placement of the wire is by use of ultrasonography, but many impalpable lesions (especially microcalcifications) are sonographically occult. The insertion of the hookwire and needle has traditionally been performed by radiologists using a fenestrated compression plate to guide the placement of the wire. The advent of stereotactic mammographic machines permits accurate localisation of a mammographic abnormality via three dimensional coordinates that can be targeted without the need for a perforated plate.

The dye/charcoal technique

This procedure utilises a high-stability and low-dispersion dye[11] (a suspension of sterile charcoal in 3% saline) to localise an impalpable lesion. No local anaesthesia is required and the dye is injected directly into the lesion under stereotactic mammography or ultrasound guidance. A black trail is left behind, extending from the lesion towards the skin, where a small tattoo mark is visible (Figure 21.1).

The surgical approach varies depending on whether stereotactic guidance or ultrasound has been

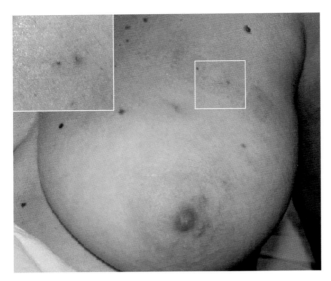

Figure 21.1 The charcoal technique skin tattoo; magnified in cartouche.

employed for the dye injection. With an ultrasound-guided technique, the tattoo corresponds exactly to the skin projection of the lesion. On the other hand, with stereotactic guidance, the skin tattoo does not correspond to the skin projection of the lesion but indicates only the position of the lesion relative to the vertical or the horizontal plane. Dissection proceeds from the skin tattoo along the track towards the end of the charcoal trail. The latter is considered to represent the centre of the lesion, and the surgeon removes this area of breast tissue with an adequate margin but avoiding excessive removal of breast parenchyma.

The stability of charcoal allows injection to be performed at the same time that fine-needle aspiration cytology (FNAC) is performed, and definitive surgery may be delayed for up to 1 month. Problems with this technique include difficulty of dye injection in patients with fibrous breasts and dispersion of the dye within the breast following core biopsies.

Stereotactic guidance/perforated plate guidance

The shortest route from the skin surface to the lesion must be determined prior to localisation. For lesions in the superior half of the breast, a craniocaudal (CC) approach is generally used, whilst for lesions in the inferior half of the breast, a lateral or medial approach is preferred.

The principle of stereotaxis involves taking two initial films 10°–15° in opposite directions. The position of the lesion on each view is compared with the position of a standard reference point and the coordinates describing the lesion's location within the breast are calculated. There are three coordinates, which collectively define the position of the lesion. The x-axis coordinate (the position in the horizontal plane) is calculated automatically by the intrinsic software of the stereotactic equipment and is a mean value of the x-axis coordinates between the stereotactic pair of films. The y-axis coordinate (the position in the vertical plane) is set by the radiologist and is coincident on both stereo-tactic images. The z-axis refers to the depth of the lesion within the breast and is also calculated by the software.

The patient is positioned and a scout image is first obtained with the lesion lying central. The stereo-tactic pair of films is then taken and the correct positioning of the needle determined from coordinate measurements. Following insertion of the needle and hookwire together, the needle is subsequently removed and a final pair of images (CC and true lateral) is taken to confirm the location of the wire relative to the lesion.

An alternative method uses a perforated compression plate (which replaces the standard mammographic compression plate), which is placed against the skin surface at the site where the needle will be inserted. As with stereotactic guidance, the site of the needle insertion needs to be determined prior to localisation. An image is obtained that indicates the location of the lesion relative to the landmarks on the compression plate. The grid system (letters or numbers) allows the appropriate perforation on the plate to be selected, and the needle and hookwire is inserted through it. An image is usually taken at this stage to confirm that the needle placement is satisfactory in relation to the lesion. The needle is removed, leaving the hookwire in situ and a final pair of images is taken.

With both of these techniques, the needle is inserted through breast tissue that is compressed between mammographic plates in either a CC or a lateral position, depending on the site of the lesion. The needle is advanced in a direction parallel to the chest wall and the wire may enter the skin at a site that is remote from the lesion. If the surgical incision is centred around the entry point of the wire then extensive dissection along the wire may be necessary. This can lead to removal of a large volume of tissue with a poor cosmetic result, and is not recommended. Prior to making any skin incision, the surgeon must estimate the location of the lesion in the breast by measuring the distance of the lesion from the nipple in both the horizontal plane (medial or lateral) on the CC film and in the vertical plane (above and below nipple) on the true lateral mammogram. This method of triangulation is described in further detail below. The skin incision should be made over the skin projection of the lesion. The aim of surgery is to excise the lesion with clear radial margins while avoiding excessive removal of tissue. It is preferable that the dissection be commenced at the margin from which the wire approaches the lesion. For instance, if the mammographic abnormality is in the upper outer quadrant of the breast then the wire will probably have been inserted via the CC route with the breast compressed in this position. Under these circumstances, if the superior margin is dissected first, the wire should be encountered within the breast tissue as it approaches the lesion. Once the wire has been identified, the remaining radial margins can be dissected systematically. For diagnostic procedures, the amount of breast tissue excised should be restricted to 20 g or less in accordance with the quality assurance guidelines of the NHS Breast Screening Programme (NHSBSP).[18] Once excised, the specimen (with wire in situ) should be carefully orientated using both sutures and ligaclips and specimen radiography performed to confirm adequacy of excision.

Technique of radiological/clinical measurements

Needle insertion is usually undertaken by radiologists using a perforated plate and is carried out in a plane parallel to the chest wall. The needle and wire are inserted while the breast is compressed between mammographic plates, and a perforated grid facilitates localisation. Depending on the precise site of the lesion, the wire can be introduced from either a CC or a lateral direction. Often, the wire enters the skin at a site that is relatively distant from the skin projection of the mammographic abnormality and tends to follow a course parallel to the chest wall

due to the compression of the breast. This is particularly the case for lesions lying centrally and close to the chest wall which are associated with wire entry at the extreme periphery of the breast. We do not favour this technique, as the surgeon is obliged either to tunnel along the wire for a relatively long distance (which may jeopardise cosmesis) or to guess the location of the lesion and make a surgical incision overlying the tip of the needle. The latter has to be searched for and there is a risk that tumour tissue is cut through. We therefore recommend insertion of the needle perpendicular to the chest wall (Figure 21.2).

Technique of localisation

We prefer the Cook breast localisation needle hook Type B DHBL-22-9 (William Cook Europe A/S wire) for the following reasons:

- It is a fine-gauge needle and insertion is relatively pain-free.
- Local anaesthesia is not required.
- Sterile gloves need not be worn.
- Insertion is relatively easy and takes only seconds.
- The needle can be easily replaced if necessary.
- A selection of introducing needles is available (18–23G).
- It is graduated, permitting recognition of distance from the tip.
- Two sets of needles and wires are available, with lengths suited for either small or large breasts.

A combination of radiological and clinical measurements are used to permit accurate insertion of the hookwire. The distance of the lesion from the nipple is measured on two mammographic views (true lateral and CC) (Figure 21.3). These measurements

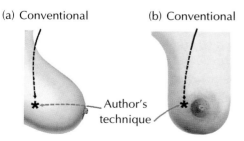

Figure 21.2 (a) True lateral view of the breast showing the direction of the wire with the conventional technique and that of the present authors. (b) View of the breast and the point of entry of the wire with the two methods of wire insertion.

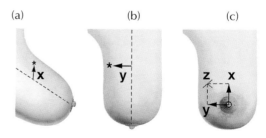

Figure 21.3 Radiological clinical measurement. (a) Measurement of distance (x) of lesion from the nipple plane on true lateral view. (b) Measurement of distance (y) of lesion from nipple plane on craniocaudal view. (c) The two measurements x and y are transferred on the patient's breast: the resulting point (z) is the skin projection of the lesion.

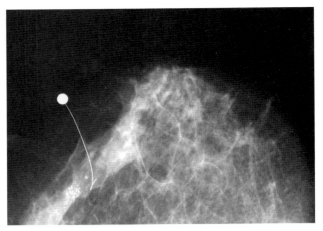

Figure 21.5 Postlocalisation film: craniocaudal view.

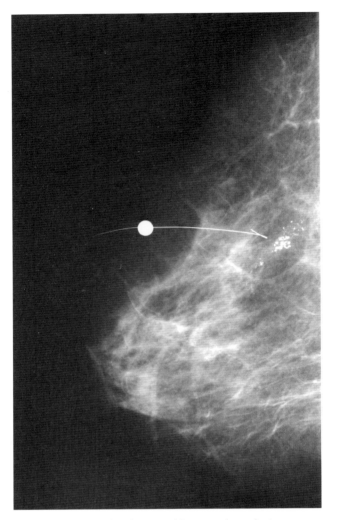

Figure 21.4 Postlocalisation film: true lateral view.

are subsequently translated into anatomical measurements on the breast itself. The resulting point of intersection represents the skin projection of the lesion. This point is critical because it provides the surgeon with the closest and most direct access to the breast lesion and corresponds to the site where the surgical incision would have been made had the lump been palpable. This is therefore the point where the hookwire is inserted, and the procedure is carried out without local anaesthesia and minimal discomfort is experienced by the patient.

With the patient lying supine and with arms elevated, the needle is inserted through the predetermined point at an angle that follows the line of the two planes of intersection with a direction perpendicular to the chest wall. Women with large pendulous breasts that tend to fall laterally are asked to turn slightly to the opposite side so that the breast lies more medially on a flat surface. Following wire insertion, films are taken (CC and true lateral) to

ascertain the position of the wire in relation to the lesion (Figures 21.4 and 21.5). It is generally considered acceptable if the wire lies within a radial distance of 2 cm for malignant lesions and 1 cm for diagnostic biopsies (a more limited volume of tissue is excised).

Excision of these impalpable lesions is carried out via an incision that passes through or lies in proximity to the point of entry of the localising wire, bearing in mind the extent of surgery. If for cosmetic reasons the incision is placed close to the wire, the latter can be delivered into the surgical field by undermining the skin edge in the direction of the wire. The dissection is carried out with a scalpel; scissors can cut the wire and should be avoided. Similarly, contact between the diathermy lead and the wire can produce burn injuries, and electrocautery should be used sparingly and with caution.

The precise technique for surgical excision depends on whether the wire traverses the lesion or passes alongside it. If the wire is not through the lesion, breast tissue is dissected to expose the whole length of the wire, which creates one of the planes of excision. Having done this, knowing the direction and distance of the lesion from the wire, the lesion can be excised with relative ease when its direction and distance from the wire are known (Figure 21.6).

If the wire traverses the lesion then it is excised with an appropriate amount of breast tissue around it that will contain the lesion (Figure 21.7). In the case of diagnostic biopsies, dissection is continued along the wire until proximity to the lesion is judged to have been reached. Dissection is then extended around the wire, which will avoid removing excessive amounts of normal breast tissue (the weight of the specimen should not exceed 20 g). Once the specimen has been excised, it is orientated using

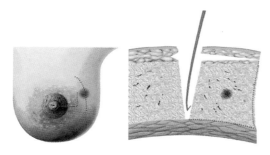

Figure 21.6 Removal of an impalpable lesion with the wire near the lesion. The skin incision is made in proximity to the wire, possibly over the impalpable lesion; the wire is found in the subcutaneous tissue and brought into the wound; breast tissue is dissected so as to expose all the length of the wire down to the pectoral fascia. This creates one of the planes of excision. Once this has been done, knowing the direction and the distance of the lesion from the wire, the lesion can easily be excised.

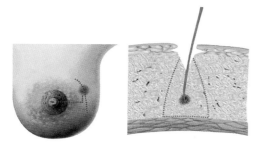

Figure 21.7 Removal of an impalpable lesion with the wire in situ. The skin incision is made through the point of entry of the wire. The wire itself is excised with an appropriate amount of breast tissue around it.

sutures and/or ligaclips. We use a black silk suture to mark the skin surface and a nylon suture to mark the nipple margin. Specimen radiography is performed in all cases and comparison made with current mammograms to confirm adequacy of excision. Specimen radiographs should be checked by a radiologist while the patient is still under general anaesthesia and further excision undertaken if necessary.

Results and complications

We have used this technique in a total of 1100 cases of impalpable breast lesions and have successfully performed localisation in the majority of cases. The localising wire was repositioned in 31 cases (2.8%). The lesion was excised at the first attempt in 1090 cases (99.1%), at the second in 7 cases (0.6%) and

Table 21.1	**Results of excision of impalpable breast lesions (1100 cases)**	
Wire repositioned	31	2.8%
Lesion excised at first biopsy	1090	99.1%
Lesion excised at second biopsy	7	0.6%
Lesion excised at third biopsy	3	0.3%
Migration of wire	2	0.2%
Transection of wire	0	0
Pneumothorax	0	0

at the third in 3 cases (0.3%) (under the same general anaesthetic). In particular, no patient had to be woken up without the lesion having been removed (Table 21.1). Migration of the wire occurred in 2 cases, requiring retrieval from the lateral breast and the posterior triangle of the neck.[17] Migration has been reported into the left pleural space[19] and the posterior paracervical region.[20] Both pneumothorax[21] and transection of the wire[22] have been reported in the literature.

The ROLL technique

The ROLL (radioguided occult lesion localisation) method[23,24] involves the injection of technetium-99m (^{99m}Tc)-labelled colloid particles of human serum albumin into an impalpable lesion, which permits localisation using a hand held γ-probe (Neoprobe Neo2000, Navigator GPS Power Probe, Scintiprobe MR 100, G-Track System or Gamma IV Europrobe). The diameter of the particles ranges between 10 and 150 μm (Macrotec, Amersham Sorin, Saluggia, Italy) and they are labelled with 3.7 MBq (0.1 mCi) of ^{99m}Tc to yield a specific activity of 74 MBq/mg.

Tracer (0.05 mg) is injected under stereotactic or ultrasound-guided control the day before surgery and the breast is scanned with a γ-camera immediately post injection and after an interval of 5 hours. Planar scintigraphy images are obtained in frontal and lateral views (Figures 21.8–21.11).

At operation, the lesion appears as a 'sphere' with multidirectional emission radioactive signals that are detected by the γ-probe. The highest signal intensity ('hot spot') corresponds to the centre of the lesion, with progressive attenuation on moving the probe towards the periphery. The rapid fall-off of signal intensity indicates that a satisfactory margin of resection has been reached. The absence of residual emission of γ-rays in the tumour cavity confirms that excision of the lesion is complete (Figure 21.12).

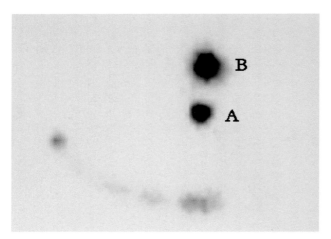

Figure 21.8 Frontal scintigraphic image. A, nipple; B, 'hot spot'.

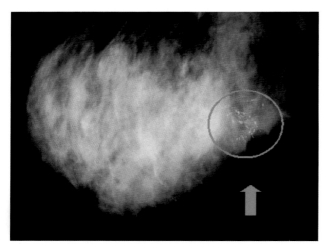

Figure 21.9 Craniocaudal mammography, non-palpable lesion (circle).

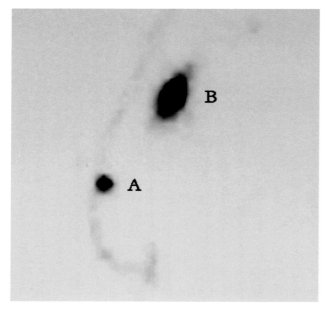

Figure 21.10 Lateral scintigraphic image. A, nipple; B, 'hot spot'.

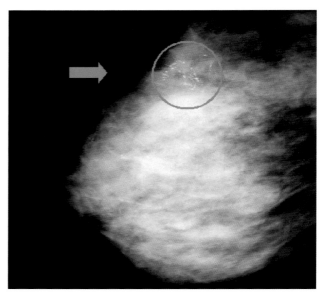

Figure 21.11 Lateral–medial mammography, impalpable lesion (circle).

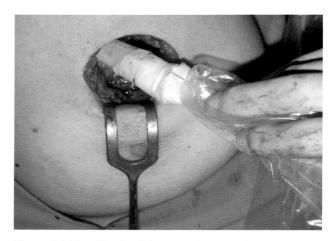

Figure 21.12 Check of the resection margins.

This is an awkward procedure to perform, and its success is linked to several different variables, such as the size of the lesion, the resection margins, and the volume and concentration of the tracer. In particular, the volume and/or concentration of tracer and the width of resection margins will vary depending on the size of the lesion.

In patients with a proven invasive impalpable cancer, it is possible to use a single tracer (Nanacoll, Amersham Sorin, Saluggia, Italy) for both tumour localisation and sentinel node biopsy.[24] However, the Nanacoll particles useful for sentinel node biopsy are smaller, and this can result in a much larger radiation field at the tumour site, with problems of 'shine through'. Under these circumstances, the ROLL technique may not be as reliable for assessing the clearance of resection margins.

Conclusion

The management of impalpable breast lesions should be considered carefully. The majority of cases are asymptomatic women called for further assessment following a routine screening mammogram. Some will have benign lesions, while others will have minimal and potentially curable breast cancer. Efforts should be made to avoid unsightly scars and significant breast deformity consequent to surgery.

Close cooperation between surgeon, radiologist and pathologist is essential to achieve an optimum outcome for the patient.

References

1. Dodd GD, Fry K, Delany W. Pre-operative localization of occult carcinoma in the breast. In: Nealon TF, ed. Management of the Patient with Cancer. Philadelphia: WB Saunders, 1966; 88–113.

2. Threatt B, Appelman H, Dew R, O'Rourke T. Percutaneous needle localization of clustered mammary microcalcifications prior to biopsy. Am J Roentgenol Radium Ther Nucl Med 1974; 121: 839–42.

3. Libshitz HI, Feig SA, Fetouh S. Needle localization of non palpable breast lesions. Radiology 1976; 121: 557–60.

4. Schwartz GF, Feig SA, Rosenberg AL et al. Localization and significance of clinically occult breast lesions. Experience with 469 needle guided biopsies. Rec Res Cancer Res 1984; 90: 125–32.

5. Marrujo G, Jolly PC, Hall MH. Non-palpable breast cancer: needle localized biopsy for diagnosis and consideration for treatment. Am J Surg 1986; 151: 599–602.

6. Frank HA, Hall FM, Steer ML. Pre-operative localization of non palpable breast lesions demonstrated by mammography. New Engl J Med 1976; 295: 259–60.

7. Kopans DB, DeLuca S. A modified needle-hookwire technique to simplify pre-operative localization of occult breast lesions. Radiology 1980; 134: 781.

8. Homer MJ. Nonpalpable breast lesion localization using a curved-end retractable wire. Radiology 1985; 157: 259–60.

9. Egan JF, Sayler CB, Goodman MJ. A technique for localizing occult breast lesions. CA Cancer J Clin 1976; 26: 32–7.

10. Czarnecki DJ, Feider HK, Splittgerber GF. Toluidine blue dye as a breast localization marker. AJR Am J Roentgenol 1989; 153: 261–3.

11. Canavese G, Catturich A, Vecchio C et al. Pre-operative localisation of non-palpable lesions in breast cancer by charcoal suspension. Eur J Surg Oncol 1995; 21: 47–9.

12. Luini A, Zurrida S, Paganelli G et al. Comparison of radioguided excision with wire localization of occult breast lesions. Br J Surg 1999; 86: 522–5.

13. Nordenstrom B, Zajicek J. Sterotaxic needle biopsy and preoperative indication of non-palpable mammary lesions. Acta Cytol 1977; 21: 350–1.

14. Svane G. A sterotaxic technique for pre-operative marking of non palpable breast lesions. Acta Radiol Diagn 1983; 24: 145–51.

15. Parekh NJ, Wolfe JN. Localization device for occult breast lesions: use in 75 patients. AJR Am J Roentgenol 1987; 148: 699–701.

16. Goldberg RP, Hall FM, Simon M. Preoperative localization of nonpalpable breast lesions using a wire marker and perforated mammographic grid. Radiology 1983; 146: 833–5.

17. Querci della Rovere G, Benson JR, Morgan M et al. Localization of impalpable breast lesions: a surgical approach. Eur J Surg Oncol 1996; 22: 478–82.

18. Quality Assurance Guidelines for Surgeons in Breast Disease. NHSBSP Publication 20. Sheffield: NHS Breast Screening Programme, 1992.

19. Bristol JB, Jones PA. Transgression of localizing wire into the pleural cavity prior to mammography. Br J Radiol 1981; 54: 139–40.

20. Davis PS, Wechsler RJ, Feig SA, March DE. Migration of breast biopsy localization wire. AJR Am J Roentgenol 1988; 150: 787–8.

21. Tykka H, Castren-Persons M, Sjoblom M, Roiha M. Pneumothorax caused by hook wire localization of an impalpable breast lesion detected by rnammography. Breast 1993; 2: 52–3.

22. Homer MJ. Transection of the localizing hook wire during breast biopsy. Am J Radiol 1983; 141: 929–30.

23. Gennari R, Galimberti V, De Cicco C et al. Use of technetium-99m-labelled colloid albumin for preoperative and intraoperative localisation of non-palpable breast lesion. J Am Coll Surg 2000; 190: 692–8.

24. Tanis PJ, Deurloo EE, Valdes Olmos RA et al. Single intralesional tracer dose for radio-guided excision of clinically occult breast cancer and sentinel node. Ann Surg Oncol 2001; 8: 850–5.

22 ABBI: Advanced Breast Biopsy Instrumentation

Gianantonio A Farello, Antonio Cerofolini

Introduction

The progressive lowering of the threshold for identification of abnormalities in the breast as a result of the widespread use of mammography and the development of methods for breast imaging is associated with a number of diagnostic difficulties; the increasing detection rate of breast lesions means that ever more frequently, samples of cells/tissue must be taken, since this is the only way in which morphologically non-specific lesions can be identified. Furthermore, taking cell/tissue samples from the breast is controversial at present because there are so many technical options available (including fine-needle biopsy, core biopsy and minimally invasive breast biopsy) and the indications for each, and their reliability, are still under discussion. Fine-needle biopsy and core biopsy are purely diagnostic procedures, whereas taking a sample by means of Advanced Breast Biopsy Instrumentation (ABBI) is clearly different from these two methods because its purpose is twofold, i.e. diagnostic and, especially, therapeutic.[1–3]

Fine-needle aspiration (FNA) has progressed considerably over the last decade or so, and, in expert hands, has been shown to be highly sensitive and specific. Nevertheless, operators are often reluctant to make definitive decisions on the basis of cytology, because FNA is associated with the possibility of false negatives due to sampling errors; furthermore, it is difficult, if not impossible, to discriminate between hyperplasia with atypical features, ductal carcinoma in situ (DCIS) and invasive carcinomas.

The advent of core biopsy has led, gradually and progressively, towards percutaneous mini-invasive biopsy. By comparison with FNA, core biopsy allows a more precise morphological profile of a breast lesion to be drawn; it can distinguish between benign and malignant forms and between infiltrating and in situ lesions. Core biopsy is not, however, immune from false negatives, also due to sampling errors. If, however, hyperplasia with atypical features or carcinoma in situ are found, the lesion as a whole must be examined, and so surgical biopsy is required.

From the diagnostic point of view, the characteristic features of sampling with ABBI are its high sensitivity and specificity, with a predictive value similar to that of open surgical biopsy (there are no artefacts in the sample, which is readily legible even at the periphery), and the fact that much less breast tissue is removed.[4]

Lesions of the breast can be classified into three groups: those that are definitely benign, those that are definitely malignant and borderline lesions (ductal hyperplasia with or without atypical features, lobular atypical hyperplasia and lobular carcinoma in situ (LCIS)) that increase the risk of developing a cancer in the future. In non-palpable lesions, ABBI resolves the diagnostic problem accurately.[5]

The system

The ABBI system consists of permanent apparatus and a disposable 'trocar'. The permanent apparatus consists of:

- a table
- a control console
- a system for calculating the coordinates

The table (Figure 22.1) consists of a flat padded area that supports the patient during the procedure; the breast is brought through a circular opening 25 cm in diameter into the operating area, which is below

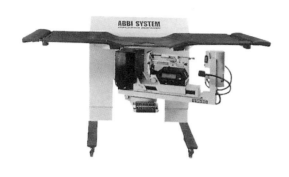

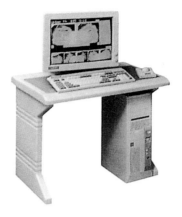

Figure 22.1 The table consists of a paddle area with a circular opening 25 cm in diameter.

Figure 22.2 The computer for calculating the coordinates.

Figure 22.3 The disposable trocar.

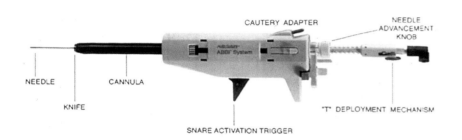

CAUTERY ADAPTER
NEEDLE ADVANCEMENT KNOB
NEEDLE
CANNULA
KNIFE
"T" DEPLOYMENT MECHANISM
SNARE ACTIVATION TRIGGER

the flat part of the table. At each end, there is a support that can be pulled out so that the patient can be positioned with her head to one side or the other and so that either breast can be approached from any direction (360°).

This feature means that the breast can also be entered from below, which shortens the computed track of the needle through the gland. The prone position reduces the danger of vagal reactions and allows the doctor to work out of the patient's line of sight so that she is not subjected to unnecessary anxiety-inducing stimuli. In the operating area below the flat part of the table, there is a C-shaped arm supporting the tube that produces the X-rays, the image recorder, the apparatus for stereotactic direction finding and the breast compressor.

The X-ray tube and the compressor can be rotated together around the central axis of the table from 0° to 180°. The direction-finding apparatus is used to position the tip of the needle in accordance with the coordinates calculated by the computer. The digital system for image recording means that images of the breast can be acquired without the use of film. An image is passed to the computer in 5 s for processing. The use of digital images reduces the overall duration of the operation. The controls for regulat-

ing the X-ray tube are located on the control console.

The system for calculating the coordinates consists of a computer (Figure 22.2) with a screen on which the operator can show the site of the lesion directly. The computer calculates the coordinates in three spatial planes and then transmits them to the direction-finding system. Images can also be memorised, recalled and stored.

The disposable trocar (Figure 22.3) is placed on the direction-finding device and comprises a cannula (available in various diameters: 5, 10, 15 and 20 mm) containing a narrow circular blade, a snare at the distal end to which an electrical diathermy device can be attached and a central coaxial needle at the tip with a T-shaped arrester. The trocar allows removal of a cylinder of tissue at the centre of which is the lesion identified by the T-piece on the needle.

The operation is carried out on an outpatient basis under local anaesthesia and lasts for 25 minutes on average. Recovery is immediate and the patient can be discharged within a couple of hours.

The site of the lesion, which has been localised previously by mammography, governs the point of entry and the direction of the trocar. The breast is

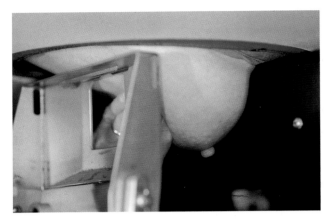

Figure 22.4 The breast is compressed and immobilised.

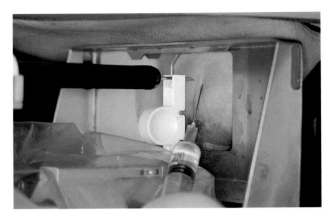

Figure 22.6 Moderate local anaesthesia is inserted at the point at which the needle is to be inserted.

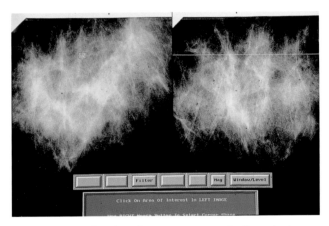

Figure 22.5 The digital system automatically calculates the *x*-, *y*- and *z*-coordinates of the lesion with an accuracy of ±1 mm.

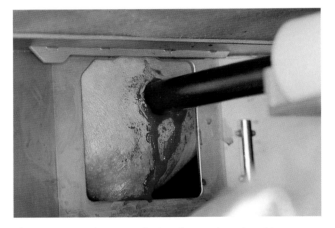

Figure 22.7 The cannula is advanced to the skin incision and guided by the surgeon to the required depth.

compressed and immobilised (Figure 22.4). A sterile transparent cover is placed over the working area to maintain sterility during use of the manual controls. Stereotactic imaging is used to check the site of the lesion. The surgeon identifies the target area on the monitor. The digital system automatically calculates the *x*-, *y*- and *z*-coordinates of the lesion with an accuracy of ±1 mm (Figure 22.5). These coordinates are passed to the guidance system on which the trocar is fixed. The guidance system operates automatically on the *x*-, *y*- and *z*-coordinates to line up with the area of interest on horizontal and vertical axes. Moderate local anaesthesia is inserted at the point at which the needle is to be inserted (Figure 22.6).

A small incision is made in the skin with the blade and the needle is inserted to the required depth. A stereotactic image is taken to establish the position of the needle, at which point the T-shaped guidewire is advanced to stabilise the tissue. At this stage, local anaesthesia must be extended to the

deeper layers. The skin incision is lengthened to permit insertion of the trocar. The cannula is advanced to the skin incision and guided by the surgeon to the required depth (Figure 22.7).

The instrument isolates the piece of tissue within the cannula by slight oscillation of the surgical blade. A stereotactic image is used to check that the snare is beyond the point of insertion of the T-shaped guidewire. The diathermy on the snare is then used for cutting. The cannula and the whole sample of tissue are carefully removed. Pressure with a piece of gauze at the site of insertion prevents any blood loss. The piece of tissue is taken out of the cannula and sent for histology (Figure 22.8).

The needle with the T-shaped guidewire allows correct pathological orientation (Figure 22.9).

The patient is rolled over onto her back. Any bleeding can be controlled by the application of pressure, diathermy and/or suturing by hand (Figure 22.10).

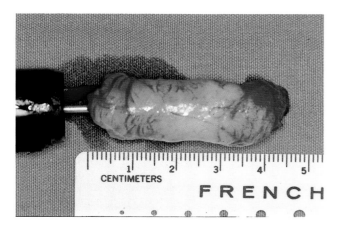

Figure 22.8 The piece of tissue is taken out of the cannula and sent for histology.

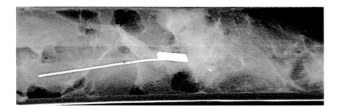

Figure 22.9 The needle with the T-shaped guidewire allows correct pathological orientation.

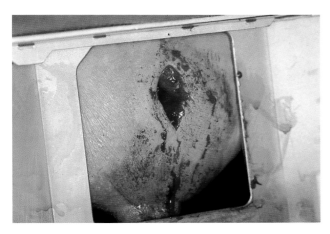

Figure 22.10 Any bleeding can be controlled by the application of pressure, diathermy and/or suturing by hand.

The small incision in the skin is sutured with a few stitches. A pressure dressing is applied.[6,7]

Results

In the period September 1996–August 2002, we treated 351 patients with impalpable breast lesions using the ABBI system. Their average age was 51.2 (range 23–89). The average duration of the procedure was 27 minutes (range 15–150 minutes). The local anaesthetic was lidoocaine (2–15 cm^3, average 8 cm^3).

In an additional 37 patients (10.5%), the ABBI procedure was not feasible for the following reasons:

- lesion undetectable with the ABBI digital instrumentation (16 patients)
- non-accessible site (13 patients)
- dislocation of lesion with excessive local anaesthetic (1 patient)
- breast too thin on compression (7 patients)

The mammographic lesions were as follows:

- microcalcifications with or without a mass (272 cases; 77.4%)
- solid lesions (73 cases; 20.7%)
- parenchymal distortions (6 cases; 1.7%)

Table 22.1

Lesion diameter (mm)	No. of patients
<5	181
5–10	141
10–15	26
>15	3

Trocar size (mm)	No. of patients
5	3
10	39
15	147
20	162

Table 22.2

Histopathology	No. of patients
Cystic mastopathy	23
Papilloma	1
Lymph node	3
Fibroadenoma	11
Hyperplasia without atypia	81
Hyperplasia with atypia	69
Lobular carcinoma in situ	11
Ductal carcinoma in situ	40
Invasive lobular carcinoma	17
Invasive ductal carcinoma	95

Table 22.3   Excision margins after ABBI excision of cancer (total 163 patients with malignant lesions)

	Status of margins after ABBI	Status of margins after surgical biopsy	Further foci of cancer at distance from margins	Surgical margins
Positive[a]	114 (69.9%)	51 (31.3%)	41 (25.2%)	9 (5.5%)
Negative	49 (30.1%)	49 (30.1%)	17 (10.4%)	0 (0%)

[a]Cancer <1 mm from or at the margin of excision.

To attempt complete excision of the mammographic lesions, we have always used trocars larger than the maximum diameter of the lesion (Table 22.1).

In 80 patients the ABBI system was the only intervention required, as either a diagnostic or a therapeutic procedure (Table 22.2).

The excision margins of the ABBI specimens were as follows: in 114 cases (69.9%), margins were involved or less than 1 mm. Of those patients, 51 (44.7%) had no residual disease on surgical re-excision of margins. In 41 patients (35.9%), there were residual foci of cancer at a distance from the margins, and in 9 cases (7.8%), even the surgical biopsy margins were positive, requiring further surgical intervention (Table 22.3).

The high percentage of positive margins after ABBI excisions[8–12] is due to the lack of correlation between the size of the microcalcifications and the size of the cancers and to the irregularities of the lesions.[13,14] To increase the chances of clear margins, one must use trocars of at least 20 mm (25 mm trocars will soon be available).[15]

Our results and the frequent presence of multifocal lesions make the ABBI system at present unsuitable for therapeutic purposes. In the future, perhaps, larger trocars (30 mm) associated with intraoperative radiotherapy may overcome this problem.[7,16,17]

Patients were sent home after an average time of 2.5 hours with a pressure dressing and were reviewed in the outpatient department 1 week later.

Small trocars (5 and 10 mm) can cause displacement of the target area and have more technical problems, such as malfunction of the diathermy snare, of the blade or of the T-shaped guidewire (12.4%).[18–20]

In 4 patients (1.1%), the specimen X-ray failed to show the presence of microcalcifications; in 3 of those patients, the procedure was carried out successfully with larger trocars, whereas in 1 case, an open biopsy was required.

One patient developed a large haematoma; smaller haematomas of 1–2 cm were more frequent, but all resolved spontaneously without further complications. Follow-up mammography, even more than 4 years after ABBI intervention, showed no significant scarring or difficulties with radiological interpretation of the images.[21–24]

Discussion

The ABBI system has many advantages:

- It removes the whole piece of tissue in one operation (localisation is no longer necessary).
- It allows correct orientation of the specimen.
- It identifies accurately the objective to within ±1 mm, so that the surgeon has to remove a smaller amount of healthy tissue (13–17 cm^3 versus 26–32 cm^3).
- The smaller incision results in a better cosmetic result,[25] and scars and disfigurement are avoided.
- There is less anxiety with minimal emotional and physical trauma, since an operation is avoided.
- It reduces operating theatre costs: in Italy, the costs are core biopsy 480 Euros, ABBI 1650 Euros and surgical biopsy 3000 Euros.[26,27]

On the other hand, the procedure is not always appropriate, because although digital imaging heightens contrast and facilitates the identification of microcalcifications, localising small solid nodules can be more difficult because the definition is poorer.[28] Deep-seated lesions close to the pectoral muscle and peripheral lesions or those in the axillary extension, especially in patients with small breasts, are difficult to aim at.[29]

The complications of ABBI are relatively few; haematomas may occur, especially if the lesion is deep, the breast large and the course of the trocar particularly long.

Conclusions

This is a new and extremely promising method,[8,30] which looks likely to change the treatment of non-palpable lesions of the breast in the future.[31,32] It cannot, however, at present be regarded as a therapeutic procedure.[33-35]

References

1. Winzer KJ, Filimonow S, Guski H et al. [Stereotactic tumor biopsy and tumor excision]. Langenbecks Arch Chir Suppl Kongressbd 1998; 115: 374–8 (in German).

2. Winzer KJ, Filimonow S, Frohberg HD et al. [Three-dimensional breast biopsy and surgery]. Chirurg 1999; 70: 384–93 (in German).

3. Yang JH, Lee SD, Nam SJ. Diagnostic utility of ABBI(R) Advanced Breast Biopsy Instrumentation) for nonpalpable breast lesions in Korea. Breast J 2000; 6: 257–62.

4. Ammann M, Haid A, Breitfellner G. [Advanced Breast Biopsy Instrumentation (ABBI). Histopathologic evaluation of a new investigation method]. Pathologe 2000; 21: 234–9 (in German).

5. Atallah N, Karam R, Younane T, Aftimos G. [Stereotaxic excisional biopsy of non-palpable breast lesions by the ABBI (Advanced Breast Biopsy Instrumentation) technique. Advantages. Disadvantages. Indications. Apropos of 67 cases]. J Med Liban 2000; 48: 70–6 (in French).

6. D'Angelo PC, Galliano DE, Rosemurgy AS. Stereotactic excisional breast biopsies utilizing the Advanced Breast Biopsy Instrumentation system. Am J Surg 1997; 174: 297–302.

7. Ferzli GS, Hurwitz JB. Initial experience with breast biopsy utilizing the Advanced Breast Biopsy Instrumentation (ABBI). Surg Endosc 1997; 11: 393–6.

8. Schwartzberg BS, Goates JJ, Keeler SA, Moore JA. Use of Advanced Breast Biopsy Instrumentation while performing stereotactic breast biopsies: review of 150 consecutive biopsies. J Am Coll Surg 2000; 191: 9–15.

9. Smathers RL. Advanced Breast Biopsy Instrumentation device: percentages of lesion and surrounding tissue removed. AJR Am J Roentgenol 2000; 175: 801–3.

10. Vargas HI, Agbunag RV, Khaikhali I. State of the art of minimally invasive breast biopsy: principles and practice. Breast Cancer 2000; 7: 370–9.

11. Wedegartner U, Otto U, Buitrago-Tellez C et al. [Percutaneous stereotactic biopsy of non-palpable breast lesions using the Advanced Breast Biopsy Instrumentation (ABBI) system: critical evaluation of indication strategies]. Rofo Fortschr Geb Rontgenstr Neuen Bildgeb Verfahr 2001; 173: 224–8 (in German).

12. Wi GA, El-Zein YR, Haddad MC. The epitaph of the Advanced Breast Biopsy Instrumentation (ABBI). J Med Liban 2001; 49: 129; discussion 129–30.

13. Gubaidullin KhM, Khasanov RSh, Sigal EI et al. [Biopsy of non-palpable tumors of the breast]. Khirurgiia (Mosk) 2001; 2: 7–8 (in Russian).

14. Guenin M. Wherefore ABBI? Advanced Breast Biopsy Instrumentation. AJR Am J Roentgenol 1999; 173: 1410–1.

15. Marti WR, Zuber M, Oertli D et al. Advanced Breast Biopsy Instrumentation for the evaluation of impalpable lesions: a reliable diagnostic tool with little therapeutic potential. Eur J Surg 2001; 167: 15–18.

16. Ferzli GS, Hurwitz JB, Puza T, Van Vorst-Bilotti S. Advanced breast cancer biopsy instrumentation: a critique. J Am Coll Surg 1997; 185: 145–51.

17. Ferzli GS, Puza T, Vanvorst-Bilotti S, Waters R. Breast biopsies with ABBI(R): experience with 183 attempted biopsies. Breast J 1999; 5: 26–8.

18. Haj M, Kniaz D, Eitan A, et al. Three years of experience with Advanced Breast Biopsy Instrumentation (ABBI). Breast J 2002; 8: 275–80.

19. Hergan K, Haid A, Turtscher M et al. [Advanced Breast Biopsy Instrumentation (ABBI) experiences and critical comments]. Rofo Fortschr Geb Rontgenstr Neuen Bildgeb Verfahr 2001; 173: 893–7 (in German).

20. Insausti LP, Alberro JA, Regueira FM et al. An experience with the Advanced Breast Biopsy Instrumentation (ABBI) system in the management of non-palpable breast lesions. Eur Radiol 2002; 12: 1703–10.

21. LaRaja RD, Saber AA, Sickles A. Early experience in the use of the Advanced Breast Biopsy Instrumentation: a report of one hundred twenty-seven patients. Surgery 1999; 125: 380–4.

22. Liberman L. Advanced Breast Biopsy Instrumentation (ABBI): analysis of published experience. AJR Am J Roentgenol 1999; 172: 1413–16.

23. Leibman AJ, Frager D, Choi P. Experience with breast biopsies using the Advanced Breast Biopsy Instrumentation system. AJR Am J Roentgenol 1999; 172: 1409–12.

24. Lifrange E, Dondelinger RF, Fridman V, Colin C. En bloc excision of nonpalpable breast lesions using the Advanced Breast Biopsy Instrumentation system: an alternative to needle guided surgery? Eur Radiol 2001; 11: 796–801.

25. Chun K, Velanovich V. Patient-perceived cosmesis and satisfaction after breast biopsy: comparison of stereotactic incisional, excisional, and wire-localized biopsy techniques. Surgery 2002; 131: 497–501.

26. Damascelli B, Frigerio LF, Patelli G et al. [Diagnosis of non-palpable lesions of the breast with stereotactic excisional biopsy with cannula. Advanced Breast Biopsy Instrumentation (ABBI) with fine diameter of 20 mm]. Radiol Med (Torino) 1998; 95: 437–44 (in Italian).

27. Damascelli B, Frigerio LF, Lanocita R et al. Stereotactic excisional breast biopsy performed by interventional radiologists using the Advanced Breast Biopsy Instrumentation system. Br J Radiol 1998; 71: 1003–11.

28. Bloomston M, D'Angelo P, Galliano D et al. One hundred consecutive Advanced Breast Biopsy Instrumentation procedures: complications, costs, and outcome. Ann Surg Oncol 1999; 6: 195–9.

29. Denton ER, Michell MJ, Wilson AR, Britton P. Stereotactic excisional breast biopsy performed by interventional radiologists using the ABBI system. Br J Radiol 1999; 72: 828–9.

30. Sheth D, Wesen CA, Schroder D et al. The Advanced Breast Biopsy Instrumentation (ABBI) experience at a community hospital. Am Surg 1999; 65: 726–9; discussion 729–30.

31. Portincasa G, Lucci E, Navarra GG et al. Initial experience with breast biopsy utilizing the Advanced Breast Biopsy Instrumentation (ABBI). J Surg Oncol 2000; 74: 201–3.

32. Rebner M, Chesbrough R, Gregory N. Initial experience with the Advanced Breast Biopsy Instrumentation device. AJR Am J Roentgenol 1999; 173: 221–6.

33. Matthews BD, Williams GB. Initial experience with the Advanced Breast Biopsy Instrumentation system. Am J Surg 1999; 177: 97–101.

34. Oertli D, Zuber M, Muller D et al. [The Advanced Breast Biopsy Instrumentation (ABBI), a system for stereotactic excision of mammographically suspect nonpalpable findings in the breast]. Schweiz Med Wochenschr 1998; 128: 811–16 (in German).

35. Perelman VS, Colapinto ND, Lee S et al. Experience with the Advanced Breast Biopsy Instrumentation system. Can J Surg 2000; 43: 437–41.

23 The Fischer table, Mammotome and Site Select

Michael Michell

Introduction

The Fischer table and stereotactic equipment is a dedicated breast biopsy system that can be used with several sampling methods, including automated 14G needle biopsy, vacuum-assisted breast biopsy (Mammotome; Ethicon Endo-surgery, Inc., Cincinnatti, OH) and the Site Select device.

The Fischer table and stereotactic equipment

The patient lies in the prone or prone oblique position, and the breast to be biopsied is passed through a round aperture near the head of the table (Figure 23.1). The aperture is large enough to allow the arm and shoulder girdle to be passed through, which permits access to lesions that are positioned very posteriorly or in the axillary tail. The X-ray tube is mounted below the table and can move through a 180° arc. A lesion can therefore be approached from any direction within the arc. The biopsy apparatus is positioned between the X-ray tube and the breast.

The angle of approach is selected by examining the craniocaudal and lateral views – usually the shortest route is selected, and there should be sufficient breast tissue distal to the lesion to ensure that there is no danger of the tip of the needle or sampling device hitting the surface of the image acquisition device. Thus, for a lesion in the upper outer quadrant, a supero-inferior or a lateromedial approach may be used, while for a lesion in the lower inner quadrant, a mediolateral approach is used.

The biopsy procedure is carried out below the table and out of sight of the patient; the patient is in a stable position and there is negligible risk of a vasovagal episode.

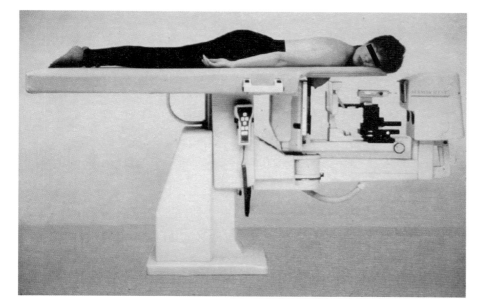

Figure 23.1 The Fischer prone stereotactic breast biopsy table.

The breast is compressed between a small compression plate with a 5 cm × 5 cm aperture and the surface of the image acquisition device. The digital imaging system allows images to be displayed approximately 5 s following X-ray exposure. The contrast and brightness of the digital images are adjusted on the computer console – black/white reversal and magnification facilities are also available and are routinely used for microcalcification. Targeting is carried out on the console and may be done by using the stereotactic image pair or by using the straight scout image and one of the stereotactic pair. When targeting has been carried out at the computer console, the information is transferred to the biopsy device holder, which moves to the appropriate angle. The apparatus is calibrated according to the type of sampling device being used – the correct depth is set by adjusting a millimetre scale on the biopsy device holder.

Sampling methods

14G core biopsy (Figure 23.2)[1–3]

An automated core biopsy device is used. After targeting of the lesion on the computer console as described above, the skin is cleaned, the core biopsy device is mounted on the biopsy device holder, and the breast tissue, where sampling is to take place, is infiltrated with local anaesthetic. For superficial anaesthesia, 5 ml of 1% lidocaine buffered with 0.5 ml of sodium bicarbonate is used; for the deeper tissues, 5–10 ml of bupivacaine with adrenaline is used. A 2 mm skin nick is made with a scalpel blade and the biopsy needle is then introduced to the depth determined by the targeting procedure and set manually. A check pair of images is obtained, and repositioning may be carried out if required. When the positioning is satisfactory, up to eight further 'offset' targets are selected on the computer console. The needle is withdrawn 3–5 mm so that the tip lies just proximal to the lesion. The needle is then fired and a check pair of images may be taken. Further samples are then acquired from the 'offset' targets. The needle is withdrawn following each pass and the specimens are delivered into normal saline. A final 'straight' post-biopsy image is obtained and is compared with the pre-biopsy image to ensure that the appropriate area has been effectively sampled. Some or all of the microcalcification in a small cluster may be absent on the post-biopsy film. For microcalcification, the core samples are X-rayed to confirm that calcification has been removed. Following the procedure, manual compression is applied for 5 minutes to the biopsy site and the skin nick is dressed with Steristrips.

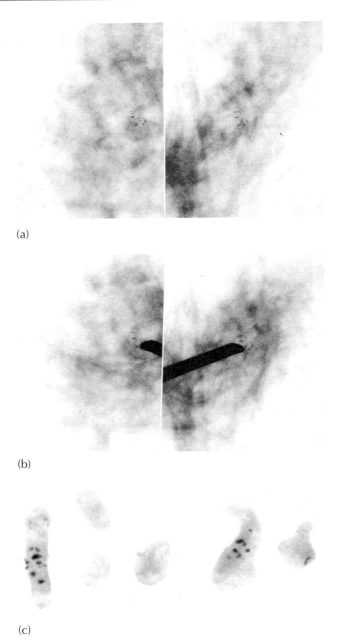

(a)

(b)

(c)

Figure 23.2 14G core biopsy of a small cluster of microcalcification. (a) The microcalcification is seen on the stereotactic images. (b) The needle tip is positioned just proximal to the microcalcification prior to firing. (c) The specimen X-ray confirms that the core samples contain microcalcification.

Vacuum-assisted core biopsy: the Mammotome

The Mammotome biopsy device consists of a hollow needle-tipped probe with a side aperture and a separate channel, which transmits negative pressure (Figure 23.3a,b).[4] Tissue is pulled into the aperture by the negative pressure and the biopsy specimen is then separated from the adjacent breast tissue by a rotating cutting cylinder that passes down within

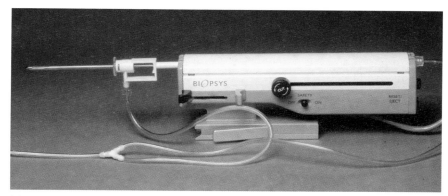

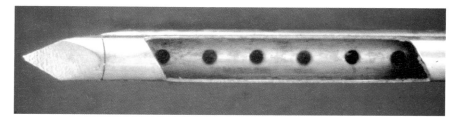

(a)

(b)

Figure 23.3 Breast biopsy sampling devices. (a) The Mammotone vacuum-assisted core biopsy device. (b) The vacuum core biopsy probe, showing the holes in the base of the biopsy port leading to the vacuum. (c) The Site Select device. (d) The blades and cannula of the Site Select device.

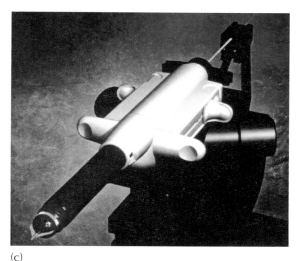

(c)

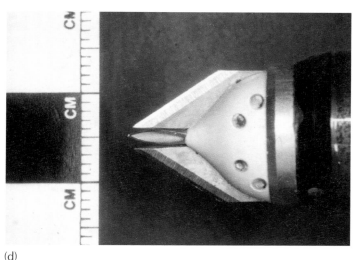

(d)

the probe – the specimen is then delivered by withdrawing the cutting cylinder and applying negative pressure while the probe remains within the breast (Figure 22.4). Any haematoma that collects in the biopsy cavity is rapidly evacuated by the vacuum.

14G, 11G and 8G Mammotome probes are available, but most work is carried out with the 11G device, which is not associated with any additional complication rate compared with the smaller 14G device. Most published results on the Mammotome device describe its use with prone digital stereotactic apparatus, although it may be used with upright stereo systems and can be used for sampling under ultrasound guidance.

Positioning and targeting are carried out in the same way as for 14G core biopsy. The probe may be either 'fired' or advanced into position. The tip of the sampling probe should be positioned just proximal to the target lesion before firing – the position of the probe may be adjusted if necessary by changing the target coordinates on the computer console and reinserting the probe. Firing the probe into the sampling position is the preferred method, because advancing the probe tends to push the lesion further distally. A check pair of images is obtained to ensure that the biopsy port is traversing the target area (Figure 23.5). Sequential samples are then obtained by rotating the biopsy probe within the breast so that the biopsy port is aligned with the chosen site for sampling. In practice, samples are taken from

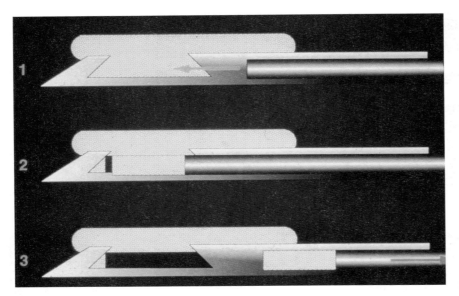

Figure 23.4 Vacuum-assisted core biopsy: mechanism of action. (1) Tissue is pulled into the biopsy aperture by the vacuum. (2) The cutting cylinder separates the tissue specimen from the surrounding breast tissue. (3) The tissue specimen is withdrawn within the cutting cylinder.

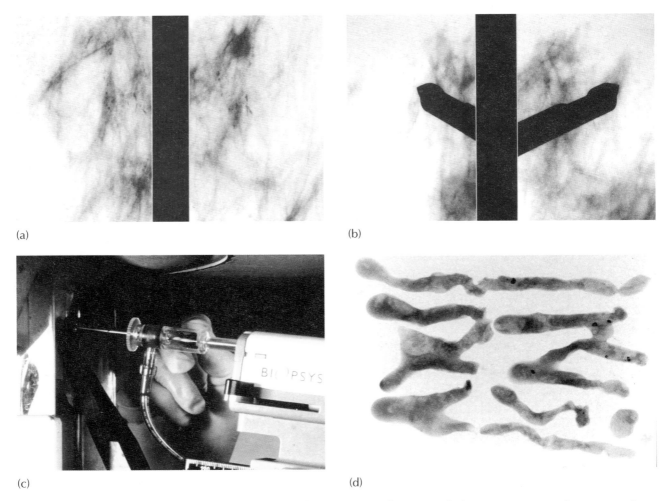

(a)

(b)

(c)

(d)

Figure 23.5 Vacuum-assisted core biopsy of microcalcification. (a) The microcalcification is seen on the stereotactic images. (b) The biopsy probe is in position. (c) Core specimens are obtained. (d) A specimen X-ray confirms the presence of microcalcification.

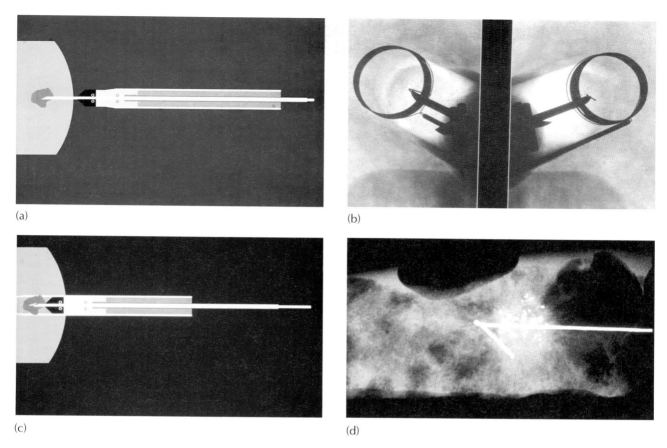

(a)

(b)

(c)

(d)

Figure 23.6 Site Select biopsy. (a) The localisation wire is deployed. (b) The stylet is translated into the breast. (c) The cutting cannula rotates and translates into the breast, coring the target tissue. (d) The specimen is withdrawn.

sequential sites around the clockface: 12 o'clock, 2 o'clock, 4 o'clock, etc. Two or more 360° rotations may be made and small clusters of microcalcification measuring up to 5 mm diameter will be removed completely. If the probe is positioned adjacent to the target area rather than across it, the direction of sampling can be selected appropriately. Post-biopsy check images and specimen radiographs are obtained in the same way as for 14G core biopsy. In cases where the whole mammographic marker has been removed, a small metal marker clip is introduced through the biopsy probe and deployed at the biopsy site – this acts as a marker for localisation should subsequent surgical excision be indicated.

Site Select

The Site Select biopsy device consists of a 15 mm diameter cylindrical sampling cannula that enables a single large specimen to be removed (Figure 23.3c,d).[5,6] The lesion is targeted using stereotaxis as described above. A 16G localising needle is first positioned under local anaesthesia with the tip just distal to the lesion. When the position is satisfactory, the needle is anchored by deploying a localising wire

with the hook in the breast tissue just distal to the needle tip. After further deep infiltration with local anaesthetic, a 22 mm skin incision is made to allow insertion of the 15mm diameter biopsy cannula. The stylet blades on the leading edge of the cannula allow insertion along the line of the guide needle until the device is positioned just proximal to the target lesion. The blades are withdrawn and the biopsy cannula is rotated and advanced 28 mm to encapsulate the lesion. The lesion is then separated from the remaining breast by activating a garrotte wire that cuts through the tissue at the end of the cannula. The biopsy device and specimen are then withdrawn from the breast and haemostasis is obtained by direct compression. A specimen X-ray is obtained to confirm that the target lesion has been excised (Figure 23.6).

Dedicated prone biopsy table versus upright add-on stereotaxis

The principal advantage of the dedicated prone table for breast biopsy is the stable position that is provided for the patient with no risk of vasovagal reaction and consequently a stable position for the breast undergoing biopsy. This, together with digital imaging, allows for very accurate targeting of small lesions and better access for lesions in difficult positions (e.g. near the chest wall or in the axillary tail). The design of the apparatus and the position of the patient mean that there is ample space for the radiologist and assistant to work in – this is particularly important for the more invasive procedures described above. The disadvantages of the dedicated prone system compared with the standard upright machine are related to space and cost – the prone system requires a dedicated room and costs more than the upright systems. It would therefore be impractical for every breast diagnostic centre to have a dedicated prone system. A regional network of such dedicated facilities, however, would ensure that effective diagnostic procedures could be offered to patients in whom lesions could not be satisfactorily sampled using upright apparatus.

Indications, contraindications and complications (Table 23.1)

All suspicious mammographic lesions should undergo a thorough diagnostic work-up prior to biopsy in order to characterise the imaging features and thereby determine the level of suspicion for malignancy – for microcalcification, the work-up should include fine-focus magnification views. Ultrasound is the imaging method of choice for biopsy of most soft tissue lesions, but some small masses in fatty breasts may be difficult or impossible to visualise satisfactorily, particularly if they are situated posteriorly in a large beast – these lesions are more satisfactorily sampled under stereotactic guidance.

Table 23.1	**Indications for stereotactic breast biopsy**

- Suspicious microcalcification
- Suspicious mass lesion not visible or not accessible for ultrasound-guided biopsy
- Architectural deformity/parenchymal distortion

Contraindications and complications are related mainly to the risk of bleeding. Patients who are taking warfarin or who have a bleeding diathesis should have their clotting time measured. The biopsy procedure can be carried out when the clotting time is satisfactory (e.g. after stopping warfarin). Provided that adequate compression over the site of the biopsy and needle track is maintained for approximately 5 minutes following the procedure, haematoma formation is not a problem in clinical practice.

If the compressed breast thickness is less than 4 cm, stereotactic biopsy using the standard approach may not be possible because of the risk of the tip of the needle/probe hitting the image receptor surface. A lateral arm attachment is available that allows a lateral approach – the needle/probe passes in a direction 90° to the direction of the straight scout X-ray beam.

Choice of sampling method

There is now published evidence showing that for some non-palpable mammographic lesions – particularly moderately suspicious calcification clusters and areas of architectural distortion – higher levels of both sensitivity and specificity and fewer equivocal results are achieved if larger volumes of tissue are provided for the histologist to examine.[7,8]

Larger volumes of tissue can be removed for examination using vacuum-assisted biopsy compared with 14G automated core biopsy and this can be shown to be associated with lower rates of underdiagnosis of ductal carcinoma in situ (DCIS) where only atypical ductal hyperplasia (ADH) is found on needle biopsy or underdiagnosis of invasive carcinoma where only DCIS is found.[9,10] The additional advantages of vacuum-assisted biopsy include single insertion of the probe (compared with multiple insertions for 14G automated core biopsy) and immediate evacuation of any haematoma that collects at the biopsy site during the procedure – this ensures that good-quality core tissue specimens are obtained throughout the procedure. Because of the use of the vacuum, lesions can be sampled successfully even if they lie several millimetres from the probe – with automated 14G core biopsy, tissue is only acquired if it lies directly in the line of the needle.

Studies have confirmed higher rates of successful calcium retrieval from clusters of microcalcification using vacuum-assisted biopsy compared with automated 14G core biopsy.[11,12]

The theoretical advantage of the Site Select device and the Advanced Breast Biopsy Instrumentation (ABBI) system (see Chapter 22) is the ability to obtain a single specimen containing a small lesion, allowing the histopathology to be examined in continuity rather than in multiple fragments. This theoretical advantage is outweighed, however, by the invasive nature of the procedures, requiring a 2 cm skin excision, the high complication rate, the high cost and the high frequency of involvement of the excision margin by tumour.

Clinical management

Following stereotactic needle biopsy, further patient management is decided at a multidisciplinary meeting, where the imaging findings and biopsy histology findings are discussed by the radiologist, histopathologist and surgeon.[13] In order to reach a definitive diagnosis upon which management can be based, there must be concordance between the biopsy findings and the differential diagnosis suggested by the imaging. For lesions that are highly suspicious of malignancy, such as pleomorphic branching microcalcification, needle biopsy is used to confirm the diagnosis of malignancy and to demonstrate the presence of invasive tumour, so that definitive surgery may be planned.[14] In such cases, if a benign or equivocal needle biopsy result is obtained, repeat needle biopsy or diagnostic surgery is planned. For areas of localised architectural distortion – stellate lesions with no central mass – where there is 50% chance of malignancy on surgical excision, a positive preoperative diagnosis of malignancy can be obtained for most cancers, allowing therapeutic surgery to be performed. Diagnostic surgical excision may not be required for cases where needle biopsy shows evidence of a benign lesion such as a radial scar, provided that no evidence of atypia is shown on histology.

For lesions with a lower probability of malignancy, such as a localised cluster of microcalcification showing slight pleomorphism, the radiologist and pathologist must be confident that an adequate sample has been obtained and that a benign histological diagnosis can be made that is compatible with the imaging findings – for microcalcification, calcium must be demonstrated radiologically within the core biopsy specimens. Cases where an inadequate or equivocal result is obtained should be offered either repeat needle biopsy or diagnostic surgery. When the needle biopsy shows features of ADH, diagnostic surgical excision should be offered, because surgical histology will demonstrate the presence of either in situ or invasive carcinoma in 30–40% of cases.[15,16]

References

1. Parker SM, Lovin JD, Jobe WE et al. Stereotactic breast biopsy with a biopsy gun. Radiology 1990; 176: 741–7.
2. Parker SM, Jobe WE, eds. Percutaneous Breast Biopsy. New York: Raven Press, 1993.
3. Parker SM, Lovin JD, Jobe WE et al. Non-palpable breast lesions: stereotactic automated large core biopsies. Radiology 1991; 180: 403–7.
4. Myer JE, Smith DN, Di Pino PJ et al. Stereotactic breast biopsy of clustered microcalcifications with a directional, vacuum-assisted device. Radiology 1997; 204: 575–6.
5. Denton ERE, Mitchell MJ, Nash RM, Bingham M. Use of the Site Select percutaneous breast biopsy device. Breast 2000; 9: 107–9.
6. Liberman L. Centennial dissertation. Percutaneous image-guided core breast biopsy: state of the art at millennium. AJR Am J Roentgenol 2000; 174: 1191–9.
7. Liberman L, Dershaw BD, Rosen PP et al. Stereotactic 14G breast biopsy; how many specimens are needed? Radiology 1994; 192: 793–5.
8. Rich PM, Michell MJ, Humphreys S et al. Stereotactic 14G core biopsy of non-palpable breast cancer: What is the relationship between the number of core samples taken and the sensitivity for the detection of malignancy? Clin Radiol 1999; 54: 384–9.
9. Burbank F. Stereotactic breast biopsy of atypical ductal hyperplasia and ductal carcinoma in-situ lesions: improved accuracy with a directional, vacuum-assisted biopsy instrument. Radiology 1997; 202: 843–7.
10. Jackman RJ, Burbank F, Parker SH et al. Atypical ductal hyperplasia diagnosed at stereotactic breast biopsy: improved reliability with 14G directional, vacuum-assisted biopsy. Radiology 1997; 204: 485–8.
11. Liberman L, Smolkin JM, Dershaw DD et al. Calcification retrieval at stereotactic 11G vacuum-assisted breast biopsy. Radiology 1998; 208: 251–60.
12. Burbank F, Parker SM, Fogarty TJ. Stereotactic breast biopsy: improved tissue harvesting with the Mammotome. Am Surg 1996; 62: 738–44.
13. Michell MJ, Dixon JM, eds. FNAC and Core Biopsy of Impalpable Lesions in Breast Cancer: Diagnosis and Management. Amsterdam: Elsevier Science, 2000.
14. Liberman L, Dershaw DD, Rosen PP et al. Stereotactic core biopsy of breast carcinoma: accuracy at predicting invasion. Radiology 1995; 194: 379–81.
15. Moore MM, Marge HC, Hanks JB et al. Association of breast cancer with findings of atypical ductal hyperplasia at core breast biopsy. Am Surg 1997; 225: 726–33.
16. Liberman L, Dershaw DD, Glassman J et al. Atypical ductal hyperplasia diagnosed at stereotactic core biopsy of breast lesions: an indication for surgical biopsy. AJR Am J Roentgenol 1995; 164: 1111–13.

24 The normal breast and benign breast lesions

Kusum Agarwal

Introduction

Mammary glands are distinguishing features of mammals. The term 'mammal' is derived from the Latin word *mamma*, the breast. The mammary gland and breast are not synonymous: the latter includes the connective tissue and fat that surround and support the gland. The human species is unusual in that the female breast develops without the stimulus of copulation or pregnancy. Although present in both sexes, the breast remains rudimentary in the male.

Embryology

The breasts are highly specialised apocrine sweat glands developed from ectoderm, and as down growth from the skin they first appear at the 8 mm embryo stage (the 5-week human fetus) when there is bilateral longitudinal thickening along the ventral body wall from the axillae to the medial aspect of the proximal part of the thigh; these are known as mammary lines – milk lines. In humans, they regress and disappear except in the area of the thoracic region, and, in the 20 mm embryo stage, only one persists at the definite site of the adult nipple and is the precursor of the future mammary gland.

In the 5th or 6th month of fetal life, the cords of epithelium extend into the underlying mesoderm as solid epithelial columns comprising 15–20 branches that form the outline of lactiferous ducts. These are surrounded by invading mesenchyme, which later develops into the fat and connective tissue. During the last 8 weeks of fetal life, these epithelial cords become canalised and acquire lumina. The epidermis at the point of origin of the gland forms a depression, which is called 'the mammary pit', into which these lactiferous ducts open.

At the time of birth, this pit evaginates to form the nipple, and the epithelium responds to the circulating maternal hormones with occasional secretion of milk, i.e. witch's milk. Congenital anomalies can be explained by these developmental processes.

Anatomy

The adult human female breast has a distinctive and uniquely protuberant form; it extends from the 2nd or 3rd rib to the 6th rib below. Its medial border extends to the lateral edge of the sternum and its lateral border extends up to the mid-axillary line. It is important also to note that the breasts extend superolaterally as a projection into the axillae. The breast includes glandular tissue, which is concentrated in the centre and upper outer half. The glandular tissue is composed of milk-producing lobular units, a system of branching ducts that are connected to the nipple–areola complex. Adipose and connective tissue surround these functional units and form the bulk of the breast. Dense connective tissue bands extend from the underlying pectoral fascia to the skin; these ligaments (Cooper's ligaments) hold the breast upwards, and their lengthening is responsible for ptosis of the breast with age. In the centre, is the nipple, which is elevated and pink in colour in nulliparous women, surrounded by the areola.

Development of the breast

The life cycle of the breast consists of three main periods: development (and early reproductive life), mature reproductive life and involution.

The female human breast undergoes two separate phases of growth and maturation. The first occurs

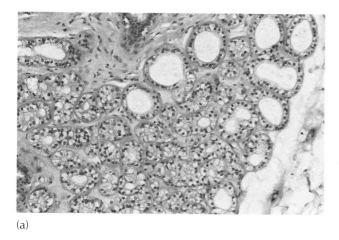

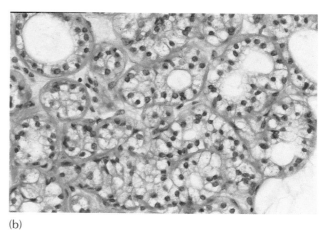

(a)

(b)

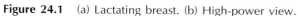

Figure 24.1 (a) Lactating breast. (b) High-power view.

during fetal development, resulting in the formulation of a rudimentary organ consisting of simple branched ducts. The breasts are identical in boys and girls in childhood, are inactive and consist of sparse ducts lying in stroma. The second period of growth occurs at puberty in females, when the ducts elongate, divide and form specialised terminal structures, i.e. terminal duct lobular units. The onset of puberty varies among different races, although in the Western world it can start from the age of 9–10 onwards.

The breasts are integral parts of the reproductive system, and with the onset of puberty, major changes take place in the female breast, in both size and shape as well as morphologically. There is enlargement of the breast, with increase in volume of connective tissue and fat. There is elongation, reduplication, branching and budding of the epithelial ducts with the formation of new lobules. The nipple and areola alter in shape and pigmentation.

All of these changes are hormone-induced, particularly related to the release and production of oestrogen and progesterone, both of which stimulate and promote growth in the breast parenchyma and are released after the onset of ovulation along with general growth hormones. By the onset of menstruation, the breasts are often well developed and a normal adolescent protuberant form takes shape.

After the breast has developed, it undergoes regular changes in relation to the menstrual cycle, and responds to repeated hormonal stimuli. In recent years, several authors have commented on and described subtle underlying changes taking place.[1]

During the luteal phase, the ductules are small and surrounded by condensed intralobular stroma containing plasma cells. In the secretory phase,

there is an increase in the size of lobules and ductules, and the stroma becomes loose and oedematous. There is vacuolation of the basal cells in the late secretory phase. In the premenstrual phase, there is a peak in the number of mitoses, lymphocytic infiltration and apoptosis following the onset of menstruation.[2]

Fully functional differentiation is said not to occur until the breast is subject to the stimulus of pregnancy. Pregnancy results in a series of changes in the breast that culminate in the fully differentiated state of lactation. Changes occur in the external appearance, with enlargement, vascularity and pigmentation of the areola and nipple and doubling of weight at term.[3]

In the breast parenchyma, there is marked proliferation and enlargement of the lobules in pregnancy, with diminution of the intralobular as well as the interlobular stroma. Secretory activity starts with supranuclear vacuolation in the early stages, proceeding to collection of colostrums in the lumen and an abundance of lipid inclusions, fat globules and vesicles in the later stages. The myoepithelial cells show slight elongation.

With the onset of lactation, there is even greater distension of the glandular lumina, with obliteration of the stroma (Figure 24.1). Interlobular ducts and lactiferous sinuses are markedly dilated. These changes are not uniform, some acini showing minimal activity.

After pregnancy and lactation, involutionary changes take place, the rate and degree varying between individuals. After a period of 3 months or so, the breast returns to the 'resting phase'.[4] The term 'involution' is used specifically, however, to describe postmenopausal atrophic changes in the

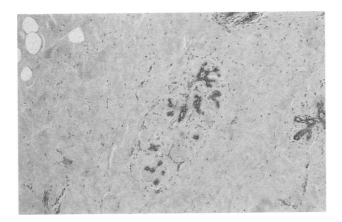

Figure 24.2 Normal atrophic lobules.

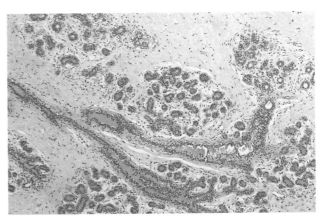

Figure 24.3 Normal lobules and terminal duct–lobular units.

breast that involve the lobules, ducts and stroma. In nulliparous women, these changes begin after the age of 30. There is a gradual decrease in the lobular component, with both stroma and epithelium being involved. The stroma converts into dense hyaline collagen and resembles ordinary connective tissue. The basement membrane of acini becomes thickened, the epithelium shrinks and becomes flattened, and the luminal space becomes narrow, almost obliterated, with cessation of secretions (Figure 24.2). Some acini may coalesce, with the formation of small cysts (microcysts), which may later shrink and be replaced by fibrous tissue. The interlobular ducts are also affected: some disappear, while some show shrinkage with irregular loss of elastic tissue and the prominent myoepithelial layer. These changes are not uniform, and may vary from segment to segment. The stroma is replaced by fat, and the breast becomes less radiodense, softer and droopy – hence more amenable to mammographic screening and examination.

It is extremely important to be familiar with and to appreciate the various changes that affect breast parenchyma in order to understand those breast conditions that occur during specific periods of life and are so common that they are best considered as aberrations rather than disease. This is particularly true when considering benign fibrocystic disease.[4]

Histology: normal structure of the breast

The functional unit of the breast is the terminal duct–lobular unit (TDLU; Figure 24.3), which is composed of lobules (Figure 24.4) and terminal ducts, which drain via a branching duct system to the nipple.

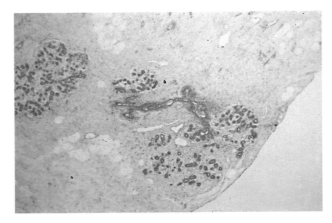

Figure 24.4 Normal lobules.

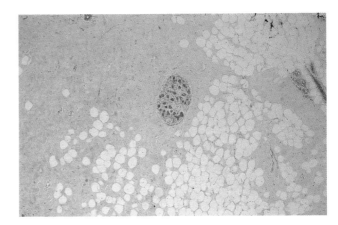

Figure 24.5 Normal lobule.

Under the microscope, the lobule is seen to consist of a collection of small blind-ending epithelial structures variously termed acini, alveoli or ductules and embedded in connective tissue stroma. The number of acini in a normal lobule varies from less than 15

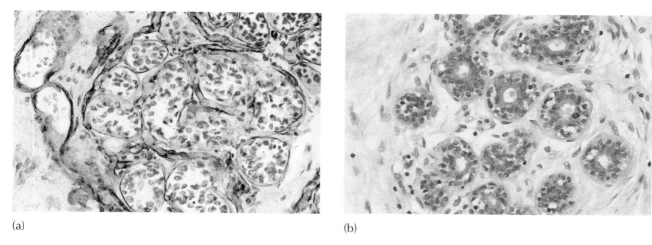

(a)

(b)

Figure 24.6   Normal lobule: (a) staining for basement membrane; (b) high-power view showing double cell layer and basement membrane.

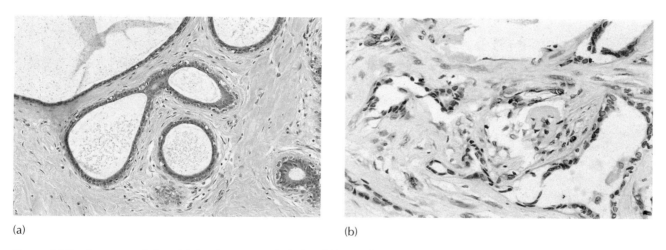

(a)

(b)

Figure 24.7   Immunostaining: (a) for the myoepithelial cell layer; (b) for myoepithelial cells.

to more than 100 (Figure 24.5). The acini are lined by two cell layers: an inner luminal layer consisting of epithelium (either cuboidal or columnar in type) and an outer layer consisting of myoepithelial cells, which lie beneath the epithelium and are discontinuous (hence some epithelial cells reach the basement membrane). The myoepithelial cells are spindle-shaped and contain small nuclei and clear cytoplasm (Figure 24.6). These cells can be difficult to demonstrate in haematoxylin and eosin (H&E) preparations; however, the immunohistochemical stains facilitate the identification of these cells. Epithelial cells can be stained by antibodies to epithelial membrane antigen (EMA) and by anticytokeratin antibodies (especially to low-molecular-weight cytokeratins). Myoepithelial cells can be demonstrated by various stains in fresh tissue and in formalin-fixed paraffin-embedded tissue (Figure 24.7). Smooth muscle actin is a useful marker. S100 protein can also be localised in these cells.

The lobular stroma is very distinct from the periductal stroma, both in type and in cellularity. It is highly specialised and richly vascular, and contains fine collagen fibres and abundant reticulin. It also constitutes the major bulk of the lobule and is mucoid and more cellular. A mixture of cells, including lymphocytes, histiocytes, plasma cells and mast cells, is found in addition to blood vessels and nerves.

In contrast, the extralobular stroma is more compact and contains elastic tissue, which becomes more abundant with ageing, and lobules of fat, which make up the bulk of breast tissue (Figure 24.8). This stroma also contains supplying blood vessels, lymphatics and nerves of the breast.

The extralobular terminal ducts lead to larger ducts, eventually to segmental ducts and ultimately to collecting ducts (Figure 24.9). The proximal part of

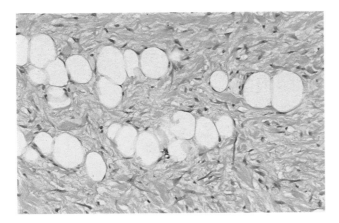

Figure 24.8 Fat, stroma and fibroblasts.

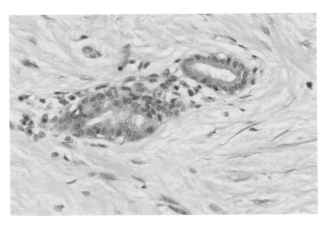

Figure 24.9 Ductal system in fibrous stroma.

the collecting ducts is lined by stratified squamous epithelium that is continuous with the skin, but the distal part shows an abrupt transition and is lined by two cell layers like the rest of the glandular epithelium, the only difference being that the myoepithelial layer is continuous.

The collecting ducts are continuous with the lactiferous sinuses. It is important to note that in the resting state there is marked papillary infolding of the wall of the lactiferous sinus, and to distinguish this normal appearance from intraductal papilloma or papillomatosis.

About 15–20 collecting ducts converge under the areola onto the surface of a nipple through separate orifices. Nipple and areola have distinctive histological appearances, the nipple being covered by stratified squamous keratinised epithelium, while the subcutaneous tissue contains irregularly arranged smooth muscle fibres, which have an erectile function (Figure 24.10). The areola has numerous sebaceous glands, many of which are not associated with hair follicles and discharge directly onto the nipple. Apocrine sweat glands are also normally present, and should not be mistaken for apocrine metaplasia arising in breast lobules.

Non-neoplastic conditions (miscellaneous benign conditions)

There are several conditions that are poorly understood but are clinically of great importance as they mimic carcinoma although they are benign in nature.

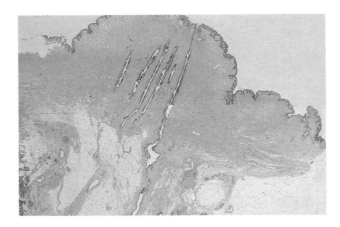

Figure 24.10 Normal nipple and major ducts.

Duct ectasia

The major subareolar ducts dilate and shorten during involution, and a minor degree of such change is commonly seen in breast biopsies as an incidental finding. Postmortem findings have indicated that this is present in almost 40–50% of women aged 60 or more.

The term 'duct ectasia', i.e. dilatation of ducts, coined by Haagensen in 1951,[5] is a poorly understood condition that is also variously known as plasma cell mastitis, comedo mastitis and obliterating chronic mastitis. Its aetiology is unknown: some suggest that the dilatation is the primary event, with the inflammation being secondary, perhaps due to a leak of the contents; others suggest that the inflammation is the primary process leading to fibrosis and duct dilatation with destruction of periductal elastic tissue.

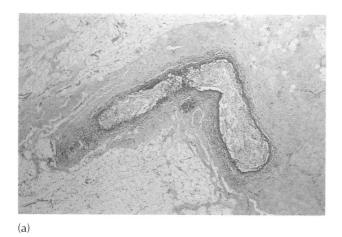

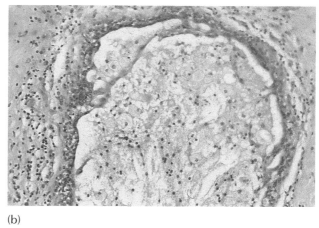

(a)   (b)

Figure 24.11   (a) Dilated duct with reactive macrophages in the lumen. (b) High-power view.

Clinically, duct ectasia is a disease of mature women, who present with nipple discharge, nipple retraction or a palpable mass that may be hard or doughy. The discharge is usually cheesy, which may cause eczematous reaction, and the nipple retraction is 'slit-like' classically. These features may clinically mimic carcinoma or Paget's disease. Mammographically, features such as calcification of the ducts in duct ectasia may resemble the pattern of calcification seen in comedo ductal carcinoma in situ.

Pathologically, the subareolar zone is firm, and the ducts are dilated and filled with greenish brown tenaceous fluid or more commonly paste-like material.

Duct ectasia is a ductal disease, its hallmark being dilated ducts filled with pasty material, periductal inflammation and fibrosis. In the early stages, the dilated ducts contain amorphous eosinophilic debris, some lipid-filled foamy cells and occasional crystalline material (Figure 24.11).

The epithelium may be attenuated, deformed or absent. There may be replacement by granulation tissue that also contains giant cells, foamy cells and myofibroblasts. There is a periductal inflammatory cellular infiltrate, which consists mainly of plasma cells, lymphocytes and histiocytes.

In the later stages, there is predominant periductal fibrosis, which may be irregular, resulting in distortion and obliteration of the ducts. Finally, there may be calcification.

Fat necrosis

Traumatic fat necrosis is another uncommon benign condition that is frequently mistaken for carcinoma.

It is most commonly encountered in elderly women, with voluminous pendulous breasts. It is post-traumatic, and a history of trauma can be elicited in 50% of cases. Focal ischaemia is a possible aetiological factor.

Clinically, fat necrosis can present as a firm ill-defined, indurated mass with pain, redness of the overlying skin and cutaneous retraction.

Macroscopically, the breast tissue shows an indurated zone with a bright yellow/opaque area of fat necrosis that is quite different from the adjacent unaffected fat. In some patients, it can form a cystic mass. In advanced cases, there may be fibrosis and calcification.

Histologically, there is necrosis of adipose tissue, with an inflammatory cell infiltrate that is rich in lymphocytes, plasma cells and histiocytes. There is release of fat from adipose tissue, with empty spaces being surrounded by macrophages, with foamy cells and multinucleated giant cells of foreign body type.

In the later stages, the granulomatous and fibroelastic reactions progress, resulting in fixation to the overlying skin. Granules of lipofuscin and haemosiderin pigment can be demonstrated by special stains. Sclerosis progresses and calcification can occur.

Aberration of normal development and involution (ANDI)

Benign non-neoplastic conditions of the breast show a wide variety of proliferative and regressive

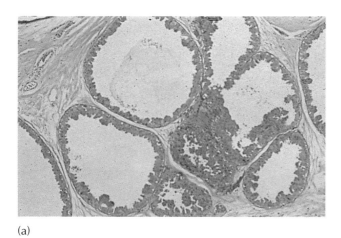

(a)

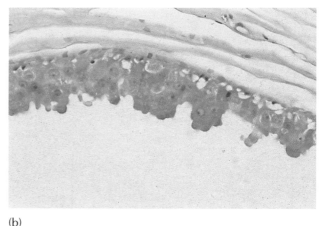

(b)

Figure 24.12 Apocrine metaplasia: (a) low-power view. (b) high-power view.

changes in the breast parenchyma, epithelial elements and stroma; some form distinct entities, but most have been grouped together and various terms have been used in the past to describe these changes collectively. These include chronic mastitis, interstitial mastitis, benign mammary dysplasia, mazoplasia, cystic mastopathy, fibroadenosis, Reclus' disease, Schimmelbusch's disease, and (most commonly) fibrocystic disease. Fibrocystic disease refers clinically to a condition of painful nodularity, and histologically to a picture of fibrosis, adenosis, apocrine metaplasia, epithelial hyperplasia, and cyst formation.

Cyclic pain and nodularity is extremely common in women of reproductive age and is regarded as physiological rather than pathological. Focal nodularity is seen in women of all ages and is the most common cause of a breast lump. Yet when excised and examined, a normal evolutionary process in the form of fibrosis or sclerosis is seen, and no pathological abnormality is found. Similarly, these changes have been found in the breasts of women without any clinical disease in autopsy studies. All of these observations have led to questions regarding the designation of 'disease' in this context, and the term 'fibrocystic change' has been suggested as being more appropriate. As already mentioned, fibrocystic change histologically includes cysts, apocrine metaplasia, adenosis and epithelial hyperplasia. In addition, to encompass all of the clinicopathological changes, the concept of aberration of normal development and involution (ANDI) has been proposed as a framework to classify benign breast disorders – a concept that is comprehensive, based on pathogenesis and important for rational management.[6]

The spectrum of change for each disorder varies from normal to mild abnormality, and only in some cases is there progression to disease.

Apocrine metaplasia

Apocrine change/metaplasia denotes the presence of pink apocrine cells that resemble apocrine sweat glands (Figure 24.12a). The cells are large and mostly columnar in shape, and contain abundant granular eosinophilic pink cytoplasm and basal nuclei. They show apical snouts, i.e. rounded protrusions (Figure 24.12b).

The cytoplasmic granules stain with Sudan black B and are periodic acid–Schiff (PAS)-positive after diastase digestion. The nuclei are round, basal and show prominent nucleoli. Nuclear pleomorphism is a common feature, but is not regarded as atypical (indeed, the presence of apocrine change denotes benignity). The apocrine change may present as a single layer of cells, but most commonly they form papillary projections. These changes are most frequently seen in the cysts and lobules.

Adenosis

Adenosis is a term used to describe an increase in the number of acini or ductules in a lobule, thus resulting in expansion of the lobule and alteration in its architecture. Two forms are recognised: blunt duct adenosis and microglandular adenosis.

Blunt duct adenosis

In blunt duct adenosis, the acini show marked dilatation and an irregular outline. Two cell layers are present. There is hypertrophy of the epithelium as well as the myoepithelium (Figures 24.13 and 24.14). The inner epithelial cells exhibit apocrine snouts. There is an increase in the specialised stroma; these changes are described as organoid lobular hypertrophy. Some acini show considerable dilatation resulting in microcysts.

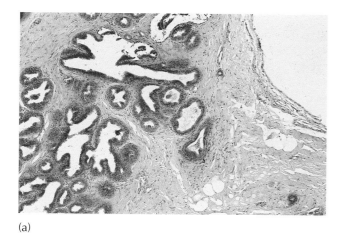

(a)

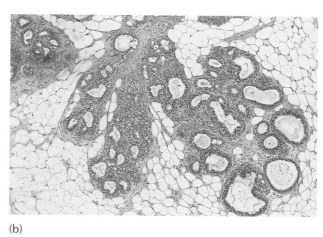

(b)

Figure 24.13 (a,b) Blunt duct adenosis.

Microglandular adenosis

This is a rare condition that histologically can be mistaken for a well-differentiated carcinoma, particularly tubular carcinoma. It can be an incidental finding in a biopsy or can present as a lump. The diameter can vary from 0.3 cm to 1.3 cm.

Microscopically, there are foci of numerous small rounded acinar/glandular structures infiltrating and present in breast adipose tissue. The acini are lined by a single layer of uniform small cells, many containing PAS-positive material. No myoepithelial cells are present, but basement membrane is present and can be demonstrated by reticulin stain and with type IV collagen. The stroma consists mainly of adipose tissue.

Epithelial hyperplasia

Epithelial hyperplasia is described as a benign, non-papillary intraluminal epithelial proliferation that can affect any part of the glandular system, but most frequently involves the TDLU or the interlobular ducts (Figure 24.15). Larger ducts are rarely involved.

The affected structures are expanded. There is multilayering (>4 cells in thickness), but there is no cytological atypia. Two-cell-type differentiation is present. The epithelial cells are uniform and cohesive and often appear syncitial. The nuclei are normochromatic and vesicular, and nucleoli are inconspicuous. Mitotic activity is usually low and no abnormal forms are seen. Myoepithelial cells are present, intermingling with proliferating epithelial cells, and can be demonstrated by the special stains mentioned above. Epithelial hyperplasia is described as mild, moderate or florid, depending on the degree of proliferation.

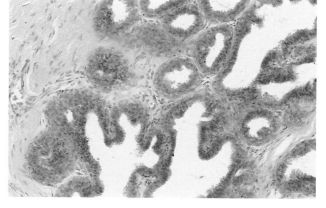

Figure 24.14 Blunt duct adenosis and ductal hyperplasia.

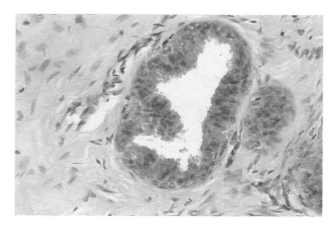

Figure 24.15 Ductal hyperplasia (usual type).

Fibroadenomatoid hyperplasia

This term is used to describe a fibroadenoma-like change in individual lobules; occasionally, these lobules may be loosely coalescent, forming an ill-

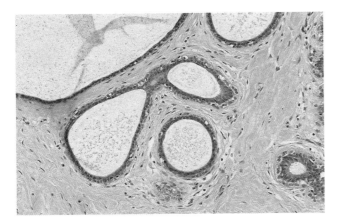

Figure 24.16 Early stage of cyst formation.

defined irregular mass. Depending on the size, fibroadenomatoid hyperplasia may or may not be clinically detectable. Macroscopically, as well as microscopically, there is no clear demarcation between the lobules showing fibroadenomatoid hyperplasia and the surrounding breast tissue. Very often, the nearby breast tissue shows fibrocystic change.

Cysts

Cysts are round or spherical structures derived from lobules, and are defined by the presence of a walled space filled with fluid. Cysts are often multifocal and bilateral and are usually found in clusters. Small cysts (microcysts) seen in breast biopsies represent an involutionary process, but several microcysts may expand and coalesce to form a solitary large cyst (Figure 24.16).

Large cysts (macrocysts) commonly present as discrete, palpable, smooth, sometimes painful lumps, which may or may not be fluctuant. Cysts constitute up to 15% of all discrete breast lumps and are common in pre- and perimenopausal women, the median age being 40–60. They are uncommon after the age of 60 (but are important because of associated intracystic papilloma).

They vary in size and can measure up to several centimetres, but cysts less than 1 cm are not usually palpable. They are readily diagnosed by ultrasound and mammography. The diagnosis is confirmed by aspiration of contents and cytology. Cytology is indicated only if the aspirated fluid is uniformly blood stained (intracystic papilloma or carcinoma). Larger cysts have rounded contours and a bluish colour (blue domed cysts). The cyst fluid can be thin and yellow, but more often is turbid, thick and vary in colour from dark green to brown, occasionally being blood-stained.

The cysts are usually lined by epithelium, which may be flattened, attenuated or even absent, particularly if the contents are under pressure. However, myoepithelial cells can be demonstrated by special stains. Many cysts are lined by an apocrine type of epithelium that forms small papillae.

Rupture of the cyst results in an inflammatory response, with collection of lymphocytes, plasma cells and histiocytes in the adjacent stroma. Foamy macrophages can be seen in the lumen as well as in the wall, with dense fibrosis.

Aberration of stromal involution

Aberration of stromal involution includes the development of localised areas of excessive sclerosis. These lesions, although benign, have the capacity to infiltrate locally, but are not known to metastasise or have any premalignant potential. However, they are of clinical importance as they cause diagnostic problems both clinically and mammographically. Excision biopsy is usually required to make a definite diagnosis. Two separate conditions belong to this group: sclerosing adenosis and radial scar/complex sclerosing lesions.

Sclerosing adenosis

This is the most widely recognised form of organoid lobular proliferation, in which the increased number of acini show elongation and distortion with spiky infiltrative margins. The lobular proliferation is multifocal, and, with coalescence of lobules, can present as a painful palpable mass. The term 'adenosis tumour' has been used to describe such lesions. The condition affects pre- or perimenopausal women, is most common in the age group 30–45, and is thought to recede after the menopause. The incidence of sclerosing adenosis has been described as between 12.5% and 25% of all benign biopsies.

Macroscopically, it can form a mass with well-defined borders and is firm (not hard) in consistency. On slicing, it can mimic carcinoma, particularly when yellow streaks of elastosis are present.

Microscopically, characteristic changes are present on low-power examination, which is of great value in making the correct diagnosis. Enlarged nodular units show a whorled pattern of compressed tubules. Normal lobular architecture is retained, although there is myoepithelial and stromal hyperplasia. An early proliferative and a later fibrotic/sclerotic phase can be recognised. The proliferative process involves the epithelial and myoepithelial cells, and results in

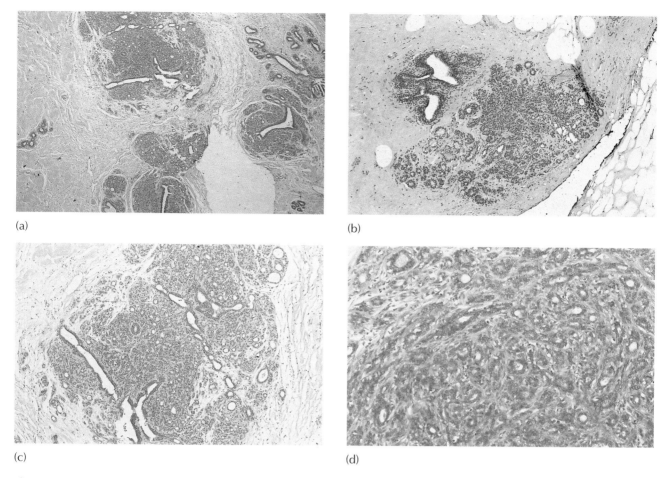

(a)

(b)

(c)

(d)

Figure 24.17 (a–d) Sclerosing adenosis.

compression and distortion of ductules, with obstruction of the lumen (Figure 24.17).

However, normal two-cell population (double cell layers) can be recognised in the tubules, there is no cytological atypia, cells have uniform small nuclei, and no abnormal mitotic figures are seen. Myoepithelium is abundant in the proliferative phase and can be demonstrated by special staining (i.e. PAS) or by immunocytochemical methods (Figure 24.18). Proliferating units extend and infiltrate not only stroma but also the nerves and vessels, but two-cell layers can be demonstrated, confirming the benign nature of the condition. The incidence of vascular and perineural infiltration varies and has been described as being between 3.9% and 10%. Apocrine metaplasia is seen in some areas.

In the later stages, there is evidence of elastosis, and the lumina of tubules contain calcispherules (Figure 24.18).

The main differential diagnosis is with carcinoma of the breast, including tubular carcinoma, from which

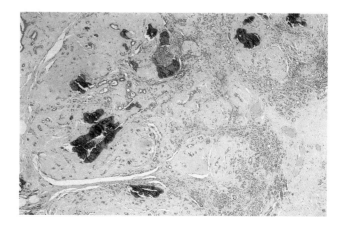

Figure 24.18 Sclerosing adenosis and microcalcifications.

sclerosing adenosis can easily be differentiated by a lack of cytological atypia, a normal organoid lobular pattern and the presence of a normal two-cell layer in the acini.

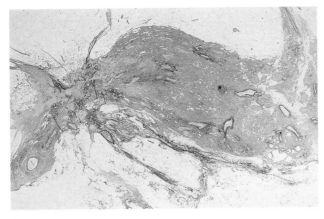

(a)

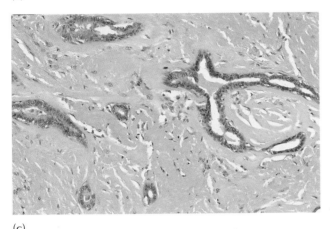

(c)

(b)

Figure 24.19 (a) Radial scar. (b) Low-power view. (c) High-power view.

Radial scar/complex sclerosing lesion

Radial scar

Radial scar (RS) is yet another proliferative lesion with a pseudo-infiltrative growth pattern. Over the years, these lesions have been described under several names, including infiltrative epitheliosis, sclerosing papillary proliferation, complex compound heteromorphic lesion, benign sclerosing ductal proliferation, non-encapsulated sclerosing lesion, rosette-like lesion, indurative mastopathy, radial sclerosing lesion and proliferation.

Radial scars are usually less than 1 cm in diameter; lesions larger than 1 cm are termed complex sclerosing lesions (CSL). They rarely present as a palpable mass. The reported incidence varies between 1.7% of benign surgical biopsies to as much as 28%, but they are becoming more and more common since the implementation of mammography as a diagnostic tool for screening women for cancer.

They present as a stellate mammographic abnormality, but their greatest importance is due to their ability to mimic carcinoma mammographically and even histologically. Macroscopically, small lesions may be difficult to see, but if viewed by a hand lens an irregular stellate shaped area is seen. Yellow streaks and flecks of calcification may be apparent, and again these features may mimic a malignant lesion.

The histological changes depend on the stage of development and maturation. The mature fully developed lesion consists clinically of a central area of fibroelastic tissue that shows entrapped tubules with proliferating epithelial elements radiating out at the periphery. This appearance has been described as 'flower-head', 'daisy head' or floret manner (Figures 24.19 and 24.20).

The dense fibroelastic tissue in the central core stains pink with H&E and black with the Weigert stain, but also shows entrapped tubules that are angulated randomly and distributed in a non-organoid manner. It is this pattern than can mimic a well-differentiated tubular carcinoma. The epithelial tubules in RS still show a normal two-cell layer. The myoepithelial layer as well as the basement membrane can be demonstrated both by conventional staining (PAS) or by immunocytochemical staining. The epithelial element at the periphery

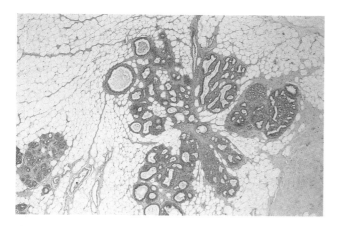

Figure 24.20 Radial scar and blunt duct adenosis.

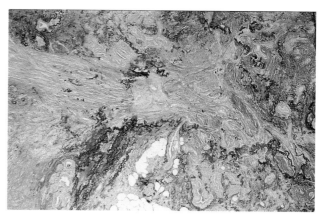

Figure 24.21 Complex sclerosing lesion (stained with EVG).

shows variable proliferative changes. There is epithelial hyperplasia, which may be papillary, solid or cystic and may contain intraluminal calcispherules. There is no cytological atypia.

Complex sclerosing lesions

CSLs are larger than 1 cm and have all the features of RS, although on a greater scale. Macroscopically, they may appear as a nodular mass with a central area of fibrosis, although occasionally they give the impression of a mass, which is due to the coalescence of several small adjacent sclerosing lesions. Like RS, they may mimic carcinoma on naked eye examination.

Besides being larger than RS, these lesions show in addition greater disturbance of structure and other additional changes, namely apocrine metaplasia, papilloma formation and sclerosing adenosis at the periphery resulting in nodule formation. As with RS, epithelial atypia is lacking, and the two-cell layer and basement membrane are present and can be demonstrated by special stains (Figure 24.21).

As with other lesions, the most important differential diagnosis is from tubular carcinoma. The epithelial tubules in carcinoma are lined by a single cell layer, the basement membrane is absent and there is infiltration of fat.

Benign tumours

Fibroadenoma

Fibroadenomas (FA) are benign circumscribed tumours of the breast, composed of varying amounts of epithelial and stromal components (Figure 24.22). Although described as benign tumours, these lesions

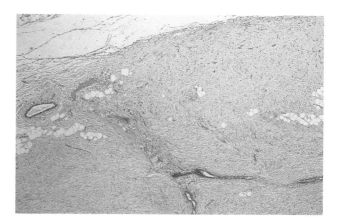

Figure 24.22 Fibroadenoma.

are thought to be a benign malformation/aberration of normal development. They arise from a single lobule rather than from a single cell, and, are under the same hormonal control as the rest of the breast – they lactate during pregnancy and undergo involution in the perimenopausal stage and may be calcified. Their incidence is variable; overall they account for 13% of all palpable breast lumps, although the relative incidence in different age groups varies, accounting for 60% in the younger age group (15–25 years) but only 15% in women aged 30–40. They are found much less frequently in the breasts of older women. The autopsy incidence varies from 9% to 28% in different series. FA are said to occur more frequently in Afro-Carribean populations. They are usually solitary, but sometimes can be multiple and bilateral.

Clinically, FA present as palpable breast lumps. The majority are located in the upper outer quadrant of the breast. Classically, the lump is discrete, smooth, mobile and not painful. The clinical diagnosis of FA must be confirmed by aspiration cytology.

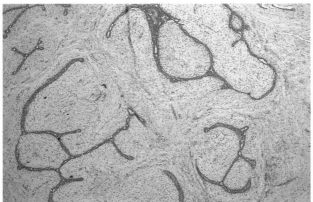

Figure 24.23 Fibroadenoma: high-power view.

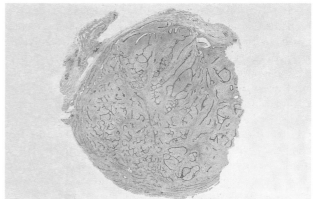

Figure 24.25 Fibroadenoma: pericanalicular type, with some leaf-like structures (on the right-hand side).

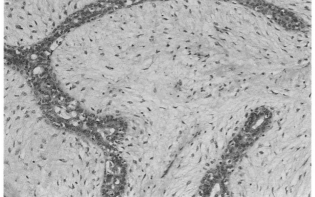

Figure 24.24 Fibroadenoma with ductal hyperplasia (usual type).

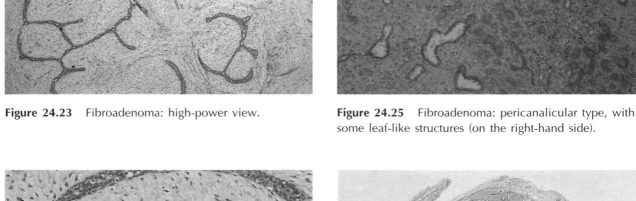

Figure 24.26 Fibroadenoma: intracanalicular type.

Most FA grow to a size varying from 1 to 3 cm, some stay stationary in size, but many regress and even disappear; a few grow larger (giant FA). Several follow-up studies have confirmed this behaviour, and this is why, after confirming the diagnosis of fibroadenoma, many hospitals and units allow the patient the choice of excision or observation. However, if there is an increase in size or other unusual features, they are excised and examined histologically.

Four separate clinical entities have been described:

- common fibroadenoma
- giant fibroadenoma
- juvenile fibroadenoma
- phyllodes tumour.

FA exhibit a wide variety of histological and cytological changes, as already mentioned, both epithelial and stromal components being present. The epithelium usually has two cell layers, but may be multilayered (Figures 24.23 and 24.24).

The stroma is rather loose and myxoid, and consists of spindle cells. Rarely, other mesenchymal elements (fat, muscle and, rarely, bone) are present. Two types of growth pattern are described: pericanalicular and intracanalicular (Figures 24.25 and 24.26).[7]

In the pericanalicular type, the epithelial component consists of rounded duct-like structures surrounded by stroma arranged in a concentric manner. In the intracanalicular type, the epithelial element shows considerable thinning, elongation and distortion, with prominent intervening stroma. In any FA, usually both patterns are present.

Older lesions show atrophy of epithelium, hyalinisation and sometimes calcification of the stroma. They can undergo infarction.

As FA arise from lobules, other histological changes that affect the lobule (apocrine metaplasia, epithelial hyperplasia and sclerosing adenosis), can also be seen. Rarely, in situ malignant changes can also be seen.

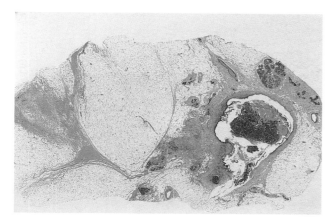

Figure 24.27 Intraductal papilloma (low power).

Papilloma

Papilloma is a term that refers to a distinct villous lesion with an arborescent fibrovascular stroma covered by a double layer of epithelium: an outer myoepithelial layer and an inner epithelial layer. Papillomas can be microscopic or macroscopic (Figure 24.27).

Solitary papillomas occur centrally and are found most frequently in large collecting ducts beneath the nipple. They are relatively uncommon and can appear at any age – they may be seen in adolescents or in elderly women – but occur most commonly in middle age. They are the commonest cause of nipple discharge, with 80% of patients presenting clinically with this symptom. The discharge can be serosanguinous or blood-stained. A mass can sometimes be felt, but nipple retraction is uncommon. Papillomas can be revealed by galactography.

Papillomas can be small, a few millimetres in diameter, when they appear as an elongated structure extending along a major duct and are only seen on microscopic examination. However, they can be larger, forming soft and friable spheroidal masses. If such a mass is present in a major duct, this may result in dilatation and distension of the duct, and the papilloma may assume a cyst-like appearance (hence the name intracystic papilloma) and may be filled with blood. Even when large, papillomas are rarely more than 3 cm in diameter.

Sections show a true papilloma with a stalk attached to the duct wall. It has a distinct arborescent configuration with branching fibrovascular stroma, usually well developed, and contains blood vessels and collagenous elements. These are covered by epithelium. The epithelium has the normal two cell layers (an essential feature of a benign papilloma): an outer myoepithelial layer and an inner luminal epithelial layer.

The cells are either cuboidal or columnar, and their nuclei are vesicular with inconspicuous nucleoli and normochromatic. The nuclear/cytoplasmic ratio is low, mitoses are usually infrequent, and no abnormal forms are seen (Figure 24.28).

There may be foci of epithelial hyperplasia, which is without atypia.

Other features are also seen: apocrine metaplasia is a frequent finding; squamous metaplasia is also sometimes seen, particularly near areas of infarction. Haemorrhage and sclerosis are very common. Periductal fibrosis and sclerosis may result in entrapped epithelium, which may be distorted and may be mistaken for infiltration or invasion. In spite of this appearance of pseudo-infiltration, the two-cell-layer structure is retained and myoepithelial cells can be demonstrated by special stains, particularly by α smooth muscle actin antibody.

All of the features present in a lesion should be taken into account to confirm the diagnosis of a benign papilloma.

Multiple papillomas are found at the periphery, distant from the nipple; they involve the TDLU and are an integral part of the fibrocystic change.

Phyllodes tumour (cystosarcoma phyllodes)

Cystosarcoma phyllodes is a tumour with the basic structure of a fibroadenoma but is characterized by marked proliferation of connective tissue stroma and has potential for local recurrence and metastasis. The name cystosarcoma phyllodes was given to the tumour by Müller in 1938, describing a large fleshy tumour with a papillary 'leaf-like' appearance on the cut surface.[8]

These tumours have been called giant fibroadenomas, adenomyxomas, pseudosarcomatous adenomas and papillary cystofibromas. As most of the tumours are benign, the use of the term 'sarcoma' has caused considerable confusion. The World Health Organization (WHO) classification has adopted the term phyllodes tumour, which is widely used nowadays. The biological behaviour of these tumours is unpredictable; even the histological appearance is not a good prediction of subsequent behaviour, but many authors classify them as neither benign nor malignant.

The tumours appear in middle-aged women, with the maximum incidence being in the fifth decade, although they have been reported in adolescent as well as in elderly women. The most common age of appearance of phyllodes tumour is 10 years later than that of fibroadenoma.

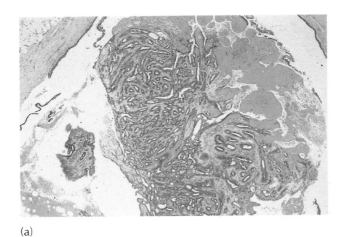

(a)

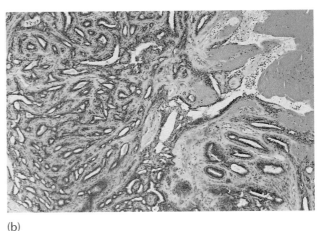

(b)

Figure 24.28 Sclerosing intraductal papilloma: (a) low-power view; (b,c) high-power views.

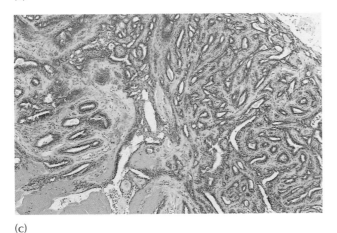

(c)

Characteristically, phyllodes tumours grow slowly at first, then rapidly attain a large size. Although they are usually larger than fibroadenomas, size is not an acceptable criteria for diagnosis. Clinically, a large spherical well-circumscribed tumour is present in the breast. It can be up to 10–20 cm in diameter. Cutaneous ulceration may be present, but is a late manifestation. Bilateral tumours are very rare.

The tumour is well-circumscribed, grey to white in colour, firm and generally more than 5 cm in diameter. The cut surface shows clefts and cystic spaces, and loose myxoid areas may be seen. Larger tumours are soft, fleshy and may show areas of haemorrhage or necrosis.

Sections show a tumour with the basic growth pattern of an intracanalicular fibroadenoma. There are leaf-like epithelial-lined papillary projections into the cystic spaces (Figure 24.29). The main changes are seen in the stroma, which is abundant and prominent, and shows both increased cellularity as well as variation in appearances within the same tumours.

The cells may show the appearances of uniform spindle-shaped fibroblasts, as well as nuclear hyper-

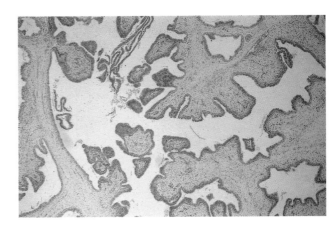

Figure 24.29 Benign phyllodes tumour.

chromasia, marked pleomorphism and mitotic activity. The stromal cells usually aggregate around the epithelium and sometimes around blood vessels. The cellularity of the stroma may vary from a cellular fibroma to a fibrosarcoma (Figure 24.30). Hyalinisation and myxoid change are common. Adipose tissue, smooth muscle cartilage and bone may be seen.

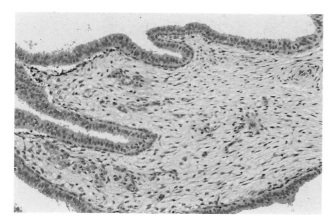

Figure 24.30 Benign phyllodes tumour: double cell layer and cellular stroma.

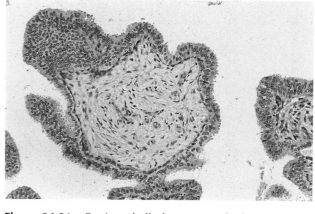

Figure 24.31 Benign phyllodes tumour: high-power view.

The epithelium is composed of two cell layers, and may show hyperplasia (Figures 24.30 and 24.31). Other changes (e.g. apocrine metaplasia and sclerosing adenosis) are not commonly seen in phyllodes tumour. Phyllodes tumours must be differentiated from fibroadenomas because of their different clinical behaviour and surgical treatment.

References

1. Rudland PS, Barraclough R, Fernig DG, Smith JA. Growth and differentiation of the normal mammary gland and its tumours. Biochem Soc Symp 1998; 63: 1–20.

2. Rosen PP, Oberman HA. Atlas of Tumour Pathology: Tumours of the Mammary Gland. Washington, DC: Armed Forces Institute of Pathology, 1992.

3. Rosen PP. Rosen's Breast Pathology. Philadelphia: Lippincott-Raven, 1997.

4. Bland KI, Coleland EM. The Breast. Philadelphia: WB Saunders, 1991.

5. Haagensen CD. Mammary-duct extasia; a disease that may simulate carcinoma. Cancer 1951; 4: 749–61.

6. Hughes LE, Mansel RE, Webster DJT. Benign Disorders and Diseases of the Breast. London: Balllière Tindall, 1989.

7. Harris JA, Lippman ME, Morrow M, Hellman S. Diseases of the Breast. Philadelphia: Lippincott-Raven, 1996.

8. Müller J. Uber den feinern Bau und die Formen der Krankhaften Geschwulste. Berlin: G Reimer, 1838: 54–60.

25 Histological risk factors, prognostic indicators and staging

Sarah E Pinder, Ian O Ellis

Risk factors

Risk factors may be defined as those characteristics that impart a greater chance of developing a disease over the risk of the general population. The biological risk factors for the development of breast cancer are complex and multifactorial and still remain poorly understood. Several risk factors for breast cancer are well recognised, including family history of breast cancer, reproductive hormone and radiation exposure, diet/nutrition, together with morphological factors within the breast itself. However, it is not appropriate to cover all of these in this chapter, which will concentrate on histopathological risk factors.

It is clear that epithelial proliferative diseases, including usual and atypical ductal epithelial hyperplasias and lobular neoplasia, confer an increased risk of developing breast cancer. These lesions may be discovered coincidentally in histopathology breast screening practice. Much of the work on risk associated with histopathological lesions has been performed by Page and Dupont, and their criteria for atypical proliferative diseases in particular must be adhered to if risk estimates are to be extrapolated.[1,2] Fibrocystic changes are no longer believed to be a true disease, but there is a minimally increased risk of cancer in patients with usual type epithelial hyperplasia amounting to 1.5–2.0 times that of a reference population during the subsequent 10–15 years after diagnosis.[3] A 4.6-fold increased risk is found for patients with atypical ductal hyperplasia (ADH), although it is important to note that this risk falls after 10–15 years towards that of a control population.[4] However, if there is an associated family history (at least one first-degree relative), the risk associated with ADH doubles.[4] Atypical lobular hyperplasia confers a 4- to 5-fold-increased relative risk and lobular carcinoma in situ (LCIS) an 8- to 10-fold-increased risk.[5]

Other benign conditions, such as sclerosing adenosis and fibroadenomas are said to be associated with a minor increased relative risk of breast carcinoma (1.7-fold[6] and 2.17-fold that of the general population respectively), but this increases to 3.10-fold in 'complex' fibroadenomas with foci of sclerosing adenosis or papillary apocrine change.[7]

These epithelial proliferative lesions may be excised coincidentally, for example in association with a lesion noted symptomatically or detected in a breast screening programme, but may, if sufficiently high a risk is conferred, warrant follow-up. The risk incurred by the patient with these lesions and the lifetime risk for an 'average' woman (which is reported as 1 in 8 for women in the USA[8]) must be interpreted with care by clinicians. The *relative risk* indicates the number of patients who develop breast cancer compared with that of the general population over a given period of time, but the *absolute risk* of developing breast cancer reflects the probability of developing breast cancer for that patient and is related to the women's age, the age-specific incidence of carcinoma and deaths from other causes, as well as the relative risk of that individual, and is thus a more useful concept for the patient. Thus the relative risk of a 40-year-old woman with ADH of 4.5 is reflected in an absolute risk of about 8–10% of developing invasive breast carcinoma in the following 18–20 years, but for a 60-year-old with ADH, the chance is 25% within 20 years. Thus it may be easier for a patient to understand her true individual risk of developing breast carcinoma in terms of *absolute risk*. It is also important that the relative risks described associated with epithelial proliferative diseases may not be long-lasting; the increased risk associated with ADH lasts only 10–15 years, therefore indefinite follow-up at a high-risk clinic for patients with some of these lesions (and no family history) may not be justified and induce unnecessary anxiety.

Prognostic indicators

Prediction of the behaviour of breast carcinoma by the use of prognostic indicators is essential; breast cancer is not a single disease entity and does not behave in a standard fashion. In particular, the range of treatment choices for patients with breast cancer has widened considerably (and continues to do so), including variation in extent of surgery from breast conservation to mastectomy, variation in extent of axillary surgery (sentinel node, biopsy sampling or clearance) and differing adjuvant local and systemic therapies.

Prognostic factors have been described as having three major functions.[9] The first purpose is to identify patients whose prognosis is so good that they require no further adjuvant treatment. The second reason is to identify patients whose prognosis is so poor that an aggressive approach to treatment may be required. The third function is to identify patients who may respond or be resistant to specific therapies, thus acting as predictive agents. Treatment strategies for individual patients can and should therefore be tailored, based on the prediction of behaviour of each breast tumour. Although historically the major role of the pathologist lay in providing an accurate diagnosis, it is now well recognised that much prognostic information can be obtained from careful examination of well-fixed resected tumour and regional lymph nodes.

Tumour size

Clinical measurement of breast tumours is inaccurate; a correlation between surgical and pathological assessment of tumour size was found in only 54% of cases by the Yorkshire Breast Cancer Group.[10] Ultrasound measurement is more useful if an estimate of clinical tumour size is required for treatment planning. Tumour size can be assessed in the fresh state and in the fixed specimen, when the margins of the tumour may be better defined. However, it is particularly important for accurate size determination of small lesions, pure in situ cancers and cases where there is extensive in situ

disease on tissue sections using the Vernier scale on the microscope stage.

A multitude of studies have confirmed the prognostic significance of breast cancer size;[11] patients with small tumours have better long-term survival. Rosen and Groshen[12] reported a 20-year relapse-free survival rate of 88% for patients with tumours less than 10 mm in diameter and 73% for women with cancers measuring 11–13 mm, falling to 65% and 59% for 14–16 mm and 17–22 mm lesions respectively. It is well recognised that breast screening programmes identify smaller tumours than can be found in symptomatic practice.[13]

The terms 'minimal breast cancer' and 'minimal invasive breast carcinoma' have been used by different groups to represent lesions of varying sizes, but there is little doubt that lesions that, for example, measure 10 mm or less are at an earlier stage than larger tumours; lymph node positivity was seen in approximately 15–20% compared with 40% in lesions greater than 15 mm in diameter by Rosen and Groshen.[12] Because of the recognition of the prognostic importance of tumour size, this parameter has become an important quality assurance measure for radiologists in the UK National Health Service Breast Screening Programme (NHSBSP), with a recommendation that a target of 15 minimal invasive carcinomas per 10 000 women screened should be detected.

Histological grade and type

Differentiation of a breast carcinoma may be assessed by the determination of tumour type and histological grade. Both factors can be assessed by microscopic examination of routinely stained tissue sections, although it is essential that samples be well fixed, and well-defined criteria must be used and adhered to.[14] Ideally, specimens should be sent to the laboratory in the fresh state, incised immediately and placed in fixative to obtain optimum preservation of morphological details and mitotic figures.

Histological grade is well recognised as a prognostic indicator, and several studies have refuted earlier suggestions of lack of reproducibility if strict criteria are maintained.[15,16] Two main methods for histological grading have evolved. One is based on nuclear features alone and the other on both architectural and tumour cell features. The latter has been modified to give greater objectivity[17] and has been adopted for use in the NHSBSP,[14] much of Europe and the USA.[18,19] This method of histological grading assesses the three features of tubule formation, nuclear size/pleomorphism and mitotic count; each of these elements is scored 1–3 and the sum of the scores is used to categorise the tumour. If less than 10% of the carcinoma is forming luminal structures, a score of 3 is given, those with 10–75% score 2, and if more than 75% of the cancer is forming tubules, a score of 1 is given. A score for tumour cell pleomorphism/size is given as 1, 2 or 3 according to whether mild pleomorphism/small cell size, moderate pleomorphism/medium size or highly pleomorphic/large nuclear size is seen. As noted above, good fixation is essential for reliable assessment of mitotic count. A score for this component is given according to the field area of the high-power lens used. Although included in the technique of Bloom and Richardson[20] for determination of histological grade, hyperchromatic (and apoptotic) nuclei should be discounted in the modified system – only nuclei with definite features of metaphase, anaphase or telophase are included. An overall sum of the three component scores of 3, 4 or 5 indicates a grade 1 cancer, a score of 6 or 7 a grade 2 tumour, and a score of 8 or 9 a carcinoma of histological grade 3.

Histological grade is a strong indicator of patient survival (Figure 25.1). Patients with grade 1 carcinomas have an 85% 10-year survival rate, compared with a rate of less than 45% for patients with grade 3 tumours. A greater proportion of grade 1 carcinomas are found in screening programmes compared with symptomatic practice.

In addition, histological grade provides information on prediction of response to therapy, and in this way can also be regarded as a predictive factor in both the adjuvant[21] and advanced breast cancer settings.[22]

Breast carcinomas show a great variation in morphological appearance, and some forms of primary breast cancer, the so-called 'special types', carry a significantly better prognosis than the more common 'no special type' (NST)/ductal tumours. Other tumour types with varying prognoses can be recognised, however, and up to 15 categories of invasive tumour type are used in the Nottingham unit, excluding the in situ and microinvasive classes.[23] If a large number of mixed types are recorded, a smaller proportion of lesions will be classified as NST/ductal (only approximately 50% of breast carcinomas in our unit); tumours that include areas of NST with additional foci of 'special-type' morphology are categorised separately. In our hands, we have found that these groups of tumours behave differently, with a 64% 10-year survival rate in tumours of NST when combined with foci of special type carcinoma, compared with a 47% 10-year survival rate of 'pure' NST breast carcinomas.[23] An increased proportion of the good-prognosis 'special types' is seen in screening compared with symptomatic practice.

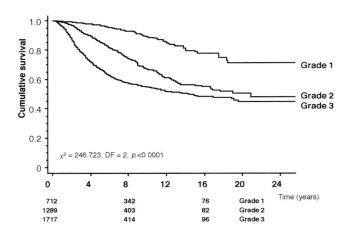

Figure 25.1 Long-term overall survival in the Nottingham Tenovus Primary Breast Carcinoma Series by histological grade.

The complexities of invasive breast tumour classification will not be outlined in this chapter, but for prognostication purposes several tumour types can be amalgamated into four prognostic groups according to the demonstrated 10-year survival rate from the Nottingham Tenovus Primary Breast Cancer Series (NTPBCS).[24] Those tumour types with an excellent prognosis (>80% 10-year survival rate) include tubular, invasive cribriform, mucinous and tubulolobular carcinomas. Tumours with a good prognosis (68–80% 10-year survival rate) include tubular mixed, alveolar lobular and mixed ductal/NST with special type. A 58–60% 10-year survival rate is seen with medullary, invasive papillary and classical lobular carcinomas and a poor prognosis (<50% 10-year survival rate) with lesions of mixed lobular, NST, solid lobular and mixed ductal with lobular types.

Tumour type group alone provides important biological information, but is not in our opinion as valuable as histological grade for predicting any individual patient's likely prognosis. This is not only true for tumours of NST/ductal morphology, in which the importance of histological grade is well recognised, but is of value for all invasive breast cancers. Previously, pathologists may have only assessed the histological grade of tumours of ductal/NST morphology, but it should be remembered that although, for example, the majority of invasive lobular carcinomas are of grade 2 morphology (scoring 3 for tubules, 2 for pleomorphism and 1 for mitoses), rarer subgroups of either histological grade 1 or grade 3 may be identified with better and worse survivals respectively (Figure 25.2). Thus we would recommend grading all invasive breast carcinomas.

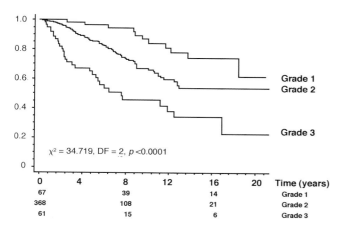

Figure 25.2 Long-term overall survival in the Nottingham Tenovus Primary Breast Carcinoma Series for lobular carcinoma (all subtypes) by histological grade.

It has been suggested that histological grade was not a reproducible technique for providing prognostic information, but the same potential difficulties regarding reproducibility apply to accurate histological typing of some lesions. Although some histological tumour types, such as mucinous carcinoma, may be determined reproducibly,[25] problems of typing are compounded by the larger number of type categories that must be selected from by the reporting pathologist. Issues of reproducibility may to some extent explain the variation in patient survival reported in the literature for some types of invasive breast cancer; for example, medullary carcinomas do not have as good survival in the NTPBCS[24] that is reported in some other studies.[26,27] This variation in survival of patients with medullary carcinoma is likely to be, at least in part, a reflection of the difficulties in establishing robust diagnostic criteria for this breast carcinoma type.[28,29] While criteria for grading carcinomas are now strictly defined, this is less true for breast tumour typing.

Despite the difficulties described, it should be noted that both histological type and grade provide important complementary prognostic information. While in multivariate analysis, grade is of much greater importance in predicting survival than type, tumour typing provides additional information on behaviour. For example, lobular carcinomas, particularly those of alveolar lobular type, are often oestrogen receptor (ER)-positive,[30] show different expression of markers such as E-cadherin and the catenins,[31] and may also demonstrate a different pattern of metastatic disease to tumours of no special type.[32]

Staging

Staging of breast cancer is essential in the assessment of a patient's prognosis and selection of treatment options. Staging may be purely clinical, or pathological by examination of the tumour and axillary tissue and, when appropriate, material from other sites such as internal mammary nodes. The TNM staging method incorporates an assessment of the primary tumour size (T), the regional lymph nodes (N) and distant metastases (M). Although initially proposed in 1954, several modifications have since been made (see Table 25.1 for the 'N' part of the classification).[33] When clinical determination alone is used, the system is notoriously inaccurate; lymph nodes may be enlarged due to reactive changes, while nodes bearing metastatic tumour may be impalpable. Reliable staging of invasive breast carcinoma is imperative and a careful histological examination of lymph nodes should be carried out.

Questions over whether lymph nodes should be sampled or whether the axilla should be cleared remain unresolved, and arguments have been presented for both clearance[32] and sampling[34] procedures. Steele et al[34] found no difference in the incidence of cases of lymph node positivity in patients with sampling or clearance and argued that, provided that at least four nodes were examined, sufficient prognostic information could be provided by sampling. The greater number of nodes obtained by clearance is associated with increased postoperative morbidity, including lymphoedema and reduced shoulder mobility. Conversely, sampling or low axillary clearance may potentially 'understage' the axilla. There is no consensus on the number of nodes that should be examined to ensure accurate staging. Numerous studies have shown that patients with involved lymph nodes have a poorer prognosis than those with no metastases in the locoregional nodes and that prognosis is also related to the absolute number of involved lymph nodes; the greater the number of nodes with metastatic tumour, the poorer the prognosis.[35] There is evidence that the anatomical level of involvement is also important[36,37] Some studies have found that the proportion of 'negative' axillae decreases as more nodes are sampled,[38–40] but this is not a consistent finding.[41] While this could be interpreted as indicating that more nodes should be sampled, the sentinel lymph node technique is increasingly being utilised to target nodal retrieval.

The sentinel lymph node is the first node that drains the tumour and is thus potentially the site of initial metastasis.[42] Whether the sentinel lymph node is involved or not should therefore reflect the nodal status of the axilla and thus the patient's prognosis. The sentinel node concept has been validated for breast cancer;[43–46] if only one node is involved with metastatic carcinoma, this is almost always the sentinel node and moreover, this is frequently the only site of metastasis.

Table 25.1	**TNM pathological classification for regional lymph node stage**[33]
pNX	Regional lymph nodes not assessable
pN0	No metastasis and no additional examination performed
pN0(i–)	No regional node metastasis, negative immunohistologically
pN0(i+)	No regional node metastasis, positive immunohistologically but no cluster > 0.2 mm
pN0(mol–)	No regional node metastasis, negative molecular findings (RT–PCR)
pN0(mol+)	No regional node metastasis, positive molecular findings (RT–PCR)
pN1mi	Micrometastasis (> 0.2 mm, but ≤2 mm in greatest dimension)
pN1	Metastasis in 1–3 ipsilateral axillary lymph nodes, and/or in internal mammary nodes with microscopic metastasis detected by sentinel lymph node dissection but not clinically apparent
pN1a	Metastasis in 1–3 axillary lymph nodes (including at least one that is >2 mm, i.e. not micrometastatic)
pN1b	Metastasis in internal mammary lymph nodes with microscopic metastasis detected by sentinel lymph node dissection but not clinically apparent
pN1c	Metastasis in 1–3 axillary lymph nodes *and* internal mammary lymph nodes with microscopic metastasis detected by sentinel lymph node dissection but not clinically apparent
pN2	Metastasis in 4–9 ipsilateral axillary lymph nodes, or in clinically apparent ipsilateral internal mammary lymph nodes in the absence of axillary lymph node metastasis
pN2a	Metastasis in 4–9 axillary lymph nodes (including at least one that is >2 mm, i.e. not micrometastatic)
pN2b	Metastasis in clinically apparent internal mammary lymph nodes in the *absence* of axillary lymph node metastasis
pN3	Metastasis in ≥10 ipsilateral axillary lymph nodes or in infraclavicular lymph nodes or in clinically apparent ipsilateral internal mammary lymph nodes in the *presence* of one or more positive axillary lymph nodes; or in >3 axillary lymph nodes with clinically negative, microscopic metastasis in internal mammary lymph nodes; or in ipsilateral supraclavicular lymph nodes
pN3a	Metastasis in ≥10 axillary lymph nodes (at least one >2 mm) *or* metastasis in infraclavicular lymph nodes
pN3b	Metastasis in clinically apparent internal mammary lymph nodes in the *presence* of one or more positive axillary lymph nodes; or metastasis in >3 axillary lymph nodes and in internal mammary lymph nodes with microscopic metastasis detected by sentinel lymph node dissection but not clinically apparent
pN3c	Metastasis in ipsilateral supraclavicular lymph nodes

If determined using a sentinel node technique alone, stage is designated '(sn)', e.g. pN0 (i–)(sn).
RT–PCR, reverse transcriptase polymerase chain reaction.

The robust evidence that axillary nodal status provides prognostic information is largely based on studies in which a single slice from each axillary node was examined using routinely stained sections. A weakness of some of the sentinel lymph node studies is that the sentinel node is examined more intensively than the other nodes, which may mean that metastases in non-sentinel nodes are missed or that small deposits in the sentinel node are more likely to be reported compared with previous conventional studies in the established medical literature.[47–50] Additional laboratory techniques, including complete embedding of the node or assessment of step sections, immunohistochemistry and even reverse transcriptase polymerase chain reaction (RT–PCR), can be used to increase the sensitivity of detection of metastases. Complete embedding of each node and/or serial, step sectioning increase the chance of identifying metastases, as more of the node is examined.[51–53] Immunohistochemistry increases detection,[52,54,55] in part by making small metastases more visible. RT–PCR examines all the tissue submitted with a very sensitive method that is theoretically capable of identifying a single tumour cell.[56,57]

From the point of view of the histopathologist, whatever the surgical extent and technique, all of the excised nodes must be examined microscopically. Whether the lymph nodes received are taken as part of an axillary sampling or as a sentinel node technique, blocks are taken by serial slicing of each node along the long axis in approximately 3 mm slices, thus providing the largest area of lymph node and peripheral sinus possible in one section. Ideally, each node should be examined in a separate cassette, and the majority of lymph nodes can be entirely embedded in slices in this way, although large non-sentinel lymph nodes may have alternate slices embedded.

There has been debate over the prognostic significance of micrometastases; it has previously proven impossible to agree unequivocally a definition of the maximum size of these lesions, and different methods of examination have been used to identify these tumour deposits in reported series. Some groups have suggested that micrometastases identified by serial sectioning of lymph nodes are prognostically significant.[51] Other authors have found that micrometastases identified by immunohistochemical techniques are not prognostically significant in lobular carcinomas but are associated with recurrence in ductal/NST tumours.[58] It is undoubtedly true that immunohistochemical examination using anti-cytokeratin antibodies can identify a small number of cases that have not been found with routine stains, but these appear to have no prognostic significance.[59] Thus the true prognostic significance of occult or very small metastases is unknown. Although there are no prospective studies on prognosis of occult metastases in either sentinel lymph node biopsies or conventional axillary specimens, the TNM staging system has recently been revised.[33] It now includes a regional lymph node stage classification that incorporates small deposits and those detected by additional laboratory tests, and may bring some clarity to the prognostic significance of micrometastatic disease (Table 25.1).

It should be noted, however, that, there is a significant increase in workload and cost entailed in examining every case either immunohistochemically or by serial sectioning. Guidelines in the UK for pathology specimen handling and reporting in breast cancer screening do not recommend routine use of immunohistochemistry, step sectioning or indeed RT–PCR for examination of lymph nodes from patients with breast cancer.[14] A few cases where features suspicious of metastatic disease are seen may be assessed immunohistochemically with anti-cytokeratin antibodies.

Vascular invasion

Apart from tumour size, histological grade and type and lymph node stage, the other variable that in multivariate analysis is found to be of independent significance in predicting for survival in the NTPBCS is the presence or absence of vascular (blood vessel or lymphatic space) invasion. However, there remains a strong association with lymph node involvement.[60] Although some studies have suggested that the assessment of vascular invasion can be used, and provides information as

powerful as lymph node examination,[61] this is not widely accepted. We believe that this feature is perhaps more important in the prediction of either local recurrence in patients who have had wide local excision[60] and flap recurrence in patients who have had mastectomy and in prediction of prognosis in node negative patients.[62] Other groups have not found similar correlations, and a wide variation in the incidence of this feature has been reported. This may be related to the difficulties in adhering to strictly defined criteria and obtaining good fixation of specimens, which must be optimal to avoid the difficulties of retraction artefacts mimicking tumour emboli.

While special techniques have been used to assess vascular invasion in breast carcinoma, these have a role to play predominantly in distinguishing artefactual shrinkage from true vascular spaces. Elastic stains are of little help in distinguishing ducts from vessels, and neither lymphatics nor small capillaries have elastic lamina. At present, we report vascular invasion in three categories: absent, definite or probable. Probable vascular invasion is reported when an unequivocal endothelial lining cannot be seen but when possible tumour emboli are seen in the tissue adjacent to the invasive tumour; for therapeutic purposes, this category is grouped with tumours showing no vascular invasion.

Multivariate analyses have shown that in the NTPBCS, the features that predicted for local recurrence in patients who had had wide local excision (without any selection criteria for surgery) included tumour size, the presence of vascular invasion and young age.[63] As a result of this analysis, it is now our practice to advise patients with tumours larger than 3 cm clinically or radiologically against conservation surgery, especially if they are younger than 40 years of age. Postoperatively, completion mastectomy is advisable if the tumour is larger than 2 cm, histological grade 3, node-positive and shows definite vascular invasion. Thus the importance of the presence of vascular invasion in patient management lies in the prediction of local recurrence and should be routinely reported in excision specimens.

Use of prognostic indicators

Several factors provide prognostic information in patients with primary breast cancer, and no single indicator is universally recognised to be of overall importance. The time-dependent factor of lymph node stage has been most consistently used as a guide for stratification in most centres for patient treatment and entry into clinical trials. It should be noted, however, that nodal stage is of relatively poor

Table 25.2 **Proportion of patients and overall survival in the Nottingham Tenovus Primary Breast Carcinoma Series by Nottingham Prognostic Index (NPI) group – updated analysis based on over 3700 women with primary operable breast cancer aged less than 71 years**

	NPI group (NPI values)				
	Excellent (<3)	Good (<3.4)	Moderate I (3.4–4.5)	Moderate II (4.4–5.4)	Poor (>5.4)
Number of cases	475	744	1001	891	590
Proportion of cases	13%	20%	27%	24%	16%
5-year survival rate	97%	93%	85%	75%	42%
10-year survival rate	91%	82%	73%	55%	26%
15-year survival rate	84%	74%	63%	46%	18%

discriminatory value; neither a group of patients with close to 100% mortality nor a group with almost normal survival can be identified by the presence or absence of lymph node metastases alone. The intrinsic biological 'aggressiveness' of the tumour is also of prognostic importance, and is assessed by histological grade. For each individual patient, benefit may be gained from a combination of the time-dependent and biological features of the tumour in attempts to predict prognosis.

It has long been recognised that a combination of lymph node stage and differentiation is more useful than either alone in the prediction of the behaviour of many epithelial malignancies. Variables that are of independent prognostic significance in multivariate analyses can be combined into a prognostic index to obtain the best prediction of survival for each individual patient. The factors of greatest prognostic importance in primary operable breast carcinoma have been found to be histological grade, lymph node stage and tumour size. These have been combined, with appropriate weighting from the β^2-value of multivariate analyses to form the Nottingham Prognostic Index (NPI): (0.2 × tumour size (in cm)) + histological grade (scored 1–3) and lymph node stage (scored 1–3). This index was initially derived from a series of 387 patients by entry of 9 separate variables in multivariate analysis and has been confirmed prospectively.[64] Further confirmation of the value of the NPI has come from other large and multicentre series.[65–68]

The NPI is used to determine patients' probable prognosis (Table 25.2 and Figure 25.3) and thus to select the appropriate treatments for patients with primary operable breast cancer. Patients with a NPI <3.4 have a survival comparable to that of aged-matched controls and thus receive no systemic

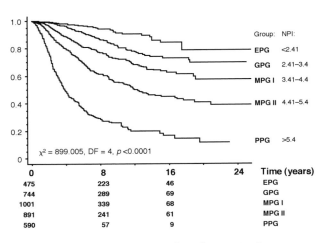

Figure 25.3 Long-term survival in the Nottingham Tenovus Primary Breast Carcinoma Series by Nottingham Prognostic Index (NPI) group: EPG, excellent; GPG, good; MPG I, moderate I; MPG II, moderate II; PPG, poor.

adjuvant treatment. Conversely, patients with a higher score receive systemic treatment based on additional data such as ER status. Although in multivariate analyses this is not of independent significance in survival, ER status is routinely assessed by immunohistochemical means on paraffin-fixed tissue sections (in many units).[69] Hormone treatment can thus be given to patients who are most likely to respond to it, while those who have a poor chance of responding to tamoxifen can be given other treatments without delay.

The quantitative assessment of ER immunoreactivity may be performed in several ways. In its simplest form, the percentage of tumour cells that show positive immunostaining is determined, while other

Table 25.3	**Response to tamoxifen according to oestrogen receptor (ER) status assessed with the 1D5 antibody (Dako) on paraffin sections[69]**		
	ER-negative (H-score <50)	ER-positive (H-score >50)	Total
Response (UICC 1+2)	2	18	20
Static disease (UICC 3)	1	17	18
Progression (UICC 4)	37	15	52
Total	40	50	90

$\chi^2 = 35.7$, DF = 3, p <0.0001.

techniques also include an assessment of the degree of positivity.[69,70] The modified histochemical score (H-score) is one such method, incorporating a semiquantitative assessment of both the percentage and the degree of tumour cell immunoreactivity, scored from negative (0) to strong (3) into a formula: (0 × % of negative cells) + (1 × % of weakly positive cells) + (2 × % of moderately stained tumour cells) + (3 × % strongly positive tumour cell nuclei). Thus the H-score ranges from 0 to 300. ER status provides a good prediction of response to hormone therapy (Table 25.3). Many screen-detected breast carcinomas, however, show good prognostic features and have a NPI <3.4, and so, despite often showing ER positivity, patients may choose to receive no further systemic treatment. Groups have suggested that, in addition to ER status, progesterone receptor (PgR) status or other oestrogen-inducible molecules should be examined in patients with breast carcinoma to assess the functioning of the ER pathway and to determine whether PgR positivity is present in ER-negative lesions. This is not uniformly assessed in all laboratories; indeed, we do not ourselves routinely perform PgR immunohistochemistry on all invasive breast cancers and rely on ER examination to predict response to hormone treatment at this time.

Although subsequent analyses have demonstrated that tumour type and the presence of vascular invasion are of independent prognostic significance in primary operable breast cancer, the effects of these additional factors are small in comparison with the weight of histological grade, lymph node stage and tumour size. The NPI is simple to calculate and is derived from data that is relatively easy to obtain from routine careful histological examina-

tion of sections of tumour and lymph nodes. Thus additional components have not been included that might make the index more cumbersome and difficult to calculate. The NPI may also be used to compare groups of patients, and the prognosis of symptomatic and screen-detected breast carcinomas can be compared with this technique. Seventy-six percent of screen-detected carcinomas in the Nottingham unit fall within the excellent and good prognostic groups, compared with only 29% of symptomatic breast cancers. Conversely, only 4% of screening cancers are in the poor-prognosis group, compared with 17% of symptomatic tumours.

Other morphological and molecular markers of prognosis

A number of other morphological factors have been suggested as useful prognostic indicators, including angiogenesis, peritumoral lymphoid infiltrate, tumour necrosis, stromal fibrosis, stromal elastosis and stromal giant cells. The former feature is of particular interest. However, although the hypothesis that breast cancer growth and metastasis are angiogenesis-dependent is logical, attractive and supported by some studies, others have failed to confirm an association with prognosis. The neovascularisation of the tumour periphery provides an increased surface area for adherence and entrance of tumour cell emboli to the circulation, but the development of new vessels may occur around foci of ductal carcinoma in situ (DCIS).[71] The growth of new vessels at the periphery of a neoplasm may thus be an early event in tumour development rather than a rate-limiting step. The assessment of angiogenesis in breast carcinomas requires the identification of so-called 'hot spots' and immunohistochemical staining of these areas with subsequent counting of new vessel formation. The lack of association with prognosis in several series, including a study performed in Nottingham, may be a failure to identify these areas of highest neovascularisation.[72] The role of angiogenesis and angiogenetic factors in breast carcinoma may prove to be more important and interesting as a therapeutic target rather than as a prognostic factor.

The significance of other morphological features is unclear; tumour necrosis has been reported predominantly in breast carcinomas of no special type. The criteria and techniques for the assessment of tumour necrosis have varied among studies, making comparison of results difficult, but the overall impression is that this is a poor prognostic feature. Both early treatment failure and reduced overall survival have been reported and further investigation with strict reproducible criteria and evaluation of extent is required.

Many invasive tumours show no or minimal associated DCIS, while a small proportion (approximately 10% of cases) are associated with abundant DCIS. The presence of extensive in situ carcinoma (EIC) has been reported to be of prognostic significance. Matsukuma et al[73] reported that tumours with less than 20% invasive component had significantly fewer lymph node metastases and a better overall 10-year survival than tumours with a greater invasive element, but other series have noted an association between a prominent in situ component and lower histological grade;[74] it may be histological grade rather than EIC that is the significant feature. Multivariate analyses are required to determine if the presence of abundant DCIS is of independent significance.

The main risk factor for local relapse after breast-conserving surgery is residual tumour burden. Although there are data indicating that the extent of extratumoral DCIS may be a predictor of prognosis in primary operable breast carcinoma treated by breast-conserving surgery,[75] we believe that the importance of the extent of DCIS around an invasive carcinoma lies more in determining local recurrence risk and management after conservation treatment. EIC has been defined by Schnitt et al[76] as the presence of DCIS amounting to 25% or more of the overall tumour mass of an invasive carcinoma and extending beyond the confines of the infiltrating component. This latter group reported that tumours with EIC had a higher local relapse rate than those without EIC.[77] Assessing the completeness of excision histologically of DCIS, either in a 'pure' form or in association with invasive carcinoma, is notoriously difficult. This is supported by the finding that the presence of EIC predicts for residual disease in re-excision specimens.[78,79] The residual disease is frequently DCIS.[80] None of 30 patients with an EIC-positive tumour developed recurrence at the site of previous excision within 5 years if the margins were negative or close, but 50% did so when the margins were more than focally positive,[81] and subsequently the same group reported that among patients treated with breast-conserving therapy and radiotherapy to the tumour bed, those with focally positive margins had a considerably lower risk of local recurrence than those with more than focally positive margins.[82] These data all indicate that the value of EIC in predicting outcome is very closely related to adequacy of tumour excision. They suggest that breast carcinomas with EIC are difficult to assess histologically to ascertain whether excision is complete and that pathologists should be particularly thorough in the examination of specimen margins in these cancers. Other features have been shown to be more powerful predictors of local recurrence in multivariate analyses in some series, including patient age, nodal status, tumour size and the presence of vascular invasion.[63]

Many potential molecular and genetic markers of prognosis have been described in recent years.[83] These include the proliferation fraction marker Ki67 (and its paraffin equivalent MIB1[84]), as well as the more technically complex assessment of thymidine labelling, S-phase fraction and bromodeoxyuridine labelling of tumours. While these appear to be of significance in univariate analyses, in stepwise multivariate analysis, histological grade, which includes mitotic count as a proliferation component, appears to be more important. Other molecular markers, including growth factors and their receptors (e.g. epidermal growth factor receptor (EGFR), HER-2/neu (c-ErbB-2) and c-RrbB-3), proteases (e.g. cathepsin D), cell adhesion markers (e.g. E-cadherin), tumour suppressor genes (e.g. p53) and a multitude of other factors, do not consistently show independent prognostic significance in primary breast carcinoma when morphological markers such as histological grade and type, tumour size, and lymph node stage are included. Although these latter parameters appear to be rather simple and old-fashioned, histological grade and tumour type are measurements of tumour morphology reflecting a variety of complex biological changes within the tumour, including cell adhesion and structure, DNA content, and proliferation index. Thus it is perhaps not surprising that individual biological markers cannot replace or surpass these well-recognised morphological prognostic factors at present.

The place of molecular markers in the future appears to be to determine treatment choices, with specific molecules reflecting a probable response or resistance to a particular therapy. Indeed, the value of the ER in predicting response to hormone therapy is incontrovertible, and the selection of suitability of a patient for trastuzumab therapy relies on the reliable and reproducible determination of the HER2/neu status of an invasive breast cancer.[85,86] Other targets are on the horizon. It is possible that other non-specific biological features such as tumour angiogenesis may prove to be directly useful in anticancer treatment. It is certain that the examination of the expression of many molecular pathways will augment our understanding of the biology of breast cancer and thus should not be ignored.

References

1. Page DL, Dupont WD, Rogers LW, Rados MS. Atypical hyperplastic lesions of the female breast. A long-term follow-up study. Cancer 1985; 55: 2698–708.
2. Page DL, Rogers LW. Combined histologic and cytologic criteria for the diagnosis of mammary atypical hyperplasia. Hum Pathol 1992; 23: 1095–7.

3. Page DL, Dupont WD. Anatomic markers of human premalignancy and risk of breast cancer. Cancer 1990; 66: 1326–35.

4. Page DL, Jensen RA. Evaluation and management of high risk and premalignant lesions of the breast. World J Surg 1994; 18: 32–8.

5. Page DL, Kidd T Jr, Dupont WD et al. Lobular neoplasia of the breast: higher risk for subsequent invasive cancer predicted by more extensive disease. Hum Pathol 1991; 22: 1232–9.

6. Jensen RA, Page DL, Dupont WD, Rogers LW. Invasive breast cancer risk in women with sclerosing adenosis. Cancer 1989; 64: 1977–83.

7. Dupont WD, Page DL, Parl FF et al. Long-term risk of breast cancer in women with fibroadenoma. N Engl J Med 1994; 331: 10–15.

8. Feuer EJ, Wun LM, Boring CC et al. The lifetime risk of developing breast cancer. J Natl Cancer Inst 1993; 85: 892–7.

9. Clark GM. Do we really need prognostic factors for breast cancer? Br Cancer Res Treat 1994; 30: 117–26.

10. Yorkshire Breast Cancer Group. Critical assessment of the clinical TNM system in breast cancer. BMJ 1980; 281: 134–6.

11. Galea MH, Blamey RW, Elston CW et al. The Nottingham Prognostic Index in primary breast cancer. Breast Cancer Res Treat 1992; 22: 207–19.

12. Rosen PP, Groshen S. Factors influencing survival and prognosis in early breast carcinoma (T1N0M0–T1N1M0). Assessment of 644 patients with median follow up of 19 years. Surg Clin North Am 1990; 70: 937–62.

13. Jansen JT, Zoetelief J. MBS: a model for risk benefit analysis of breast cancer screening. Br J Radiol 1995; 68: 141–9.

14. Pathology Reporting of Breast Disease. Sheffield: NHS Breast Screening Programme No 58, 2005.

15. Robbins P, Pinder S, de Klerk N et al. Histological grading of breast carcinomas. A study of interobserver agreement. Hum Pathol 1995; 26: 873–9.

16. Frierson H Jr, Wolber RA, Berean KW et al. Interobserver reproducibility of the Nottingham modification of the Bloom and Richardson histologic grading scheme for infiltrating ductal carcinoma. Am J Clin Pathol 1995; 103: 195–8.

17. Elston CW, Ellis IO. Pathological prognostic factors in breast cancer. I. The value of histological grade in breast cancer: experience from a large study with long-term follow-up. Histopathology 1991; 19: 403–10.

18. Page DL, Ellis IO, Elston CW. Histologic grading of breast cancer. Let's do it. Am J Clin Pathol 1995; 103: 123–4.

19. Fitzgibbons PL, Page DL, Weaver D et al. Prognostic factors in breast cancer. College of American Pathologists Consensus Statement 1999. Arch Pathol Lab Med 2000; 124: 966–78.

20. Bloom HJG, Richardson WW. Histological grading and prognosis in breast cancer. A study of 1409 cases of which 359 have been followed for 15 years. Br J Cancer 1957; 11: 359–77.

21. Pinder SE, Murray S, Ellis IO et al. The importance of histological grade in invasive breast carcinoma and response to chemotherapy. Cancer 1998; 83: 1529–39.

22. Robertson JF, Ellis IO, Pearson D et al. Biological factors of prognostic significance in locally advanced breast cancer. Breast Cancer Res Treat 1994; 29: 259–64.

23. Ellis IO, Galea M, Broughton N et al. Pathological prognostic factors in breast cancer. II. Histological type. Relationship with survival in a large study with long-term follow-up. Histopathology 1992; 20: 479–89.

24. Pereira H, Pinder SE, Sibbering DM et al. Pathological prognostic factors in breast cancer. IV: Should you be a typer or a grader? A comparative study of two histological prognostic features in operable breast carcinoma. Histopathology 1995; 27: 219–26.

25. Sloane JP, Amendoeira I, Apostolikas N et al. Consistency achieved by 23 European pathologists from 12 countries in diagnosing breast disease and reporting prognostic features of carcinomas. Virchows Arch Int J Pathol 1999; 434: 3–10.

26. Richardson WW. Medullary carcinoma of the breast. A distinctive tumour type with a relatively good prognosis following radical mastectomy. Br J Cancer 1956; 10: 415–23.

27. Moore OS Jr, Foote FW Jr. The relatively favourable prognosis of medullary carcinoma of the breast. Cancer 1949; 2: 635–42.

28. Lidang Jensen M, Kiaer H, Andersen J et al. Prognostic comparison of three classifications for medullary carcinomas of the breast. Histopathology 1997; 30: 523–32.

29. Gaffey MJ, Mills SE, Frierson HF et al. Medullary carcinoma of the breast: interobserver variability in histopathologic diagnosis. Mod Pathol 1995; 8: 31–8.

30. Domagala W, Markiewski M, Kubiak R et al. Immunohistochemical profile of invasive lobular carcinoma of the breast: predominantly vimentin and p53 protein negative, cathepsin D and oestrogen receptor positive. Virchows Arch (A) Pathol Anat Histopathol 1993; 423: 497–502.

31. Gonzalez MA, Pinder SE, Wencyk PM et al. An immunohistochemical examination of the expression of E-cadherin, α- and β/δ-catenins and α_2- and β_1-integrins in invasive breast cancer. J Pathol 1999; 187: 523–9.

32. Lamovec J, Bracko M. Metastatic pattern of infiltrating lobular carcinoma of the breast: an autopsy study. J Surg Oncol 1991; 48: 28–33.

33. Singletary SA, Allred C, Ashley P et al. Revision of the American Joint Committee on Cancer Staging system for breast cancer staging. J Clin Oncol 2002; 20: 3628–36.

34. Steele RJC, Forrest APM, Gibson T et al. The efficacy of lower axillary sampling in obtaining lymph node status in breast cancer: a controlled randomised trial. Br J Surg 1985; 72: 368–9.

35. Fisher ER, Sass R, Fisher B. Pathologic findings from the National Surgical Adjuvant Project for Breast Cancers (Protocol No. 4). X. Discriminants for tenth year treatment failure. Cancer 1984; 53: 712–23.

36. Canavese G, Catturich A, Vecchio C et al. Prognostic

role of lymph-node level involvement in patients undergoing axillary dissection for breast cancer. Eur J Surg Oncol 1998; 24: 104–9.

37. Veronesi U, Galimberti V, Zurrida S et al. Prognostic significance of number and level of axillary node metastases in breast cancer. Breast 1993; 2: 224–8.

38. Axelsson CK, Mouridsen HT, Zedeler K. Axillary dissection of level I and II lymph nodes is important in breast cancer classification. Eur J Cancer 1992; 28A: 1415–18.

39. Kutiyanawala MA, Sayed M, Stotter A et al. Staging the axilla in breast cancer: an audit of lymph-node retrieval in the U.K. regional centre. Eur J Surg Oncol 1998; 24: 280–2.

40. Mathiesen O, Carl J, Bonderup O, Panduro J. Axillary sampling and the risk of erroneous staging of breast cancer. Acta Oncol 1990; 29: 721–5.

41. Fisher B, Wolmark N, Bauer M et al. The accuracy of clinical nodal staging and of limited axillary dissection as a determinant of histologic nodal status in carcinoma of the breast. Surg Gynecol Obstet 1981; 152: 765–72.

42. Lee AHS, Ellis IO, Pinder SE et al. Pathological assessment of sentinel lymph node biopsies in patients with breast cancer. Virchows Arch (A) Pathol Anat 2000; 436: 97–101.

43. Albertini JJ, Lyman GH, Cox C et al. Lymphatic mapping and sentinel node biopsy in the patient with breast cancer. JAMA 1996; 276: 1818–22.

44. Giuliano AE, Kirgan DM, Guenther JM, Morton DL. Lymphatic mapping and sentinel lymphadenectomy for breast cancer. Ann Surg 1994; 220: 391–401.

45. Nwariaku FE, Euhus DM, Beitsch PD et al. Sentinel lymph node biopsy, an alternative to elective axillary dissection for breast cancer. Am J Surg 1998; 176: 529–31.

46. Rubio IT, Korourian S, Cowan C et al. Sentinel lymph node biopsy for staging breast cancer. Am J Surg 1998; 176: 532–5.

47. Borgstein P, Pijpers R, Comans EF et al. Sentinel lymph node biopsy in breast cancer: Guidelines and pitfalls of lymphoscintigraphy and gamma probe detection. J Am Coll Surg 1998; 186: 275–83.

48. Giuliano A, Dale P, Turner R et al. Improved axillary staging of breast-cancer with sentinel lymphadenectomy. Ann Surg 1995; 222: 394–401.

49. Giuliano A, Jones R, Brennan M, Statman R. Sentinel lymphadenectomy in breast cancer. J Clin Oncol 1997; 15: 2345–50.

50. Veronesi U, Paganelli G, Viale G et al. Sentinel lymph node biopsy and axillary dissection in breast cancer: results in a large series. J Natl Cancer Inst 1999; 91: 368–73.

51. International Breast Cancer Study Group. Prognostic importance of occult axillary lymph node micrometastases from breast cancers. Lancet 1990; 335: 1565–8.

52. Nasser IA, Lee AKC, Bosari S et al. Occult axillary lymph node metastases in 'node-negative' breast carcinoma. Hum Pathol 1993; 24: 950–7.

53. Wilkinson EJ, Hause LL, Hoffman RG et al. Occult axillary lymph node metastases in invasive breast carcinoma: characteristics of the primary tumor and significance of the metastases. Pathol Ann 1982; 17: 67–91.

54. Hainsworth PJ, Tjandra JJ, Stillwell RG et al. Detection and significance of occult metastases in node-negative breast cancer. Br J Surg 1993; 80: 459–63.

55. McGuckin MA, Cummings MC, Walsh MD et al. Occult axillary node metastases in breast cancer: their detection and prognostic significance. Br J Cancer 1996; 73: 88–95.

56. Noguchi S, Aihara T, Nakamori S et al. The detection of breast carcinoma micrometastases in axillary lymph nodes by means of reverse transcriptase–polymerase chain reaction. Cancer 1994; 74: 1595–600.

57. Schoenfeld A, Luqmani Y, Smith D et al. Detection of breast cancer micrometastases in axillary lymph nodes by using polymerase chain reaction. Cancer Res 1994; 54: 2986–90.

58. de Mascarel I, Bonichon F, Coindre JM, Trojani M. Prognostic significance of breast cancer axillary lymph node micrometastases assessed by two special techniques: reevaluation with longer follow-up. Br J Cancer 1992; 66: 523–7.

59. Galea MH, Athanassiou E, Bell J et al. Occult regional lymph node metastases from breast carcinoma: immunohistological detection with antibodies CAM 5.2 and NCRC-11. J Pathol 1991; 165: 221–7.

60. Pinder SE, Ellis IO, Galea M et al. Pathological prognostic factors in breast cancer. III. Vascular invasion: relationship with recurrence and survival in a large series with long-term follow-up. Histopathology 1994; 24: 41–7.

61. Bettelheim R, Penman HG, Thornton-Jones H, Neville AM. Prognostic significance of peritumoral vascular invasion in breast cancer. Br J Cancer 1984; 50: 771–7.

62. O'Rourke S, Galea MH, Morgan D et al. Local recurrence after simple mastectomy. Br J Surg 1994; 81: 386–9.

63. Locker AP, Ellis IO, Morgan DA et al. Factors influencing local recurrence after excision and radiotherapy for primary breast cancer. Br J Surg 1989; 76: 890–4.

64. Todd JH, Dowle C, Williams MR et al. Confirmation of a prognostic index in primary breast cancer. Br J Cancer 1987; 56: 489–92.

65. Brown JM, Benson EA, Jones M. Confirmation of a long-term prognostic index in breast cancer. Breast 1993; 2: 144–7.

66. Balslev I, Axelsson CK, Zedelev K et al. The Nottingham Prognostic Index applied to 9,149 patients from the studies of the Danish Breast Cancer Cooperative Group (DBCG). Breast Cancer Res Treat 1994; 32: 281–90.

67. Sundquist M, Thorstenson S, Brudin L, Nordenskjold B. Applying the Nottingham Prognostic Index to a Swedish breast cancer population. South East Swedish Breast Cancer Study Group. Breast Cancer Res Treat 1999; 53: 1–8.

68. D'Eredita G, Giardina C, Martellotta M et al. Prognostic factors in breast cancer: the predictive value of the Nottingham Prognostic Index in patients with a long-

term follow-up that were treated in a single institution. Eur J Cancer 2001; 37: 591–6.

69. Goulding H, Pinder S, Cannon P et al. A new immunohistochemical antibody for the assessment of estrogen receptor status on routine formalin-fixed tissue samples. Hum Pathol 1995; 26: 291–4.

70. Harvey JM, Clark GM, Osborne CK, Allred DC. Estrogen receptor status by immunohistochemistry is superior to the ligand-binding assay for predicting response to adjuvant endocrine therapy in breast cancer. J Clin Oncol 1999; 17: 1474–85.

71. Lee AHS, Happerfield LC, Bobrow LG, Millis RP. Angiogenesis and Inflammation in ductal carcinoma in situ of the breast. J Pathol 1997; 181: 200–6.

72. Goulding H, Nik Abdul Rashid NF, Robertson JF et al. Assessment of angiogenesis in breast cancer. An important factor in prognosis? Hum Pathol 1995; 26: 1196–200.

73. Matsukuma A, Enjoji M, Toyoshima S. Ductal carcinoma of the breast. An analysis of proportions of intraductal and invasive components. Pathol Res Pract 1991; 187: 62–7.

74. Silverberg SG, Chitale AR. Assessment of the significance of the proportion of intraductal and infiltrating tumor growth in ductal carcinoma of the breast. Cancer 1973; 32: 830–7.

75. Crombie N, Rampaul RS, Pinder SE et al. Extent of ductal carcinoma in situ within and surrounding invasive primary breast carcinoma. Br J Surg 2001; 88: 1324–9.

76. Schnitt SJ, Connelly JL, Harris JR et al. Pathologic predictors of early recurrence in stage I and stage II breast cancer treated by primary radiation therapy. Cancer 1984; 53: 1049–57.

77. Schnitt SJ, Connolly JL, Khettry U et al. Pathologic findings on re-excision of the primary site in breast cancer patients considered for treatment by primary radiation therapy. Cancer 1987; 59: 675–81.

78. Beron PJ, Horwitz EM, Martinez AA et al. Pathologic and mammographic findings predicting the adequacy of tumour excision before breast-conserving therapy. AJR Am J Roentgenol 1996; 167: 1409–14.

79. Campbell ID, Theaker JM, Royle GT et al. Impact of an extensive in-situ component on the presence of residual disease in screen detected breast cancer. J R Soc Med 1991; 84: 652–6.

80. Wazer DE, Schmidt RK, Schmid CH et al. The value of breast lumpectomy margin assessment as a predictor of residual tumour burden. Int J Radiat Oncol Biol Phys 1997; 38: 291–9.

81. Schnitt SJ, Abner A, Gelman R et al. The relationship between microscopic margins of resection and the risk of local recurrence in patients with breast cancer treated with breast conserving surgery and radiation therapy. Cancer 1994; 74: 1746–51.

82. Gage I, Schnitt SJ, Nixon AJ et al. Pathologic margin involvement and the risk of recurrence in patients treated with breast-conserving therapy. Cancer 1996; 78: 1921–8.

83. Mirza AN, Mirza NQ, Vlastos G et al. Prognostic factors in node-negative breast cancer: a review of studies with sample size more than 200 and follow-up more than 5 years. Ann Surg 2002; 235: 10–26.

84. Pinder S, Wencyk P, Sibbering DM et al. Assessment of the new proliferation marker MIB1 in breast carcinoma using image analysis: associations with other prognostic factors and survival. Br J Cancer 1995; 71: 146–9.

85. Hanna W, Kahn HJ, Trudeau M. Evaluation of HER-2/*neu* (*erb*B-2) status in breast cancer: From bench to bedside. Mod Pathol 1999; 12: 827–34.

86. Goldhirsch A, Coates AS, CastiglioneGertsch M, Gelber RD. New treatments for breast cancer: breakthroughs for patient care or just steps in the right direction? Ann Oncol 1998; 9: 973–6.

26 Premalignant and borderline lesions: ductal and lobular carcinoma in situ

Catherine N Chinyama, Clive A Wells

Background

A premalignant condition is one that has a potential to develop into malignancy, and can subsequently pose a threat to life.[1] Premalignant lesions of the breast were investigated by Foote and Stewart[2] as early as 1945 in a comparative study that attempted to assess the risk of developing invasive carcinoma when certain types of epithelial proliferations were present in both cancerous and non-cancerous biopsies. Epithelial proliferations, sometimes associated with cytological atypia, were five times more common in breasts containing cancer than in non-cancerous breasts. This was not followed up until 30 years later, when, by meticulous subgross analysis of sections, Wellings et al[3] demonstrated that most epithelial abnormalities and carcinomas arise from the terminal duct–lobular unit (TDLU) rather than from the major ducts.

When assessing premalignant epithelial proliferations or non-invasive carcinoma of the breast, it is clinically useful to estimate the probability of progression to invasive carcinoma. Page[1] provided useful criteria in assessing non-invasive breast proliferations by calculating the relative risk of developing invasive carcinoma. The notion of risk factors enables the clinician to take into account the histologically assessed risk of subsequent malignancy, in addition to age, family history of breast cancer and reproductive history, and to plan suitable patient management.[4] Screening mammography is effective in detecting non-palpable architectural abnormalities or calcifications. Biopsies of these lesions yield very small invasive carcinomas, carcinoma in situ and atypical or benign epithelial proliferations. Carcinoma in situ and various epithe-

lial proliferations are more frequently encountered nowadays than in the premammographic era. Consequently, the need to assess the risk factors for developing invasive carcinoma has never been greater in order to give patients and clinicians more information so that the most suitable treatment can be instituted. Advances in molecular pathology will also assist the clinician in making a more accurate prediction of patients at risk of developing cancer by combining genetic susceptibility and abnormal epithelial proliferations.

Pathological assessment of biopsies

There is no place for frozen-section examination in the management of mammographically detected impalpable lesions, because of the risk of false-positive diagnosis in the assessment of benign lesions such as sclerosing adenosis or radial scars. It is also important to properly assess these lesions as a whole, because they are usually small and sampling for frozen section analysis may interfere with the final diagnosis. Biopsy specimens should be submitted to the laboratory fresh and fixed for 24 hours for optimum processing. A radiograph is essential prior to processing of the specimen. This enables the radiologist and surgeon to assess the adequacy of excision of the area of microcalcification or architectural distortion noted in vivo. The radiograph also helps the pathologist to select the appropriate area for histological examination. The biopsy specimen is painted with Indian ink or any similar substance to aid histological assessment of margins. The specimen is sliced along its long axis and the slices re-X-rayed if no macroscopic lesion is

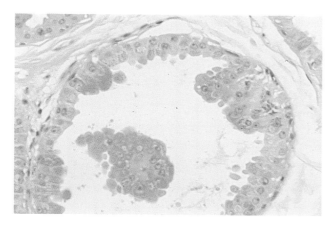

Figure 26.1   Apocrine epithelium in fibrocystic change illustrating granular cytoplasm and apical snouts. (H&E, ×20.)

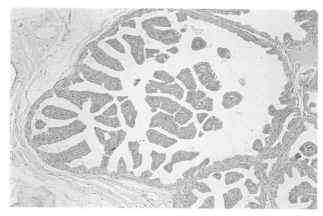

Figure 26.2   Florid apocrine papillary hyperplasia. (H&E, ×20.)

identified. After description of any gross abnormality, tissue blocks are taken. The whole lesion is sampled if it is small, or a minimum of four blocks including margins are taken. Microcalcification present in the specimen radiograph must be confirmed on histology. At all stages, cooperation between radiologist, surgeon and pathologist is vital.[5]

Lesions of doubtful malignant potential

Fibrocystic change and apocrine metaplasia

Apocrine epithelium is found lining the sweat glands of the vulva and axilla. Its presence in the breast is thought either to be of similar embryological origin to the sweat glands or to arise due to metaplasia.[6] The latter view is widely held. However, apocrine metaplasia has been detected in fetal tissue, which supports the view that the epithelium is native to the breast tissue.[7] Apocrine metaplasia is an integral part of fibrocystic change or gross cystic disease (Figure 26.1). The cells are large, with eosinophilic granular cytoplasm and basally located nuclei with or without apical 'snouts'. Fibrocystic change often presents as an ill-defined palpable mass generally between the ages of 35 and 50.

There is conflicting evidence as to whether apocrine epithelium is premalignant or not. In 1932, Dawson identified apocrine epithelium in both cancerous and non-cancerous breasts,[6] but was unable to demonstrate carcinoma arising directly in apocrine epithelium, and concluded that this was unlikely to be a premalignant condition. These findings were disputed by Haagensen,[8] who followed up patients whose biopsies had revealed apocrine metaplasia in

gross cystic disease. His patients had a fivefold risk of developing carcinoma. The significant apocrine metaplasia in Haagensen's series had mainly a papillary configuration. Although some apocrine proliferations can be florid, cytological atypia is unusual (Figure 26.2).

Using subgross analysis Wellings et al[9] demonstrated that apocrine metaplastic change occurred in the TDLU, the site of premalignant proliferation, and that it was a marker for increased risk of breast cancer. This conclusion was based on the fact that apocrine metaplasia was more prevalent in cancerous than in non-cancerous breasts – hence apocrine metaplasia was a manifestation of an unstable epithelium. In an earlier study, Page et al[10] suggested that patients over the age of 45 with papillary apocrine metaplasia had twice the relative risk of developing invasive carcinoma. Seven years later, in a separate study, Dupont and Page[11] concluded that cysts and apocrine epithelium per se did not increase the risk of carcinoma. However, the presence of cysts in a patient with a family history of breast cancer elevated the risk slightly to 2.7 times higher than that of women without this risk factor.

Dixon et al[12] followed up 1300 women with palpable cysts aspirated between 1981 and 1987. They reported that the overall incidence of breast cancer was three times higher than that in the general population. Younger women below the age of 45 were 6 times more likely than the general population to develop cancer, compared with a relative risk of 1.7 in women aged over 55. A possible explanation of this age difference was that in younger women the breast epithelium was more susceptible to malignant change due to the proliferative activity involved in cyst formation and associated high oestrogen levels. Complex apocrine papillary hyperplasia has been associated with a small increased relative risk of 2.4 of subsequent malignancy. However, 20% of the complex apocrine hyperplasia had associated atypical ductal hyperplasia (ADH). In the absence of ADH, the risk was not significant.[13]

Following complaints from women who were paying high insurance premiums after the diagnosis of 'fibrocystic disease', a consensus meeting was held in New York in 1985 by the Cancer Committee of the College of American Pathologists.[14] They agreed to assign the term to fibrocystic change and concluded that cysts and apocrine metaplasia alone were not premalignant. If the general term 'fibrocystic change' is to be used, the associated epithelial components must be specifically defined to allow an accurate assessment of the risk of subsequent cancer. This concept was reaffirmed with an updated consensus in 1998.[15]

Molecular biological studies have demonstrated loss of heterozygosity (LOH) in apocrine epithelium. Washington et al[16] demonstrated LOH in 10 out of 19 cases of apocrine epithelium not related to malignancy, and 7 out 14 cases of apocrine epithelium adjacent to carcinoma. In all 7 cases, the carcinoma and apocrine epithelium shared LOH in one or more loci. In a separate study,[17] multiple chromosomal losses and gains were present in apocrine epithelium at a similar frequency to apocrine DCIS. Earlier, Agnantis et al[18] demonstrated immunohistochemical expression of the c-Myc, p66 and p21 Ras oncoproteins. These studies suggest that apocrine metaplasia may serve as a putative precursor of apocrine carcinoma – albeit a rare one.

Radial scar

The radial scar or complex sclerosing lesion is a benign lesion, which mammographically and histologically mimics tubular carcinoma (see Chapter 13). The genesis of a radial scar is thought be to a secondary reaction to an unknown injurious agent, possibly vascular, which heals with central fibrosis and elastosis, resulting in the characteristic stellate configuration. Despite the benign nature of this lesion, carcinomas (in particular tubular carcinomas) have been reported to arise in association with radial scars. In an extensive study of these lesions, Linnell et al[19] concluded that radial scars were premalignant. This view was further supported by Jacobs et al,[20] who carried out a case–control study of 1396 women with benign breast disease, 225 of whom subsequently developed cancer. The women with radial scars associated with atypical hyperplasia had a 5.8 relative risk of developing carcinoma, compared with 3.8 for those patients without a radial scar. From this study, Jacobs et al[20] concluded

that radial scars were an independent histological risk factor for developing breast cancer. However, it appears that the atypical epithelial hyperplasia was the main risk factor rather than the radial scar per se. Andersen and Gram[21] followed up 32 women with excised radial scars without atypical proliferation for a mean of 19.5 years, and only 1 developed breast cancer. In a subsequent study, Sloane and Mayers[22] reported a high association of large radial scars (>7 mm) with atypical hyperplasia in women aged over 50. A similar follow-up study by Jacobs et al[20] reported the development of cancer in 32% (32 of 99) of women with radial scars compared with 17% (223 of 1297) of the control group without radial scars. The women with radial scars who developed cancer tended to be older than 45.

In an attempt to prove the link between radial scar and tubular carcinoma, Jacobs et al[23] performed molecular tests on the stromal elements of the two lesions. In situ hybridisation detected similarities in the pattern of expression of mRNA of the stromal and vascular elements in radial scars and tubular carcinomas, suggestive of similar disturbances in the stromal–epithelium interaction. Although these studies are inconclusive, most authorities would agree that local excision of a radial scar without associated atypical hyperplasia is curative and the patients' risk of developing breast cancer is comparable to that of the general population. However, because of the difficulty in differentiating radial scars from carcinoma radiologically, all radial scars must be excised for histological examination.

Lesions with a premalignant potential

Sclerosing adenosis (SA)

Jensen et al[24] defined sclerosing adenosis (SA) as a benign lobulocentric lesion with a disordered increase in acinar, myoepithelial and connective tissue elements. The enlargement of the lobular units due to an increase in the number of acini with concomitant fibrosis often distorts the lobular architecture (Figure 26.3). The significance of SA lies in its ability to mimic invasive cancer clinically, mammographically, macroscopically and microscopically, especially when perineural invasion is present. SA is most prevalent in perimenopausal women and its tendency to calcify makes mammographic detection easy. Jensen et al[24] followed up patients with SA and calculated the relative risk for developing invasive breast cancer to be 2.1, regardless of the presence of atypical hyperplasia. The risk decreased to 1.7 when patients with atypical hyperplasia were excluded and increased to 6.7 when

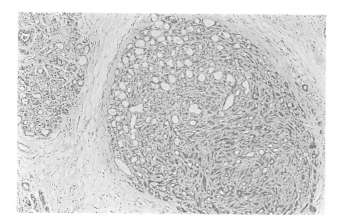

Figure 26.3 Sclerosing adenosis characterised by increased lobular units and fibrosis. (H&E, ×10.)

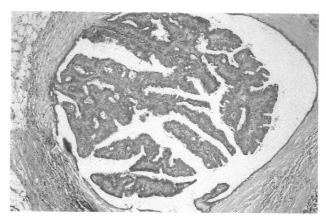

Figure 26.4 Intraductal papilloma consisting of a fibrovascular core covered by two layers of cells. (H&E, ×10.)

patients with atypical hyperplasia and SA were analysed. Consequently, SA qualifies to be included in the category of proliferative breast disease without atypia, with an overall cancer risk of 1.5–2 times that of the general population. A positive family history of breast cancer in the absence of atypical hyperplasia did not significantly elevate the risk for invasive cancer. In the same study, there was a positive association of SA and atypical lobular hyperplasia (ALH), which elevated the relative risk for developing invasive cancer to 7.6. Oberman and Markey[25] and Fechner[26] independently reported an association of lobular carcinoma in situ (LCIS) and SA, although they did not consider SA a risk factor for lobular neoplasia. This association of lobular proliferations with SA should alert the pathologist to search for lobular neoplasia in the presence of sclerosing adenosis.

Apocrine adenosis, defined as the presence of apocrine cytology in a recognisable lobular unit, which may or may not be deformed, is sometimes detected on screening mammography due to the presence of microcalcification or in association with a SA or radial scar. Because the cells are large and pleomorphic, there is a risk of misdiagnosis of cancer both on cytological and an histological examination.[27,28] The architectural and cytological atypia in these lesions justifies the use of the term atypical apocrine adenosis. Seidman et al[29] followed 37 patients with atypical apocrine adenosis for an average of 8.7 years, and 4 patients developed carcinoma after a mean of 5.6 years, with a relative risk of 5.5. All patients were aged over 60. The authors suggested that apocrine adenosis may represent carcinoma in situ, which is difficult to diagnose because of the unusual architectural and cytological features. Apocrine adenosis has been reported to express abnormal c-ErbB-2 oncoprotein, further highlighting the malignant potential of this lesion.[30,31]

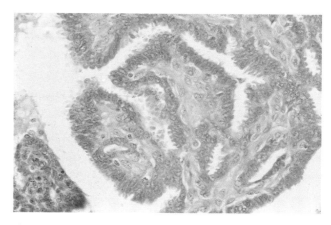

Figure 26.5 Papillary fronds showing a basal myoepithelial and a luminal epithelial layer. (H&E, ×40.)

Intraductal papillomas

Papillomas are an intraductal proliferation of villous-like or arborescent structures with a central fibrovascular core covered by a basal myoepithelial and luminal epithelial cell layer (Figures 26.4 and 26.5). Multiple papillomas may be indistinguishable from fibrocystic change clinically. Ohuchi et al[32] demonstrated by three-dimensional (3D) reconstruction that multiple papillomas arise peripherally from the TDLUs. In 24% of cases, carcinoma in situ – mainly of ductal type – was discovered incidentally during the reconstruction. 3D reconstructions also revealed that carcinomas with multifocal origin in the TDLUs were connected with peripheral papillomas. In contrast, none of the patients with solitary papillomas, which arose centrally from the nipple major ducts, had concomitant carcinoma. Central papillomas usually present with nipple discharge, while peripheral papillomas present with multiple nodules.

The premalignant nature of multiple papillomas was first illustrated by Muir[33] in 1941 in his article on the evolution of carcinoma of the breast, in which relatively young women aged 50 and below had developed carcinoma in association with multiple papillomas. The carcinomas were mostly of cribriform type, either invasive or in situ. Multiple papillomas are an infrequent condition, with only 53 cases retrieved from Haagensen's files over a period of 39 years.[8] The majority of the patients were aged 40 or younger, and 6 out of 53 developed breast cancer after a follow-up of 19 years. Again, in this study, Haagensen emphasised the difference between central solitary papillomas and multiple peripheral papillomas. Central papillomas tend to have a lower premalignant potential. Because of the frequent association of multiple papillomas with ductal hyperplasia of usual type, it is difficult to accurately ascertain the risk for developing invasive cancer in patients with multiple papillomas.

In a case–control study of 368 women with intraductal papillomas, Page et al[34] reported a relative risk of invasive carcinoma of 3.5 times that of the general population. The lesions tended to be micropapillomas (3 mm) and the risk was irrespective of family history, the presence of atypical hyperplasia nor other proliferative epithelium. Papillomas larger than 3 mm had a risk 1.8 times that of the population. Page et al[35] did not assess the significance of multiple versus single papillomas. Progression to malignancy can be identified by the presence of atypical papillomas. These show a mixed population of cells (two cell types) as well as monomorphic cells resembling intracystic papillary carcinoma. However, the use of molecular markers has been reported to differentiate benign intraductal papillomas from intracystic carcinoma by LOH in chromosome 16q in the latter.[35] Although the premalignant nature of multiple papillomas was disputed in the past, it was agreed at a consensus meeting in New York that the relative risk for developing carcinoma is comparable to that of epithelial hyperplasia of usual type, which is 1.5–2 times that of the general population.[11] Haagensen's experience with these lesions, however, would suggest that the risk is higher than this, and our anecdotal experience is in agreement.[8]

Epithelial hyperplasia

Normal breast ducts and lobular units are lined by two cell types, consisting of an outer myoepithelial layer and an inner epithelial layer. Epithelial hyperplasia denotes an increase in the number of cells to more than two cell layers above the basement membrane.[36] Like most forms of breast proliferation, hyperplasia originates from the TDLUs, and this varies from mild through florid to atypical proliferation, which may be virtually indistinguishable from carcinoma in situ. The relative risk for developing invasive carcinoma escalates numerically according to the degree of atypia. This was demonstrated in a large study by Dupont and Page[11] who followed up over 10 000 women who had undergone biopsy for clinically benign breast disease. The histological slides were reviewed, and the features present in biopsies of women who subsequently developed cancer were compared with those who did not. It was this work by Page and colleagues that led to the classification of ductal epithelial proliferations into mild, moderate or florid proliferative disease without atypia (PDWA) and ADH. These proliferations may be identified incidentally in biopsies removed for palpable abnormalities or screen-detected architectural distortion with or without calcification. ADH may also be detected as developing microcalcification in the incident round of breast cancer screening. Although all epithelial proliferations arise from the TDLUs, the most prevalent pattern is known as 'usual ductal hyperplasia' to distinguish it from ALH.

Mild ductal hyperplasia

Mild hyperplasia is present within a duct when three or four layers of epithelium are seen above the basement membrane.[36] The proliferation may be diffuse or focal (Figure 26.6). The latter gives rise to a corrugated luminal appearance. It is important not to label tangentially cut ducts as hyperplasia. Mild hyperplasia is classified as a non-proliferative disease and carries the same risk of subsequent breast cancer as the general population. Its presence or absence in biopsies is not critical to patient management.[4] A family history of breast cancer does not increase the risk of subsequent cancer in patients with mild hyperplasia.

Usual ductal hyperplasia

The World Health Organization (WHO) defined usual ductal hyperplasia (UDH) as a 'benign ductal

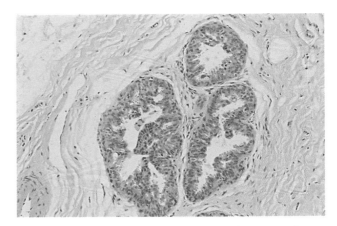

Figure 26.6 Mild ductal hyperplasia with an irregular epithelial proliferation. (H&E, ×10.)

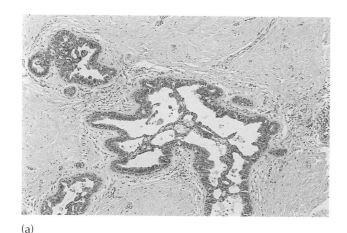

(a)

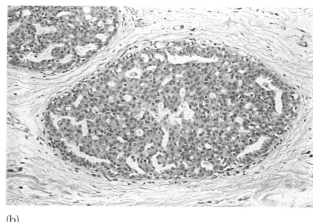

(b)

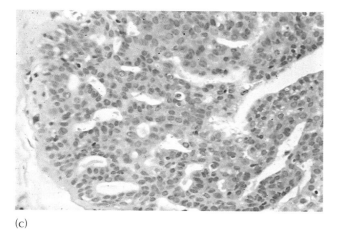

(c)

Figure 26.7 (a) Usual ductal hyperplasia (UDH): epithelial proliferation is present at the periphery of the duct with formation of bridges (H&E, 10x). (b) UDH without atypia: the duct is completely filled by epithelial cells with serpiginous slits at the periphery. (H&E, ×20.) (c) Two cell types in UDH without atypia. (H&E, ×20.)

proliferative lesion typically characterised by secondary lumens and streaming of proliferative cells'.[37] Page and Rogers[36] termed this process proliferative disease without atypia. The cells of usual hyperplasia may be confined to the periphery of the duct and may form papillae with bridges across the ductal lumen (Figure 26.7a). The papillae do not have the 'rigid' appearance of micropapillary or cribriform ductal carcinoma in situ (DCIS) and the cells lack the monotony of in situ carcinoma. Florid hyperplasia is due to expansion of the ducts by epithelial proliferation, which almost completely fills the lumen, with residual serpiginous slit-like lumina at the periphery (Figure 26.7b).

The cytomorphology of UDH is variable, and it is important not to make a diagnosis of atypical hyperplasia or DCIS. The nuclei are bland, with a delicate nuclear chromatin pattern, and may be mildly hyperchromatic with small or inconspicuous nucleoli (Figure 26.7c). Mitoses may be present, but are infrequent. The cytoplasm may be pale or eosinophilic, and the cells may merge into an apocrine pattern with luminal 'snouts'. The cells can be arranged parallel to each other – a phenomenon that Azzopardi termed 'streaming' or 'swirling'. Malignancy should not be diagnosed in the presence

of this architectural pattern. The presence of apocrine change within the lesion or peripheral slit-like spaces are also positive signs of benignity. Occasionally, central necrosis occurs in florid hyperplasia, and this should not be interpreted as comedo carcinoma.

UDH is usually associated with invasive cancer or DCIS, and other benign proliferations such as fibrocystic change, intraductal papillomas or radial scars. It has always been assumed that the UDH is the initial step in the pathogenesis of invasive cancer in a stepwise progression: UDH→ ADH→ DCIS→ invasive carcinoma. This model was challenged by Boecker et al,[38] who demonstrated that UDH and DCIS were biologically different lesions. Using double immunofluroresence, they demonstrated that UDH was a CK5/14+ progenitor cell lesion and DCIS expressed a different phenotype and was CK8+ and CK18+. Based on these findings, UDH is not considered to be a risk factor for subsequent malignancy. The WHO[37] also support this view that there is insufficient genetic evidence to classify UDH as a precursor lesion. The updated consensus statement on benign breast diseases assesses the risk of subsequent breast cancer of moderate or florid hyperplasia without atypia to be 1.5–2.0 times that of the general population.[39]

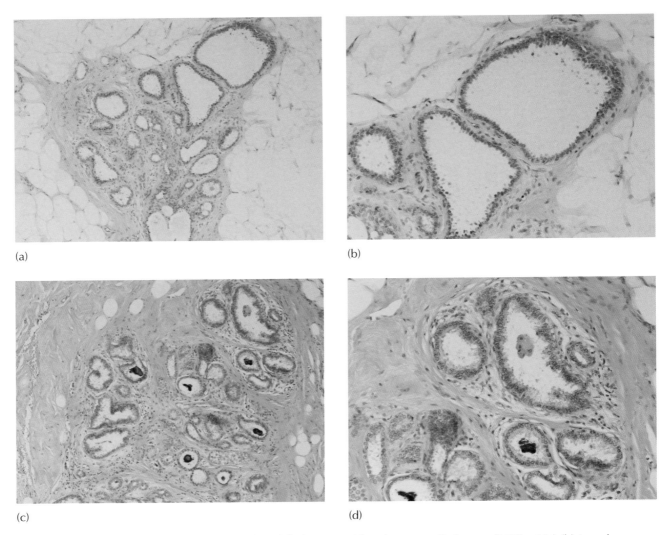

(a) (b)

(c) (d)

Figure 26.8 (a) A slightly dilated terminal duct–lobular unit with columnar cell change. (H&E, ×10.) (b) In columnar cell change, the units are lined by a single layer of epithelium with apical snouts. There is no atypia. (H&E, ×20.) (c) Screen-detected columnar cell hyperplasia with psammomatous calcification. (H&E, ×10.) (d) In columnar cell hyperplasia, there is mild nuclear stratification but no cytological atypia. (H&E, ×20.)

Columnar cell lesions

Although recently recognised as an entity, columnar cell lesions have been previously described by pathologists under different terminology.[40–42] The blunt duct adenosis of Foote and Stewart[2] is a variant of columnar cell lesion. Similar to DCIS, the high prevalence of columnar cell lesions has been highlighted by the use of screening mammography and needle core biopsies. Columnar cell lesions can exist independently of or in association with other benign lesions. The majority of mammographically detected lesions tend to calcify. Columnar cell lesions have been classified into two main categories: columnar cell change and columnar cell hyperplasia.[43]

Columnar cell change consists of variably dilated TDLUs lined by two cell layers. The cells are arranged perpendicular to the basement membrane, and apical cytoplasmic snouts are present on the luminal aspect, but are not prominent (Figure 26.8a,b). Nucleoli are inconspicuous. Luminal secretions and calcifications may or may not be present. In columnar cell hyperplasia, there is prominent epithelial proliferation, with nuclear stratification and exaggerated apical snouts, and psammomatous calcification is invariably present (Figure 26.8c,d). Cytological atypia can arise in both lesions. In columnar cell change, the cytological atypia is low-grade, and these lesions were previously termed clinging carcinoma.[44]

Columnar cell hyperplasia with atypia exhibits complex architectural patterns associated with nuclear stratification. Cytological atypia is usually low-grade and may resemble tubular carcinoma.[43] Schnitt[44] has emphasised that high nuclear grade is

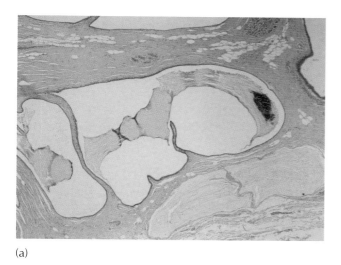

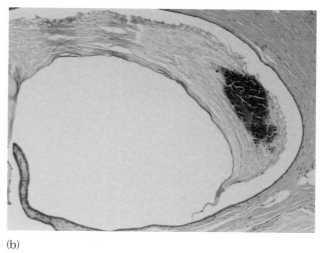

(a)

(b)

Figure 26.9 (a) Screen-detected mucocoele-like lesion with mucin extravasastion and amorphous microcalcification. (H&E, ×4.) (b) The mucin-filled duct is lined by a simple layer of epithelium. There is no atypia. (H&E, ×20.)

not a feature of columnar cell lesions – and if it is present then the appropriate diagnosis is DCIS. Columnar cell lesions have been reported in association with lobular neoplasia[45] and tubular carcinoma.[46] Because of the latter association, columnar cell lesions have been assumed to be precursors of tubular carcinoma.

In a study of a columnar cell lesion that they termed columnar alteration with prominent apical snouts (CAPSS), Fraser et al[42] reported the coexistence of CAPSS and low-grade DCIS in 38% of patients. As there are no long-term studies to guide clinicians on the true biological behaviour of columnar cell lesions, Schnitt[43] has advised that there be no further pathological work-up if columnar cell change and columnar cell hyperplasia are identified in needle core biopsies. Further levels and excision biopsies are recommended if there is associated cytological atypia. If atypia is present in excision biopsies, a careful search for ADH or DCIS is warranted, which may require processing of the tissue in its entirety. The presence of a columnar cell lesion with cytological atypia in association with DCIS should not prompt further excision, which would result in overtreatment of a lesion whose biological behaviour is still to be determined.

Mucocoele-like lesions

Mammary mucocoele-like lesions (MCLs) were first described by Rosen[47] in 1986. These lesions are characterised by mucinous distension of duct–lobular units associated with mucin extravasation into the surrounding stroma analogous to salivary gland lesions. MCLs constituted 3% of the cases in

a study of 1297 screen-detected and symptomatic breast lesions carried out by Chinyama and Davies.[48] Twelve cases were mammographically detected on account of microcalcification. Evaluation of the MCLs revealed a spectrum of benign mucin-filled ducts with or without calcification similar to the illustration above (Figure 26.9), mucinous ADH and low-grade mucinous DCIS. Mucinous ADH was present in 8 of the screen-detected cases. Combined mucin-filled ducts with or without extravasation, mucinous ADH and mucinous DCIS were associated with 11 of the 30 mucinous carcinomas. This study suggested that mucin-filled ducts were possible precursors of mucinous carcinoma. In a similar study, Weaver et al[49] also concluded that mucinous lesions of the breast were a pathological continuum, ranging from benign mucin-filled ducts to frank carcinoma. Detection of an MCL on a needle core biopsy associated with mammographic abnormality should prompt an excision biopsy to exclude mucinous carcinoma.

Borderline lesions

Atypical ductal hyperplasia (ADH)

ADH is the most controversial topic in breast pathology, and scores of papers have been dedicated to the subject. This is due to the lack of definite histopathological criteria, as illustrated in the following definition of 'having both architectural and cytological atypia which approximates, but falls short of that seen in carcinoma in situ'.[4] This rather ambiguous definition was felt to be unacceptable by Azzopardi,[50] who stated that '...the clinician should

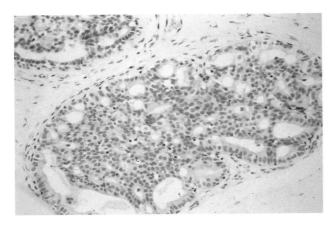

Figure 26.10 Atypical ductal hyperplasia with a cribriform pattern, showing partial involvement of the duct with atypical cells. (H&E, ×10.)

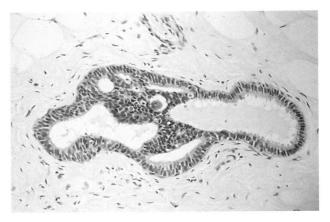

Figure 26.11 Atypical ductal hyperplasia with atypical cells centrally and normal epithelium at the periphery. (H&E, ×20.)

be told as unequivocally as possible whether the pathologist considers that the lesion is benign or malignant. Terms like .... "atypical hyperplasia" should be avoided as far as possible ... as such terms frighten surgeons into performing unnecessary mastectomies'. Over the years, however, pathologists have come to recognise a borderline epithelial proliferation that architecturally and cytologically does not qualify for the diagnosis of carcinoma in situ.

In their impressive follow up study of 10 542 women, 3.6% of whom had atypical epithelial proliferations, Page et al[51] illustrated that the term 'atypical hyperplasia' was appropriate for those lesions where the pattern or the cytological criteria of carcinoma in situ are partially met but not fully expressed. In that study, they outlined criteria for identifying ADH, which Page and Rogers[52] later improved. In making a diagnosis of ADH, the criteria must be based on cytological features, histological pattern and anatomical extent. ADH exhibits partial involvement of basement membrane-bound spaces by a cell population similar to non-comedo type DCIS (cribriform). These atypical cells are evenly spaced and uniform, with oval to round nuclei. The cytoplasm is pale with distinct intercellular borders. The non-atypical cells are columnar and are arranged radially at the periphery of the duct, just above the basement membrane. The histological pattern is variable. This includes secondary spaces with smooth rounded 'punched-out' borders of cribriform architecture with or without rigid non-tapering bars (Figures 26.10 and 26.11). Micropapillary structures may also be present. To qualify for ADH, the uniform cells must not completely involve two membrane-bound spaces; if they do then DCIS is the appropriate diagnosis. ADH is usually 2–3 mm in diameter.[53] The schematic

diagram in Figure 26.12 illustrates the different features of DCIS, florid hyperplasia without atypia (FHWA) and ADH.

In spite of these criteria, there is still much interobserver variation in the reporting of ADH, as Rosai[54] disovered when he distributed cases to five prominent breast pathologists in the USA. There was no consensus in the diagnosis of ADH versus DCIS. The root of all this disagreement lies in the fact that it may be virtually impossible to distinguish ADH from small cell (low-grade) DCIS of cribriform type. For this reason, the consensus statement[14] asserted that only cases of severe atypia should be classified as ADH. Similarly, the UK guidelines[53] advocate that the pathologist should only make the diagnosis of ADH where a diagnosis of DCIS is seriously considered. ADH can be detected as mammographic calcification, and its presence in a needle core biopsy should prompt an excisional biopsy to exclude DCIS or invasive carcinoma. ADH is a rare lesion, which often coexists with fibrocystic change, sclerosing adenosis or multiple papillomas and is identified in 2% of non-screening biopsies.[53] The figure is much higher in screen-detected lesions – up to 12% in some series.[55]

In a 15-year follow-up study of women with ADH, Page and associates demonstrated a fourfold relative risk of developing invasive carcinoma of the breast compared with the general population. Translating this to absolute risk, approximately 10% of women with ADH would develop invasive cancer within 10–15 years of biopsy in the ipsilateral or contralateral breast. The relative risk doubles to 8–10 times if there is a family history of breast cancer (mother, sister or daughter) and the absolute risk is elevated to 20% at 15 years.[56] Annual mammographic follow-up is advisable for patients with ADH.

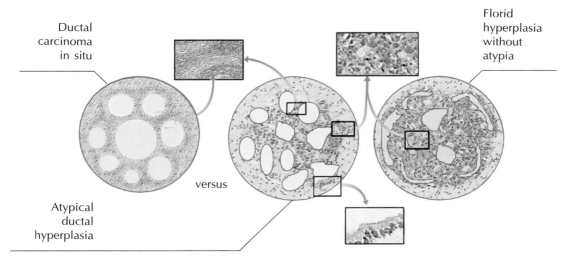

Figure 26.12 Ductal carcinoma in situ (DCIS) versus atypical ductal hyperplasia (ADH) versus florid hyperplasia without atypia (FHWA): cytology and histology. DCIS features smooth, punched-out luminal borders within an involved basement membrane-bound space. The cytological features are regular and present throughout the entire population of at least two basement membrane-bound spaces. FHWA is the most densely cellular and extensive of the lesions classed as proliferative disease without atypia (PDWA) – also called 'papillomatosis'. There are ragged, often slit-like, luminal borders. The nuclei throughout the involved area show the variability and tendency to a swirling pattern, as illustrated. ADH has features predominantly of non-comedo, cribriform DCIS, but also some features of proliferative disease without atypia or normally polarised cells within the same basement membrane-bound space. (Reproduced with permission from Dr DL Page, Dr LW Rogers and WB Saunders Publishers, from Human Pathology 1992; 23: 1095–7.)

Lobular neoplasia

Haagensen et al[57] applied the term lobular neoplasia to classify collectively proliferations currently separated into lobular carcinoma in situ (LCIS) and atypical lobular hyperplasia (ALH). LCIS and ALH differ architecturally in the degree by which the cells expand the lobular units, but they are cytologically identical. Because of inter- and intra-observer variation, this distinction is considered by some authorities to be arbitrary, and therefore the use of 'lobular neoplasia' to encompass the whole range of proliferations would improve reproducibility.[58] However, this concept has not been fully embraced by pathologists.[5] Rosen[59] has proposed that the term lobular neoplasia should be reserved for a spectrum of proliferations ranging from mild atypia to ALH to fully developed LCIS. Whenever possible, LCIS should be distinguished from ALH as they possess different risk factors. As both LCIS and ALH do not present with clinical or radiological abnormalities, Jacobs et al[60] have advocated that if these lesions are discovered as incidental findings, then follow-up rather that local excision is advisable. Both LCIS and ALH can be present in biopsies removed for clinically benign conditions such as fibrocystic change. Further excision is advisable in the following situations:[58]

- if another lesion such as ADH or DCIS is present
- if there is clinical radiological and pathological discordance
- if a mass lesion or an area of architectural distortion is present
- there is pleomorphic LCIS
- there is ALH or LCIS with mixed histological features indistinguishable from DCIS.

Atypical lobular hyperplasia (ALH)

The histological criteria for ALH are met when there is partial distension of the acini in a lobular unit by a population of cells identical to those seen in LCIS with residual intercellular spaces.[51] The resemblance to LCIS is striking but the acini are not uniformly distended in more than 50% of the lobular units (Figure 26.13a). ALH cells are bland and uniform, with small or inconspicuous nucleoli. Pagetoid spread of atypical cells along ducts is sometimes seen in ALH as in LCIS. The latter diagnosis should not be made purely on the basis of this criterion without taking other features into consideration. Small clear spaces sometimes containing mucin may be present within the cells, and these intracytoplasmic lumina or 'private acini' are not true glandular lumina but represent dilated Golgi apparatus.

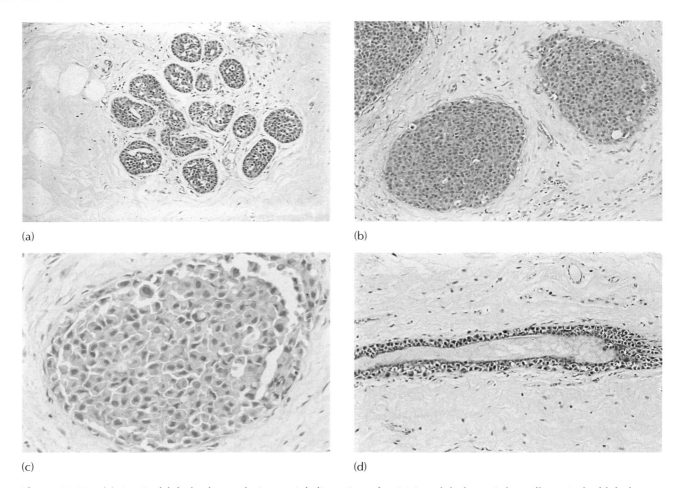

(a)

(b)

(c)

(d)

Figure 26.13   (a) Atypical lobular hyperplasia: partial distension of acini in a lobular unit by cells typical of lobular neoplasm. (H&E, ×10.) (b) Lobular carcinoma in situ (LCIS), showing completely distended acini with neoplastic cells. (H&E, ×10.) (c) Cells of LCIS, some of which show eccentrically displaced nuclei and an occasional intracytoplasmic vacuole. (H&E, ×40.) (d) Pagetoid spread within a duct by lobular neoplastic cells. (H&E, ×10.)

ALH is more common in perimenopausal women, with an average age of 46.[51,57] The relative risk for developing invasive carcinoma with ALH is four times that of the general population, and this risk doubles when associated with a family history of breast cancer. The absolute risk for developing invasive cancer is 10% at 15 years. The cancers associated with ALH are mainly lobular, although ductal carcinoma can also develop and the contralateral breast is equally at risk.

Lobular carcinoma in situ (LCIS)

LCIS was first recognised as an entity by Foote and Stewart[61] as early as 1941. LCIS is distinguished from ALH by the complete distension of more than 50% of the acini in a lobular unit by a uniform population of neoplastic lobular cells (Figure 26.13b). The cells are arranged in a regular pattern with no intercellular spaces, but intracellular lumina (private acini) may be present, displacing the rather hyperchromatic nuclei

eccentrically (Figure 26.13c). Pagetoid spread along ducts is more prevalent in LCIS than in ALH (Figure 26.13d). Seventy percent of women with LCIS are premenopausal and the condition is present in 1% of screen-detected lesions.[62]

LCIS tends to be multifocal and bilateral and predisposes to invasive cancer, even after a long interval. In a 15-year follow-up study of 39 patients with LCIS, Page et al[63] calculated the relative risk for developing invasive cancer to be 10–11 times that of the general population. The absolute risk of developing invasive cancer in patients with LCIS is 25–30% at 15–20 years. This risk of cancer is apportioned 50–60% in the same breast and 40–50% in the contralateral breast.[62] Seventy percent of the cancers are of lobular type and the remainder mixed or ductal of no special type.

In contrast to atypical hyperplastic lesions, a family history of breast cancer does not appear to have any further predictive value in identifying women who develop invasive carcinoma.[63] The effect of exogenous oestrogen in postmenopausal women is not known. However, the risk for subsequent invasive disease is higher with more extensive disease.

Ductal carcinoma in situ (DCIS)

As early as 1932, Broders[64] recognized carcinoma in situ of the breast as a neoplastic epithelial proliferation confined to the ducts and acini without migration beyond the basement membrane. Using subgross analysis, Wellings et al[3] demonstrated that carcinomas as well as other preneoplastic proliferations arise from the TDLUs and that the histological appearance of DCIS is due to 'unfolding' of the lobules. According to this theory, during epithelial proliferation, the ductules of a lobule enlarge and the interlobular part ceases to exist. The ductules continue to dilate and incorporate themselves in a single lumen, with resultant loss of the lobular architecture, which is termed 'unfolding'.

Traditionally, these structures have been called ducts and the term *ductal* carcinoma in situ is used to differentiate the lesion from *lobular* carcinoma in situ. In the premammographic era, DCIS made up only 1–5% of symptomatic carcinoma.[65] In contrast to LCIS, which mainly affects premenopausal women, 70% of patients with DCIS are postmenopausal.[62] DCIS presents symptomatically as an ill-defined mass, nipple discharge or Paget's disease or as an incidental finding in a clinically benign lump. However, since the introduction of breast screening mammography, DCIS has been more frequently identified as a non-palpable, usually calcifying lesion, with figures ranging from 10% to 20%, depending on the breast screening unit.[66] Traditionally, DCIS has been classified according to its architectural pattern into comedo and non-comedo types, disregarding cytomorphology.[36] The non-comedo type was further subclassified into cribriform, micropapillary, solid and papillary types. Although this is a useful pathological classification in terms of pattern recognition for diagnosis, it has little therapeutic or prognostic implication. Patchefsky et al[67] noted the heterogeneous nature of DCIS both pathologically and in biological behaviour, and classified DCIS according to nuclear grade.

Investigations using biological markers, three-dimensional studies, mammographic analysis and follow up of patients demonstrated that the simple classification of DCIS according to architecture did not always correspond to the biological behaviour. Holland et al[68] proposed a classification of DCIS based on nuclear morphology rather than on architecture and the presence or absence of necrosis. Using these criteria, DCIS is divided into well, moderately and poorly differentiated types. The only problem with using this terminology is that clinicians may misinterpret 'differentiated' as invasive carcinoma. Similarly, the UK Coordinating Group for Breast Screening Pathology classified DCIS according to nuclear grade into high, intermediate and low grades.[53] Cytonuclear grade gives less interobserver variation than architectural differentiation. However, there is often cytological and architectural overlap of features in the same breast, and the in situ carcinomas must be graded according to the worst area. Both the architectural and cytological features of DCIS will be discussed in relation to radiological appearance, expression of biological markers and biological behaviour.

High-grade DCIS

High-grade DCIS with comedo necrosis is the most prevalent type of DCIS, constituting up to 85% of high-grade lesions.[67] This presents clinically with an ill-defined mass or Paget's disease of the nipple. Radiologically, there is often a linear, branching or granular pattern of microcalcification. On cut surface, breast tissue containing comedo carcinoma in situ reveals large ducts filled by yellow necrotic semisolid debris, which is easily expressed like a 'comedone'. Histologically, high-grade DCIS has variable architectural differentiation or cellular polarisation. The most common pattern consist of solid sheets of neoplastic cells, which line the ducts with central comedo necrosis (Figure 26.14). Necrosis is present in most cases, but not exclusively. Conversely, not all cases with comedo necrosis are high-grade. Pure solid DCIS is rare and is usually confined to nipple ducts in cases associated with Paget's disease. The mammographic calcification has an amorphous histological pattern (Figure 26.15). Sometimes, the neoplastic ducts accumulate foamy macrophages, simulating necrosis (Figure 26.16). The cells may lack the solid pattern, forming a pseudocribriform or micropapillary configuration (Figure 26.17). Periductal fibrosis and lymphocytic infiltration are often associated with this type of DCIS.

The cells show marked variations in nuclear size and shape (pleomorphism), with a high nuclear-to-cytoplasmic ratio and condensation of chromatin. They are usually large, with pale or eosinophilic cytoplasm (Figure 26.18). The luminal layer of the epithelium is often retracted away from the necrotic debris. This distinguishes comedo necrosis from that occasionally seen in benign lesions such as juvenile papillomatosis, nipple adenoma and hyperplasia of usual type.[4] Mitoses are often evident, and high-grade DCIS frequently demonstrates individual cell necrosis. Pleomorphic cells often involve recognisable lobular units, in 'cancerisation' of lobules (Figure 26.19).

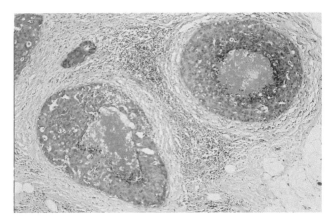

Figure 26.14 High-grade DCIS with central necrosis. (H&E, ×10.)

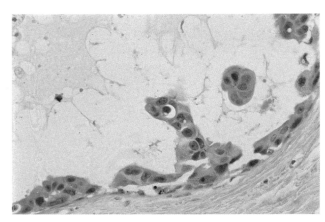

Figure 26.17 High-grade micropapillary DCIS. (H&E, ×20.)

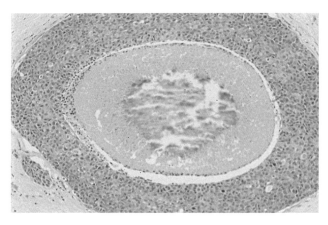

Figure 26.15 Amorphous calcification of comedo high-grade DCIS. (H&E, ×20.)

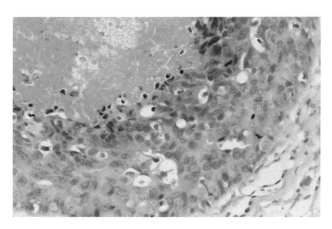

Figure 26.18 Cytological features of high-grade DCIS: pleomorphic large nuclei within eosinophilic abundant cytoplasm. Abnormal mitoses are common. (H&E, ×40.)

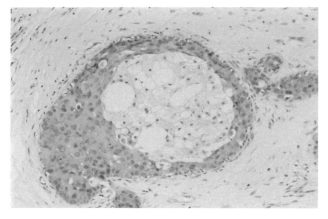

Figure 26.16 High-grade DCIS with central accumulation of foamy macrophages, simulating necrosis. (H&E, ×20.)

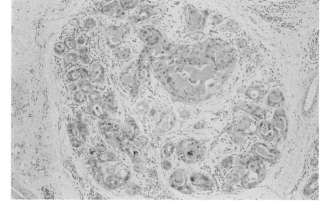

Figure 26.19 Cancerisation of lobules in high-grade DCIS. (H&E, ×20.)

Low-grade DCIS

Low-nuclear grade DCIS rarely presents with a palpable mass, and is usually identified incidentally in a biopsy for a clinically benign lesion. Mammographic calcification is mostly granular, and this is reflected histologically, with a laminated crystalline pattern resembling psammoma bodies

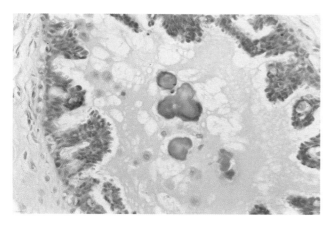

Figure 26.20 Laminated calcification usually associated with low-grade DCIS with a micropapillary architecture. (H&E, ×20.)

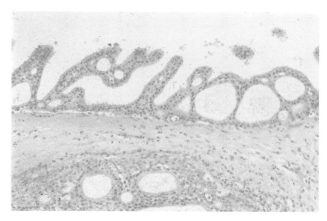

Figure 26.22 Low-grade DCIS showing 'Roman bridges'. (H&E, ×20.)

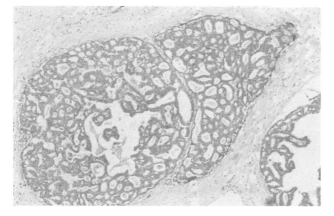

Figure 26.21 Low-grade DCIS with characteristic cribriform pattern. (H&E, ×10.)

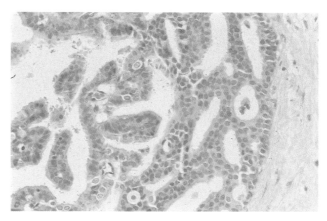

Figure 26.23 The cells of low-grade DCIS are uniform, with small nucleoli. (H&E, ×40.)

(Figure 26.20). In contrast to high-grade DCIS, low-grade DCIS tends to show architectural differentiation or cellular polarisation, resulting in cribriform or micropapillary carcinoma. The cribriform pattern consists of an intraductal proliferation of neoplastic cells separated by round or oval lumina (Figure 26.21). This must be distinguished from collagenous spherulosis and adenoid cystic carcinoma. The papillae of micropapillary DCIS are devoid of fibrovascular cores and are held rigidly and perpendicular to the basement membrane. Sometimes, anastomosing arcades give rise to 'Roman bridges' (Figure 26.22). Occasionally, a single layer of neoplastic cells lines the duct lumen without projections, a pattern Azzopardi termed 'clinging carcinoma'. In cases where this is the only pattern, this would now be classified as ADH or columnar cell change with cytological atypia. The cells of low-grade DCIS are small and monomorphic, with round or oval nuclei. The nuclear membrane is smooth and the nucleolus is small or inconspicuous (Figure 26.23). Mitoses are infrequent and individual cell

necrosis is not a feature.[68] Luminal necrosis is uncommon, but can occur. Figure 26.24 illustrates clearly necrosis in low-grade cribriform DCIS, which would probably be termed comedo carcinoma in the old classification. Rarely, low-grade DCIS exhibits a solid proliferation mimicking LCIS.

Intermediate-grade DCIS

This group of DCIS cannot be easily assigned into either the high- or low-grade categories. The architecture is variable and there is cellular polarisation with micropapillae, but this is not as marked as in low-grade DCIS (Figure 26.25). Solid areas with intercellular spaces may also be present. The cytomorphology of intermediate grade lies midway between that of high- and low-grade DCIS. The cells show moderate variations in nuclear size and shape. The chromatin pattern is coarse and the nucleoli are small. Calcification may be of mixed pattern, showing both amorphous and psamommatous

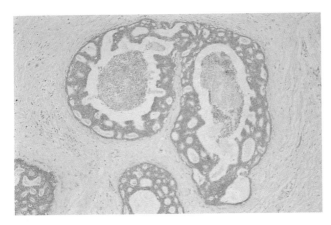

Figure 26.24 Low-grade DCIS with central necrosis. (H&E, ×20.)

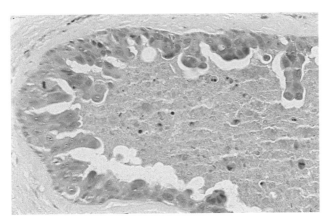

Figure 26.25 Intermediate-grade DCIS, showing partial architectural differentiation. (H&E, ×20.)

features in different ducts. Necrosis may or may not be present.[68] Biological markers justified the inclusion of this third category of DCIS.[69] Clear cell and apocrine DCIS are usually of intermediate nuclear grade.

Intracystic papillary carcinoma (encysted papillary carcinoma)

Intracystic papillary carcinoma is a form of DCIS that involves a grossly dilated duct varying in size from 1 to 3 cm.[36] Irrespective of the size, the important factor is that these lesions are non-invasive. Grossly, the tumour may appear solid, or a dilated duct filled with haemorrhagic debris may be evident. Histologically, the tumours may show a thick fibrous wall from which papillary excrescences arise (Figure 26.26a). The papillae consist of a fibrovascular core covered by a layer of epithelium without intervening myoepithelial cells. The cells are small, monomorphic and reminiscent of those seen in low-grade DCIS (Figure 26.26b). Some lesions are so well differentiated that when Betsill et al[70] reported papillary intraductal carcinoma, he used the term 'low-grade and well-differentiated carcinoma', which would fit into the current classification of DCIS. Cribriform-type DCIS is sometimes present outside the 'cystic' wall, where foci of micro-invasion occasionally lurk. Carter et al[71] followed 29 women who had had mastectomy for intracystic carcinoma, and none of them developed metastatic carcinoma after 5 years of follow-up. LOH on chromosome 16q in intracystic papillary carcinomas was reported to differentiate these lesions from intraductal papillomas.[35]

Prognostic implication of DCIS

Because of the heterogeneous nature of DCIS, classification using cytomorphology and biological markers attempts to predict the behaviour of the different lesions. There is no long-term prospective study of the behaviour of mammographically

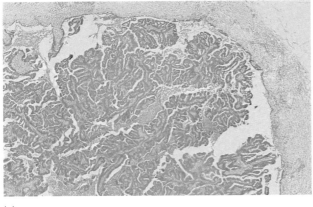

(a)

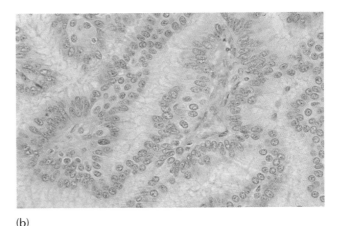

(b)

Figure 26.26 (a) Intracystic papillary carcinoma. (H&E, ×4.) (b) Papillary fronds of intracystic carcinoma with low-grade cells devoid of a myoepithelial layer. (H&E, ×40.)

detected DCIS, and the information available is on retrospective studies of radiologically detected, symptomatic or incidental in situ carcinomas. Page et al[72] followed up 28 patients with non-comedo DCIS identified incidentally in clinically benign lumps and treated by biopsy alone. This study predicted that 28% of women treated with biopsy alone for incidental DCIS would develop invasive carcinoma in approximately 15 years. Clinically significant invasive carcinoma tends to occur proximal to the site of the original biopsy.

The calculated risk factor for developing invasive cancer following a diagnosis of DCIS is 10–11 times that of the general population.[72] The overall absolute risk of developing invasive carcinoma for both comedo and non-comedo DCIS is 30–50% at 10–18 years, with 99% of the carcinomas occurring in the ipslateral breast.[62] Invasive carcinoma occurring after mastectomy for DCIS is rare.[73] Lagios et al[66] followed up 79 women with mammographically detected DCIS treated by local excision alone (tylectomy). They classified the in situ carcinomas into four types – type I representing large cell comedo carcinoma and type IV the other end of the spectrum of small cell cribriform/micropapillary DCIS, with two intermediate grades. The overall recurrence rate was 10% at 4 years. DCIS with high nuclear grade was more likely to recur than the cases with low nuclear grade, and seven out of the eight recurrences were high-grade comedo DCIS. None of the small cell DCIS recurred, while a single case of intermediate grade DCIS recurred. Price et al[74] recorded a higher recurrence figure of 55% at 7 years in patients with DCIS treated by local excision alone. Both invasive and in situ carcinomas were counted as recurrence.

Multicentricity and incompleteness of excision are usually incriminated as the underlying causes of recurrence of invasive carcinoma from residual DCIS. While an occult focus of invasive carcinoma may be responsible for the development of subsequent invasive carcinoma, the majority of cases evolve from residual DCIS.[72] Rosen et al[75] demonstrated residual carcinoma in 56% of mastectomy specimens performed immediately after biopsy, and 33% of these were present in quadrants other than the biopsy site. In the study by Patchefsky et al,[67] micropapillary DCIS had a high propensity for multicentricity, with more ducts involved than in any other type. Multicentric DCIS is defined as tumour foci separated by uninvolved glandular tissue of 4 cm or more.[76] In the past, multicentricity of DCIS was used as a justification for mastectomy.[72] Contrary to the widely held belief, DCIS is not always multicentric. Faverly et al[76] studied 60 mastectomy specimens using three-dimensional imaging and only 8% of the cases of DCIS were multicentric. Using radiological and pathological mapping, they demonstrated that

DCIS generally does not have a multicentric but rather a unicentric (segmental) distribution. DCIS tends to grow continuously by extending through the glandular tree, but may also have a discontinuous or multifocal growth pattern. The latter is defined as at least two foci of tumour separated by an uninvolved portion of duct of any length less than 4 cm.[76] In this study, 90% of high-grade DCIS had a continuous growth pattern, compared with a multifocal distribution in 70% of low-grade cases.

In spite of the rare occurrence of multicentricity, DCIS tends to be extensive – hence completeness of excision is not always attainable, which is demonstrated by the frequency of recurrence following local excision.[66,74] Theoretically, the assessment of margins should be more reliable in high-grade DCIS, which tends to have a continuous growth pattern as opposed to the multifocal nature of low-nuclear-grade in situ carcinoma. At the time of excision, at least a 1 cm rim of normal breast tissue should be included. This approach surgically removes nearly 90% of unifocal in situ carcinoma, irrespective of histological type.[76] The use of both clinical and specimen radiographs is invaluable in assessing adequacy of excision, as is the use of shaved (en face) excision margin assessment.

DCIS and micro-invasion

Micro-invasion is defined as the presence of an invasive carcinoma no more than 1 mm in diameter (2 high-power fields) outside the confines of membrane-bound lobular units, where the dominant lesion is carcinoma in situ.[5] Micro-invasion indicates the presence of a clone of cells with a propensity to metastasize, putting the patient at risk of a life-threatening disease. Definite micro-invasion consists of irregularly shaped and variably sized nests of cells surrounded by a 'fresh' fibroblastic proliferation that is not well oriented around individual epithelial nests.[4] However, lesions that fulfil this criterion are rare, and if there is any doubt then a diagnosis of DCIS should be made. Disruption of the stromal–epithelial interface per se does not indicate micro-invasion. A prominent lymphocytic infiltrate should lead to a search for micro-invasion.[4] Basement membrane stains using immunocytochemistry can aid in the assessment of micro-invasion. In the study by Pachefsky et al,[67] 29% of patients with DCIS had micro-invasive carcinoma, the majority being associated with comedo-type DCIS (high-grade). None of the solid or cribriform variants had micro-invasion. Multiple sections may reveal a focus of micro-invasion. Overall, patients with high-grade DCIS are at risk of harbouring micro-invasion with subsequent metastases.

The difficulty faced by the breast surgeon when dealing with patients who have DCIS with micro-invasion is whether or not to perform axillary dissection. Zavostsky et al[77] examined sentinel lymph nodes in 14 patients with DCIS (mostly high-grade) and micro-invasion. Two patients had sentinel lymph node micrometastasis, with no further metastasis on completion axillary dissection. Sentinel lymph node sampling could be a useful tool in the management of patients with DCIS and micro-invasion.

DCIS in invasive carcinoma

DCIS is commonly associated with invasive carcinoma of no special type and is not a component of medullary carcinoma. The presence of in situ lesions in invasive carcinoma confirms their premalignant nature. Lampejo et al[78] demonstrated a positive correlation between the different grades of invasive and in situ carcinomas, which was prognostically significant. Low-grade DCIS was usually associated with grade 1 invasive carcinoma, intermediate-grade DCIS with grade 2 invasive carcinomas, and high-grade DCIS with either grade 2 or grade 3 cancers.

The type of DCIS associated with the invasive component was predictive of the outcome. None of the patients with tumours containing low-grade DCIS developed recurrence after a median follow-up of 13 years. Cancers containing high-grade DCIS had the worst prognosis. In addition to assessing the type of DCIS present in the invasive carcinoma, it is also of clinical significance to determine the extent of DCIS outside the invasive component. The Boston group defined extensive DCIS as that consisting of more than 25% of the main invasive tumour mass and extending beyond it into the surrounding breast tissue or a tumour that shows foci of invasion within a predominantly in situ carcinoma.[79] It was agreed at a European Organization for Research on Treatment of Cancer (EORTC) consensus meeting that the principal risk factor for local relapse following conservative surgery is a large residual burden of DCIS found adjacent to 10–15% of invasive carcinoma.[80] DCIS is commonly present beyond mammographically detected microcalcification, and it is important to sample the apparently normal breast tissue to detect any extensive in situ component.

DCIS and expression of biological markers

Histological grade, lymph node status and the application of biological markers have been used in combination to evaluate prognosis in invasive carcinomas. The commonly studied biological markers are the c-ErbB-2 and p53 proteins, and oestrogen and progesterone receptors (ER and PgR). These markers have also been applied to non-invasive carcinomas in an attempt to predict their behaviour.

The c-erbB-2 gene (also known as HER2/neu) encodes a transmembrane glycoprotein (c-ErbB-2) with tyrosine kinase activity that is homologous to but distinct from the epidermal growth factor receptor (EGFR).[81] The gene is located on chromosome 17q and its amplification is associated with over-expression of the protein product, which can be detected by immunohistochemistry as cell membrane staining. Overexpression of c-ErbB-2 in 20% of invasive carcinomas is associated with poor prognosis, with most of the tumours being poorly differentiated grade 3 carcinomas.[82] Approximately 60–80% of high-grade DCIS strongly express the c-ErbB-2 protein[83] (Figure 26.27). None of the low-grade DCIS express the c-ErbB-2 oncoprotein, while approximately 23% of intermediate-grade lesions do.[69]

The TP53 (p53) tumour suppressor gene is the most commonly deleted gene in human cancers.[84] It has been mapped to the short arm of chromosome 17 (17p13).[85] TP53 encodes a nuclear phosphoprotein, p53. Mutant p53 has a longer half-life than the wild type and can be detected by immunocytochemistry,[86] giving rise to positive nuclear staining. Sixty percent of high-grade DCIS show positive nuclear staining for p53 protein, compared with 4% of intermediate grade and none of the low-grade cases.[69]

Poller et al[87] demonstrated an inverse relationship between the expression of the c-ErbB-2 oncoprotein in DCIS and hormone receptor status. A similar pattern is seen in invasive carcinomas. The majority of high-grade DCIS and poorly differentiated invasive ductal carcinomas overexpress c-ErbB-2 and lack ER. In the study by Potter et al,[88] mostly small cell (low-grade) DCIS expressed ER and PgR. The latter is directly modulated by oestrogen, and therefore its level of expression mirrors that of ER. A separate study by Zafrani et al[88] on mammographically detected DCIS reported a higher percentage of high-grade lesions that expressed ER as well as c-ErbB-2. The presence of both ER and PgR can be demonstrated using immunocytochemistry on wax-embedded tissue. Similar to p53, steroid receptors are demonstrated by nuclear staining (Figure 26.28).

A study by Buerger et al[89] suggested that there may be at least three different pathways for the development of DCIS, with loss of the long arm of chromosome 16 being prevalent in low-grade DCIS, and gains in 17q12 and 20q13 and loss of 13q occurring

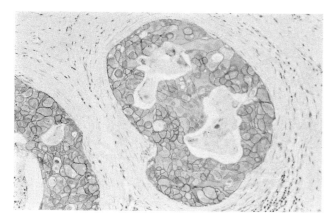

Figure 26.27 High-grade DCIS, showing membrane c-ErbB-2 overexpression with immunocytochemistry staining. (×20.)

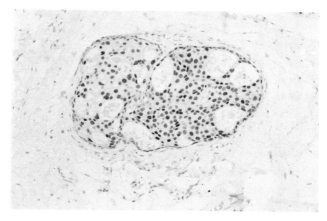

Figure 26.28 Low-grade DCIS positive for oestrogen receptors. (×20.)

in high-grade DCIS. Gain in 11q13 appears to be associated with intermediate-grade DCIS, as does loss of 11q. Loss of 16q is also a genetic alteration noted in intracystic carcinomas, which tend to be low-grade lesions. Although chromosomal abnormalities occur in both low- and high-grade DCIS, none of these molecular techniques overrides conventional histological diagnosis.

References

1. Page DL. Cancer risk assessment in benign breast biopsies. Hum Pathol 1986; 17: 871–4.
2. Foote FW, Stewart FW. Comparative studies of cancerous versus noncancerous breasts. Ann Surg 1945; 121: 6–53; 197–222.
3. Wellings SR, Jensen HM, Marcum RG. An atlas of the subgross pathology of human breast with special reference to possible precancerous lesions. J Natl Cancer Inst 1975; 55: 231–73.
4. Fechner RE, Mills SE (eds). Philosophy of risk assessment. Ductal carcinoma in situ. In: Breast Pathology, Benign Proliferations, Atypias and In Situ Carcinomas. Chicago: ASCP Press, 1990: 1–3; 107–18.
5. Sloane JP. Pathology reporting in breast cancer screening. J Clin Pathol 1991; 44: 710–25.
6. Dawson EK. Sweat gland carcinoma of the breast. A morpho-histological study. Edin Med J 1932; 39: 409–38.
7. Viacava P, Naccarato AG, Bevilicqua G. Apocrine epithelium of the breast: Does it result from metaplasia? Virchows Arch 1997; 431: 205–9.
8. Haagensen CD. Apocrine epithelium; Solitary intraductal papilloma; Multiple intraductal papillomas; Lobular neoplasia (Lobular carcinoma in situ). In: Diseases of the Breast (Harris JR, Lippman ME, Morrow M, Osborne CK, eds). Philadelphia: WB Saunders, 1986: 82–101; 136–75; 176–91; 192–241.
9. Wellings SR, Alpers CE. Apocrine cystic metaplasia: subgross pathology and prevalence in cancer associated versus random autopsy breasts. Hum Pathol 1987; 18: 381–6.
10. Page DL, Zwaag RV, Rogers LW et al. Relation between component parts of fibrocystic disease complex and breast cancer. J Natl Cancer Inst 1978; 61: 1055–63.
11. Dupont WD, Page DL. Risk factors for breast cancer in women with proliferative breast disease. N Engl J Med 1985; 312: 146–51.
12. Dixon JM, McDonald C, Miller WR. Risk of breast cancer in women with palpable cysts: a prospective study. Lancet 1999; 353: 1742–5.
13. Page DL, Dupont WD, Jensen RA. Papillary apocrine change of the breast: associations with atypical hyperplasia and risk of breast cancer. Cancer Epidemiol Biomarkers Prev 1996; 5: 29–32.
14. Hutter RV et al. Consensus Meeting: Is 'fibrocystic disease' of the breast precancerous? Arch Pathol Lab Med 1986; 110: 171–3.
15. Fitzgibbons PL, Henson DE, Hutter RV. Benign breast changes and risk of subsequent breast cancer: an update of the 1985 Consensus Statement. Cancer Committee of the College of American Pathologists. Arch Pathol Lab Med 1998; 122: 1053–5.
16. Washington C, Dalbegue F, Abreo F et al. Loss of heterozygosity in fibrocystic change of the breast: genetic relationship between benign proliferative lesions and associated carcinoma. Am J Pathol 2000; 157: 323–9.
17. Jones C, Damiani S, Wells D et al. Molecular cytogenetic comparison of apocrine hyperplasia and apocrine carcinoma of the breast. Am J Pathol 2001; 158: 207–14.
18. Agnantis NJ, Mahera H, Maounis N, Spandidos DA. Immunohistochemical study of ras and myc oncoproteins in apocrine breast lesions with and without papillomatosis. Eur J Gynaecol Oncol 1999; 13: 309–15.
19. Linnell F, Ljungberg O, Anderssen I. Breast carcinoma: aspects of early stages, progression and related problems. Acta Pathol Scand 1980; 272 (Suppl): 1–233.
20. Jacobs TW, Byrne C, Colditz G et al. Radial scars in benign breast biopsy specimens and the risk of breast cancer. N Engl J Med 1999; 340: 430–6.

21. Andersen JA, Gram JB. Radial scar in the female breast. A long-term follow-up study of 32 cases. Cancer 1984; 53: 2557–60.

22. Sloane JP, Mayers MM. Carcinoma and atypicical hyperplasia in radial scars and complex sclerosis lesions: importance of lesion size and patient age. Histopathology 1993; 23: 225–31.

23. Jacobs TW, Schnitt SJ, Tan X, Brown LF. Radial scars of the breast and breast carcinomas have similar alterations in expression of factors involved in vascular stroma formation. Hum Pathol 2002; 33: 29–38.

24. Jensen RA, Page DL, Dupont WD, Rogers LW. Invasive breast cancer risk in women with sclerosing adenosis. Cancer 1989; 64: 1977–83.

25. Oberman HA, Markey BA. Noninvasive carcinoma of the breast presenting in adenosis. Mod Pathol 1991; 4: 31–5.

26. Fechner RE. Lobular carcinoma in situ in sclerosing adenosis. A potential confusion with invasive carcinoma. Am J Surg Pathol 1981; 5: 233–9.

27. Makunura CN, Curling OM, Yeomans P et al. Apocrine adenosis within a radial scar: a case of false positive breast cytodiagnosis. Cytopathology 1994; 5: 123–8.

28. Simpson JF, Page DL, Dupont WD. Apocrine adenosis – a mimic of mammary carcinoma. Surg Pathol 1990; 3: 289–99.

29. Seidman JD, Ashton M, Lefkowitz M. Atypical apocrine adenosis of the breast: a clinicopathologic study of 37 patients with 8.7–year follow-up. Cancer 1996; 77: 2529–37.

30. Wells CA, McGregor IL, Makunura CN et al. Apocrine adenosis: a precursor of aggressive cancer? J Clin Pathol 1995; 48: 737–42.

31. Selim AG, El-Ayat G, Wells CA. c-ErbB2 oncoprotein expression, gene amplification, and chromosome 17 aneusomy in apocrine adenosis of the breast. J Pathol 2000; 191: 138–42.

32. Ohuchi N, Abe R, Kasai M. Possible cancerous change of intraductal papillomas of the breast. A 3–D reconstruction study of 25 cases. Cancer 1984; 54: 605–11.

33. Muir R. The evolution of carcinoma of the mamma. J Pathol 1941; L11(2): 155–72.

34. Page DL, Salhany KE, Jensen RA, Dupont WD. Subsequent breast carcinoma risk after biopsy with atypia in breast papilloma. Cancer 1996; 78: 258–66.

35. Tsuda H, Uei Y, Fukutomi T, Hiroshoshi S. Different incidence of loss of heterozygosity on chromosome 16q between intraductal papilloma and intracystic papillary carcinoma of the breast. Jpn J Cancer Res, 1994; 85: 992–6.

36. Page DL, Rogers LW. Epithelial hyperplasia; Carcinoma in situ (CIS). In: Page DL, Anderson TJ, eds. Diagnostic Histopathology of the Breast. Edinburgh: Churchill Livingstone, 1987: 120–56; 157–92.

37. Tavassoli FA, Hoefler R, Rosai et al. Intraductal profilerative lesions. In: Tavassoli FA, Devilee P (eds). Pathology and Genetics of Tumours of the Breast and Female Genital Organs. Lyon: IARC Press, 2003: 63–73.

38. Boecker W, Moll R, Dervan P et .al. Usual ductal hyperplasia of the breast is a committed stem (progenitor) cell lesion distinct from atypical ductal carcinoma in situ. J Pathol 2002; 198: 458–67.

39. Fitzgibbons PL, Henson DE, Hutter RVP, for the Cancer Committee of the College of American Pathologists. Benign breast changes and the risk for subsequent breast cancer. An update of Consensus Statement. Arch Pathol Lab Med 1998; 122: 1053–5.

40. Bonser GM, Dossett JA, Jull JW. Neoplastic epithelial proliferation. In: Human and Experimental Breast Cancer 1961. London: Pitman Medical Publishing, 1961: 336–43.

41. Goldstein NS, O'Malley BA. Cancerization of small ectatic ducts of the breast by ductal carcinoma in situ cells with apocrine snouts. A lesion associated with tubular carcinoma. Am J Clin Pathol 1997; 107: 561–6.

42. Fraser JL, Raza S, Chorny K et al. Columnar alterations with prominent apical snouts and secretions: a spectrum of changes frequently present in breast biopsies performed for microcalcifications. Am J Surg Pathol 1998; 22: 1521–7.

43. Schnitt SJ. Columnar cell lesions of the breast: pathological features and clinical significance. Curr Diagn Pathol 2004; 10: 193–203.

44. Azzopardi JG. Underdiagnosis of malignancy. In: Azzopardi JG (ed.) Problems in Breast Pathology. Philadelphia: WB Saunders, 1979: 192–213.

45. Brogi G, Oyama T, Koerner FC. Atypical cystic lobules in patients with lobular neoplasia: Int J Surg Pathol 2001; 9: 201–6.

46. Rosen PP. Columnar cell hyperplasia in association with lobular carcinoma in situ and tubular carcinoma. Am J Surg Pathol 1999; 23: 1561.

47. Rosen PP, Mucocele-like tumours of the breast. Am J Surg Pathol 1986; 10: 464–9.

48. Chinyama CN, Davies JD. Mammary mucinous lesions: congeners, prevalence and important pathological associations. Histopathology 1996; 29: 533–9.

49. Weaver MG, Abdul-Karim FW, Al-Kaisi N. Mucinous lesions of the breast. A pathological continuum. Pathol Res Pract 1993; 189: 873–6.

50. Azzopardi JG. Over diagnosis of malignancy. In: Azzopardi AG (ed) Problems in Breast Pathology. Philadelphia: WB Saunders, 1979: 167–91.

51. Page DL, Dupont WD, Rogers LW, Rados MS. Atypical hyperplastic lesions of the female breast: a long term follow-up study. Cancer 1985; 55: 2698–708.

52. Page DL, Rogers LW. Combined histologic and cytologic criteria for the diagnosis of mammary atypical ductal hyperplasia. Hum Pathol 1992; 23: 1095–7.

53. National Coordinating Group for Breast Screening Pathology. Pathology Reporting in Breast Cancer Screening. NHSBSP Publication 3, 2nd edn. Sheffield: NHS Breast Screening Programme, 1997.

54. Rosai J. Borderline epithelial lesions of the breast. Am J Surg Pathol 1991; 15: 209–21.

55. Owings DV, Hann L, Schnitt S. How thoroughly should needle localization breast biopsies be sampled for microscopic examination? Am J Surg Pathol 1990; 14: 578–85.

56. Page DL, Dupont WD. Indicators of increased breast

cancer risk in humans. J Cell Biochem 1992; 16G (Suppl): 175–82.

57. Haagensen CD, Lane N, Lattes R, Bodian C. Lobular neoplasia (so-called lobular carcinoma in situ) of the breast. Cancer 1978; 42: 737–69.

58. Fulford LG, Reis-Filho JS, Lakhani SR. Lobular in situ neoplasia. Curr Diagn Pathol 2004; 10: 183–92.

59. Rosen PP. Lobular carcinoma in situ and atypical lobular hyperplasia: In: Rosen's Breast Pathology. Philadelphia: Lippincott Williams and Williams, 2001: 527–38.

60. Jacobs TW, Conolly JL, Schnitt SJ. Nonmalignant lesions in breast core needle biopsies: to excise or not to excise? Am J Surg Pathol 2002; 26: 1095–110.

61. Foote FW Jr, Stewart FW. Lobular carcinoma in situ. A rare form of mammary cancer. Am J Pathol 1941; 27: 491–5.

62. Page DL, Steel CM, Dixon JM. Carcinoma in situ and patients at high risk of breast cancer. BMJ 1995; 310: 39–42.

63. Page DL, Kidd TE, Dupont WD et al. Lobular neoplasia of the breast: higher risk for subsequent invasive cancer predicted by more extensive disease. Hum Pathol 1991; 22: 1232–9.

64. Broders AC. Carcinoma in situ contrasted with benign penetrating epithelium. JAMA 1932; 99: 1670–4.

65. Rosner D, Bedwani RN, Vana J et al. Non-invasive breast carcinoma Results of a national survey of the American College of Surgeons. Ann Surg 1980; 192: 139–47.

66. Lagios MD, Margolin FR, Westdahl PR, Rose MR. Mammographically detected duct carcinoma in situ. Frequency of local recurrence following tylectomy and prognostic effect of nuclear grade on local recurrence. Cancer 1989; 63: 618–24.

67. Patchefsky AS, Schwartz GF, Finkelstein SD et al. Heterogeneity of intraductal carcinoma of the breast. Cancer 1989; 63: 731–41.

68. Holland R, Pertese JL, Millis RR et al. Ductal carcinoma in situ: a proposal for a new classification. Semin Diagn Pathol 1994; 11: 167–80.

69. Bobrow LG, Happerfield LC, Gregory WM et al. The classification of ductal carcinoma in situ and its association with biological markers. Semin Diagn Pathol 1994; 11: 199–207.

70. Betsill WL Jr, Rosen PP, Lieberman PH, Robbins GF. Intraduct carcinoma. Long term follow-up after treatment by biopsy alone. JAMA 1978; 239: 1863–7.

71. Carter D, Orr SL, Merino MJ. Intracystic papillary carcinoma of the breast: after mastectomy, radiotherapy or excisional biopsy alone. Cancer 1983; 52: 14–19.

72. Page DL, Dupont WD, Rogers LW, Landenberger M. Intraduct carcinoma of the breast: follow-up after biopsy only. Cancer 1982; 49: 751–8.

73. Millis RR, Thynne GSJ. In situ intraduct carcinoma of the breast: a long term follow up study. Br J Surg 1975; 62: 957–62.

74. Price P, Sinnet HD, Gusterton B, Walsh G, A'Hern RP, McKinna JA. Duct carcinoma in situ: predictors of local recurrence and progression in patients treated by surgery alone. Br J Cancer 1990; 61: 869–72.

75. Rosen PP, Senie R, Schottenfeld D, Ashikari R. Noninvasive breast carcinoma. Frequency of unsuspected invasion and implications for treatment. Ann Surg 1979; 189: 377–82.

76. Faverly RG, Burgers L, Bult P, Holland R. Three dimensional imaging of mammary ductal carcinoma in situ: clinical implications. Semin Diagn Pathol 1994; 11: 193–8.

77. Zavotsky F, Hansen N, Brennan MB, Turner RR, Giuliano AE. Lymph node metastasis from ductal carcinoma in situ with micro-invasion. Cancer 1999; 85: 2439–43.

78. Lampejo OT, Barnes DN, Smith P, Millis RR. Evaluation of infiltrating ductal carcinomas with a DCIS component: correlation of histologic type of the in situ component with grade of the infiltrating component. Semin Diagn Pathol 1994; 11: 215–22.

79. Schnitt SJ, Connolly JL, Harris JR et al. Pathologic predictors of early local recurrence in stage I and II breast cancer treated by primary radiation therapy. Cancer 1984; 53: 1049–57.

80. van Dongen JA, Harris JR, Peterse JL et al. In situ breast cancer: the EORTC Consensus Meeting. Lancet 1989; ii: 25–7.

81. Imamate T, Ikawa S, Akiyama T et al. Similarity of protein encoded by the human c-erbB2 gene to epidermal growth factor receptor. Nature 1986; 319: 230–4.

82. Dykins R, Corbett IP, Henry JA et al. Long term survival in breast cancer related to overexpression of c-erbB2 oncoprotein: an immunohistochemical study using monoclonal antibody NCL-CB11. J Pathol 1991; 163: 105–10.

83. Ramachandra S, Machin L, Ashley S et al. Immunohistochemical distribution of c-erbB2 in situ breast carcinoma – a detailed morphological analysis. J Pathol 1990; 161: 7–14.

84. Harris AL. Mutant p53: the commonest genetic abnormality in human cancer? J Pathol 1990; 162: 5–6.

85. Isobe M, Emmanuel BS, Giro D et al. Localization of gene for human p53 tumour antigen to band 17p13. Nature 1986; 320: 84–96.

86. Walker RA, Daring SJ, Lane DT, Valley JM. Expression of p53 in infiltrating and in-situ breast carcinomas. J Pathol 1991; 165: 203–11.

87. Poller DN, Sneak DRJ, Roberts EC et al. Oestrogen receptor expression in ductal carcinoma in situ of the breast: relationship to flow cytometric analysis of DNA and expression of the c-erbB2 oncoprotein. Br J Cancer 1993; 68: 156–61.

88. Zafrani B, Leroyer A, Fourquet A et al. Mammographically-detected ductal in situ carcinoma of the breast analysed with a new classification. A study of 127 cases: correlation with oestrogen and progesterone receptors, p53 and c-erbB2 proteins and proliferation activity. Semin Diagn Pathol 1994; 11: 208–14.

89. Buerger H, Otterbach F, Simon R et al. Comparative genomic hybridisation of ductal carcinoma in-situ of the breast – evidence of multiple genetic pathway. J Pathol 1999; 187: 398–402.

27 Invasive breast carcinoma

Salam Al-Sam, Samar N Jader, John R Benson

Introduction

Histopathologists and cytopathologists hold a key position of responsibility in the multidisciplinary management of breast cancer. They play a crucial role in the assessment of parameters upon which further treatment and prognosis are based. Histological reports are now structured and contain specific items of information, and phrases such as 'Sections of breast tissue show invasive ductal carcinoma' are no longer considered adequate. At present, pathologists follow minimum datasets and protocols and provide detailed information about tumour size and grade together with lymphatic or vascular invasion and the proximity of a tumour to excision margins. Confirmation of malignancy is followed by provision of oestrogen and progesterone receptor status and sometimes expression of HER2/*neu* (c-*erb*B-2). Pathological work-up requires a team approach and familiarity with radiological as well as surgical data and protocols. Ideally, all pathologists should have experience in cytological diagnosis, but this is not always possible and some centres are unable to provide a cytology service of appropriate quality. The mode of presentation of breast cancer to the pathologist has changed in recent years. Increasing numbers of small impalpable lesions are removed and methods of handling surgical specimens must comply with accepted guidelines (e.g. the UK National Health Service Breast Screening Programme (NHSBSP) for screen-detected lesions).[1]

All pathologists providing diagnostic cytopathology and histopathology services, both within a breast screening programme and for symptomatic breast clinics, are expected to participate in appropriate quality control programmes. Quality assurance has been an integral component of the audit and monitoring process that is an essential activity within the NHS and has been a guarantor of its success.[2]

Surgical breast specimens should be dispatched to the pathology laboratory accompanied by relevant clinical and radiological details. In the case of localisation specimens, it is mandatory that the specimen radiograph be sent to the laboratory for radiological–pathological correlation. Furthermore, where microcalcification has been retrieved on core biopsy, radiographs of both core biopsies and original mammograms must be submitted. Copies of formal radiology reports are also helpful for the pathological assessment of these impalpable lesions.

In situ carcinoma may be defined as cancer confined within ducts and lobules (ductal and lobular carcinoma in situ, DCIS and LCIS) without evidence of tumour cells having crossed the basement membrane.[3] The earliest form of invasive breast cancer is microinvasive carcinoma, which was a rarity in the past.[3] With increased detection of DCIS within the screening programme, the incidence of this form of invasive carcinoma is rising.[4] This chapter will focus on overtly invasive forms of cancer, but a short account of microinvasive carcinoma is included.

Fine-needle aspiration cytology (FNAC)

In our experience, fine-needle aspiration cytology (FNAC) remains an important investigative procedure and constitutes the first line of preoperative diagnostic work-up. It should be emphasised that the sensitivity of FNAC for detection of cancer is slightly higher than that of core biopsy in our unit. Combined FNAC and core biopsy yields a sensitivity of 92% for DCIS based on 12 years' experience within the Chelmsford Breast Screening Service. Optimum results for FNAC are obtained from the use of three stains: Giemsa, Papanicolaou (Pap), and haematoxylin and eosin (H&E).

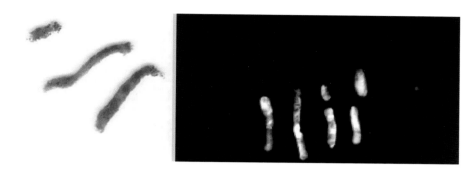

Figure 27.1   Core biopsy. Six levels are cut and determinations of oestrogen and progesterone receptor status are performed in cancer cases. Radiography is necessary in cases of microcalcification.

The success of FNAC as a diagnostic tool is dependent on the availability of a cytopathologist with expertise in the field of breast cancer.[5] The technique of FNAC is being superseded in many breast units by image-guided core biopsy.[6,7]

Core biopsies/Tru-cut biopsies

Increasing numbers of core biopsies are being performed as a means of providing tissue diagnosis before commencement of definitive treatment, whether this be surgical or some other modality of primary therapy. In some centres, core biopsy techniques have completely replaced FNAC, with the consequence that tissue evaluation during one-stop clinics is no longer possible. Core biopsies may be used for cancer patients opting for chemotherapy before surgery. Tissue samples obtained by core or Tru-cut biopsies are used to provide histological diagnosis and determination of hormonal status (Figure 27.1).

Macroscopic examination

Core biopsies/Tru-cut biopsies

Pathologists should record the number of cores submitted and provide an estimate of the total length of all cores. When the procedure is performed for microcalcification, the radiologist must submit radiographs of the cores together with a copy of the current mammogram. A comment about these films should be included in the pathology report. The macroscopic description should include details such as the colour of the cores (e.g. yellow (fat) or white (breast parenchyma)) and whether they were floating or sank to the bottom of the specimen pot. Yellow cores floating on the surface are usually composed predominantly of fat. Contact cytology from core biopsies can be a useful technique for immediate cytological assessment and verification of adequacy of the specimen.

Table 27.1	**NHS Breast Screening Programme reporting categories**[2]
B1	Normal breast tissue/or sample not representative
B2	Benign breast lesion
B3	Lesion of uncertain malignant potential. This includes atypical ductal hyperplasia, atypical lobular hyperplasia, phylloides tumour, papillary lesions, radial scar and complex sclerosing lesion
B4	Suspicious of malignancy. This includes crushed or poorly fixed cores that contain probable carcinoma but cannot provide the definitive diagnosis, neoplastic cells within blood clot outside the tissue of the core biopsy, and tiny areas of carcinoma that disappear on deeper levels for immunohistochemistry
B5	Malignant B5a Ductal carcinoma in situ (DCIS) B5b Invasive carcinoma B5c Carcinoma with no further assessment possible

The NHSBSP recommends the use of a reporting protocol with categories B1–B5 (Table 27.1).[2]

Lumpectomy and localisation specimens (Figures 27.2 and 27.3)

Details of weight, size (three-dimensional measurements) and any accompanying specimen X-ray are essential items of information that should be recorded in the macroscopic examination (Figure 27.4). In addition, the presence or absence of markers for orientating the specimen should be noted and documented in the macroscopic description. A useful method for orientation is to employ sutures to which radiopaque ligaclips are applied (Figures 27.5 and 27.6). It is conventional to place two sutures superiorly and one laterally (Figure 27.7). Details of practice vary from centre to centre, but should be consistent within a particular institu-

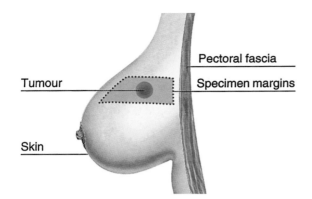

Figure 27.2 Schematic lateral view of the breast to show surgical excision margins in a segmental excision specimen. Breast tissue between the skin and the pectoral fascia is included.

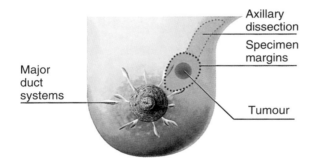

Figure 27.3 Schematic anteroposterior view of the breast to show excision margins of the upper quadrant. The nipple margin and other excision margins must be labelled by the surgeon to help the pathologist orientate the specimen.

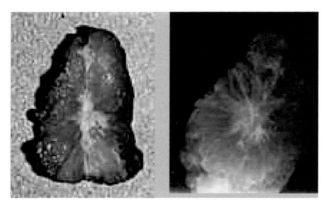

Figure 27.4 Screen-detected breast cancer: a stellate lesion with identical appearances to those seen on X-ray.

tion. Some surgeons prefer to attach the specimen to a piece of card immersed in formalin. The margins can be identified by placing V- and U-shaped cuts on the sides of the card itself. It is not advisable to

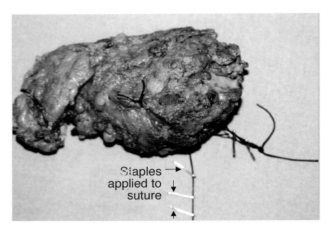

Figure 27.5 Metal staples are applied to sutures to visualise margins on X-ray films. We prefer this method, as staples applied directly to breast tissue cause difficulty in cutting specimens without disturbing margins.

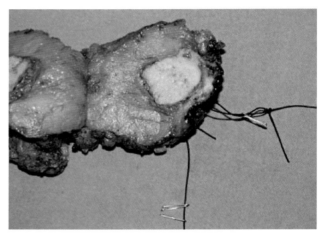

Figure 27.6 Application of sutures and staples to resection margins. Staples will aid in visualising margins on X-ray films.

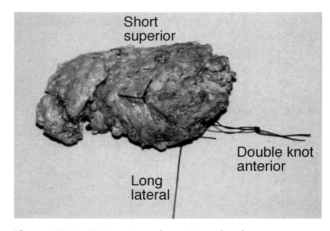

Figure 27.7 Orientation of specimen by the surgeon – three sutures: short, long and double knot.

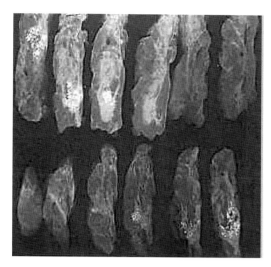

Figure 27.8 Thin slicing of the specimen and a repeat X-ray reveal important information and allow proper sampling of suspicious areas.

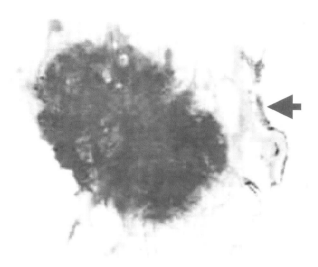

Figure 27.9 Painted margin of excision.

apply clips directly to the breast tissue for orientation, as this can present problems with processing of the specimen – the pathologist needs to ink the resection margins and may take a shave from the edge. Furthermore, when sutures are used, ligaclips should not be applied too far away from the proximal ends in order to avoid confusion when orientating the specimen for X-ray. Two films at 90° may facilitate interpretation of microcalcification in relation to DCIS and permit cutting of the specimen in the most appropriate way. Moreover, they can assist with assessing the nearest margin of excision. Labelling of the nipple margin is encouraged for all cases of suspected or confirmed DCIS and invasive carcinoma, and we prefer to take a shave sample from resection margins to assess completeness of excision. The distance of the tumour from the resection margins can still be accurately recorded even when a shave sample is taken (see Chapter 34). The overall weight of the specimen must include cavity shaves taken at the time of initial surgery but submitted in separate pots. Increasing numbers of smaller breast cancers (<5 mm) are being detected by screening mammography and can be difficult for the pathologist to identify if they are not well-defined lesions and have dense surrounding fibrous stroma. Examination of cut sections using a magnifying glass may prove useful. Specimen radiology following slicing of the tissue can also aid localisation (Figure 27.8).[8,9]

Resection margin specimens

These may be either substantial pieces of tissue or small bed biopsies. In the case of a large cavity

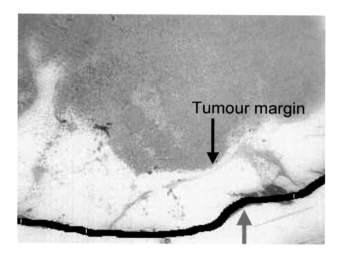

Figure 27.10 Painted margin of excision: red arrow.

shaving, it is important that the new outer excision margin be marked so that pathologists can orientate the specimen and assess this new margin for any additional in situ or invasive carcinoma (Figures 27.9 and 27.10).

Mastectomy

Mastectomy specimens should be labelled and sent to pathologists according to local protocols (Figure 27.11). A single suture laterally should suffice for orientating any mastectomy specimen (provided that the side is indicated). Pathologists must attend to these specimens immediately upon their arrival in the pathology department in order to ensure that

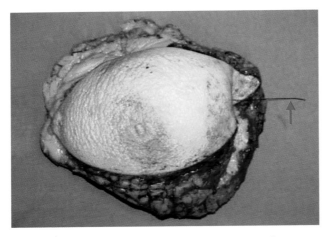

Figure 27.11 Mastectomy with long suture on the lateral aspect (arrow).

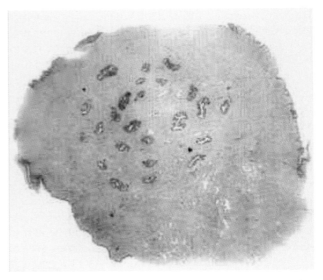

Figure 27.12 Cross-section of lactiferous ducts beneath the nipple surface, allowing assessment of all ducts in a single section. Scanning power.

tumour fixation is optimal. If the preferred method is formalin fixation then description and slicing of the specimen should be done shortly after resection, and further fixation can be undertaken subsequently.

Two methods of slicing mastectomy specimens are practised:

- *With the deep aspect of the mastectomy specimen facing the pathologist.* The specimen is sliced perpendicular to the cutting board from the posterior aspect towards the skin.
- *With the mastectomy placed with its deep aspect on the cutting board and the nipple facing the pathologist.* The breast tissue is then sliced in a plane parallel to the cutting board, which involves sectioning anatomically perpendicular to the lactiferous ducts. This allows better correlation of tumour location with the breast quadrants and the ductal system. The nipple is also cut across, with all lactiferous ducts visualised in a single section (Figures 27.12 and 27.13). The nipple surface is then processed as for any skin biopsy, with the whole tissue being embedded.

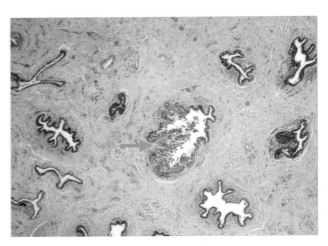

Figure 27.13 Cross-section of lactiferous ducts beneath the nipple surface. Low power. One duct shows regular epithelial hyperplasia.

Axillary clearance

It is sensible to place a ligature at the apical end of the axillary specimen to permit correct orientation by the pathologist. The yield of lymph nodes varies from approximately 10 to 30, and all nodes identified must be sampled. Each lymph node is bisected, and one section is taken from each en face cut surface and embedded. Even when the apical region is marked, the apical node may not be clear to the pathologist. It is preferable for the surgeon to dissect

the apical node and place it in a separate container. The final pathology report should state the total number of nodes in the axillary dissection and the absolute number containing metastases.

Sentinel lymph node biopsy

Pathologists must accurately number tissue blocks and indicate which of these samples contains the sentinel lymph node, as blue dye is not apparent histologically. All non-sentinel lymph nodes should be processed for histological examination. The two halves of each lymph node should be embedded, and immunohistochemistry for epithelial markers may increase the likelihood of detecting micrometastatic disease.[10] Not all units routinely undertake immunohistochemical analysis of lymph nodes, although this is often done on the sentinel node for research purposes.

It is essential that the sentinel node be assessed accurately in order to minimise false-negative rates for the technique of sentinel node biopsy. The sentinel node is scrutinised more thoroughly than any individual node in a specimen from a conventional axillary dissection. In particular, the sentinel node is subjected to serial step sectioning, sliced at a thickness of 3 mm or less perpendicular to the long axis of the lymph node. Intraoperative assessment can be undertaken either with frozen section or with touch imprint cytology. The latter method avoids the sacrifice of previous tissue and yields rapid and reliable results. Immunohistochemical techniques with staining for cytokeratins together with molecular biological techniques (polymerase chain reaction, PCR) has permitted the detection of tumour cell clusters and even isolated tumour cells in addition to micrometastases. Indeed, these ultra-sensitive techniques have prompted a redefinition of the term 'micrometastases' – this now encompasses foci measuring between 0.2 and 2 mm in diameter.[10] The clinical significance of micrometastases is uncertain, and that of submicrometastases even more so (the latter are isolated tumour cells and clusters <0.2 mm).[11,12]

Immunohistochemistry is not used for routine examination of sentinel nodes, and pathologists should report only on the presence of micrometastases detected by H&E staining. When immunohistochemistry is used for research purposes, the number of tumour cells should be quantified (≤10 cells, 11–100 cells or >100 cells).[13]

Histological types of breast carcinoma

Microinvasive carcinoma

Microinvasion represents the earliest stages of invasive breast carcinoma, and is often noted as an incidental finding during examination of biopsies for suspicious areas of microcalcification.[14,15]

Definition

Microscopic foci of malignant cells invade beyond the ductal or lobular basement membrane, and do not exceed 1 mm in size. A new TNM category,

T1*mic*, was introduced by the Union Internationale Contre le Cancer (UICC, International Union Against Cancer) in 1996 and was defined as microinvasion 1 mm or less in greatest diameter. Recent studies have attempted to correlate the clinicopathological profile of T1*mic* tumours that adhere strictly to this criterion with the use of an ocular micrometer to measure the size of individual foci and a sensitive double-immunoenzyme labelling technique to further evaluate equivocal foci of invasion. One or more foci less than 1 mm in diameter are accepted as microinvasive breast carcinoma.

Macroscopic features

This type of breast cancer has no macroscopic correlate, and the features seen on microscopic examination are those associated with either DCIS or LCIS (usually the former).

Microscopic appearances

Early invasion of a group of malignant cells beyond the boundaries of the basement membrane is seen in typically one to three foci, each measuring up to 1 mm. Microinvasion is more frequently associated with high-nuclear-grade DCIS than with low-grade types.[16]

Prognosis

The prognosis for microinvasion is difficult to predict due to inter-observer variation in reporting this condition. In a review by Padmore et al,[16] only 1 out of a total of 59 patients developed local recurrence after breast conservation surgery and no patients had involvement of axillary lymph nodes with metastases. By contrast, Schuh et al[17] reported a 20% incidence of metastatic spread to axillary lymph nodes for DCIS with microinvasive carcinoma.

Invasive ductal carcinoma of no special type (NST)

Definition

This is the most common type of infiltrating ductal carcinoma of the breast and no specific histological features are apparent. Hence it is often designated as NOS ('not otherwise specified').[18] Although the term 'no special type' (NST) has become popular to distinguish this type of invasive ductal carcinoma from the special types, approximately 70% of invasive breast cancers fall into this category, which is therefore a diagnosis by exclusion.[19] This includes lesions characterised as ductal carcinoma with productive fibrosis (previously termed scirrhous carcinoma). These tumours typically feel hard to palpation due to extensive fibrosis.

Macroscopic features

These tumours can assume various shapes, but macroscopically are mainly stellate, rounded or lobulated masses. Approximately one-third have well-circumscribed margins, while a minority have rather indistinct margins – which can pose difficulties when assessing the relationship of tumour to resection margins. It is useful for pathologists to draw a diagram of the specimen and identify sites from where tissue blocks have been taken, especially those representing resection margins.

Symptomatic invasive ductal carcinomas are usually visible to the naked eye. There is often a gritty sensation when cutting through the tumour – which has been likened to an unripe pear. The cut surface is usually solid with well-defined margins. Smaller screen-detected lesions are usually visible within the specimen, but the surgeon should send the specimen X-ray with these smaller lesions and all localisation specimens to aid identification of the exact location and to assess the resection margins. Well-circumscribed lesions are often considered to have a better prognosis. Some tumours are soft and round with a sharp outline, and can mimic benign lesions (e.g. cysts) clinically and radiologically. However, these features are more likely to be associated with a mucinous carcinoma, which is one of the special types. A significant number of invasive ductal carcinomas have calcification, which may be noted in both the specimen X-ray and histological sections. Notwithstanding these comments, small tumours found in the screened population are usually relatively easy to find in the excised specimen.

Microscopic features

The epithelial component of these tumours grows in cords, groups and tubules, with a mixture often prevailing (Figures 27.14–27.16). The central region is fibrous and the peripheral zones are more cellular.[20] Groups of malignant cells are apparent, growing in cords, nests and irregular groups of cells more than one layer thick. Formation of tubules is seen, but these differ from those seen in tubular carcinoma. Nuclear appearances vary according to the grade of the tumour. Nuclei of high-grade tumours are usually irregular in outline and vesicular in appearance, with one or more nucleoli, and

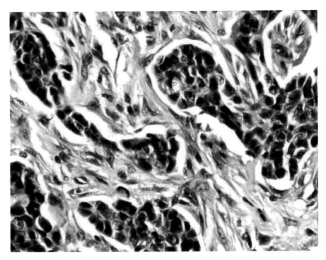

Figure 27.14   Invasive ductal carcinoma NST. (H&E, ×400.)

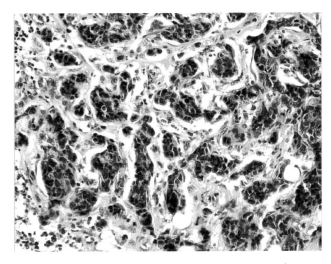

Figure 27.15   Invasive ductal carcinoma NST grade III. (H&E, ×200.)

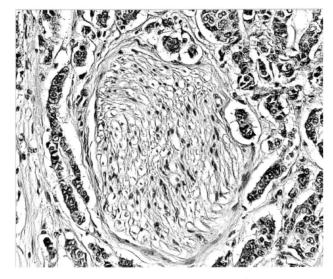

Figure 27.16   Perineural invasion of ductal carcinoma NST. (H&E, ×200.)

mitoses are frequent in higher-grade lesions. When the lesion is mounted in entirety, the characteristic fibrous stroma is often readily apparent in the centre of the tumour, with more cellular elements at the periphery, where lymphatic invasion is best demonstrated. The term 'scirrhous' carcinoma was previously applied to this type of tumour because of the densely fibrous stroma.[21] Some tumours exhibit a more anaplastic appearance, with marked cellular pleomorphism and occasionally giant cell formation.

Calcification may be present within either invasive or in situ components (or both). Up to 40% of cases of microcalcification are associated with DCIS. The grade of DCIS is almost always related to the grade of the invasive tumour. The DCIS may extend beyond the limits of the invasive component, and an aggregate measurement of both the invasive lesion and DCIS should be recorded as part of the minimum data set for pathology reporting.

Necrosis is often associated with high-grade cancers, and most lesions contain mucin-producing cells with a fibrous stroma consisting of abundant amounts of type V collagen. This contrasts with the stroma of normal breast and benign lesions. Stromal elastosis is present in more than 90% of scirrhous carcinomas, but is not as prominent as in lobular carcinoma. Elastosis is seen predominantly around vessels and ducts, but may be present more diffusely throughout the lesion.

Immunohistochemistry

Determination of oestrogen and progesterone receptor (ER and PgR) status is now mandatory before management decisions on adjuvant systemic therapy can be made in the setting of a multidisciplinary meeting attended by surgeons and oncologists (Figure 27.17).[22] Two scoring systems are available (H-score and quick score), with most departments using the quick score assessment in accordance with published NHSBSP guidelines for pathologists.[4] Most invasive ductal carcinomas NST are positive for epithelial membrane antigen (EMA) and cytokeratin, while carcinoembryonic antigen (CEA) is expressed less consistently. These tumours also stain positive for E-cadherin, pankeratin, transforming growth factor α (TGF-α), B-catenin and usually CK07.

Grade

Histological grading takes account of both the growth pattern of invasive ductal carcinomas and the cytological features of differentiation. Three parameters are assessed:

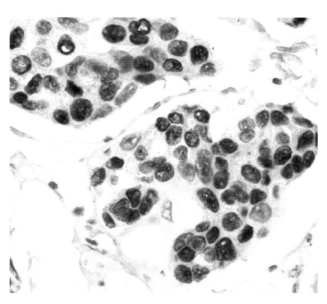

Figure 27.17 Progesterone receptor-positive invasive ductal carcinoma. (×200.)

- the extent of tubule formation
- the degree of nuclear pleomorphism
- the number of mitoses

Histological grading correlates with prognosis in breast cancer, which was first documented in a seminal paper published in 1957 by Bloom and Richardson.[23]

Prognosis

Prognosis is directly related not only to histological grade but also to tumour size and status of axillary lymph nodes. Local recurrence rates for invasive ductal carcinoma are generally lower than for invasive lobular carcinoma; this may be attributable to a higher incidence of multifocality in lobular carcinoma. Invasive ductal carcinoma NST overall has a worse prognosis than special-type carcinomas or invasive lobular carcinoma. Nodal status is the single most important determinant of prognosis, with 5-year actuarial survival rates of 100% and 77% for node-negative and node-positive patients respectively.[24] Hormone receptor status and HER2/neu expression are predictive factors and determine whether a tumour will respond to hormonal treatment or chemotherapy.[25–27]

Tubular carcinoma

Incidence and clinical features

Tubular carcinoma represents a particularly well-differentiated form of infiltrating ductal carcinoma,

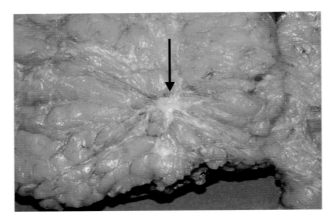

Figure 27.18 Tubular carcinoma showing a stellate lesion with a depressed cut surface.

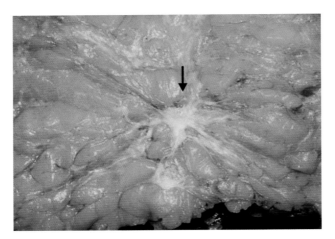

Figure 27.19 Tubular carcinoma.

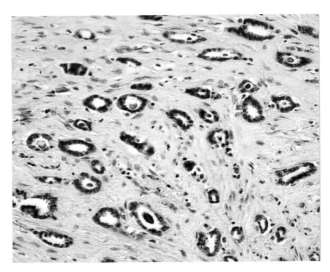

Figure 27.20 Tubular carcinoma. (H&E, ×100.)

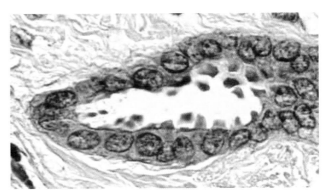

Figure 27.21 Tubular carcinoma. (H&E, ×400.)

usually measuring less than 2 cm in maximum dimension.[28] Tumour cells are typically arranged into regular or sometimes angulated tubular structures surrounded by desmoplastic stroma and elastosis. These may have a rather disorganised appearance, and tubular carcinomas may be found in association with areas of DCIS or atypical ductal hyperplasia (ADH). The incidence of this tumour type used to be low, but has increased significantly with the advent of the NHSBSP, in which up to 9% of tumours detected are tubular carcinomas. This term is applied to those tumours in which tubule formation is seen in 90% or more of their surface area, although in the past it was applied to tumours that were only 75% tubular. This new definition allows a better correlation of pure tubular lesions with behaviour, grade and prognosis. The reported frequency of contralateral carcinoma varies from 0% to 38%,[20,29] while the incidence of bilateral pure tubular carcinoma is rare. Tubular carcinomas are common in the first (prevalent) round of screening programmes, and this may reflect length bias, with slower-growing tumours existing for a longer time in the preclinical phase (see Chapter 5). Patients with pure tubular carcinoma tend to be younger than those with mixed ductal and tubular types, but otherwise no consistent clinical differences have been reported.

Macroscopic features

In the majority of cases, the lesion is a spiculate mass with or without calcification and measures 1 cm or less. It is uncommon for tumours fulfilling the criteria for this tumour type to exceed 2 cm, although tubular carcinomas of up to 4 cm in diameter have been reported. These tumours are ill-defined stellate lesions that are either firm or hard and usually retract on sectioning, leaving a slightly depressed cut surface (Figures 27.18 and 27.19).

Microscopic features

These tumours are principally composed of small tubules and glands haphazardly distributed within fibrous stroma (Figure 27.20). The tubules are lined by a single layer of neoplastic epithelium, which characteristically exhibits apical 'snouts' on the luminal side (Figure 27.21). The tubules are oval or angular in shape; this feature differentiates them from the benign condition of microglandular adenosis, which is similar in appearance. Tubular carcinoma does not have a lobulocentric configuration and the tubules are usually small with little branching or anastomosis. The glandular lumina are patent and mitoses infrequent, but microcalcification can be extensive. Tubular carcinoma may form part of a mixed tumour of ductal or lobular origin. Those lesions with more than 10% constituted of other tumour types should be classified as mixed tumours. Elastosis can be abundant, and may be associated with an adjacent intraductal component (DCIS). Mucin vacuoles may be seen in tubular carcinoma, and can result in diagnostic confusion with lobular carcinoma when FNAC is used for tissue biopsy.[30] Benign lesions that may have been mistaken for tubular carcinoma include the following:

- microglandular adenosis
- radial scar
- sclerosing adenosis

Tubular carcinoma infiltrates locally without any lobular pattern, and glandular structures are lined by a single layer of tumour cells, which are invariably EMA-positive. Examination under low-power magnification helps to differentiate this lesion from sclerosing adenosis.

Histochemistry and immunohistochemistry

Tubular carcinomas lack any basement membrane, which can be demonstrated in sclerosing adenosis and other benign lesions of similar morphology.[31] Tissue components such as laminin, type IV collagen and basement membrane proteoglycan are not detected in tubular carcinoma. Myoepithelial cells are highlighted by staining for actin and S-100 and are distributed around acini and tubules of benign lesions, but do not occur in association with tubules of breast cancer. Hormone receptors (ER and PgR) are strongly positive in most tubular carcinomas.[22] Positive staining for EMA in tubular carcinoma contrasts with its absent expression in microglandular adenosis.

Prognosis

Taking the term tubular carcinoma to be stringently applied only to tumours composed almost entirely of classical tubules, prognosis is very favourable when compared with other types of breast tumours. These pure forms of tubular carcinoma are low-grade tumours with minimal metastatic potential, and survival is largely independent of tumour size.[32] The incidence of axillary nodal metastases is about 10% for pure tubular carcinomas, but occurs in 30% of tubulolobular carcinomas.[33] This highlights the importance of distinguishing between these two types of lesion by the use of strict diagnostic criteria. Patients with unifocal pure tubular carcinomas are usually candidates for breast conservation therapy, and postoperative radiotherapy may be omitted for small tubular carcinomas excised with adequate surgical clearance, particularly in the older age group (aged over 55). Multifocal disease is often associated with extensive DCIS, which precludes breast conservation therapy. The absolute benefits of systemic adjuvant therapy are relatively small for pure tubular carcinomas less than 3 cm in diameter because of their good prognosis. The mixed form of tubular carcinoma is prognostically similar to infiltrating ductal carcinoma when matched for degree of differentiation and tumour size.

Infiltrating lobular carcinoma

Incidence and clinical features

Infiltrating lobular carcinoma is the second most frequent type of invasive breast carcinoma after the ductal type (NST), and comprises 2–15% of all invasive breast cancers.[34,35] This variation in reported incidence may be related in part to lack of concordance between diagnostic criteria, but demographic and racial differences may also be important. This tumour type may be more frequent in the UK than in the USA, and is commoner among Blacks than Caucasians. A higher incidence in later life may be related to increased detection rates in prevalent screening rounds and use of E-cadherin assays. In the past, many E-cadherin-negative tumours were erroneously labelled as invasive ductal carcinoma.[36,37] The term lobular carcinoma was introduced in 1941 in a publication by Foote and Stewart.[38] These tumours are bilateral in 30% of cases and frequently multicentric, with a tendency to metastasize to serous cavities more frequently than other breast carcinomas.[39] Increasing numbers of lobular tumours are being detected by breast screening programmes and incidence figures of up to 14% have been quoted by various investigators compared with figures of 4–5% in the past. The median age at diagnosis is between 45 and 56. Screen-detected infiltrating lobular carcinomas often present as areas of architectural distortion and symptomatic lesions as palpable masses with ill-defined margins. Many of these tumours are mammographically occult and cytological samples yield a paucity of cellular material. Magnetic

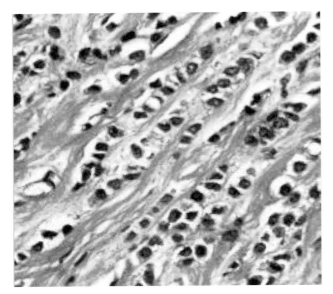

Figure 27.22   Infiltrating lobular carcinoma, classical type. (H&E, ×400.)

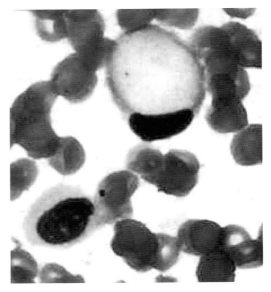

Figure 27.23   Lobular carcinoma: FNAC. (Giemsa, ×400.)

resonance imaging (MRI) is better at assessing the extent and size of these lesions than mammography. The occurrence of a satellite lesion adjacent to the main tumour is more common than for invasive ductal carcinoma NST, and this partly accounts for the higher rate of positive resection margins after breast conservation surgery for lobular carcinoma.

Macroscopic features

Infiltrating lobular carcinomas range from occult, grossly inapparent lesions of microscopic dimensions to tumours with diffuse involvement of the entire breast.[40] Typically, infiltrating lobular carcinoma is a firm to hard tumour with irregular borders, which may not be visible but may be appreciated by palpation as a firm or hard area. Lobular carcinoma is associated with extensive stromal fibrosis, which imparts to the tumour its hardness on palpation and an irregular soft tissue opacity on mammography. In a significant proportion of cases, there is diffuse infiltration among normal breast structures, which can make gross assessment of resection margins difficult. For similar reasons surgical excision of these tumours may be inadequate, with invasive lobular tumour remaining at the excision margins. There may be significant disparity between macroscopic and microscopic measurements of the lesion. The excised breast specimen may appear unremarkable except for slight firmness on palpation.

Microscopic features

Lobular carcinoma has distinct cytological features and patterns of infiltration. Six different subtypes are recognised:

- mixed
- classical
- tubulolobular
- solid
- alveolar
- pleomorphic.

Apart from the pleomorphic variant, these tumours are composed of small round uniform cells that are cytologically indistinguishable from those seen in lobular carcinoma in situ (Figure 27.22). The cells have characteristic appearances on FNAC (Figure 27.23).[41] A single cytoplasmic vacuole causing nuclear indentation is characteristic, and this feature may be seen on FNAC preparations from tubular carcinoma. Cells tend to have a relatively small nuclear volume.

The relative incidence of the different subtypes varies between series, but the following figures are representative:[42]

- mixed   40.0%
- classical   30.4%
- tubulolobular   13.5%
- solid   6.4%
- alveolar   4.1%
- pleomorphic   3.6%

Distinction between these subtypes is important, as the tubulolobular type has a particularly favourable prognosis while the solid and pleomorphic types have a worse prognosis.[43,44] The cellular features in the pleomorphic type are characteristic, with large cells and nuclei that are more hyperchromatic and irregular (Figure 27.24). All histological types of

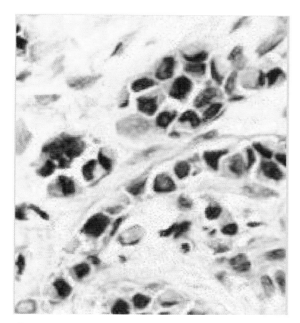

Figure 27.24   Pleomorphic variant. (H&E, ×400.)

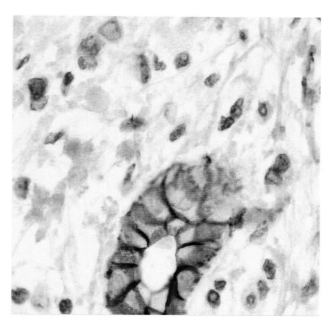

Figure 27.25   Duct-positive, lobe-negative E-cadherin negative mixed ductal–lobular carcinoma. (×400.)

lobular carcinoma are negative for E-cadherin, which is a useful marker to distinguish between lobular and ductal carcinomas.[36,37] In situ and infiltrating lobular carcinoma sometimes coexist, particularly with the classical forms of infiltrating lobular carcinoma. The classical type of infiltrating lobular carcinoma is characterised by a linear growth pattern (Indian file arrangement) with loss of cohesion between cells.[34] Moulding of nuclei is apparent, and often these show a characteristic targetoid pattern around ducts and vessels. A single cytoplasmic vacuole is often present, which tends to push the nucleus to one side, resulting in a kidney-shaped appearance (Figure 27.23).

Tumour cells spread around the periductal fibrous tissue in a concentric fashion, yielding a characteristic pattern. Individual cells have small to medium-sized nuclei that are either uniformly round or oval in outline. There is a paucity of cytoplasm, inconspicuous nucleoli and infrequent mitotic figures. In the solid type of infiltrating lobular carcinoma the tumour cells are distributed in diffuse sheets with little intervening stroma and can simulate malignant lymphoma or leukaemic infiltration in appearance. In the alveolar variant, loosely cohesive tumour cells form discrete aggregates and are surrounded by a thin fibrous stroma.

The pleomorphic variant is composed of cells with medium to large nuclei that are irregular and hyperchromatic and have an eosinophilic cytoplasm simulating rhabdomyoblasts (Figure 27.24). It is believed that pleomorphic lobular carcinoma

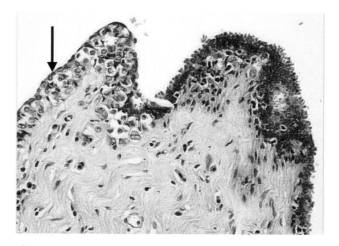

Figure 27.26   Pagetoid spread of infiltrating lobular carcinoma within a duct.

exhibits apocrine differentiation, which may be responsible for the more aggressive phenotype. In some cases, cells may show a histiocytoid appearance, which can be mistaken for invasive ductal carcinoma. Lobular carcinoma may also display a trabecular pattern, and negative staining for E-cadherin helps differentiate this type from invasive ductal carcinoma (Figure 27.25). A lymphocytic reaction may be seen with infiltrating lobular carcinoma, and Pagetoid spread can occur along major lactiferous ducts with lobular carcinoma cells infiltrating deep to the duct lining (Figures 27.26 and 27.27). Abundance of mucin secretion within lobular carcinoma cells may give rise to an appear-

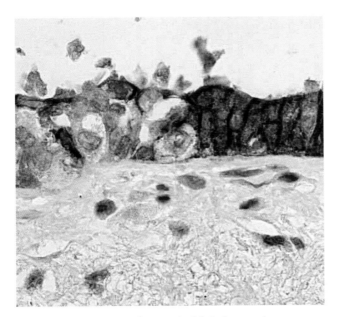

Figure 27.27 Pagetoid spread of lobular carcinoma within duct lining. (E-cadherin, ×400.)

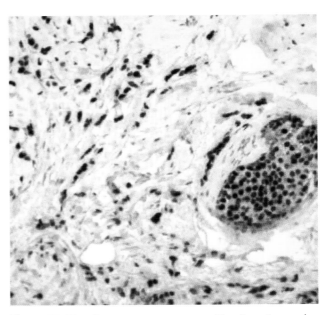

Figure 27.28 Oestrogen receptor-positive invasive and in situ lobular carcinoma.

ance that has recently been reported as signet ring breast carcinoma. This is considered to be a further variant of lobular carcinoma.[45]

Histochemistry

Alcian blue aids identification of the single mucin vacuole within the cytoplasm of lobular carcinoma cells. Grimelius-positive cells may occur in a minority of tumours.

Immunohistochemistry

Staining for ER and PgR is strongly positive in the majority of invasive lobular carcinomas (Figure 27.28). The tumours are negative for E-cadherin and positive for CEA, while chromogranin has been detected in the classical type and the pleomorphic variant of infiltrating lobular carcinomas. The HER2/*neu* gene product is rarely expressed in classical in situ or invasive lobular carcinomas.[46]

Prognosis

Patients with classical-type infiltrating lobular carcinomas have a better prognosis than those with the variant types.[29,44,47] Optimal outcomes are observed in patients with tubulolobular carcinoma.[43] There is a general consensus that the pleomorphic type is more aggressive and has a worse prognosis than other types of lobular carcinoma. The frequency of

ipsilateral breast tumour recurrence is higher for invasive lobular than ductal carcinoma. Incomplete excision due to poorly defined macroscopic margins coupled with the presence of satellite lesions may account for differences in rates of recurrence, but the lobular phenotype per se is not a contraindication to breast conservation. Lobular carcinoma overall (as a group) has a better prognosis (70–80% 5-year survival rate) than ductal carcinoma when matched for disease stage and patient age,[29] with the most important determinants of prognosis being primary tumour size and nodal status.

Mucinous carcinoma

Incidence and clinical features

Mucinous carcinoma encompasses a group of tumours variously termed colloid, mucoid or gelatinous carcinoma.[28,47–51] These tumours represent less than 5% of all breast cancers and have a wide age distribution. They can be mistaken clinically for a benign lesion on account of their smooth outline and soft consistency (due to extracellular mucin). These lesions are often categorised as R3 U3 on imaging and yield a C5 diagnosis on FNAC.[52] A significant number of women with mucinous carcinomas are aged over 50, and these tumours may be associated with microcalcification. The classical mammographic appearances are those of a rounded or lobulated breast lesion, which may have a low index of radiological suspicion.[51]

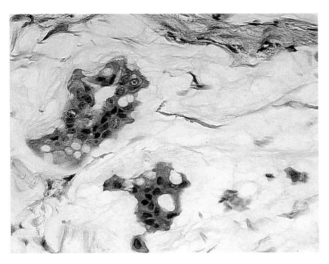

Figure 27.29   Mucinous carcinoma. (H&E, ×200.)

Macroscopic features

This tumour has characteristic gross features that serve to distinguish it from other types. It is well circumscribed but not encapsulated and abuts against adjacent normal breast tissue. The cut surface is a pale grey colour with a gelatinous consistency that imparts to the tumour a soft texture.[53] Size ranges from 1 cm to 20 cm, but the majority of excised lesions measure between 2 cm and 4 cm.

Microscopic features

Histologically, these tumours contain lakes of mucin within which nests, cords and even isolated malignant epithelial cells are seen (Figure 27.29).[43,50] The appearance of cells on FNAC preparations is similar to that in histological sections and the mucous component is readily discernible after Giemsa or Diff Quick staining.[52] The fibrous stroma constitutes a small proportion of the tumour and usually contains no or minimal elastin or lymphoid tissue. There is generally little variation in size of individual tumour cells and necrosis is not a feature.[53] DCIS may be seen in the peritumoral zone in 60–75% of lesions, and this should be carefully looked for in adjacent breast tissue. A fibroadenoma with a mucoid stroma and mucocoele-like lesions are two benign breast entities that can mimic mucinous carcinoma morphologically.

Histochemistry and immunohistochemistry

The mucin is a mixture of neutral and non-sulfated sialidase-susceptible acid type. Intracellular mucin is present in mucinous carcinoma but is absent from mucocoele-like lesions.[54]

Argyrophilic Grimelius-positive granules are detected in 25–50% of cases and at the subcellular level appear to be related to endocrine secretory granules.[55,56]

Prognosis

Mucinous carcinoma is one of the 'special types' of breast cancer and has a better prognosis than invasive ductal carcinoma NST or lobular carcinoma. The majority of these tumours do not have axillary nodal involvement, with quoted negativity rates of 70–97%.[57] The presence of microcalcification is associated with improved prognosis, and overall rates of disease-free survival at 10 years range from 85% to 87% following mastectomy. Interestingly, late distant recurrences have been reported following primary treatment with mastectomy.[57]

Papillary carcinoma

Incidence and clinical presentation

This is an uncommon type of breast carcinoma, representing only 1–2% of all invasive tumours.[58] It is important to distinguish between invasive and intracystic papillary carcinomas because of differences in their prognoses. Furthermore, there is a particular difficulty in distinguishing between benign and malignant papillary lesions on FNAC due to significant overlap in cytological features.[59,60] Papillary carcinoma occurs in an older age group compared with other types of breast carcinomas, with a median age ranging from 63 to 67 years.[61] Half of these lesions arise in the central portion of the breast and are commonly associated with nipple discharge.

Macroscopic features

The appearance of papillary tumours is variable and depends principally on the relative size of the solid and cystic components. These tumours are usually well circumscribed and may appear encapsulated. Spontaneous haemorrhage can produce bloodstaining of the tumour, and this can also be secondary to haemorrhage following FNAC or core biopsy prior to surgery.

Microscopic features

Papillary structures are readily visible microscopically in both invasive and intracystic papillary carci-

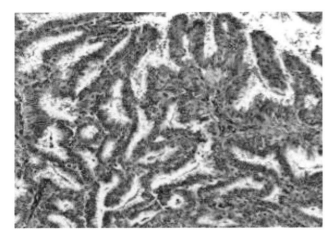

Figure 27.30 Papillary carcinoma. (H&E, ×100.)

nomas. However, a papillary pattern is less evident when cellular proliferation becomes solid and the papillary cores less conspicuous (Figure 27.30). A branching network of fibrovascular cores can be demonstrated by a combination of histochemical stains for collagen and immunohistochemical markers for endothelial cells.[62]

The tumour closely resembles papillary and cribriform DCIS. Complex papillary projections and cribriform glands consist almost entirely of epithelial cells without evidence of myoepithelial cells, and fibrovascular stalks are less prominent than those seen in a benign intraductal papilloma. The borders of the lesion are generally irregular and infiltrative.[60]

The presence of foci of papillary DCIS at the periphery of tumours can be helpful in corroborating the diagnosis of papillary carcinoma. Differentiation between papilloma and papillary carcinoma relies on careful examination of cellular morphology and demonstration of the absence of a myoepithelial component in carcinoma by immunohistochemical staining for smooth muscle actin and S-100.[62] The epithelial elements in a papilloma are arranged in an orderly fashion and mitoses are rare.

The diagnosis of an intraductal papillary carcinoma arising from a papilloma can be a challenge to the pathologist. These lesions retain areas of papilloma that appear benign or atypical, but in addition there are foci of more active cellular proliferation that support a diagnosis of carcinoma.

Histochemistry and immunohistochemistry

The cells in a minority of papillary carcinomas contain Grimelius-positive and chromogranin-positive cytoplasmic granules.

Prognosis

Intracystic papillary carcinoma is best considered as a variant form of DCIS that carries a relatively good prognosis compared with invasive carcinoma.

The frequency of axillary lymph node metastases in invasive papillary carcinoma is determined by the size of the invasive component and nuclear grade. Metastatic foci within lymph nodes tend to appear as papillary structures resembling the primary lesion.

These papillary lesions have an excellent prognosis, with a low incidence of lymph node involvement. Rates of local recurrence are very low provided that the tumour is completely excised. Longer-term outcome is similar to that of mucinous carcinoma.[61]

Invasive micropapillary carcinoma

Incidence and clinical presentation

This is a morphologically distinct type of breast carcinoma representing less than 1% of all invasive ductal carcinomas. There is no difference in age distribution compared with other types of breast carcinomas, and most cases present as a breast mass.[63–65]

Macroscopic features

The median tumour size ranges from 1.5 cm to 4.9 cm and there are no specific macroscopic features.

Microscopic features

The lesion is composed of morule-like clusters separated by fine and loose fibrocollagenous stroma.[65] The cells are cuboidal or columnar, with granular eosinophilic cytoplasm. Nuclei are rounded and vesicular and usually of intermediate or high grade (Figure 27.31). Epithelial elements are arranged into round or oval structures, some several layers thick and lacking apical 'snouts'. Microvilli are demonstrable on the outer border of cell clusters by electron microscopy. Areas of DCIS (micropapillary and cribriform types) are frequently seen adjacent to the main tumour (Figure 27.32).

Histochemistry and immunohistochemistry

Some tumours have mucinous material between the clusters of tumour cells. Micropapillary carcinoma

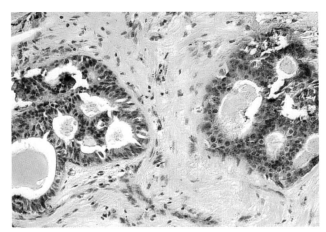

Figure 27.33   Cribriform carcinoma. (H&E, ×100.)

Cribriform carcinoma

Incidence and clinical presentation

This is an uncommon breast tumour in which the invasive component resembles cytologically that seen in cribriform DCIS but the outline of the tumour cluster is irregular.[66]

Macroscopic features

There are no specific macroscopic features of this tumour, and some cases may be multifocal.

Microscopic features

There are two basic forms: classical and mixed. The classical type is composed mainly of a cribriform pattern, while the mixed type possesses a tubular component or ductal carcinoma NST (Figure 27.33). Cribriform carcinoma is a well-differentiated variant of invasive ductal carcinoma, but the term is only applied to those tumours with at least 90% of the tumour showing a cribriform pattern.[66] The classical type has a sieve-like growth pattern, and the epithelial component is sharply outlined and present in collagenous stroma. Calcification may be present, and foci of in situ cribriform small cell type may be seen in the adjacent breast tissue. Perineural invasion is present in a small percentage of cases, but lymphatic and vascular invasion is rarely seen. Endocrine differentiation is not a feature of this tumour.

Prognosis

Clinical outcomes are generally favourable, with a prognosis comparable to that of tubular carcinoma

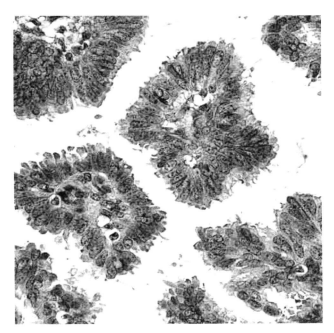

Figure 27.31   Micropapillary carcinoma. (H&E, ×200.)

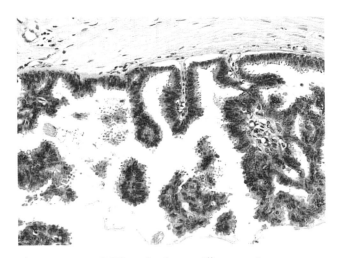

Figure 27.32   DCIS and micropapillary carcinoma. (H&E, ×100.)

is ER-positive in almost three-quarters (73%) of cases, PgR-positive in almost half (45%) and HER2/*neu*-positive in approximately one-third (36%). Tumour cells are invariably EMA-positive.

Prognosis

Lymphatic invasion can be detected in almost three-quarters (72%) of cases. The tumour should be treated as an aggressive lesion, but due to its rarity relatively little is known about its propensity for local or distant relapse. One series reported disease-related death in 50% of cases.[63–65] (especially for the classical type). Mixed cribriform carcinoma has a greater tendency to spread to axillary lymph nodes.[66]

Medullary carcinoma

Incidence and clinical presentation

This is a rare and rather controversial entity that constitutes about 3% of all invasive breast carcinomas.[67] It affects women of a lower age group than ordinary ductal carcinoma and is relatively more common in American women of African descent. There is a much greater degree of interobserver and intraobserver variation in the diagnosis of this tumour compared with other types.

Macroscopic features

This tumour was sometimes referred to as 'bulky' carcinoma in the past, due to the relatively large size at diagnosis. The tumour is well demarcated from surrounding breast tissue and has a moderately firm consistency resembling a fibroadenoma. Indeed, medullary carcinomas can be initially diagnosed as fibroadenomas on clinical examination, but are less mobile than the latter. The tumours have a characteristically pushing margin and the outer surface has a vaguely lobulated or nodular structure. It is not unusual to see haemorrhage and necrosis, even in lesions as small as 2 cm.

Microscopic features

At a microscopic level, medullary carcinoma should meet all of the following criteria:[68]

- smooth, non-infiltrative borders
- prominent lymphoplasmocytic infiltration present diffusely within the tumour and involving at least 75% of the tumour periphery
- tumour cells arranged in large solid nests and sheets with poorly defined cell borders (the so-called syncytial pattern)
- individual cells with large pleomorphic nuclei, prominent nucleoli and high mitotic activity
- limited amounts of fibrous stroma and absence of any DCIS component.

Medullary tumours with high mitotic counts and lymphocytic infiltrates are more common in patients with mutations in the tumour suppressor gene *BRCA1*. The overall features resemble lymphoepithelial carcinomas arising in sites other than the breast. Necrosis is common and may be extensive,

and the mitotic rate is often high. The stroma exhibits small amounts of fibrous tissue, and elastosis is absent.

Tumours with some but not all of these features have been labelled as atypical medullary carcinomas.[68,69]

The above features must be present in at least 75% of the tumour before a diagnosis of either typical and atypical medullary carcinoma is made.[19,28,47,69] The lymphocytic infiltration exclusively involves T cells.

Immunohistochemistry

Fewer than 10% of medullary carcinomas are ER- and PgR-positive, and this accounts for the poor response of metastatic medullary carcinoma to endocrine therapy.

The majority of medullary carcinomas express nuclear p53 but not HER2/*neu*. They have a relatively high proliferative index as determined by Ki67 immunoreactivity, and it has been suggested that the favourable prognosis of these tumours may be attributable to rapid cell turnover. Staining for both EMA and S-100 is positive in medullary carcinoma.[47]

Prognosis

Despite relatively high mitotic rates, medullary carcinomas have a favourable prognosis when compared with invasive ductal carcinoma NST and lobular carcinoma.[70,71] Only 10–12% of patients die of their disease 5 years following mastectomy or breast conservation surgery. The mortality rate at 10 years is approximately 17% and the overall survival rate at 20 years is almost 75%. Patients with medullary carcinoma tend to have lower rates of axillary lymph node metastases and better prognosis than patients with atypical medullary carcinoma and those with ductal carcinoma NST.[72]

Apocrine carcinoma

Other names applied to this tumour include oncocytic and sweat gland carcinoma.[73]

Incidence and clinical presentation

The incidence of apocrine carcinoma ranges from less than 1% to 4% in published series. The tumour

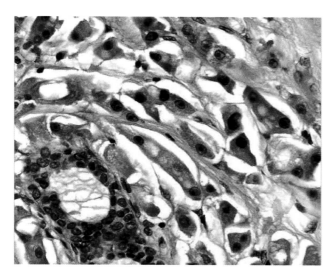

Figure 27.34 Invasive apocrine carcinoma. (H&E, ×200.)

presents clinically and radiologically in a similar manner to ductal carcinoma with a palpable breast mass. Other symptoms such as breast pain, nipple discharge and Paget's disease are rare manifestations of invasive apocrine carcinoma.

Macroscopic features

Invasive apocrine carcinomas are firm to hard tumours with infiltrating rather than pushing borders. Sectioning of these tumours reveals a grey or white cut surface.[73]

Microscopic features

The component cell of apocrine carcinoma is large with abundant eosinophilic cytoplasm and large rounded nuclei and prominent nucleoli (Figure 27.34). Apocrine differentiation is seen in pleomorphic lobular carcinoma and in papillary, intraductal and mucinous carcinomas. The tumour may colonise lobules or adjacent sclerosing adenosis and often assumes the shape of these structures.[74] The nuclei of apocrine cells may be of low, intermediate or high grade.

The cytoplasm may be either homogenous or granular. Vacuolation and clearing of cytoplasm may occur. The tumour cells grow in sheets or irregular cell clusters, and glandular formation may be apparent. Associated apocrine DCIS can be seen both within and outside the tumour and is usually of the corresponding nuclear grade.

The tumour cells show abundant granules, including mitochondria, when viewed under the electron microscope.

Histochemistry and immunohistochemistry

The cells are periodic acid–Schiff (PAS)-positive and appear red with trichrome stain. Cytoplasmic iron granules can be seen in both benign and malignant apocrine cells. The tumour cells are positive for CEA and cytokeratins but negative for S-100. p53 labelling has been demonstrated in 68.2% of invasive apocrine carcinoma but not in benign apocrine proliferation.[75]

Prognosis

In general, the prognosis of apocrine carcinoma is similar to that of invasive ductal carcinoma NST. The tumour size, nuclear grade and nodal status remain the principal determinants of prognosis.[76,77]

Metaplastic carcinoma

This tumour type is otherwise known as carcinoma with metaplasia or spindle cell carcinoma and represents a group of tumours with characteristic features of both epithelial and mesenchymal origin.[78,79]

Incidence and clinical presentation

This is a rare primary tumour of the breast, representing less than 4% of invasive tumours. It is characterised by transformation of carcinomatous glandular epithelium into spindle cells.[78] Prior to the era of immunohistochemistry, these tumours were mistaken for mesenchymal malignancies on account of the spindle-shaped cells. They commonly present with a palpable lump and the age distribution is comparable to that of other types of breast carcinoma.[78]

Macroscopic features

The size of these tumours can vary from 1 cm to 21 cm, but the mean tumour size at presentation is 3–4 cm. These are typically firm to hard tumours due to the amount of fibrous stroma induced, and can be either circumscribed, round or infiltrative. Growth patterns can be similar to that of fibromatoses. The mesenchymal component can give rise to cartilaginous or osseous differentiation.

Microscopic features

Two main types occur:

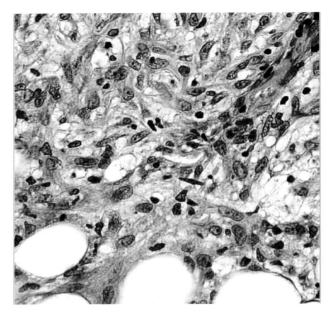

Figure 27.35 Metaplastic carcinoma. (H&E, ×200.)

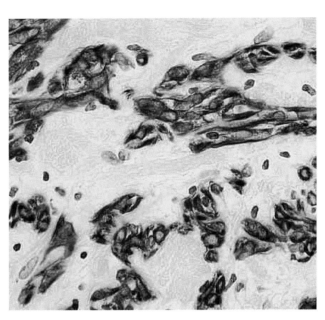

Figure 27.36 CAM5.2-positive metaplastic carcinoma. (×200.)

- spindle cell squamous carcinoma (Figure 27.35)
- Heterologous or pseudosarcomatous spindle cell carcinoma (mainly cartilage and bone components) (Figure 27.36)

The tumour tends to be bulky, and consists of poorly differentiated cells undergoing squamous spindle cell and sarcomatoid metaplasia.[80,81] The presence of cells that are morphologically diagnostic of carcinoma and positive for cytokeratin (often at the periphery) are useful features in distinguishing these tumours from true sarcomas.[82,83] These foci of carcinomatous elements often lie at the periphery of the tumour. Rarely chondroid or osseous metaplasia coexists with squamous carcinoma.[84] A storiform pattern with sprinkling of lymphocytes may be seen, which may replace the whole tumour area. Immunohistochemical markers are required to unequivocally establish the nature of this tumour and distinguish it from a sarcoma.

Histochemistry and immunohistochemistry

Without immunohistochemical stains, spindle cell and sarcomatoid components are difficult to distinguish from fibrosarcoma, leiomyosarcoma, osteosarcoma, rhabdomyosarcoma and metastatic tumours.

Some authors have observed coexpression of epithelial and mesenchymal markers in spindle cell elements of metaplastic breast carcinomas. The tumour is usually positive for cytokeratin (Figure 27.36), EMA and vimentin. The high-molecular-weight keratin K903 has been the reagent most often positive in this type of tumour. HER2/*neu* positivity is detected in 11% of cases. There is a loss of adhesion molecules, with negative staining for E-cadherin in most tumours.

Prognosis

The overall prognosis of metaplastic carcinoma is worse than that of conventional invasive ductal carcinoma, although some authors have reported similar outcomes when matched for stage. The frequency of axillary nodal metastases ranges from 6% to 31%, with disease-free survival rates ranging from 38% to 67% at 5-year follow-up.[85]

Adenoid cystic carcinoma

This tumour is also known as basaloid carcinoma and cylindroma.

Incidence and clinical features

Cases have been reported in women ranging in age between 25 and 80, but these tumours can also occur in men and children.[86–88] This is a rare tumour, accounting for less than 1% of all breast tumours, and has to be differentiated from invasive cribriform carcinoma. These tumours present clinically as a firm discrete mass. Skin dimpling, ulceration and peau d'orange have been reported in large tumours, despite the less aggressive nature and excellent prognosis of this tumour type. These tumours often arise in the region of the nipple–areola complex, which precludes breast conservation.[86]

Macroscopic features

These are well defined lesions, but 50% have infiltrative margins. Reports of tumour size range from 1 cm to 2 cm, but most are between 1 cm and 3 cm. Small cystic areas may be visible, and these tend to be more readily apparent in larger tumours.[88]

Microscopic features

An invasive tumour is seen, with features resembling cylindroma of the skin and adenoid cystic carcinoma of the salivary gland. The tumour is characterised by its solid pink cylindromatous nodules and punched-out glandular spaces containing a basophilic secretion. The solid growth pattern with a vascular stroma may resemble solid papillary breast carcinoma.[87,89] There is a tubular growth pattern and syringomatous differentiation. The neoplastic cells are small, uniform, darkly stained and basaloid in appearance. The pseudocysts punctuating the tumour cluster are composed of stromal collagen and basal lamina and are PAS-positive. A benign lesion called collagenous spherulosis bears some resemblance to this tumour.

Histochemistry and immunohistochemistry

Mucicarmine and Alcian blue can identify secretion within glands. EMA shows positivity of the epithelial lumina but not of the stromal cyst-like structures. The structural polarity of the glandular cells can be demonstrated with E-cadherin and β-catenin. Laminin and fibronectin can be demonstrated within the cylindromatous elements. Vimentin-positive cells have been referred to as myoepithelium-like or basaloid cells. These tumours are usually ER-negative.[28,47]

Prognosis

The prognosis is particularly favourable, despite the lack of ER and the high proliferative indices. Distinction from other types of breast carcinoma is therefore important. Mastectomy is potentially curative in the majority of cases, although nodal and lung metastases have been reported. Nonetheless, death from distant disease is very uncommon.

Mammary carcinoma with endocrine features

Carcinoid tumour, argyrophilic carcinoma

These comprise a heterogeneous group of neoplasms that show an endocrine growth pattern.

Incidence and clinical features

This is a rare form of invasive breast carcinoma with no specific clinical features. Less than 5% of breast carcinomas show argyrophilic cells and even fewer show a sufficient number of cells to qualify for this diagnostic label. Metastatic carcinoid tumour to the breast should be considered before a tumour is designated as a primary breast carcinoid. Neuroendocrine carcinoma of the breast is not associated with carcinoid syndrome.[90] Most tumours produce no systemic manifestation of ectopic hormonal secretion.

Macroscopic features

No specific macroscopic features are evident in this type of tumour. The tumours are moderately well circumscribed and vary in size from 1 cm to 5 cm. They are most commonly located close to the nipple–areola complex, and therefore nipple discharge is a more prominent clinical feature than for ordinary invasive ductal carcinoma.

Microscopic features

These tumours do not resemble the classical carcinoid tumour of the intestine but do show some resemblance to atypical carcinoid lesions of the bronchus. Most of these tumours are invasive ductal carcinomas with prominent endocrine differentiation in the form of argyrophilic cytoplasmic granules. The cells are arranged in solid islands or nests, and plexiform patterns can occur.[90,91] There may be nuclear pallisading around the peripheral part of the cell masses. The stroma is fibrous and there may be elastosis and foci of microcalcification. A corresponding DCIS component can often be seen around the tumour. Dense core vesicles that are characteristic of endocrine tumours are seen on electron microscopy.[92] It should be noted that not all carcinomas with an endocrine growth pattern contain argyrophilic cells.

Histochemistry and immunohistochemistry

These tumours are Grimelius-positive and chromogranin-positive. They are also reactive with lactalbumin.

Prognosis

Stage at diagnosis is the main determinant of tumour behaviour and prognosis. Patients with argyrophilic mucinous carcinomas are more likely to have axillary nodal metastases than those with Grimelius-negative tumours (48% versus 26%). They also have a higher frequency of recurrence and deaths from breast carcinoma (65% versus 33%).[91]

Secretory carcinoma

These tumours were previously known as juvenile carcinomas, but can also occur in older women.[94–96]

Incidence and clinical presentation

Secretory carcinomas are more common in the younger age group.[95] The first seven cases were described by McDivitt and Stewart in 1966 and ranged in age from 13 to 15.[96] Young males can also be affected with secretory carcinomas. The tumour may affect any part of the breast, including subareolar tissue, which can be associated with nipple discharge. The lesion is not associated with pregnancy or any abnormal hormonal imbalance.[94,95]

Macroscopic features

Mammography usually reveals a discrete opacity with an irregular border, and the tumour may be multifocal. These lesions characteristically are firm circumscribed masses that are whitish to grey in colour.

Microscopic features

The tumour exhibits solid glandular and micropapillary patterns, with microcystic areas filled with abundant pink cytoplasm. The cells exhibit microlumina and 'bubbly' cytoplasm and small round and uniform nuclei, some of which are vesicular.[97,98] Small nucleoli may be seen. A DCIS component may be seen around the tumour and signet ring cells are occasionally a feature.

Histochemistry and immunohistochemistry

Most of the tumours are ER-negative and the secretions stain with PAS.

Prognosis

The prognosis for this type of breast carcinoma is good, particularly in younger patients with tumours less than 2 cm in diameter. However, significant rates of local recurrence have been reported at 8 years following mastectomy. Axillary lymph node metastases occur, but these are usually confined to three or fewer lymph nodes. Wide local excision is an appropriate method of treatment for most of these tumours.[98]

Cystic hypersecretory carcinoma

Incidence and clinical presentation

This is a rare tumour and occurs principally as in situ forms, but invasive carcinomas have been reported. The lesion has a similar age distribution to other types of invasive breast carcinoma.[99]

Macroscopic features

These tumours vary in size from 1 cm to 10 cm. They have a typically firm but not hard consistency compared with invasive ductal and lobular carcinomas. The tumours are well defined but display numerous cystic spaces. In appearance, these tumours grossly simulate cystic hypersecretory hyperplasia, and distinction between the two lesions can only be made histologically.

Microscopic features

The cysts contain eosinophilic secretory material that resembles thyroid colloid. The spaces are lined by micropapillary structures with crowding of pleomorphic nuclei, which also exhibit mitotic activity.[99] This should be differentiated from cystic hypersecretory hyperplasia, where the cysts are lined by a single layer of flattened or low cuboidal epithelium. The nuclei of invasive carcinoma are large and vesicular and the cytoplasm is so-called 'bubbly'. These tumours may be of mixed character, with an invasive lobular component having been documented in some reports.

Histochemistry and immunohistochemistry

The majority of reported cases are ER- and PgR-negative.

Prognosis

There is a dearth of information about the clinical course of these tumours due to their rarity. Cystic hypersecretory carcinoma in situ behaves in a similar way to other types of DCIS of similar grade. More than half of invasive carcinomas have metastases to axillary lymph nodes (three out of five cases.[99]

Lipid-rich carcinoma

Incidence and clinical features

This is a rare primary tumour of the breast, constituting less than 1% of all breast cancers. It is considered to be a variant of invasive ductal carcinoma.[100]

Macroscopic features

These are poorly circumscribed tumours that are firm but not hard to palpation. The tumour size ranges from 1.5 cm to 4 cm.

Microscopic features

These tumours have large cells that show abundant foamy cytoplasm containing lipid vesicles, which may cause clearing of cytoplasm. The nuclei are small, dark and rounded, and the overall cytological appearance may be mistaken for that of a xanthomatous tumour.

Histochemistry and immunohistochemistry

The cytoplasm stains strongly for neutral lipid but weakly or negative for mucin. The cells are reactive to antibodies against EMA, cytokeratins and α-lactalbumin.

Prognosis

These are usually aggressive tumours, with axillary lymph node involvement being reported in most cases. Variable patterns of expression of ER and PgR have been described, with some positive and others negative.

Glycogen-rich carcinoma

Incidence and clinical presentation

This is a very rare breast cancer presenting as a mass in an age group similar to other more common types of breast carcinoma.

Macroscopic features

No specific gross features are attributable to this tumour.

Microscopic features

The tumour is composed of columnar and polygonal cells with small darkly stained nuclei and abundant cytoplasm. The growth pattern of the invasive component is solid cords or papillary structures, while DCIS of any type may be associated with these glycogen-rich carcinomas.[101] The cells tend to have sharply defined borders, and areas of necrosis may be seen together with mitotic figures.

Histochemistry and immunohistochemistry

Tumour cells are PAS-positive and D-PAS-negative. They are also negative for the oil-red O lipid stain but positively immunoreactive for CEA, cytokeratin and EMA. Staining is negative for α-lactalbumin, desmin and vimentin. A significant proportion of the tumours are ER-positive.

Prognosis

In general, these tumours have an unfavourable prognosis, with 30% showing metastases to axillary lymph nodes. Approximately half of patients treated by mastectomy succumb from their disease at a median follow-up of 15 months.

Inflammatory carcinoma

Incidence and clinical presentation

Inflammatory breast cancer is a locally advanced and accelerated form of breast cancer that is conventionally categorised as stage IIIb or IV (Manchester staging system). Clinical signs include a relatively rapid increase in overall breast size, which can be associated with unrelenting pruritis for which medicated creams and ointments fail to yield relief. The breast appears erythematous and may have a typical peau d'orange appearance. The redness and warmth to the touch are characteristic and are related to infiltration and blockage of dermal and subdermal lymphatic vessels with cancer cells.[102] There is thickening and induration of the skin, with the formation of ridges as a result of blockage of lymphatics by malignant cells. Mammography reveals diffuse thickening of the skin and subcutaneous tissues, with a general increase in breast

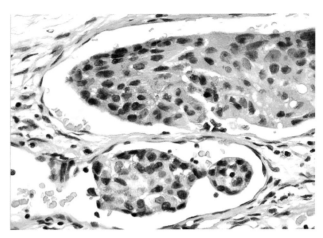

Figure 27.37 Inflammatory carcinoma with tumour present mainly within lymphatic channels. (H&E, ×200.)

density. Inflammatory carcinoma may be mistaken clinically for acute mastitis and a course of antibiotics prescribed initially by either a family or hospital doctor (ultrasound evaluation is helpful in distinguishing between these two conditions). Lack of response to such treatment should raise suspicion of more sinister pathology in younger women.[102]

Macroscopic features

These are as documented above; erythema with thickening of the skin and peau d'orange is a particularly prominent feature of this type of carcinoma, which may be mistaken for a benign inflammatory condition.

Microscopic features

Skin and breast biopsies from inflammatory breast carcinoma show tumour emboli within dermal and subcutaneous lymphatics, and there is vascular congestion (Figure 27.37). These features, however, may be seen in cases of local recurrence following treatment of breast carcinoma other than of the inflammatory type. Sometimes, clinical signs of an inflammatory carcinoma can occur without dermal lymphatic invasion, and this can lead to inconsistency and controversy with diagnosis.

Histochemistry and immunohistochemistry

Clumps of tumour cells within dermal lymphatics are positive for cytokeratins and EMA.

Prognosis

Inflammatory carcinoma is usually treated with induction chemotherapy followed by modified radical mastectomy and chest wall radiotherapy. There is a higher risk of locoregional and distant recurrence with inflammatory breast carcinoma than for other types of breast cancer, and breast reconstruction is usually contraindicated. Biopsy of recurrent lesions shows similar features to the primary lesions. Inflammatory carcinoma is the most lethal type of breast cancer, but prompt diagnosis and initiation of treatment improves survival outcome.[102,103] Chemotherapy should commence within days of diagnosis, and neoadjuvant regimens have dramatically improved 5-year survival rates. New and upcoming treatment protocols offer hope of further improvements in long-term survival.

Paget's disease of the nipple

Incidence and clinical presentation

Approximately 2% of breast carcinomas are associated with Paget's disease and occur in an age range from 26 to 88 years.[104] Paget's disease of the nipple is usually a unilateral lesion affecting one nipple only, which is an important feature serving to differentiate Paget's disease from simple eczema of the nipple. Pain and itching are accompanying symptoms, together with bleeding and possibly oozing from the surface. The condition affects primarily the nipple rather than the areola, with the surface of the former being rough, erythematous and eroded with scaling. However, the disease may extend to involve the areola.

Macroscopic features

This condition is associated with an underlying invasive or intraductal carcinoma, and the precise macroscopic features are related to this. Associated invasive lesions tend to be centrally located and close to the nipple surface, but more deeply sited tumours may occur. One or more lactiferous ducts may be involved by DCIS.

Microscopic features

Pathognomonic cells infiltrating the dermis are readily distinguished from keratinocytes, especially when large numbers are present (Figure 27.38). However, special stains or immunohistochemistry are required to demonstrate occasional cells. These Pagetoid cells simulate melanocytes, and special markers may be needed in certain cases to differentiate them from this cell type. Malignant cells occur singly or in groups and are seen infiltrating all layers of the epidermis up to the skin surface.

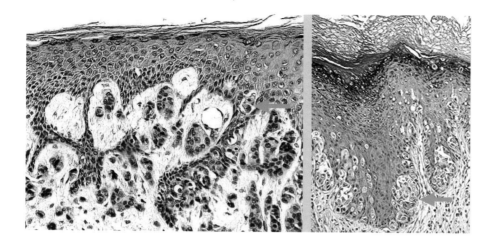

Figure 27.38 Paget's disease of the nipple with groups of tumour cells infiltrating the dermis and epidermis (arrows). (H&E, ×40.)

The underlying carcinoma is most commonly ductal, but can be lobular in type.

Histochemistry and immunohistochemistry

Paget's disease must be differentiated at the microscopic level from malignant melanoma and Bowen's disease of the nipple. This is particularly important if a biopsy of skin from the nipple is the only specimen upon which the diagnosis is based. Pagetoid cells may contain mucin, which can be highlighted by PAS or mucicarmin stains. Staining for S-100 and HMB45 is positive in melanomas, while cytokeratins are positive in both Paget's and Bowen's diseases (the latter is also positive for CK20). Pagetoid cells also stain positive for EMA, HMFG, CAM 5.2 (Figure 27.39) and CK7, while these four markers are negative in melanoma and Bowen's disease. Both ER and PgR are expressed in Paget's disease and can prove to be useful markers. Paget's disease cells are usually HER2/*neu*-positive.

Prognosis

The clinical outcome is dependent on the nature and extent of the underlying tumour. Those cases of pure DCIS have an excellent prognosis, with 10-year survival rates ranging from 82% to 100% following mastectomy. When invasive ductal carcinoma is present, the overall 10-year survival rate falls to 70%, with prognosis being principally determined by the state of the lymph nodes at diagnosis.

Mucoepidermoid carcinoma

This is a very rare primary breast tumour that is morphologically identical to those arising in salivary

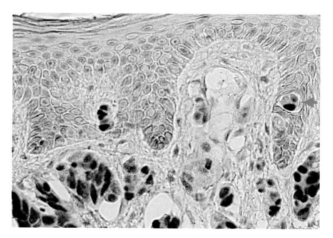

Figure 27.39 Paget's disease of the nipple, with malignant cells present within the epidermis. (CAM5.2, ×100.)

glands, with squamous differentiation and mucin production. There are few reports in the literature on the behaviour of this tumour.[105]

Squamous cell carcinoma

Incidence and clinical presentation

Breast cancers exhibiting squamous differentiation are rare, and of these only one-third are composed of pure squamous carcinoma.[106]

Macroscopic features

These are often large tumours with solid components containing cystic spaces. The solid components may show keratinisation.

Microscopic features

Tumours composed purely of squamous carcinoma vary from well- to poorly differentiated lesions, with keratin formation being evident in the well-differentiated forms. The cystic spaces may be lined by squamous epithelium, and spindle cell components can be seen. Two-thirds of these tumours contain a component of invasive ductal carcinoma. When tumours lie close to the skin surface, it is important to exclude the possibility of a primary cutaneous malignancy or a secondary deposit in the skin from a primary lesion at a distant site. Squamous differentiation often persists in any metastatic deposits.[106]

Histochemistry and immunohistochemistry

These tumours are positive for cytokeratins.

Prognosis

Squamous cell carcinomas of the breast have a similar prognosis to invasive ductal carcinoma and in the presence of distant metastases can cause diagnostic confusion.

Small cell carcinoma

Incidence and clinical picture

This is one of the least common types of breast carcinoma, and when suspected it is imperative to first exclude the possibility of secondary deposits from a primary bronchogenic carcinoma.[107]

Macroscopic features

These lesions may present clinically as a breast mass or be detected mammographically as a dense stromal opacity.

Microscopic features

Both in situ and invasive carcinomas may occur with component cells identical to those seen in small cell carcinoma of the bronchus (Figure 27.40). Accompanying solid and cribriform small cell carcinomas have been reported in association with the invasive small cell carcinoma. Tumour cells possess little cytoplasm and have dark nuclei. This tumour may coexist with other types of breast cancer, such as invasive ductal or lobular carcinomas.

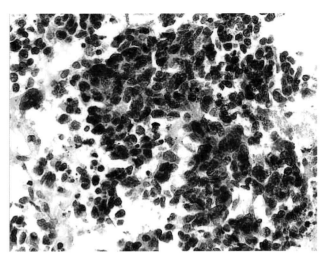

Figure 27.40　Small cell carcinoma. (H&E, ×200.)

Histochemistry and immunohistochemistry

The cells are positive for cytokeratins, CAM5.2 and CK7, in addition to NSE, chromogranin and CD56.

Prognosis

The prognosis of these small cell tumours is generally poor without treatment, but they are responsive to chemotherapy just like small cell bronchial carcinoma. Mastectomy appears to be the surgical treatment of choice, and a proportion of patients with relatively large tumours will have axillary nodal metastases.[107]

Mixed breast carcinoma

There are two types of mixed malignant tumours of the breast:

* tumours composed of more than one type of epithelial neoplasia, such as tubulolobular carcinoma or mixed mucinous and NST breast carcinoma.
* tumours composed of mixed epithelial and mesenchymal elements of malignant character

Mixed epithelial tumours

As diagnostic criteria for pure types of carcinomas are being applied more strictly, increasing numbers of these tumours are being described. The clinical behaviour of these tumours is determined by the histological subtype with the worst prognosis.[108]

Mixed epithelial and mesenchymal tumours

Two main groupings are identified: metaplastic carcinoma and true carcinosarcomas. Metaplastic carcinoma is more common and has been described earlier in this chapter. For carcinosarcomas, the mesenchymal component must fulfil the same criteria for malignancy as a pure mesenchymal neoplasm of the same histogenic type. A significant number of carcinosarcomas contain cartilage or bone, while the epithelial component frequently shows squamous differentiation.[109,110] Some of these tumours may arise from a pre-existing fibroadenoma or phyllodes tumour.

Multicentric breast carcinoma

Multicentricity may be related to multiple sites of origin or may be due to intramammary spread from a single index tumour. Some authors define multicentricity as the presence of more than one tumour focus separated by a minimum distance of 5 cm. Radiological and pathological data must be correlated in order to assess these lesions more accurately and obtain consensus on the definition of this entity.

Incidence and clinical presentation

This is an important area that requires careful presurgical assessment in the setting of a multidisciplinary breast meeting. Establishing a diagnosis of multicentric carcinoma will influence the surgical approach and facilitate selection of the most appropriate operation. The radiological findings are crucial, and a copy of the mammogram should be sent to the pathologist to aid histological assessment.

Fisher et al (1975) found microscopic evidence of multicentric foci of carcinoma in 13% of surgically resected specimens, with almost two-thirds of the additional foci being non-invasive.[111] Multicentricity is more common with infiltrating lobular carcinoma and with subareolar tumours, and less common with medullary and mucinous carcinomas. Lagios et al (1981) found multicentric carcinoma in 28% of 286 mastectomies.[112]

Macroscopic features

More than one tumour is seen within the resection or mastectomy specimens. It is important to differentiate multicentric tumours from satellite nodules lying in proximity to a main primary tumour mass.

Microscopic features

These tumours may be ductal or lobular in origin, and their microscopic appearances correspond to the descriptions given earlier in this chapter under the relevant headings. Furthermore, the tumours may be of a similar histological type or completely different and unrelated.

Prognosis

There is no correlation between multicentricity and axillary nodal involvement. However Egan and McSweeney (1984) reported that multicentric tumours were associated with a poorer prognosis than unicentric tumours.[113] Mastectomy is usually mandated for multicentric tumours and is associated with lower rates of local recurrence than attempts at breast conservation. However, overall rates of survival following wide local excision and radiotherapy are comparable to mastectomy.[114]

Centrally necrotising breast carcinoma

Incidence and clinical presentation

This is a recently reported subtype of breast cancer with an aggressive phenotype. The true incidence of this tumour type is unclear, but distinction from other types of breast cancer is important according to a report by Jimenez et al, who described 34 cases with a mean age of 57.5 ± 11.6 (median age 58.5).[115]

Macroscopic features

The mean tumour size in this series was 2.5 cm ± 1.2 cm, and all lesions were well circumscribed, with infiltrative margins. Sections of these tumours fully mounted reveal a distinct pale-coloured centre.

Microscopic features

All tumours in the series of Jimenez et al[115] consisted of a unicentric nodule with a prominent central zone that was hypocellular and surrounded by a ring-like hypercellular area with a pushing border and sharply delineated from the surrounding breast tissue. In most tumours, the majority of this central zone consisted entirely of necrotic debris (Figure 27.41). The cells tended to be arranged in small nests, with a lack of tubular structures and formation of lumina. Mitotic rates were highest at the peripheral zone of the tumour and there was an

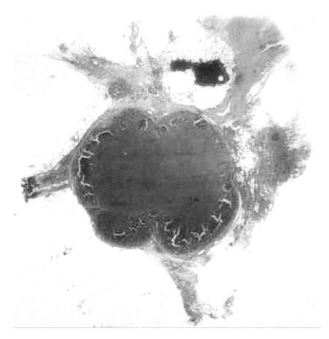

Figure 27.41 Centrally necrotising breast carcinoma. (H&E, scanning power.)

abrupt transition between the central necrotic zone and viable tumour. A notable feature of centrally necrotising breast carcinoma is the consistent and orderly nature of the central zone of necrosis, which differs from the patchy and haphazard areas of necrosis seen in other tumour types.

Prognosis

From this series of 34 patients, 21 (61%) had died at the time of analysis, with a median time interval from diagnosis to death of 22.5 months. The median interval from development of a recurrence to death was 5.2 months.

Familial/hereditary breast carcinoma

Genetic susceptibility to breast carcinoma is suggested clinically by a strong family history of breast cancer, which usually involves three or more first-degree relatives.[116,117] The number of first- and second-degree relatives together with the age of onset and bilaterality are important determinants of genetic risk. Two principal genes have been implicated in hereditary forms of breast carcinoma. These are *BRCA1* and *BRCA2*, which lie on the long arms of chromosomes 17 and 13 respectively (17q21 and 13q12.3). They account for approximately half of all cases of hereditary breast cancer.

BRCA1-associated breast carcinoma

Carcinomas associated with *BRCA1* mutations have distinctive pathological features, but these are not unique to this group of patients. Higher-grade lesions are more likely with a preponderance of invasive ductal carcinoma (grade 3) and poorly differentiated DCIS. The tumours exhibit a high proliferative rate as demonstrated by MIB1 immunostaining, and do not usually express ER or HER2/*neu*, but do exhibit p53 nuclear reactivity. High levels of angiogenesis have also been observed in these tumours. A relatively high frequency of medullary carcinoma has been reported; the frequencies of various subtypes of breast carcinoma among *BRCA1*-associated cancers compared with controls is shown in Table 27.2.

Table 27.2 Frequencies of breast carcinoma subtypes among *BRCA1*-associated cancers

Tumour subtype	Control (%)	BRCA1 (%)
Invasive ductal NST	74	74
Infiltrative lobular	10	8
Tubular	5	2
Mucinous	0	1
Medullary/atypical medullary	2	13
Ductal–lobular	3	1
Other	6	6

BRCA2-associated breast carcinoma

The frequencies of various subtypes of breast carcinoma in this group are shown in Table 27.3.

Table 27.3 Frequencies of breast carcinoma subtypes among *BRCA2*-associated cancers

Tumour subtype	Control (%)	BRCA2 (%)
Invasive ductal NST	74	76
Infiltrative lobular	10	10
Tubular	5	0
Mucinous	0	1
Medullary	2	3
Ductal–lobular	3	3
Other	6	7

Other specific genetic abnormalities have been linked to breast carcinoma, but these are usually associated with a named syndrome and confer a range of phenotypic abnormalities in addition to breast cancer. These include *TP53* (also known as *p53*) in Li–Fraumeni syndrome, *PTEN* in Cowden's syndrome and *STK11* in Peutz–Jeghers syndrome.

Interval cancers (see Chapter 6)

An interval cancer is defined as a breast carcinoma appearing during the interval between two screening rounds, with the preceding screening mammogram having been declared normal. There are two types of interval cancer:

- a true interval cancer with no evidence of any abnormality following a review of the previous mammographic films
- a false interval cancer with a lesion being evident on retrospective examination of previous films – these radiological lesions were missed at screening or were interpreted as a normal finding or non-suspicious abnormality

Causes of true interval breast cancers

These cancers may be:

- tumours developing de novo during the screening interval and becoming evident clinically (or radiologically) before the next screening round
- clinical abnormalities that were present at the time of the previous screen but were not detectable radiologically due to large breast size or high tissue density in a prospective context.

Causes of false interval breast cancers

These may be due to:

- screening error
- clerical error
- clinical/assessment error, including pathological error – for example a biopsy specimen (FNAC or core biopsy) being interpreted as benign
- poor sensitivity of mammography or ultrasound imaging

Carcinoma in accessory breast tissue

Accessory breast tissue can occur in three potential locations:

- the axillary region
- the infraclavicular region
- the epigastrium.

Malignant change within accessory breast tissue is rare but histologically resembles cancers developing within normal breast tissue. Interestingly, these tumours present clinically as subcutaneous nodules or masses that can simulate sweat gland neoplasms. Investigations to exclude coexisting breast carcinoma should include mammography, ultrasound examination and even biopsy of suspicious areas.

Radiotherapy- and chemotherapy-related breast cancers

Effects of radiotherapy

Changes induced by irradiation may mimic residual breast carcinoma and cause difficulties in interpreting FNAC and core biopsy specimens.[29,47] The major changes in normal breast tissue include:

- collagenisation of intralobular stroma
- thickening of periductal and periacinar basement membrane
- severe atrophy of acinar and ductular epithelium
- cytological atypia of residual epithelial cells
- prominent acinar myoepithelial cells
- atypical fibroblasts in the interlobular stroma

The last three of these changes can lead to problems with interpretation of samples. False-positive diagnoses can be made on FNAC and core biopsy samples. Pathological interpretation of excision specimens is more confident when relevant details of clinical history are provided and corresponding slides of pretreatment breast cancer are available for comparison.[118]

Persistent foci of in situ, lobular and ductal carcinoma following radiotherapy can cause confusion when diagnosing residual or recurrent invasive breast carcinoma. Comparison of biopsy appearances with those of pre-excision and pre-radiotherapy biopsies is essential to avoid an erroneous histological diagnosis of recurrence.

Effects of chemotherapy

Chemotherapy induces cytological and histological changes involving both normal breast tissue and any residual tumour. There is often a lack of concordance between clinical and radiological impression on the one hand and pathological findings on the other. Thus residual tumour may be confirmed histologically in situations where a complete clinical and radiological response is judged to have occurred. MRI may be a better method for radiological assessment of residual tumour. Placement of a clip at the tumour site is a useful guide to follow tumour regression, to facilitate core biopsies and ultimately to excise breast tissue following induction therapy. The histological effects of chemotherapy can be monitored and more readily assessed if samples are compared pre- and post-chemotherapy.[119]

Histological examination of tumour site samples taken shortly after chemotherapy may show residual invasive carcinoma with areas of degeneration, infarction and necrosis. There is loss of normal staining properties and disruption of architectural details. With the passage of time, degenerate tumour is absorbed, leaving distorted stroma with areas of fibrosis and oedema. There is increased vascularity, with thin-walled vessels and a chronic inflammatory cell infiltrate. DCIS and tumour emboli within lymphatics and lymph nodes possess a degree of protection from chemotherapeutic agents. Residual carcinoma contains cells with large vesicular and pleomorphic nuclei and some mitotic activity.

Proliferation rates as measured by expression of Ki67 may be increased or decreased or remain unchanged. Increased p53 and HER2/*neu* expression consequent to chemotherapy has been reported. Due to extreme effects on tumour nuclei, grading of post-chemotherapy tumours can be difficult and unreliable. Non-neoplastic breast stroma undergoes more subtle changes than those occurring within the tumour area. The size and number of normal breast lobules in the peritumoral area are decreased post chemotherapy.[119]

Carcinoma metastatic to the breast

Malignant tumours originating as primary lesions elsewhere in the body can metastasise to the breast. These include not only epithelial tumours but also malignant derivatives of mesenchymal and lymphoid tissue.[120] Melanomas arising from skin at sites other than the breast envelope can spread to the breast parenchyma and present as a breast mass. Indeed, initial presentation as a breast mass may occur in up to one-quarter of cases of melanoma, and therefore it is essential that pathologists be provided with appropriate clinical information to facilitate histopathological diagnosis. Omission of crucial clinical details can sometimes lead to erroneous conclusions.

With more efficacious cancer therapies, increasing numbers of patients are surviving long enough to develop either distant recurrences or secondary malignancies. When such patients present with a malignant breast mass, it can prove challenging to differentiate between a primary breast cancer and a metastatic lesion from a primary elsewhere. Accurate diagnosis is important, as treatment of these two entities is different. A metastatic tumour usually relates to a primary carcinoma originating outside the breast. Reported sites for primary lesions include lung (small cell carcinoma), kidney, stomach, intestine (carcinoid tumour), ovary, uterus cervix, thyroid, salivary glands and skin (including melanomas).

When submitting a diagnostic sample from patients with a known malignancy, surgeons and radiologists must provide relevant clinical information to the pathologist to avoid both confusion with and delay in diagnosis. When presented with an odd lesion, the pathologist may be obliged to carry out an extensive process of sampling and application of an exhaustive series of histochemical and immunohistochemical stains in an attempt to reach a final diagnosis.

Carcinoma of the male breast

Incidence and clinical presentation

Male breast cancer is uncommon, with between 0.5% and 1% of all breast carcinomas occurring in men.[121] The mean age at diagnosis is between 60 and 70, which is approximately 10 years older than the mean age at diagnosis of female breast cancer. Nonetheless, men of all ages can be affected with this disease. It is widely believed that male breast cancer presents with a higher incidence of axillary metastases at the time of diagnosis. This may be attributable either to late clinical presentation or to earlier lymphatic infiltration consequent to the smaller volume of breast and fatty tissue.

Predisposing risk factors include radiation exposure, oestrogen administration and diseases associated with hyperoestrogenism, such as cirrhosis of the liver and Klinefelter's syndrome. Genetic predisposition occurs in some cases of male breast cancer, with an increased incidence in patients who have a number of female relatives affected with the disease. An increased risk of male breast cancer has been reported in families for whom a mutation in the *BRCA2* gene has been identified.

Macroscopic features

Macroscopically, these tumours are similar to those of the female breast, but are more likely to infiltrate the pectoralis major muscle.

Microscopic features

Male breast cancers are most commonly of the invasive ductal type. Although intraductal carcinoma has been described, lobular carcinoma in situ is unknown or rare in males. Inflammatory varieties and Paget's disease of the nipple also occur in the male population. Lymph node involvement and haematogenous patterns of spread are similar to those observed in female breast cancer. Grading and staging of lesions correspond to those of female breast cancer.[122]

Prognosis

Prognostic factors that have been evaluated include the size of the lesion and state of the axillary lymph nodes, both of which correlate well with survival outcomes. Stage for stage, overall survival for male breast cancer is similar to its female counterpart. The impression that male breast cancer has a worse prognosis may emanate from the tendency for diagnosis to be made at a later stage.[122]

Other malignant breast lesions

Other types of tumours have been reported in both male and female breasts, including malignant lymphoma and cancers presenting within intramammary nodes. A particularly rare and unusual type of breast carcinoma with osteoclast-like giant cells has been described.

References

1. Pathology Reporting in Breast Cancer Screening, 2nd edn. National Co-ordinating Group for Breast Screening Pathology. NHSBSP Publications Sheffield: NHS Breast Screening Programme, 1995.

2. Guidelines for non-operative diagnostic procedures and reporting in breast cancer screening. NHSBSP publication 50. Sheffield: NHS Breast Screening Programme, 2001.

3. Page DL, Anderson TJ, eds. Diagnostic Histopathology of the Breast. Edinburgh: Churchill Livingstone, 1987.

4. Anderson TJ, Lamb J, Alexander F et al. Comparative pathology of prevalent and incident cancers detected by breast screening. Lancet 1986; 1: 519–22.

5. Ciatto S, Cecchiani S, Grazzini G. Positive predictive value of fine needle aspiration cytology of breast lesions. Acta Cytol 1989; 33: 894–8.

6. Britton PD. Fine needle aspiration or core biopsy. Breast 1999; 8: 1–4.

7. Burns RP. Image-guided breast biopsy. Am J Surg 1997; 173: 9–11.

8. Owings DV, Hann L, Schnitt SJ. How thoroughly should needle localization breast biopsies be sampled for microscopic examination? A prospective mammographic/pathologic correlative study. Am J Surg Pathol 1990; 14: 578–83.

9. Schnitt SJ, Wang HH. Histologic sampling of grossly benign breast biopsies. How much is enough? Am J Surg Pathol 1989; 13: 505–12.

10. Schwartz GF, Giuliano A, Veronesi U. Proceedings of the Consensus Conference on the Role of Sentinel Lymph Node Biopsy in Carcinoma of the Breast. 19–22 April 2001 Philadelphia, Pennsylvania. Cancer 2002; 94: 2542–51.

11. International (Ludwig) Breast Cancer Study Group. Prognostic importance of occult axillary lymph node micrometastases from breast cancers. Lancet 1990; 335: 1565–8.

12. Millis RR, Springall R, Lee AH et al. Occult axillary lymph node metastases are of no prognostic significance in breast cancer. Cancer 2002; 86: 396–401.

13. Goyal A and Mansel RE. Sentinel lymph node biopsy in breast cancer: facts and controversies. Advances in Breast Cancer 2004; 1: 11–15.

14. Prasad ML, Osborne MP, Giri DD, Hoda SA. Microinvasive carcinoma (T1mic) of the breast: clinicopathologic profile of 21 cases. Am J Surg Pathol 2000; 24: 422–8.

15. Connolly J, Schnitt SJ. Extent of invasive disease. In: Page DL, Anderson TJ, eds. Diagnostic Histopathology of the Breast. Edinburgh: Churchill Livingstone, YEAR? pp 278–9.

16. Padmore RF, Fowble B, Hoffman J et al. Microinvasive breast carcinoma: clinicopathologic analysis of experience of a single institution. Cancer 2000; 88: 1403–9.

17. Schuh ME, Nemoto T, Penetrante RB et al. Intraductal carcinoma: analysis of presentation, pathologic findings and outcome of disease. Arch Surg 1986; 121: 1303–7.

18. Azzopardi JG, Chepick OF, Hartmann WH et al. Histologic typing of breast tumours, 2nd edn. World Health Organisation, Geneva. Am J Clin Pathol 1981; 78: 806–16.

19. Wellings SR, Jensen HM, Marcum RG. An atlas of subgross pathology of human breast. J Natl Cancer Inst 1975; 55: 231–73.

20. Rosen PP, Oberman HA. Tumors of the Mammary Gland. In: Atlas of Tumor Pathology, 3rd Series, Fascicle 7. Washington DC: Armed Forces Institute of Pathology, 1992.

21. Richter GO, Dockerty MB, Clagett OT. Diffuse infiltrating scirrhous carcinoma of the breast. Special consideration

of the single-filing phenomenon. Cancer 1967; 20: 363–70.

22. Masood S, Barwick KW. Estrogen receptor expression of the less common breast carcinomas. Am J Clin Pathol 1990; 93: 437 (abst).

23. Bloom HJ, Richardson WW. Histological grading and prognosis in breast cancer. A study of 1049 cases of which 359 have been followed for 15 years. Br J Cancer 1957; 11: 359–77.

24. Carter CL, Allen C and Hensen DE. Relation of tumor size, lymph node status and survival in 24,740 breast cancer cases. Cancer 1989; 63: 181–7.

25. Baak JP, Van Dop H, Kurver PHJ, Hermans J. The value of morphometry to classic prognosticators breast cancer. Cancer 1985; 56: 374–82.

26. Van de Vijver MJ, Peterse JL, Mooi WJ et al. Neu-protein overexpression in breast cancer. Association with comedo-type ductal carcinoma in situ and limited prognostic value in Stage II breast cancer. N Engl J Med 1988; 319: 1239–45.

27. Wright C, Angus B, Nicholson S et al. Expression of c-erbB-2 oncoprotein: a prognostic indicator in human breast cancer. Cancer Res 1989; 49: 2087–90.

28. McDivitt RW, Boyce W, Gersell D. Tubular carcinoma of the breast. Clinical and pathological observations concerning 135 cases. Am J Surg Pathol 1982; 6: 401–11.

29. Sloane JP. Biopsy Pathology of the Breast. London: Chapman & Hall Medical, 1988.

30. Bondeson L, Lindholm K. Aspiration cytology of tubular breast carcinoma. Acta Cytol 1990; 34: 15–20.

31. Flotte TJ, Bell DA, Greco MA. Tubular carcinoma and sclerosing adenosis: use of basal lamina as a differential feature. Am J Surg Pathol 1980; 4: 75–7.

32. Carstens PH, Greenberg RA, Francis D, Lyon H. Tubular carcinoma of the breast. A long term follow up. Histopathology 1985; 9: 271–80.

33. Deos PH, Norris HJ. Well differentiated (tubular) carcinoma of the breast: a clinicopathologic study of 145 pure and mixed cases. Am J Clin Pathol 1982; 78: 1–7.

34. Dixon JM, Anderson TJ, Page DL et al. Infiltrating lobular carcinoma of the breast. Histopathology 1982; 6: 149–61.

35. Middleton LP, Palacios DM, Bryant BR et al. Pleomorphic lobular carcinoma: morphology, immunohistochemistry and molecular analysis. Am J Surg Pathol 2000; 24: 1650–6.

36. Acs G, Lawton TJ, Rebbeck TR et al. Differential expression of E-cadherin in lobular and ductal neoplasms of the breast and its biologic and diagnostic implications. Am J Clin Pathol 2001; 115: 85–98.

37. Lehr H-A, Folpe A, Yaziji H et al. Cytokeratin 8 immunostaining pattern and E-cadherin expression distinguish lobular from ductal breast carcinoma. Am J Clin Pathol 2000; 114: 190–6.

38. Foote FW Jr, Stewart FW. Lobular carcinoma in situ: a rare form of mammary cancer. Am J Pathol 1941; 17: 491–6.

39. Harris M, Howell A, Chrissohou M. et al. A comparison of the metastatic pattern of infiltrating lobular carcinoma and infiltrating duct carcinoma of the breast. Br J Cancer 1984; 50: 23–30.

40. Cooper HS, Patchefsky AS, Krall RA. Tubular carcinoma of the breast. Cancer 1978; 42: 2334 -42.

41. Howell LP. Pitfalls in the cytologic diagnosis of lobular carcinoma of the breast. ASCP Checksample C19– 4, 1991.

42. Martinez V, Azzopardi JG. Invasive lobular carcinoma of the breast: incidence and variants. Histopathology 1979; 3: 467–8.

43. Fisher ER, Gregorio RM, Redmond C, Fisher B. Tubulolobular invasive breast cancer: a variant of lobular invasive breast cancer. Hum Pathol 1977; 8: 679–83.

44. du Toit RS, Locker AP, Ellis IO et al. Invasive lobular carcinomas of the breast – the prognosis of histopathological subtypes. Br J Cancer 1989; 60: 605–9.

45. Frost A, Terahata S, Yeh I et al. The significance of signet ring cells in infiltrating lobular carcinoma of the breast. Mod Pathol 1993; 6: 15A.

46. Nesland JM, Hom R, Johannessen JV. Ultrastructural and immunohistochemical features of lobular carcinoma of the breast. J Pathol 1985; 145: 39–52.

47. Rosen PP. Rosen's Breast Pathology, 2nd edn. Philadelphia: Lippincott Williams & Wilkins, 2001.

48. Komaki K, Sakamoto G, Sugano H et al. Mucinous carcinoma of the breast in Japan. A prognostic analysis based on morphologic features. Cancer 1988; 61: 989–96.

49. Toikkanen S, Kujari H. Pure and mixed carcinomas of the breast: a clinicopathologic analysis of 61 cases with long-term follow-up. Hum Pathol 1989; 20: 758–64.

50. Rosen PP, Wang T. Colloid carcinoma of the breast. Analysis of 64 patients with long-term follow-up. Am J Clin Pathol 1980; 73: 304.

51. Rosen PP, Lesser ML, Kinne DW. Breast carcinoma at the extremes of age: a comparison of patients younger than 35 years and older than 75 years. J Surg Oncol 1985; 28: 90–6.

52. Renshaw AA. Can mucinous lesions of the breast be reliably diagnosed by core needle biopsy? Am J Clin Pathol 2002; 118: 82–4.

53. Andre S, Cunha F, Bernardo M et al. Mucinous carcinoma of the breast: a pathologic study of 82 cases. J Surg Oncol 1995; 58: 162–7.

54. Ro JY, Sneige N, Sahin AA et al. Mucocele-like tumor of the breast associated with atypical duct hyperplasia or mucinous carcinoma. A clinicopathologic study of seven cases. Arch Pathol Lab Med 1991; 115: 137–40.

55. Saponi A, Righi I, Cassoni P et al. Expression of apocrine differentiation markers in neuroendocrine breast carcinomas of aged women. Mod Pathol 2001; 14: 768–76.

56. Shousha S, Coady AT, Stamp T et al. Oestrogen receptors in mucinous carcinoma of the breast: an immunohistochemical study using paraffin wax sections. J Clin Pathol 1989; 42: 902–5.

57. Rasmussen BB, Rose C, Christensen IB. Prognostic factors in primary mucinous breast carcinoma. Am J Clin Pathol 1987; 87: 155–60.

58. Murad TM, Swaid S, Pritchett P. Malignant and benign papillary lesions of the breast. Hum Pathol 1977; 8: 379–90.

59. Tiltman AJ. DNA ploidy in papillary tumours of the breast. South Afr Med J 1989; 75: 379–80.

60. Michael CW, Buschmann B. Can true papillary neoplasms of breast and their mimickers be accurately classified by cytology? Cancer 2002; 96; 92–100.

61. Carter D, Orr SL, Merino MJ. Intracystic papillary carcinoma of the breast after mastectomy, radiotherapy or excisional biopsy alone. Cancer 1983; 52: 14–19.

62. Papotti M, Eusebi V, Gugliotta P, Bussolati G. Immuno-histochemical analysis of benign and malignant papillary lesions of the breast. Am J Surg Pathol 1983; 7: 451–61.

63. Siriaunkgul S, Tavassoli FA. Invasive micropapillary carcinoma of the breast. Mod Pathol 1993; 6: 660–2.

64. Lunamore S, Gonzalez B, Acedo C et al. Invasive micropapillary carcinoma of the breast – a new special type of invasive mammary carcinoma. Pathol Res Pract 1994; 190: 668–74.

65. Middleton LP, Tressera F, Sobel ME et al. Infiltrating micropapillary carcinoma of the breast. Mod Pathol 1999; 12: 499-504.

66. Page DL, Dixon JM, Anderson TJ et al. Invasive cribriform carcinoma of the breast. Histopathology 1983; 7: 525–36.

67. Bloom HJ, Richardson WW, Fields JR. Host resistance and survival in carcinoma of the breast: a study of 104 cases of medullary carcinoma in a series of 1411 cases of breast cancer followed for 20 years. BMJ 1970; iii: 181–8.

68. Rapin V, Contesso G, Mouriesse H et al. Medullary breast carcinoma. A reevaluation of 95 cases of breast cancer with inflammatory stroma. Cancer 1988; 61: 2503–10.

69. Harris M, Lessells AM. The ultrastructure of medullary, atypical medullary and non-medullary carcinomas of the breast. Histopathology 1986; 10: 405–14.

70. Rosen PP, Lesser ML, Senie RT, Duthie K. Epidemiology of breast carcinoma IV: Age and histologic tumor type. J Surg Oncol 1982; 19: 44–51.

71. Rubens JR, Lewandrowski KBB, Kopans DB et al. Medullary carcinoma of the breast: overdiagnosis of a prognostically favorable neoplasm. Arch Surg 1990; 125: 601–4.

72. Ridolfi RL, Rosen PP, Port A et al. Medullary carcinoma of the breast: a clinicopathologic study with 10 year follow-up. Cancer 1997; 40: 1365–85.

73. Shivas AA, Hunt CT. Cultural characteristics of an apocrine variant of human mammary carcinoma. Clin Oncol 1979; 5: 299–303.

74. Eusubi V, Betts C, Haagensen DE et al. Apocrine differentiation in lobular carcinoma of the breast: a morphologic, immunologic and ultrastructural study. Hum Pathol 1984; 15: 134–40.

75. Armin A, Connelly EM, Rowden G. An immunoperoxidase investigation of S-100 protein in granular cell myoblastomas:evidence for Schwann cell derivation. Am J Clin Pathol 1983: 79: 37–44.

76. D'Amore ES, Terrier-Lacombe MJ, Travagli JP et al. Invasive apocrine carcinoma of the breast: a long term follow-up study of 34 cases. Breast Cancer Res Treat 1988; 12: 37–44.

77. Abati AD, Kimmel M, Rosen PP. Apocrine mammary carcinoma. A clinicopathologic study of 72 cases. Am J Clin Pathol 1990; 94: 371–7.

78. Oberman HA. Metaplastic carcinoma of the breast. Am J Surg Pathol 1987; 11: 918–29.

79. Eusebi V, Cattani MG, Ceccarelli C, Lamovec J. Sarcoma-toid carcinomas of the breast: an immunocytochemical study of 14 cases. Prog Surg Path 1989; 10: 83–99.

80. Wargotz ES, Norris HJ. Metaplastic carcinoma of the breast. I. Matrix-producing carcinoma. Hum Pathol 1989; 20: 628–35.

81. Wargotz ES, Deos PH, Norris HJ. Metaplastic carcinomas of the breast. II Spindle cell carcinoma. Hum Pathol 1989; 20: 732–40.

82. Wargotz ES, Norris HJ. Metaplastic carcinomas of the breast. III. Carcinosarcoma. Cancer 1989; 64: 1490–9.

83. Kaufman MW, Marti JR, Gallager HS, Hoehn JL. Carcinoma of the breast with pseudosarcomatous metaplasia. Cancer 1984; 53: 1908–17.

84. Wargotz ES, Norris HJ. Metaplastic carcinomas of the breast. IV. Squamous cell carcinoma of ductal origin. Cancer 1990; 65: 272–6.

85. Ahmad A, Hanby AM, Poulson R et al. Stromelysin 3; an independent prognostic factor for relapse-free survival in node-positive breast cancer and demonstration of novel breast carcinoma expression. Am J Pathol 1998; 152: 721–8.

86. Anthony PP, James PD. Adenoid cystic carcinoma of the breast: prevalence, diagnostic criteria and histogenesis. J Clin Pathol 1975; 28: 647–55.

87. Rosen PP. Adenoid cystic carcinoma of the breast: a morphologically heterogenous neoplasm. Pathol Annu 1989; 24: 237–54.

88. Hjorth S, Magnusson PH, Blomquiste PJ. Adenoid cystic carcinoma of the breast. Report of a case in a male and review of the literature. Acta Chir Scan 1977; 143: 155–8.

89. Shin SJ, Rosen PP. Solid variant of mammary adenoid cystic carcinoma with basaloid features. Am J Surg Pathol 2002; 26: 413–20.

90. Cubilla AL, Woodruff JM. Primary carcinoid tumor of the breast. A report of eight patients. Am J Surg Pathol 1977; 1: 283–92.

91. Azzopardi JG, Muretto P, Goddeeris P et al. Carcinoid tumors of the breast: the morphological spectrum of argyrophil carcinomas. Histopathology 1982; 6: 549–69.

92. Sariola H, Lehtonen E, Saxen E. Breast tumors with a solid and uniform carcinoid pattern. Ultrastructural and immunohistochemical study of two cases. Pathol Res Pract 1985; 179: 405–11.

93. Clayton F, Sibley RK, Ordonez NG, Hanssen G. Argyrophilic breast carcinomas: evidence of lactational differentiation. Am J Surg Pathol 1982; 6: 323–33.

94. Tavassoli FA, Norris HJ. Secretory carcinoma of the breast. Cancer 1980; 45: 2404–13.

95. Norris JH, Taylor HB. Carcinoma of the breast in women less than 30 years old. Cancer 1970; 26: 953–9.

96. McDivitt RW, Stewart FW. Breast carcinoma in children. JAMA 1966; 195: 144–6.

97. Oberman HA. Secretory carcinoma of the breast in adults. Am J Surg Pathol 1980; 4: 465–70.

98. Rosen PP, Cranor ML. Secretory carcinoma of the breast. Arch Pathol Lab Med 1991; 115: 141–4.

99. Rosen PP, Scott M. Cystic hypersecretory duct carcinoma of the breast. Am J Surg Pathol 1984; 8: 31–41.

100. Ramos CV, Taylor HB. Lipid-rich carcinoma of the breast. A clinicopathologic analysis of 13 examples. Cancer 1974; 33: 812–19.

101. Fisher ER, Tavares J, Bulatao IS et al. Glycogen-rich, clear cell breast cancer: with comments concerning other clear cell variants. Hum Pathol 1985; 16: 1085–90.

102. Robbins GF, Shah J, Rosen PP et al. Inflammatory carcinoma of the breast. Surg Clin North Am 1974; 54: 801–10.

103. Guerin GM, Gabillot M, Mathieu MC et al. Structure and expression of cerbB-2 and EGF receptor genes in inflammatory and non-inflammatory breast cancer: prognostic significance. Int J Cancer 1989; 43: 201–8.

104. Wertheim U, Ozello L. Neoplastic involvement of nipple and skin flap in carcinoma of the breast. Am J Surg Pathol 1980; 4: 543–9.

105. Patchefsky AS, Frauenhoffer CM, Krall RA, Cooper HS. Low grade mucoepidermoid carcinoma of the breast. Arch Pathol Lab Med 1979; 103: 196–8.

106. Wargotz ES, Norris HJ. Metaplastic carcinomas of the breast. IV. Squamous cell carcinoma of ductal origin. Cancer 1990; 65: 272–6.

107. Shin SJ, DeLellis RA, Rosen PP. Small cell carcinoma of the breast – additional immunohistochemical studies. Am J Surg Pathol 2001; 25: 831–2.

108. Kaufman MW, Maerti JR, Gallager HS, Hoehn JI. Carcinoma of the breast with pseudosarcomatous metaplasia. Cancer 1984; 53: 1908–17.

109. Gonzales-Licea A, Yardley JH, Hartmann WH. Malignant tumour of the breast with bone formation studies of light and electron microscopy. Cancer 1967; 20: 1234–47.

110. Smith BH, Taylor HB. The occurrence of bone and cartilage in mammary tumours. Am J Clin Pathol 1969; 51: 610–18.

111. Fisher ER, Gregorio R, Redmond C et al. Pathologic findings from the national surgical adjuvant breast project (protocol No 4). I. Observations concerning the multicentricity of mammary cancer. 1975; 35: 247–54.

112. Lagios MD, Westdahl PR, Rose MR. The concept and implications of multicentricity in breast carcinoma. Pathol Annu 162: 83–102.

113. Egan RL, McSweeney MB. Multicentric breast carcinoma. Recent Results Cancer Res 1984; 90: 28–35.

114. Harris JR, Hellman S, Kinne DW. Limited surgery and radiotherapy for early breast cancer. N Engl J Med 1985; 313: 1365–8.

115. Jimenez RE, Wallis T, Visscher DW. Centrally necrosing carcinomas of the breast. A distinct histological subtype with aggressive clinical behaviour. Am J Surg Pathol 2001; 25: 831–2.

116. Claus EB, Risch N, Thompson WD, Carter D. Relationship between breast histopathology and family history of breast cancer. Cancer 1993; 71: 147–53.

117. Marcus JN, Watson P, Page DL et al. Hereditary breast cancer: Pathobiology, prognosis and BRCA1 and BRCA2 gene linkage. Cancer 1996; 77: 697–709.

118. Girling AC, Hanby AM, Millis RM. Radiation and other pathological changes in breast tissue after conservation treatment for carcinoma. J Clin Pathol 1990; 43: 152–6.

119. Rasbridge SA, Gillett CE, Seymour A-M et al. The effect of chemotherapy on morphology, cellular proliferation, apoptosis and oncoprotein expression in primary breast carcinoma. Br J Cancer 1994; 70: 335–41.

120. Hajdu SI, Urban JA. Cancers metastatic to the breast. Cancer 1972; 29: 1691–6.

121. Visfeldt J, Shieke O. Male breast cancer. I. Histologic typing and grading of 187 Danish cases. Cancer 1973; 32: 985–90.

122. Heller KS, Rosen PP, Schottenfeld D et al. Male breast cancer: a clinicopathological study of 97 cases. Ann Surg 1978; 188: 60–5.

28 Molecular investigation of breast disease

Chris Jones, Sunil R Lakhani

Introduction

The increasing use of mammographic screening over the last decade has led to an increased detection of preinvasive breast disease and highlighted the deficiencies in the pathological classification and our understanding of the biology of breast cancer. The development of quality assurance schemes (EQA) has led to considerable improvements in the standardisation of criteria and the reduction of inter-observer variability amongst pathologists.[1,2] However, some types of proliferation within the breast, such as atypical hyperplasia, remain problematic. There is a hope that the new molecular techniques will help to provide a classification that is more robust and clinically useful.

Technological advances over the last two decades have resulted in the development of techniques such as loss of heterozygosity (LOH),[3] comparative genomic hybridisation (CGH),[4] high-throughput mutational analysis, DNA sequencing and micro-arrays.[5] These techniques have made it easier to identify cancer-causing alterations, as well as changes in patterns of gene expression and protein function. Researchers are now in a position to investigate and quantify the many complex changes that occur during tumorigenesis. What are these techniques and how will they help in patient management?

Loss of heterozygosity (LOH)

In 1971, Knudson[6] proposed his 'two-hit' hypothesis for the presence of cancer-causing genes that we now refer to as tumour suppressor genes (TSG). The recognition that the second mutation that leads to inactivation of the gene is usually in the form of a large deletion led to the development of the technique of LOH by Cavenee et al[3] in 1983. The technique relies on the observation that markers (microsatellites) that are heterozygous and near the TSG would become homo- or hemizygous in the tumour compared with normal tissue. This was confirmed in the case of retinoblastoma, where markers close to the gene were seen to exhibit LOH in both sporadic and familial cancers.[3]

Since the introduction of the technique by Cavenee et al,[3] there have been numerous studies looking at LOH in invasive breast cancers as well as the putative precancerous lesions. LOH has been identified at almost all chromosomal locations within the genome, with high frequencies of LOH as loci on chromosomes 1p, 1q, 3p, 6q, 8p, 11q, 13q, 16q, 17p, 17q and 22q.[7] Although patterns of LOH have been reported in some series as being of prognostic significance, this information has not yet been translated into routine practice.

LOH has also been used extensively to investigate precancerous lesions in the hope that patterns of LOH would help to stratify lesions into 'benign' and 'malignant'. It has been apparent that many lesions traditionally thought of as 'benign' are monoclonal and that there is considerable overlap in LOH between these lesions and those accepted as 'malignant' (i.e. DCIS) – hence, at present, there are no robust profiles using LOH that help to definitively distinguish such lesions in clinical practice.[8–10]

Because the LOH technique requires extraction of DNA, and analysis of only a small number of microsatellites may be carried out at a time, it is a labour-intensive technique. The information is very specific for a chromosomal location; however, in order to get detailed information about any region, many microsatellites have to be investigated. The use of in situ hybridisation and the modifications of these techniques have gone some way to addressing this problem.

Comparative genomic hybridisation (CGH)

CGH is a fluorescent in situ hybridisation (FISH) technique capable of determining changes in DNA copy number between differentially labelled test (e.g. tumour) and reference (e.g. normal) samples. Unlike LOH analysis, which gives information at a very specific locus on a chromosomal arm, CGH analysis provides information from the entire genome. This has the advantage that a single experiment can give an idea about the many changes on all the different chromosomes – data that would require hundreds of experiments using LOH analysis. Traditionally, CGH has been done using competitive hybridisation to normal metaphase chromosomes – hence its resolution is poor, and it is only capable of detecting high-level amplifications of around 2 Mb, and deletions of the order of 10 Mb. Hence there is a compromise between global information and identifying very specific location of the change. Figure 28.1a,b show a classical CGH profile from an invasive breast cancer. As can be seen, numerous gains and losses of DNA material are identified in malignant epithelial cells.

Many investigators have used CGH analysis to understand the changes in DNA copy number in invasive cancer as well as in precancerous lesions.[11,12] As yet, specific profiles that are of prognostic significance or predict for response to therapy have not been developed for routine use, but clearly there is a hope that such a profile may be developed in time. One of the most significant contributions has been in delineating the pathways for the development of cancer from preinvasive breast disease. CGH analysis has contributed considerable data in recognising that low-grade DCIS and low-grade invasive breast cancers arise via a separate pathway from high-grade DCIS and high-grade invasive carcinoma.[12,13] Hence the traditional concept of 'de-differentiation' of cancers with time appears to be wrong.

The application of array technology to CGH[14] has markedly improved the resolution of the technique. The main platform developed for array-based CGH involves the spotting of DNA sequences in the form of BAC (bacterial artificial chromosome) clones (large genomic bacterial clones) onto glass slides.[15] An array of 3000 BAC clones evenly spaced throughout the genome gives a resolution of the order of 1 Mb. As more defined BAC clones become available, the resolution will increase considerably

to a few hundred kilobases. The technique again relies on the hybridisation of differentially labelled test and reference samples to the slide, and a line plot of array ratios from across the genome can be generated, identifying amplifications and deletions from defined cytogenetic locations (Figure 28.1c). Microarray technology based on the spotting of cDNA clones corresponding to specific genes, developed for the profiling of gene expression at the mRNA level (see below), may also be utilised for genomic profiling on a gene-by-gene level by CGH.[14]

CGH arrays could play an important role in understanding the biology of breast cancer, and in tumour classification by a number of means. There is a considerable amount of data indicating that specific amplicons, such as the c-erbB-2 (HER2/neu) gene encoding the receptor tyrosine kinase HER2 (c-ErbB-2), have prognostic significance or are predictive of response to therapy.[16] The ability to identify such amplicons quickly and from formalin-fixed material would allow use in routine pathology practice. Already, FISH-based detection of c-erbB-2 amplification on paraffin sections has begun to make an impact in clinical management decisions.[17] This type of approach may be superior to immunohistochemistry, which continues to have problems of specificity and sensitivity. Array-based CGH profiling has the ability to identify copy number changes across the whole genome in a single experiment, and the power associated with the measurement of multiple oncogenic markers should provide a far greater specificity for the development of new diagnostic and prognostic approaches. Because this procedure involves DNA rather than RNA, can be performed on small samples microdissected from archival material[18] and is highly reproducible, it will be useful in the study of putative precancerous lesions. The identification of CGH profiles could in theory play a major role in subdividing precancerous lesions into those that need treatment versus those that require follow-up only.

Although the initial data derived from CGH arrays may not provide complete information about the cellular abnormalities of a tumour, it could be followed up by a more detailed array analysis, by LOH analysis, FISH or direct sequencing of candidate genes. Recently, a large number of single-nucleotide polymorphisms (SNPs)[19] have also been identified in the human genome. These polymorphisms may well be associated with differences in disease pathogenesis and outcome, and may also be used to indicate the most appropriate treatment for subtypes of cancer. Large-scale studies investigating these associations are awaited with interest, and may form an important adjunct to pathological analysis.

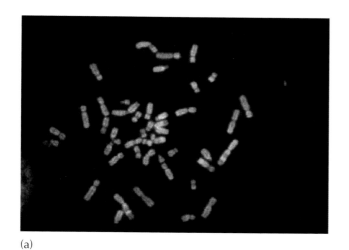

(a)

Figure 28.1 Comparative genomic hybridisation (CGH) of invasive ductal carcinoma. (a) Multiple fluorescence image showing regions of amplification (green) and deletion (red) in the tumour. (b) A number of metaphase spreads are analysed, allowing for the calculation of mean fluorescence ratios and confidence limits across the whole genome; almost all chromosomes have regions of increased or decreased copy number changes. (c) Array CGH profile of invasive ductal carcinoma; fluorescence ratios are calculated for bacterial artificial chromosome (BAC) clones aligned in order across the genome, highlighting regions or amplification and deletion, as shown here on chromosome 2.

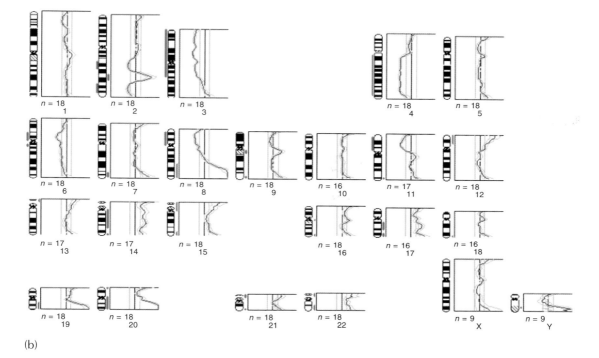

(b)

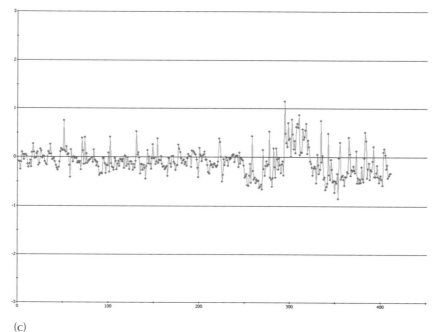

(c)

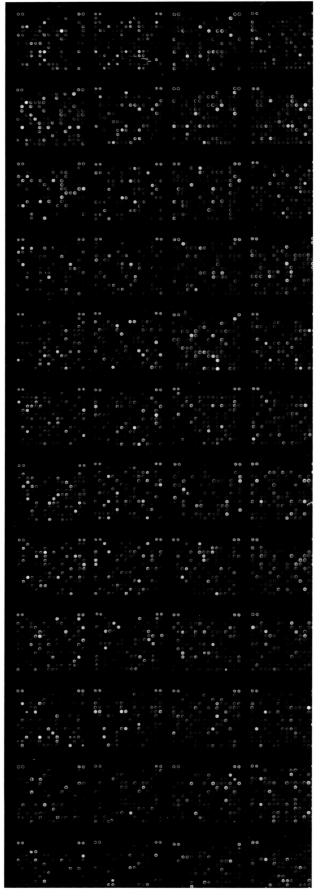

(a)

Expression arrays

As well as cataloguing the amplifications, deletions and complex rearrangements at the genomic (DNA) level, analysis of changes in the profiles of gene expression (mRNA) may give clues to the underlying molecular events in breast tumorigenesis. Two main platforms are available for the analysis of gene expression by microarrays. The first involves the construction of high-density oligonucleotide arrays by photolithography directly onto the solid support, as developed by Affymetrix.[20] These GeneChips may consist of tens of thousands of short (25-mer) probes, and may be utilised for mutational analysis, detection of SNPs and sequencing, as well as expression profiling.

The second technique used for measuring transcript levels is cDNA microarrays, pioneered by Pat Brown and colleagues.[21] These consist of thousands of sequences complementary to transcripts of known genes or expressed sequence tags (ESTs) robotically arrayed onto a glass slide. Analogous to CGH, two-colour hybridisation experiments may be carried out using RNA reverse-transcribed and labelled with fluorescent dyes such as Cy3- and Cy5-dCTP (Figure 28.2a,b). The samples are mixed and co-hybridised

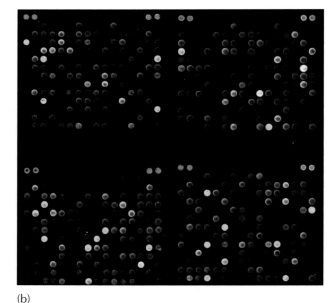

(b)

Figure 28.2 (a) A glass slide containing 10 000 cDNA spots following hybridisation of a tumour sample. A higher-power view is shown in (b). The yellow dots represent genes that are expressed equally in both channels (tumour and reference). Genes differentially expressed between the two samples are represented by red and green spots The top row of each subarray contains a number of control genes that are included on the slide for quality control.

to the arrays in a competitive manner, and the resulting fluorescence values reveal the relative levels of each RNA transcript in the test sample compared with the reference sample. Mathematical algorithms (Figure 28.3) are used by bioinformaticians to probe differences in expression patterns between sample sets. These may involve the use of hierarchical clustering, principle components analysis, artificial neural networks, support vector machines and others. Expression profiles generated by cDNA arrays can reveal similarities and differences that are not necessarily evident from traditional approaches, such as morphological or immunohistochemical analysis.

The power of this technique has been elegantly demonstrated in a number of papers.[22–24] The first showed that within the morphologically homogeneous category of large B-cell lymphoma, two subtypes exist with differing patterns of gene expression.[22] The second paper examined the expression profiles of 65 breast cancers using an array containing 8102 genes and also identified various subtypes, including an oestrogen receptor (ER)-negative group with basaloid features (tumours showing expression of markers seen in basal/myoepithelial cells, which are a normal constituent of the ductal-lobular system of the breast).[23,24]

These findings are not only interesting, but also reassuring. Although pathologists have been aware of basaloid breast cancer subsets, these are not currently treated as a distinct entity in clinical practice. Studies have already been published to suggest that basaloid tumours have different gene expression and metastatic patterns, and should therefore have a different prognosis compared with ductal carcinomas of no special type.[25–27] Array-based technologies may now be used to identify specific markers that will refine this subset of breast cancers. A paper by van't Veer et al[28] has further demonstrated the power of the new technology by identifying an expression signature that predicts for metastatic disease. This type of analysis will pave the way for future clinical applications.

However, a number of important issues must be addressed before expression profiling becomes a commonplace tool in the pathologist's laboratory. Expression profiling relies on the preservation of mRNA species from the tissue of interest. Traditional formalin fixation used in routine histopathology leads to degradation of RNA, so fresh-frozen material is required. Alternatively, ethanol-based fixatives may be used. Obtaining frozen material is not difficult. Freezing, however, produces artefacts by distorting the cellular architecture and cytological

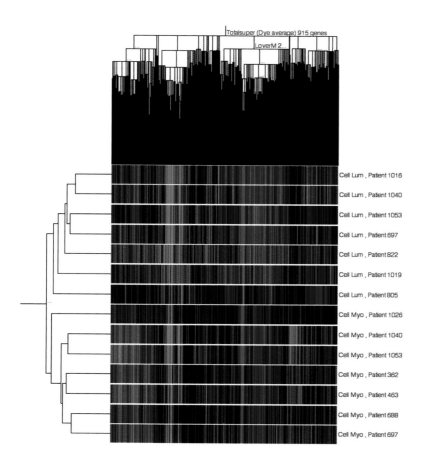

Figure 28.3 Hierarchical clustering algorithms can be used to subclassify samples after expression array analysis. In this case, the expression of genes in purified normal luminal epithelial and myoepithelial cells is shown. Each row represents a sample, while each column represents a gene. It is easy to appreciate that the samples are separated into the two cell types by their patterns of gene expression.

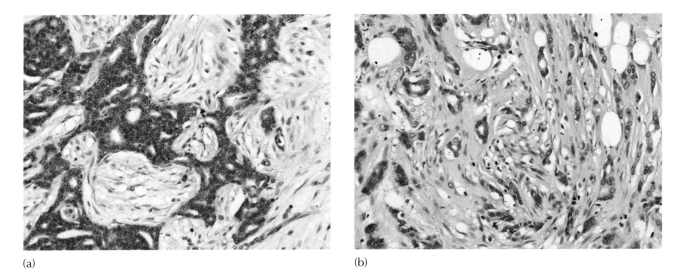

(a)　　　　　　　　　　　　　　　　　　　　　　(b)

Figure 28.4 Both of these tumours were from the same histological section and adjacent to each other. (a) is a ductal cancer with cribriform growth pattern, while (b) is a tubular carcinoma.

features that are used to classify precancerous lesions. Laser capture microdissection can be used to obtain defined cell populations; however, the primary diagnosis of the lesions (hyperplasia, atypical hyperplasia or in situ carcinoma) is difficult on frozen sections. Hence, although microarray technology is producing new and valuable insights into tumour biology, we will have to await further technological development before it can be used routinely in evaluating precancerous lesions, which are now diagnosed with increasing frequency due to improved screening programmes.

The second problem in using gene expression profiles to categorise tumours is one of tissue heterogeneity. Normal tissues are made up of many different cell types, including endothelium, different types of stromal cells and inflammatory cells. Cancer cells within a tumour are also heterogeneous. The use of clustering algorithms that allow in silico subtraction of normal tissue elements should make a significant contribution to solving the problem of contamination with normal tissue. However, this technology will not necessarily solve the problem of intratumour heterogeneity, as these data are presented as a composite of the whole population, providing an average snapshot.

It will be difficult to determine whether a gene that has been observed to increase expression in a tumour is upregulated in every cell of the tumour or whether its transcription is only activated in specific subclones. Figure 28.4(a,b) illustrate a case of breast cancer where two apparently distinct tumours exist side by side. If the whole tumour were excised, made into RNA and analysed by expression profil-

ing, the data would not reflect the heterogeneous nature of this tumour. Should these be treated as two separate tumours and analysed separately?

Currently, the technology does not readily lend itself to formalin-fixed, archival material, and thus to microdissection strategies to address these problems. However, advances in linear RNA amplification methodology are such that in the near future we can expect to be able to accurately profile the transcripts of small numbers of cells identified by routine histopathological analysis, and begin to answer some of the questions regarding intratumoral heterogeneity and tumour–stromal interactions as well as the relationship between the overt cancerous cells and their benign putative precursor lesions.

An additional problem is one of data comparison between experiments and laboratories. Data derived from experiments involving oligonucleotides are not directly comparable with those involving cDNAs. Furthermore, there is no universally consistent standard sample that can be used to normalise data. At present, there is little agreement about the number of replicates or the statistical rigour to which the data should be subjected. These issues are currently being addressed and doubtless will be solved in the future.

Protein arrays

Protein molecules, rather than DNA or RNA, carry out most cellular functions. Direct measurement of protein levels and activity within the cell is likely to be the best determinant of overall cell function.

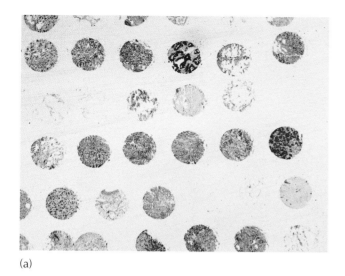

(a)

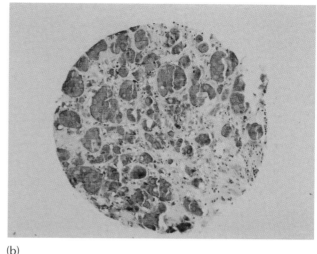

(b)

Figure 28.5a,b (a) Low-power (×10) view of a tissue array. Numerous 0.6 mm cores of breast cancers are embedded into a paraffin block to create the array. Molecules identified as differentially expressed in the array experiments can then be tested on the tissue arrays to evaluate their significance in a large number of human breast cancers. (b) High-power view (×400) of one such core.

Techniques are being developed to quantify the levels of all the proteins within a cell and compare protein levels between different cell types. Proteomic analysis, consisting of two-dimensional gel electrophoresis (2D-PAGE) and tandem mass spectrometry, has been used to map protein profiles in normal[29] and tumour cells. As would be expected, the studies have highlighted differences in protein profiles between subsets of normal cells (luminal versus myoepithelial cells), and these will form the basis for future comparisons between the tumour and normal cells. It is unlikely that the 'proteome' is stable over time, as the cell's requirements are constantly changing as it adapts to its environment. Any proteomic data is therefore likely to represent only a snapshot of the 'proteome'.

At present, the technique is labour-intensive and requires large amounts of purified samples. It is therefore not yet appropriate for use in clinical practice. However, the use of this technology will undoubtedly lead to the identification of new cancer-associated proteins. These proteins could then be validated on a larger number of samples using tissue arrays (Figure 28.5a,b),[30,31] and eventually developed as molecular markers for cancer diagnosis or prognosis. This will necessitate the development of specific antibody or in situ hybridisation probes. At present, the technology allows the identification of 2000–3000 gene products per experiment; this is less than 10% of the cell's total proteome, and a much smaller proportion of all different isoforms of individual proteins.

Advances in technology such as non-gel-based fractionation systems should allow resolution of most cellular proteins, including isoforms, in the future. Within the next few years, a protein chip may well be developed for use in clinical diagnostic practice. It would contain several hundred or thousand antibodies that could be used to measure cellular protein levels in an automated fashion.

Conclusion

Pathological assessment of tissues has remained the linchpin of diagnostic practice for over a hundred years. It has become the core science of clinical medical practice, providing data for clinical management and a framework for future correlation of new markers and new therapies. In light of the new technologies, will histopathology disappear as a speciality? Some pathologists worry that one day, the surgeon will take a small biopsy of the tumour and array analysis will produce a 'unique fingerprint'. The patient will receive individualised treatment based on the data. The pathologist may as well pack his bag.

We believe that this is an unlikely scenario, at least for the next 10–20 years. The array-based technology will undoubtedly add to and modify current pathological classifications. It will also modify or replace the current methods of grading tumours. But since the existing classifications are the basis for validation of the new techniques, it is more likely that the two will develop a symbiotic relationship, the new data refining the current classifications, which in turn will allow further correlation and validation of the new techniques. It is clear from preliminary molecular analysis of tumours and their preinvasive lesions that they share many genetic abnormalities. It is not easy to distinguish various types of in situ carcinomas from the invasive cancers. Hence it is difficult to see at present how the array technology will help to ascertain with absolute certainty whether a sample is a pure in situ cancer or an invasive cancer (and hence requiring different treatments). However, the developments are so fast in this area that even this problem might be solved in the near future.

It is not yet clear whether gene expression data can be used to differentiate a primary cancer from metastases. One area where this technology will play an increasing role is in the identification of 'metastases of unknown primary', which are currently treated on an empirical basis on best guess. At present, it is difficult to see how expression profile analysis will substitute for staging information such as tumour size, which has been demonstrated to have good prognostic value. Even when these problems have been addressed, we may still be limited by the availability of treatment options. If ductal carcinoma of the breast could be separated into 20 different subtypes on the basis of expression profiling but only two treatment options were available, we would not immediately realise the aim of 'individualised treatment'. Nevertheless, this subclassification itself as well as the microarray technology will facilitate the identification of an enormous number of targets for future development of new therapeutic strategies.

Over the last decade, pathologists have grasped the nettle of quality assurance. It is recognised that pathological diagnosis is subjective and standardisation is necessary to avoid the same tumour being classified differently between institutions with resultant implications for therapy. There has been an increase in litigation for 'wrong' diagnosis. Molecular techniques, which are perceived as 'scientific' rather than 'subjective', will still have to undergo a continuous period of quality control. Otherwise, a cancer patient's 'tumour fingerprint' will vary, depending on the laboratory in which the sample is analysed.

The most realistic scenario is that in the near future, researchers will use the new technologies to identify, for each tumour type, a panel of proteins that allow it to be categorised into a particular subtype. Tumours can then be further characterised using immunohistochemistry on tissue sections. In the longer term, the resection or biopsy sample will still go to the pathologist, who will examine and assess the specimen by conventional means. A sample will also be used for array-based genomic, transcription and even protein analysis. The combined data, perhaps in combination with neural networks,[32] will produce a 'unique tumour fingerprint'; however, the patient will likely receive one of a small number of available treatments. Over a longer time period (perhaps 10 years plus), microarray technology may result in translation of more therapeutic options into the clinic.

With the current explosion of technology and data, it is important for pathologists and other clinical specialists to embrace and incorporate these changes into their training and practice. Molecular biologists will also benefit from a closer interaction with pathologists. It is, however, difficult to be dogmatic about any of these issues, given the pace of progress.

Acknowledgements

We are grateful to Alan MacKay, Dr Peter Simpson and Professor Michael O'Hare for allowing us to use some data from the experiments using cDNA microarrays and tissue arrays and to Dr Alsam for histological figures of tissue heterogeneity.

References

1. Sloane JP, Ellman R, Anderson TJ et al. Consistency of histopathological reporting of breast lesions detected by screening: findings of the U.K. National External Quality Assessment (EQA) Scheme. Eur J Cancer 1994; 30A: 1414–19.

2. Sloane JP, Amendoeira I, Apostolikas N et al. Consistency achieved by 23 European pathologists from 12 countries in diagnosing breast disease and reporting prognostic features of carcinomas. European Commission Working Group on Breast Screening Pathology. Virchows Arch 1999; 434: 3–10.

3. Cavenee WK, Dryja TP, Phillips RA et al. Expression of recessive alleles by chromosomal mechanisms in retinoblastoma. Nature 1983; 305: 779–84.

4. Kallioniemi A, Kallioniemi OP, Sudar D et al. Comparative genomic hybridization for molecular cytogenetic analysis of solid tumors. Science 1992; 258: 818–21.

5. Schena M, Shalon D, Davis RW, Brown PO. Quantitative monitoring of gene expression patterns with a complementary DNA microarray. Science 1995; 270: 467–70.

6. Knudson AJ. Mutation and cancer: statistical study of retinoblastoma. Proc Natl Acad Sci USA 1971; 68: 820–3.

7. Devilee P, Cornelisse CJ. Somatic genetic changes in human breast cancer. Biochim Biophys Acta 1994; 1198: 113–30.

8. Stratton MR, Collins N, Lakhani SR, Sloane JP. Loss of

heterozygosity in ductal carcinoma in situ of the breast. J Pathol 1995; 175: 195–201.

9. Lakhani S, Collins N, Sloane J, Stratton M. Loss of heterozygosity in lobular carcinoma in situ of the breast. J Clin Pathol: Mol Pathol 1995; 48: M74–8.

10. Lakhani SR, Collins N, Stratton MR, Sloane JP. Atypical ductal hyperplasia of the breast: clonal proliferation with loss of heterozygosity on chromosomes 16q and 17p. J Clin Pathol 1995; 48: 611–15.

11. Tirkkonen M, Tanner M, Karhu R et al. Molecular cytogenetics of primary breast cancer by CGH. Genes Chromosomes Cancer 1998; 21: 177–84.

12. Buerger H, Otterbach F, Simon R et al. Comparative genomic hybridization of ductal carcinoma in situ of the breast – evidence of multiple genetic pathways. J Pathol 1999; 187: 396–402.

13. Vos CB, ter Haar NT, Rosenberg C et al. Genetic alterations on chromosome 16 and 17 are important features of ductal carcinoma in situ of the breast and are associated with histologic type. Br J Cancer 1999; 81: 1410–18.

14. Pollack JR, Perou CM, Alizadeh AA et al. Genome-wide analysis of DNA copy-number changes using cDNA microarrays. Nat Genet 1999; 23: 41–6.

15. Pinkel D, Segraves R, Sudar D et al. High resolution analysis of DNA copy number variation using comparative genomic hybridization to microarrays. Nat Genet 1998; 20: 207–11.

16. Cobleigh MA, Vogel CL, Tripathy D et al. Multinational study of the efficacy and safety of humanized anti-HER2 monoclonal antibody in women who have HER2-overexpressing metastatic breast cancer that has progressed after chemotherapy for metastatic disease. J Clin Oncol 1999; 17: 2639–48.

17. Cell Markers and Cytogenetics Committees College Of American Pathologists. Clinical laboratory assays for HER-2/neu amplification and overexpression. Arch Pathol Lab Med 2002; 126: 803–8.

18. Simone NL, Bonner RF, Gillespie JW et al. Laser-capture microdissection: opening the microscopic frontier to molecular analysis. Trends Genet 1998; 14: 272–6.

19. Sapolsky RJ, Hsie L, Berno A et al. High-throughput polymorphism screening and genotyping with high-density oligonucleotide arrays. Genet Anal 1999; 14: 187–92.

20. Lipshutz RJ, Fodor SP, Gingeras TR, Lockhart DJ. High density synthetic oligonucleotide arrays. Nat Genet 1999; 21: 20–4.

21. Brown PO, Botstein D. Exploring the new world of the genome with DNA microarrays. Nat Genet 1999; 21: 33–7.

22. Alizadeh AA, Eisen MB, Davis RE et al. Distinct types of diffuse large B-cell lymphoma identified by gene expression profiling. Nature 2000; 403: 503–11.

23. Perou CM, Jeffrey SS, van de Rijn M et al. Distinctive gene expression patterns in human mammary epithelial cells and breast cancers. Proc Natl Acad Sci USA 1999; 96: 9212–17.

24. Perou CM, Sorlie T, Eisen MB et al. Molecular portraits of human breast tumours. Nature 2000; 406: 747–52.

25. Jones C, Foschini MP, Chaggar R et al. Comparative genomic hybridization analysis of myoepithelial carcinoma of the breast. Lab Invest 2000; 80: 831–6.

26. Jones C, Nonni AV, Fulford L et al. CGH analysis of ductal carcinoma of the breast with basaloid/myoepithelial cell differentiation. Br J Cancer 2001; 85: 422–7.

27. Tsuda H, Takarabe T, Hasegawa F et al. Large, central acellular zones indicating myoepithelial tumor differentiation in high-grade invasive ductal carcinomas as markers of predisposition to lung and brain metastases. Am J Surg Pathol 2000; 24: 197–202.

28. van 't Veer LJ, Dai H, van de Vijver MJ et al. Gene expression profiling predicts clinical outcome of breast cancer. Nature 2002; 415: 530–6.

29. Page MJ, Amess B, Townsend RR et al. Proteomic definition of normal human luminal and myoepithelial breast cells purified from reduction mammoplasties. Proc Natl Acad Sci USA 1999; 96: 12 589–94.

30. Kononen J, Bubendorf L, Kallioniemi A et al. Tissue microarrays for high-throughput molecular profiling of tumor specimens. Nat Med 1998; 4: 844–7.

31. Camp RL, Charette LA, Rimm DL. Validation of tissue microarray technology in breast carcinoma. Lab Invest 2000; 80: 1943–9.

32. Khan J, Wei JS, Ringner M et al. Classification and diagnostic prediction of cancers using gene expression profiling and artificial neural networks. Nat Med 2001; 7: 673–9.

29 Cytological and histological correlation in breast cytopathology

Peter Trott

Introduction

In the preoperative 'triple assessment' of breast lesions, needle aspiration was formerly the more widely used technique compared with core biopsy, in combination with clinical examination and radiographic findings. Recently, needle core biopsy is being increasingly used,[1] a major factor being the introduction of the biopsy 'gun', which relies on a firing action and is less painful than the Tru-cut needle.

Both techniques have their supporters and both have advantages and disadvantages.[2] Needle aspiration is in many ways a more convenient technique that is less painful for the patient and provides a fast answer. This is the diagnostic method used in 'one-stop clinics' in which the triple assessment is applied to provide a diagnosis during the clinic morning or afternoon session.

The disadvantage of the fine-needle aspiration technique concerns specificity, i.e. the ability to exclude carcinoma when absent, in which generally the core biopsy technique is the more accurate. However, both methods are very specific, with positive predictive values of more than 98%.[3] The core technique is not suitable for the identification of small and impalpable lesions, for which the wider sampling of the fine-needle approach has advantages.

The core biopsy is a histological diagnosis, so that distinguishing in situ from invasive carcinoma is possible, as is an attempt at histological grading. Furthermore, the specimen can be radiographed in cases presenting with microcalcification, and immunohistochemistry for estrogen receptors (ER) and other markers is more easily undertaken.

It is thus clear that the aspiration and core biopsy techniques are complementary and that the choice of technique should depend on clinical circumstances. In one centre, the frequency with which preoperative diagnoses could be made on screen-detected lesions increased from 72% using needle aspiration alone to 90% using the two techniques in combination.[4] These investigators also found that one or the other investigation was positive in 97% of patients found to be suitable for primary medical therapy.[5]

The findings of the aspiration or core biopsy techniques are particularly important when investigating solid breast masses in younger patients (under 35). Mammography is often unsatisfactory at this age because of the denseness of the breast, and the clinician is often inclined to discount a diagnosis of cancer in view of its rarity. Fibroadenomas, which are common in this age group, can be conclusively diagnosed by both the aspiration and the core biopsy techniques, as can the unexpected carcinoma. In a review by Yelland et al[6] of 150 women with breast cancer aged less than 35, needle aspiration was more effective in diagnosing carcinoma than clinical examination and mammography.

Although cytopathologists involved in breast fine-needle aspiration cytodiagnosis are less concerned with histopathological classifications than with the diagnosis of malignancy, a thorough understanding of the histopathological appearances of breast disease is essential for correct cytological interpretation.[7]

This is partly because individual cells in benign lesions can have alarming appearances and also because of the heterogenous nature of breast carcinoma, so that it is easy to imagine how a misdiagnosis of malignancy might be made.

Specificity and sensitivity

The cytological appearances of breast aspirates are related to the definitive histopathological appearances, and the accuracy of the cytological diagnosis is compared in this way. By dividing all breast pathology into benign or malignant, the accuracy of the cytology can be determined. Unfortunately, the statistical methods of analysis of this information vary considerably in published papers, and some reports, for example, take into account equivocal or suspicious diagnoses when assessing positive predictive value while others only include definitive or certainly positive diagnoses. It is therefore appropriate to list definitions of the terms used commonly in published material to evaluate the efficacy of breast aspiration cytodiagnosis.

Absolute sensitivity

This refers to the number of carcinomas unequivocally diagnosed, expressed as a proportion of the total number of carcinomas aspirated. In other words, it is an expression of the ability of the test to give a positive result when cancer is present.

Complete sensitivity

Complete sensitivity is the number of carcinomas diagnosed positively, including those with equivocal appearances, expressed as a proportion of the total number of carcinomas aspirated. This figure has particular relevance in stereotactic aspiration cytodiagnosis when detection rather than diagnosis is more important.

Specificity

Specificity is the number of correctly identified benign lesions expressed as a proportion of the total number of benign lesions aspirated. It is the corollary of sensitivity and demonstrates the ability to give a negative finding when cancer is absent.

Positive predictive value

Surgeons are particularly interested in the positive predictive value, as it indicates the degree of confidence with which they can regard a positive cytology result. When it is 100%, the clinician will know categorically that a positive (C5) diagnosis of cancer has always meant malignancy and therefore probably always will. If the analysis includes equivocal diagnoses then this should be made clear. A positive predictive value of an unequivocal positive result is the number of positive results minus those that are falsely positive expressed as a proportion of the total number of true-positive results.

False-negative rate

The false-negative rate is the number of falsely negative results expressed as a proportion of the total number of carcinomas aspirated.

Table 29.1 shows a list of comparative reporting data from seven large series. So far as it is possible, the same data have been extracted from each paper and presented in tabular form and a similar statistical analysis has been undertaken. These are the calculations of the absolute and complete sensitivities, specificity and positive and negative predictive values. The largest series is from Franzen and Zajicek,[8] who reported on 3119 cases. All the carcinomas were verified histologically and the specimens were taken by cytopathologists in the cytology clinic. Their results of 76% for absolute and 78% for complete sensitivity can be compared with those of the smaller series of Brown et al,[9] in which the aspirates were also performed by pathologists. Their sensitivity figures are also very high; indeed, the highest figure of complete sensitivity of 94% is in the Brown series and indicates in statistical terms the advantages of the pathologist aspirating the tumour.

Many papers show a positive predictive value of 100% and others show a value in the high 90s. This indicates the level of the diagnostic threshold that should be geared towards, only providing a diagnosis of carcinoma when this is certain. The phrase 'the interpreter should feel at ease in making such a diagnosis'[10] aptly sums up the diagnostic pathologist's attitude in this regard. Giard and Hermans[11] have highlighted the difficulties in attempting to compare the reported results of breast aspiration cytodiagnosis papers. They reviewed 29 articles, in which there were a total of 31 340 aspirations. As well as sensitivity and specificity, they included the likelihood ratios of four different results: definitely malignant, suspicious, benign and unsatisfactory. Their analysis showed striking differences between series in the diagnostic accuracy of aspiration cytodiagnosis. For example, patients with breast cancer had a chance of obtaining a 'definitely malignant' cytological diagnosis, with a positive predictive value ranging from 35% to 92%. It is hoped that, with more training and experience, the positive predictive value will rise universally.

False-positive rate

So far as false-positive reports are concerned, Jatoi and Trott[12] found four misdiagnoses of carcinoma in

Table 29.1	**Comparative reporting data**							
		Reference						
		29	**30**	**9**	**31**	**32**	**8[a]**	**14**
Total number of cases	a	1671	793	1002	480	1283	3119	1181
Total with carcinoma	b	1539	228	356	276	689	1099	1014
Cytology positive	c	1031	158	295	219	481	832	500
Suspicious	d	335	26	40	9	88	30	372
Negative	e	166	31	21	6	48	206	142
Total without carcinoma	f	132	565	646	204	594	2020	167
Cytology positive	g	0	0	0	0	2	1	2
Suspicious	h	27	3	10	0	53	23	19
Negative	i	46	470	636	129	338	1464	146
Inadequate rate (%)		23	13	0	42	21	12	0
Absolute sensitivity (%)	c/b	0.67	0.69	0.83	0.79	0.69	0.76	0.49
Complete sensitivity (%)	c+d/b	0.89	0.81	0.94	0.83	0.83	0.78	0.86
Specificity (%)	i/f	0.35	0.83	0.98	0.63	0.57	0.72	0.87
Positive predictive value (%)	c–g/c	1.00	1.00	1.00	1.00	0.995	0.998	0.998

[a]Includes cases of benign cysts.

an analysis of 1104 cases of positive breast aspirates seen consecutively over a 4-year period. This is an incidence of 0.36% and represents a positive predictive value of 99.6%. The benign conditions that led to false-positive diagnosis were radiation, granulomatous mastitis and fibroadenoma.

Grading

Following the establishment and recognition that histopathological grading has prognostic value and is reproducible, attempts have been made to grade breast carcinoma in needle aspirates. Mouriquand et al[13] devised three grades in smears stained by the Papanicolaou technique using six parameters: cell pattern, naked nuclei, nuclear pleomorphism, nuclear size, chromasia and mitotic figures. This analysis was compared with the TNM stage of disease, and appeared to have little advantage when this was taken into account. Using the same method, Ciatto et al[14] came to similar conclusions. There appeared to be rather more value in the method devised by Zajdela et al,[15] who measured the nuclear size with a micrometer in Giemsa-stained smears and related this to the stage of the disease. In the Netherlands, techniques using image analysis morphometry have shown that a division of cases can be achieved that correlates with histological diagnosis and survival.[16]

The advent of primary (neoadjuvant) chemotherapy has prompted a need for cytological grading as a replacement for histological grading, which may only become possible after therapy. A Nottingham scheme[17] relies on three cytological features that can easily be assessed in routinely prepared air-dried Giemsa-stained smears: the measurement of nuclear diameter compared with the diameter of a red blood cell, nuclear pleomorphism and abnormal nucleoli. Cases are divided into low-grade and high-grade tumours, and the method is effective in the identification of high-grade histological tumours (grade 3) but has poor discrimination for histological grades 1 and 2.

In Guildford, Robinson et al[18] have established three cytological grades using several diagnostic parameters: extent of cell dissociation, cell size and uniformity and the appearance of nucleoli, the nuclear margin, and chromatin. In an analysis of 28 invasive ductal carcinomas, they showed that the grading matched well with conventional histological grading. They used wet-fixed smears stained by the Papanicolaou technique.

These observations are potentially extremely important because in patients undergoing primary chemotherapy or endocrine therapy, the histological features relating to prognosis are compromised in that tumour size and the lymph node status and histological grade are unknown before therapy is given.[19] Any clue to the biological nature of the tumour that can be derived before treatment from a cytological aspirate specimen may prove to be of great value.

The methods of evaluation have been outlined by Dowsett et al,[20] who described how the treatment of primary breast cancer by medical therapy prior to surgery has provided an opportunity to collect multiple samples of tumour using Tru-cut core biopsies and fine-needle aspirates. The Tru-cut sample, in which tissue architecture is retained, provides a core of tissue that can be snap-frozen for frozen-section examination or embedded in paraffin wax. The needle aspirate sample[21] is obtained into 2 ml of medium and cytocentrifuged in a Shandon cytospin using all 12 chambers. Thus 12 slides of cells are obtained from one needle aspirate sample. Studies of validation and precision have been carried out assessing ER and PgR, showing that the results are comparable with conventional staining techniques using tissue frozen sections or histology slides. c-ErbB-2 (HER2/*neu*), Bcl-2, Ki67 and TGF-β1 have all been successfully demonstrated in these samples as well as ER and progesterone receptors (PgR). Furthermore, the residual suspension can be used for proliferation indices using flow-cytometric analysis to measure DNA index and S-phase fraction. Although in some cases there was difficulty in obtaining a sufficiently cellular sample, aspiration cytology is comparatively painless and may be used sequentially to monitor response to treatment.

Correlation with histological types

Benign lesions

Breast cysts can be recognised in needle aspirates not only from the macroscopic appearance of fluid but also from the presence of foamy macrophages (Figure 29.1) and apocrine cell clusters within the deposit.[22] Furthermore, the deposit from many cysts shows a diffuse granular appearance (Figure 29.2) that can be mistaken for polymorphs. These are fine granules that may have originated from apocrine cells. Thus a cytopathologist can confidently diagnose a benign breast cyst.

Fibroadenomas have very characteristic appearances, consisting of a combination of three features.[23] The epithelial sheets often spread in a 'stag horn' shape, and large numbers of myoepithelial cells, both singly and in pairs (Figure 29.3), are present between them. The third component is the recognition of the specialised stroma found in these lesions, which stains pale pink with Giemsa (Figure 29.4). The

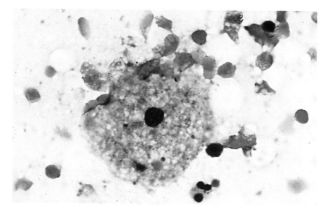

Figure 29.1 Foamy macrophage from the spun deposit of breast cyst fluid. (Giemsa, ×100.)

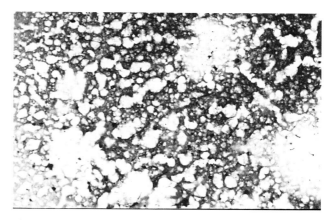

Figure 29.2 Granular proteinaceous material from a benign cyst fluid. These appearances may be mistaken for polymorphs. (Giemsa, ×25.)

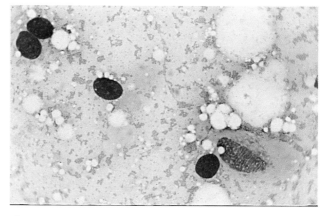

Figure 29.3 Five nuclei from an aspirate from a fibroadenoma. Four are myoepithelial nuclei, the top left showing characteristic pair formation. A duct epithelial cell is present at bottom right. (Giemsa, ×100.)

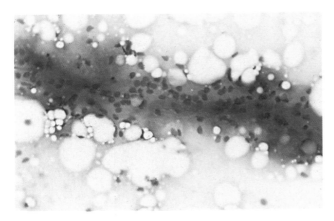

Figure 29.4 Stroma aspirated from a fibroadenoma staining a characteristic metachromatic purple colour. (Giemsa, ×25.)

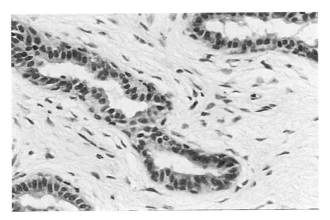

Figure 29.5 Histological section from a fibroadenoma showing epithelial clefts lined by hyperplastic cells. (H&E, ×40.)

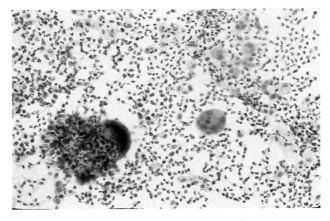

Figure 29.6 Pus aspirated from a breast abscess. Note two multinucleated histiocytes. (Papanicolaou, ×25.)

identification of these three features, particularly in aspirates from lumps from young women, will provide an almost certain diagnosis of fibroadenoma. It is important to note that fibroadenomas are often misdiagnosed in needle aspirates as carcinoma. The reason for this is the extremely hyperplastic nature of the epithelial component (Figure 29.5), which can be composed of pleomorphic irregular nuclei and can include mitotic figures. The key to the diagnosis is the recognition of myoepithelial cells, which are easily identified when they appear as pairs.

It is not possible, and probably not useful, to attempt to separate the other varieties of benign breast changes that can produce lumps and diffuse nodularity. There are reports of the description of the cytological appearances of radial scars,[24] but these studies are retrospective and are directed more at research into the natural history of these lesions rather than the diagnostic ability of a needle aspirate. Aspirate samples containing a variety of inflammatory cells are often sent to the laboratory. These include sheets of polymorphs, usually with cell debris and fibrinous streaks (frank pus) from a breast abscess (Figure 29.6). This is a straightforward cytological diagnosis that has important clinical implications. If unsuspected, a further sample can be taken and sent for microbiological analysis. Polymorphs and other inflammatory cells are commonly seen mixed with foam cells and apocrine cells in benign cyst fluids. These may indicate an inflammatory component to the lesion.

Chronic inflammation with or without multinucleated histiocytes (Figure 29.7) is quite common, and aspirates from granulomatous mastitis are often very cellular and the reactive fibroblasts can be mistaken for malignancy.[12] To avoid this, the diagnosis should be considered, especially in young women of childbearing age, even without the telltale multinucleated histiocytes. Single epithelioid cells have a characteristic bean-shaped nucleus with a single nucleolus, and typical examples should be searched for in the slide. Occasionally, exotic microorganisms are aspirated, including worms and ova in countries where these diseases are endemic.

Aspirates from intramammary lymph nodes (Figure 29.8) consist mainly of mature lymphocytes, but include occasional histiocytes, monocytes and macrophages. These lesions are usually present in the upper outer quadrant of the breast, but may occur elsewhere and can present with a palpable lump, especially in women with small breasts. The cytological diagnosis is usually clear-cut.

Malignant lesions

Between 70% and 80% of infiltrating ductal carcinoma is described as NOS (not otherwise specified).

In these lesions, there is a variety of infiltrating patterns, but no subtype other than grade is recognised. In these cases, the cytopathology will be distinctive only in so far as the diagnostic criteria of carcinoma is concerned. Of the special subtypes of carcinoma, mucoid (mucinous) carcinoma is usually easily diagnosed in needle aspirates.[25]

In these lesions, the mucin is recognised most easily in Giemsa preparations, in which it stains a pale pink colour (Figure 29.9). In the Papanicolaou-stained slides, it is not so easily seen and there may be difficulty in the diagnosis as the cells are usually small and not obviously 'malignant'. However, when mucin is identified, there is seen to be a relationship between atypical small cells and the mucin, in which the cells appear to line up in rows alongside the mucin. The histological diagnosis of mucoid carcinoma (Figure 29.10) depends on 90% of the lesion being of this type, and only those pure tumours have a good prognosis.[26] Furthermore, it should not be forgotten that some mucinous carcinomas are high-grade lesions consisting of clusters and single pleomorphic cells with a mucoid background.

Medullary carcinoma is rarer than mucoid carcinoma, but can be distinctive in needle aspirate samples (Figure 29.11). The large pleomorphic poorly differentiated carcinoma cells with prominent nucleoli are often seen singly and in fragmented clusters together with the lymphoid stroma in which plasma cells can be identified. When these features are seen in samples, which are occasionally cystic,[27] it is important to alert the clinician to the possibility of medullary carcinoma, as these lesions can be mistaken for cysts radiologically because of their regular borders.

Papillary carcinomas are found usually deep to the nipple in postmenopausal women, but they can occur in any part of the breast. The needle aspirates are often cystic and blood-contaminated; the cells may be in papillary clusters (Figure 29.12), and myoepithelial cells are absent. In practice, identification is usually difficult and an equivocal diagnosis may be the only one possible.

Sarcoma

Malignant mesenchymal tumours of the breast are divided into those with an epithelial component (malignant phyllodes tumour) and those without. Sarcomas without an epithelial component are less common and are usually fibrosarcomas. The diagnosis is made histologically after thorough sampling, as sarcomatous metaplasia is common in carcinomas in which the epithelial components may be focal

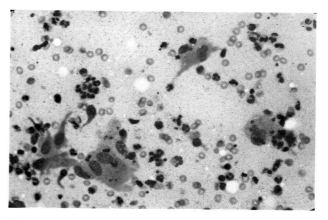

Figure 29.7 Breast aspirate showing evidence of chronic inflammation. Several histiocytes are present, with a background of lymphocytes and occasional polymorphs. (Giemsa, ×40.)

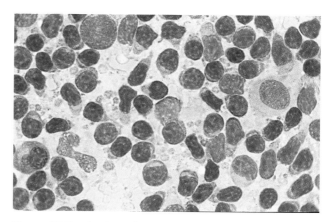

Figure 29.8 Aspirate from an intramammary lymph node. Note the variety of mature and immature lymphoid cells. (Giemsa, ×100.)

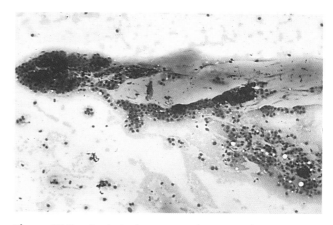

Figure 29.9 Aspirate from a mucinous carcinoma. Note the purple staining extracellular mucus with adjacent carcinoma cells. (Giemsa, ×10.)

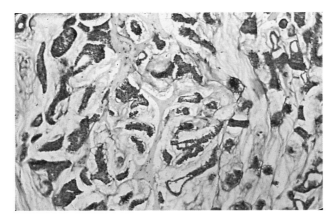

Figure 29.10 Histological section of a mucinous carcinoma. Note the islands of carcinoma floating in mucus. (H&E, ×25.)

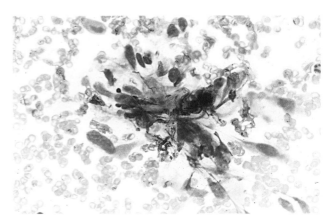

Figure 29.13 Aspirate from a fibrosarcoma. The cells present a spindly appearance. (Giemsa, ×40.)

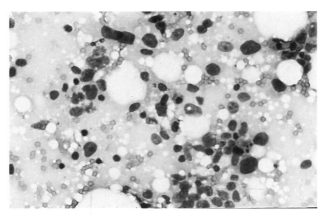

Figure 29.11 Aspirate from a medullary carcinoma. Note the scattered large carcinoma cells with prominent nucleoli. There is a background of lymphoid stroma in which a plasma cell is seen centrally. (Giemsa, ×40.)

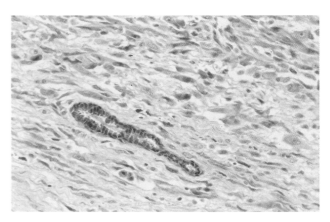

Figure 29.14 Histological section from a breast fibrosarcoma. An elongated breast duct is surrounded by a spindle cell malignant neoplasm. (H&E, ×40.)

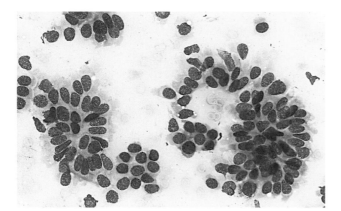

Figure 29.12 Aspirate from an intracystic papillary carcinoma. The carcinoma cells appear palisaded in papillary clusters. (Giemsa, ×40.)

and widespread. Only in the absence of evidence of carcinoma can the diagnosis of sarcoma be made confidently, and confirmation may be necessary using appropriate immunohistochemistry. Consequently, the cytodiagnosis of breast sarcoma (Figures 29.13 and 29.14) is fraught with difficulties even when good-quality samples containing spindle cells typical of sarcoma seen in other body sites are obtained.

The only situation where sarcoma can be confidently diagnosed in a breast aspirate is in recurrent sarcoma in which the primary tumour has been properly sampled and assessed histopathologically.

Lymphoma

Lymphoma of the breast usually occurs in association with known generalised lymphoma, but

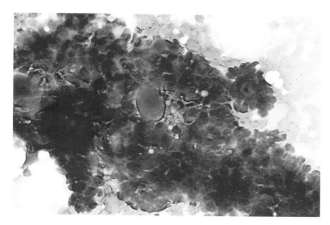

Figure 29.15   Aspirate from an adenoid cystic carcinoma. Note the blobs of pink-staining mucin surrounded by small pleomorphic irregular cells. (Giemsa, ×40.)

occasionally primary breast lymphoma occurs or the breast is the site of the first presentation of more generalised disease. The majority of cases are B-cell non-Hodgkin lymphomas (NHL), although occasional reports of T-cell NHL have appeared.[28] Cytodiagnosis is comparatively easy if the pathologist is aware of the condition. The usual disassociated round cells with scanty cytoplasm are seen, with nuclear configurations with or without nucleoli. The appearances may be difficult to differentiate from small cell carcinoma, in which the cells are also largely disassociated. However, careful hunting will reveal a few clusters of cells with an epithelial pattern.

Lymphomas of the breast are usually high-grade, but in doubtful cases immunocytochemical staining for lymphoid markers may be necessary.

There are many reports in the literature of the cytological appearances of rarer forms of breast malignancy, but these descriptions are unhelpful in prospective diagnosis. Adenoid cystic carcinoma (Figure 29.15) appears similar to the lesions aspirated from the head and neck area, so that it is important to remember the diagnosis when confronted with a case that is difficult to interpret and perhaps offer the diagnosis in the description. The main purpose of breast fine-needle aspiration cytodiagnosis is to differentiate between malignant and benign lesions. Many cytopathologists think this is hard enough without attempting refinements.

References

1.   Britton PD. Fine needle aspiration or core biopsy. Breast 1999; 8: 5–11.

2.   Britton PD, McCann J. Needle biopsy in the NHS Breast Screening Programme 1996/97: how much and how accurate? Breast 1999; 8: 5–11.

3.   Sloane JP. Biopsy Pathology of the Breast, 2nd edn. London: Arnold, 2001: Chap 4.

4.   Pinder SE, Elston CW, Ellis IO The role of pre-operative diagnosis in breast cancer. Histopathology 1996; 28: 563–6.

5.   Poole GH, Willsher PC, Pinder SE et al. Diagnosis of breast cancer with core-biopsy and fine needle aspiration cytology. Aust NZ Surg 1996; 66: 592–4.

6.   Yelland A, Graham MD, Trott PA et al. Diagnosing breast carcinoma in young women. BMJ 1991; 302: 618–20.

7.   Trott PA. Breast Cytopathology: A Diagnostic Atlas. London: Chapman & Hall, 1996

8.   Franzen SL, Zajicek J. Aspiration biopsy in diagnosis of palpable lesions of the breast. Critical review of 3479 consecutive biopsies. Acta Radiol 1968; 7: 241–62.

9.   Brown LA, Coghill SB, Powis SAJ. Audit of diagnostic accuracy of FNA cytology specimens taken by the histopathologist in a symptomatic breast clinic. Cytopathology 1991; 2: 1–7

10.   The Royal College of Pathologists Working Group. Guidelines for Cytology Procedures and Reporting in Breast Cancer Screening, revised edition. NHSBSP Publication 22. Sheffield: NHS Breast Screening Programme, 1993.

11.   Giard RWM, Herman JO. The value of aspiration cytologic examination of the breast: a statistical review of the medical literature. Cancer 1992; 69: 2104–11.

12.   Jatoi I, Trott PA. False positive reporting in breast fine needle aspiration cytology: incidence and causes. Breast 1996; 5: 270–3.

13.   Mouriquand J, Gozlan-Fior M, Villemain D et al. Value of cytoprognostic classification in breast carcinomas. J Clin Pathol 1986; 39: 489–96.

14.   Ciatto S, Cecchiani S, Grazzini G. Positive predictive value of fine needle aspiration cytology of breast lesions. Acta Cytol 1989; 33: 894–8.

15.   Zajdela A, DeLaRiva L, Ghossein N. The relation of prognosis to the nuclear diameter of breast cancer cells obtained by cytologic aspirations. Acta Cytol 1984; 23: 75–80.

16.   Van Driest PI, Baak IPA. The morphometric prognostic index is the strongest prognosticator in premenopausal lymph node negative and lymph node positive breast cancer patients. Hum Pathol 1991; 22: 326–30.

17.   Hunt CM, Ellis IO, Elston CW et al. Cytological grading of breast carcinoma – a feasible proposition? Cytopathology 1990; 1: 287–95.

18.   Robinson IA, McKee G, Nicholson A et al. Prognostic value of cytological grading of fine-needle aspirates from breast carcinomas. Lancet 1994; 343: 947–9.

19.   Trott PA. Pathological assessment in patients receiving primary medical therapy for breast cancer. Cytopathology 1996; 7: 75–7.

20.   Dowsett M, Johnston SRD, Detre S et al. Cytological evaluation of biological variables in breast cancer

patients undergoing primary medical treatment. In: Motta M, Serio M (eds). Sex Hormones and Antihormones in Endocrine Dependent Pathology: Basic and Clinical Aspects. Amsterdam: Elsevier Science, 1994: 329–36.

21. Fernando IN, Powles TJ, Dowsett M et al. Determining factors which predict response to primary medical therapy in breast cancer using a single fine needle aspirate with immunocytochemical staining and flow cytometry. Virch Arch 1995; 426: 155–61.

22. Ciatto S, Cariaggi P, Bulgaresi P. The value of routine cytologic examination of breast cyst fluids. Acta Cytol 1997; 31: 301–4.

23. Trott PA. Aspiration cytodiagnosis of the breast. Diagn Oncol 1991; 1: 79–87.

24. Lamb J, McGoogan E. Fine needle aspiration cytology of breast carcinoma of tubular type and in radial scar/complex sclerosing lesions. Cytopathology 1994; 5: 17–26.

25. Stanley M.W, Tani EM, Skoog L. Mucinous breast carcinoma and mixed mucinous infiltrating ductal carcinoma: a comparative cytologic study. Diagn Cytopathol 1989; 5: 134–8.

26. Clayton F. Pure mucinous carcinomas of breast; morphologic features and prognostic correlates. Hum Pathol 1986; 17: 34–8.

27. Howell LP, Kline TS. Medullary carcinoma of the breast; a rare cytologic finding in cyst fluid aspirates. Cancer 1990; 65: 277–82.

28. Peltinato G, Manivel JC, Petrella G, De Chiara A. Primary multilobated T-cell lymphoma of the breast diagnosed by fine needle aspiration cytology and immunocytochemistry. Acta Cytol 1991; 35: 294–299.

29. Eisenberg AJ. Preoperative aspiration cytology of breast tumours. Acta Cytol 1986; 30: 135–46.

30. Powles TJ, Trott PA, Cherryman G. Fine needle aspiration cytodiagnosis as a prerequisite for primary medical treatment of breast cancer. Cytopathology 1991; 2: 7–12.

31. Smallwood J, Herbert A, Guyer P. Accuracy of aspiration cytology in the diagnosis of breast disease. Br J Surg 1985; 72: 841–3.

32. Barrows GH, Anderson TJ, Lamb JL, Dixon JM. Fine needle aspiration of breast cancer. Cancer 1986; 58: 1493–8.

30 Radio-pathological correlations

Stefano Ciatto, D Ambrogetti, S Bianchi

Introduction

The appearance of breast lesions on mammography is strictly correlated with their macro- and microscopic pathological features. A description of such correlations may help in understanding the limits of mammography in the differential diagnosis of breast carcinoma and the occurrence of radiological false-negative/benign or false-positive reports.

Radio-pathological correlations that may justify radiological false-negative/benign reports

Invasive lobular carcinoma

This histological type may present diagnostic difficulties on radiological examination and is currently reported to be associated with a high rate of false-negative reports on mammography. The explanation of such a finding depends on the peculiar growth pattern of the typical invasive lobular carcinoma variant, which is characterised by small cells diffusely infiltrating the mammary stroma, sometimes with no tendency to form a well-defined mass as it produces a poor desmoplastic reaction (Figure 30.1). Such a growth pattern may result in some abnormality at palpation, such as an indeterminate area of increased consistency, but does not lead to radiological opacity; mammography is often completely normal, especially if a dense parenchymal pattern is present (Figure 30.2). On sonography, the evidence is also often negative, or sometimes a vague non-specific hypo-echoic area is appreciated, which allows no reliable diagnostic conclusion to be drawn.

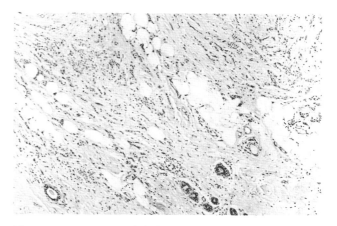

Figure 30.1 Invasive lobular carcinoma: histology. Classical variant – the tumour cells infiltrate the mammary stroma with a linear growth pattern, entrapping normal structures. There is no desmoplastic reaction. (H&E, ×1000.)

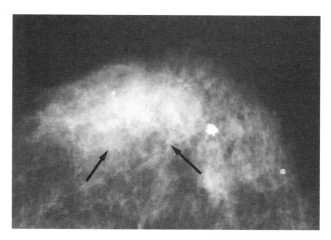

Figure 30.2 Invasive lobular carcinoma: mammography. A 2 cm palpable lesion in the upper central quadrant (arrows) is not associated with any mammographic abnormality.

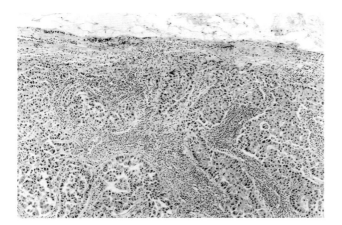

Figure 30.3 Invasive medullary carcinoma: histology. The lesion is well defined with pushing sharp margins. (H&E, ×40.)

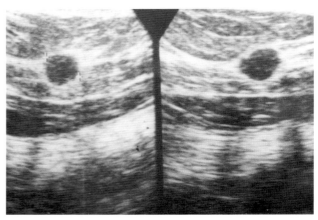

Figure 30.5 Invasive medullary carcinoma: sonography. An 8 mm non-palpable lesion appears with regular margins, a feature that might be consistent with benign fibroadenoma.

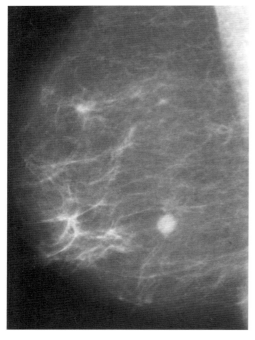

Figure 30.4 Invasive medullary carcinoma: mammography. An 8 mm non-palpable lesion in the lower central quadrant is evident as a rounded mass with sharp margins, virtually indistinguishable from a cyst or fibroadenoma.

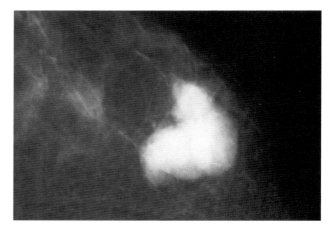

Figure 30.6 Malignant non-Hodgkin lymphoma: mammography. A rounded mass with sharp lobulated margins is visible.

Medullary carcinoma

This histological type often presents as a sharp, regular, rounded mass with well circumscribed margins (Figure 30.3), which are also evident on mammography (Figure 30.4) and sonography (Figure 30.5). This radio-pathological pattern is typical of medullary carcinoma, but may also be associated with other non-medullary invasive carcinomas (e.g. mucinous), whenever a 'pushing' rather than an 'infiltrating' growth pattern is present. A similar appearance may also occur with breast localisation of malignant lymphoma (Figure 30.6). Radiological diagnosis of carcinoma is impossible on mammography. Although carcinomas with regular margins are round, whereas fibroadenomas tend to be oval, with the major axis parallel to the skin surface, such a difference is not constant and reliable. Suspicion may arise when the lesion is reported for the first

The diffuse growth pattern of the classic variant of invasive lobular carcinoma may also result in a lower accuracy of cytology, mostly due to difficulty in aiming the needle at the lesion either freehand or guided. This condition influences to a lesser extent the accuracy of core biopsy, which is more strongly indicated than cytology (or indicated when cytology is negative) in the presence of densities/opacities with poorly defined borders, which may suggest a lesion with a diffuse growth pattern.

time in women aged over 60 (fibroadenomas are often typically calcified), especially if a negative previous mammogram is available. The accuracy of fine-needle aspiration cytology is not influenced by tumour morphology in this case and routine aspiration of isolated solid lesions with regular margins at their first appearance is recommended, particularly in postmenopausal women.

Non-comedo intraductal carcinoma

Microcalcifications are often associated with breast cancer, and their typical appearance (linear, branching, casting and grouped in an isolated cluster) is well known, being typically associated with comedo intraductal or invasive carcinomas.

Unfortunately, microcalcifications associated with carcinoma may also have a less suspicious appearance (punctuate, crystalline, granular and sparse), which occurs typically with non-comedo intraductal carcinoma (Figure 30.7). On histological examination (Figure 30.8), these calcifications appear as calcium deposits in lumina of micropapillary or cribriform ductal carcinoma in situ. Differential diagnosis on a radiological basis is very difficult, and a poor specificity (high benign-to-malignant biopsy ratio) is generally associated with attempts to achieve maximum sensitivity in these cases. Even the prediction of non-comedo intraductal carcinoma on a radiological basis is unreliable.[1] Sonography is of no help in this case, as most microcalcifications are not visualised.[2] Cytology may fail to detect abnormalities in such cases, mostly as a consequence of inadequate aiming at the cancer site, and multiple core biopsies are indicated in presence of areas of sparse calcifications of the non-comedo type.

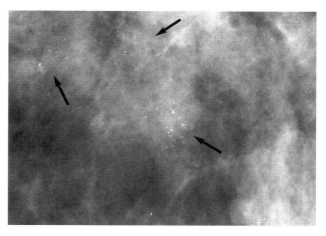

Figure 30.7 Non-comedo intraductal (cribriform) carcinoma: mammography. Sparse granular and punctuate microcalcifications (arrows) are the only radiological evidence.

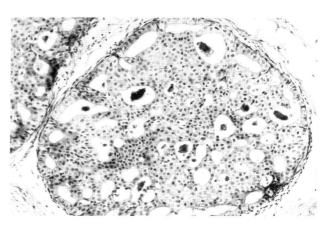

Figure 30.8 Non-comedo intraductal carcinoma: histology. Fine granular calcifications are evident within the lumina of intraductal carcinoma, cribriform variant. (H&E, ×250.)

Radio-pathological correlations that may justify radiological false-positive reports

Radial scar

Radial scar of the breast was described more than 50 years ago, but became the object of renewed interest after a report by Linell et al[3] in 1980. A number of synonyms have been used for this lesion in the recent literature (scleroelastotic lesion, proliferation centre of Aschoff, infiltrating epitheliosis, non-encapsulated sclerosing lesion and indurative mastopathy). It has a spiculated cancer-like appearance on mammography, and although some typical signs indicating its benign nature have been

described,[4,5] such as the absence of central opacity, or the presence of a radiolucent central area, and of long thin spicules radiating from the central lesion (Figure 30.9), they are not completely reliable and surgical biopsy is currently recommended. A typical radiological appearance, a negative cytological report, and the fact that the lesion is relatively large and superficial but still not palpable may justify careful surveillance in selected cases.[6]

On histological examination, diagnosis is not simple. At low magnification, the lesion is typified by a stellate or radial arrangement, with a central nucleus dominated by fibroelastosis and hyalinisation. At high magnification, haphazardly distributed and distorted, entrapped tubular structures with irregular angulated contours are evident (Figure

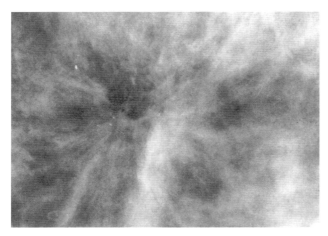

Figure 30.9 Radial scar: mammography. Typical appearance of a large stellate lesion with a radiolucent centre and thin elongated radiating spicules.

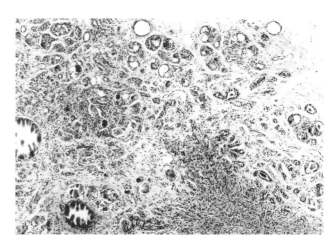

Figure 30.11 Sclerosing adenosis: histology. Lobular proliferation due to an increased number of acini shows compressed and elongated tubules. (H&E, ×100.)

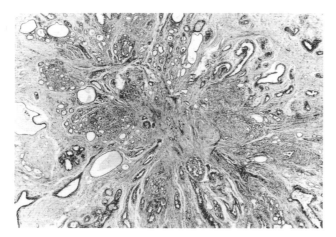

Figure 30.10 Radial scar: histology. The typical stellate arrangement with entrapped tubular structures in the central fibroelastotic zone is evident. (H&E, ×40.)

30.10). The latter finding may cause some diagnostic difficulties on microscopic examination in differentiating radial scar from tubular carcinoma. This is particularly true for core biopsies, which usually do not allow 'panoramic' evaluation of the lesion and increase the difficulty of differential diagnosis (and the risk of false positivity) with tubular carcinoma. If imaging indicates a radial scar, core biopsy is currently not recommended.

Sclerosing adenosis

Sclerosing adenosis is a lobular proliferation of both epithelial and myoepithelial cells, in which the acinus appears distorted and with pseudo-infiltrative margins. Ductules exhibit elongation and obstruction of their lumina due to compression by

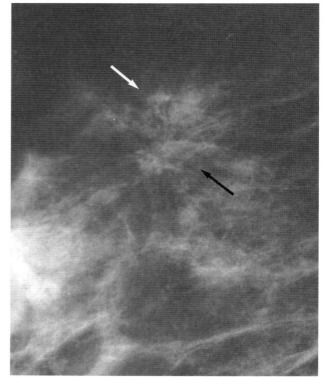

Figure 30.12 Sclerosing adenosis: mammography evidences an irregular opacity with a distorted appearance (arrows).

the prominent or hyperplastic myoepithelial cell layer (Figure 30.11).

On mammography (Figure 30.12), sclerosing adenosis may appear as an asymmetrical density with poorly defined or definitely irregular margins, and cancer should be suspected in these cases. Suspicion may be reduced by the absence of clini-

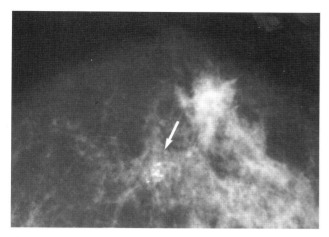

Figure 30.13 Benign calcifications: mammography. An isolated cluster of granular crystalline microcalcifications is seen (arrow).

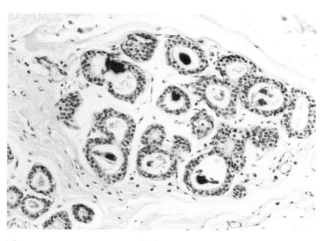

Figure 30.14 Benign calcifications: histology. Fine granular microcalcifications are evident in the ductules of a normal lobule. (H&E, ×250.)

cal and sonographic findings, or by a negative cytological report, but open biopsy is recommended in most cases, unless core biopsy provides a reliable diagnosis.

Benign calcifications

Microcalcifications are often visible on mammography of normal breasts. Although benign microcalcifications usually have a typical appearance (punctate, anular, teacup-like, diffuse, sparse and bilateral), sometimes they may assume a granular crystalline appearance, being circumscribed to a limited area (Figure 30.13).

Histological examination (Figure 30.14) shows benign microcalcifications within normal lobules, cysts or stroma. In this case, differential diagnosis with carcinoma (e.g. non-comedo intraductal type) may be very difficult, and when the decision whether to recommend open biopsy is based only on the radiological appearance, a high benign-to-malignant biopsy ratio is expected. The adoption of stereotactic fine-needle aspiration cytology as a part of the routine assessment of non-palpable lesions is a great help, and the benign-to-malignant biopsy ratio in the presence of microcalcifications with a questionably/probably benign appearance has been definitively reduced, with no appreciable impact on cancer detection rates.

The use of core biopsy is now further reducing benign biopsies in such cases: in fact, a negative finding on core biopsy with core specimen radiography demonstrating microcalcifications is much more reliable than a negative finding on cytology, which might suggest that the lesion has not been properly sampled (finding calcifications on the cytological specimen is anecdotal).

Asymmetrical parenchymal densities

The radiological density of cancer is equal to that of normal breast parenchyma, and cancers may be depicted on mammography as asymmetrical densities with non-stellate poorly defined margins. Such mammographic abnormalities may be easily suspected in older women, especially if they occur in fibroadipose breasts, or if they were not present in a previous available mammogram, but differential diagnosis between a scattered asymmetrical area of breast parenchyma (Figure 30.15a) and breast cancer (Figure 30.15b) may be difficult in a normally dense premenopausal breast. In the past, such cases were often sent for open biopsy, and histological diagnosis did usually confirm the presence of an island of normal breast parenchyma in those cases (Figure 30.16).

Since the introduction of sonography for the assessment of breast lesions, the need for histological confirmation of such mammographic abnormalities has been dramatically reduced, as regions of breast parenchyma are easily recognised, appearing as hyperechoic areas on the hypo-echoic background of the surrounding fat (Figure 30.17a). Only hypoechoic lesions (Figure 30.17b) are worth further investigation, and the benign-to-malignant biopsy ratio is thus reduced.

Spicules of cancer lesions erroneously interpreted as malignant

Breast cancer is often depicted on mammography as a nodular density with radiating spicules (Figure 30.18) – a pattern that is typical of tubular carcinoma. In these cases, it is questionable whether or not the spicules should be assumed as an expression of cancer invasion. In fact, in some cases, the

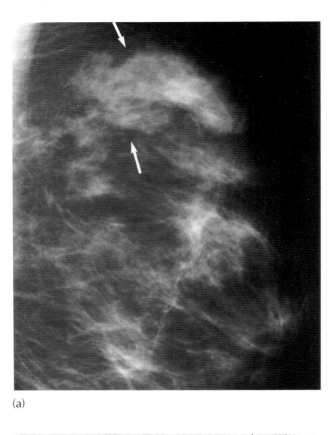

(a)

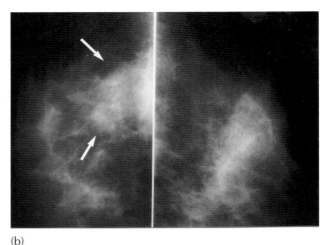

(b)

Figure 30.15 (a) Asymmetrical pseudonodular area of normal breast parenchyma: mammography. An asymmetrical density (arrows) stands out from the fatty background. The margins of the lesion are poorly defined but not frankly irregular. (b) Breast cancer: mammography. The lesion (arrows) appears as an asymmetrical density with poorly defined borders, similar to the surrounding areas of normal breast parenchyma.

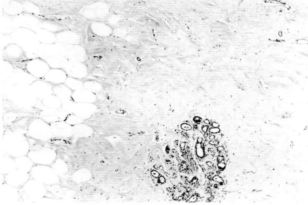

Figure 30.16 Asymmetrical pseudonodular area of normal breast parenchyma: histology. A microcystic atrophic lobule is surrounded by fibrosis and fat tissue. (H&E, ×100.)

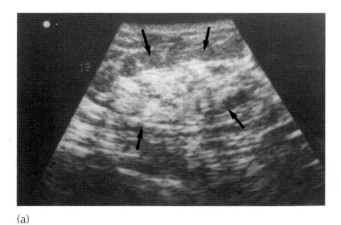

(a)

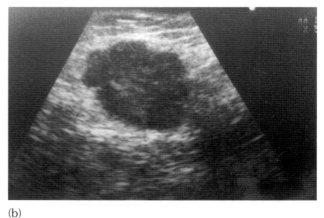

(b)

Figure 30.17 (a) Asymmetrical pseudonodular area of normal breast parenchyma: sonography. A frankly hyperechoic area, consistent with breast parenchyma, is evident on a hypo-echoic fatty background (arrows). (b) Breast cancer: sonography. A circumscribed hypo-echoic pseudonodular solid lesion is evident, surrounded by parenchyma.

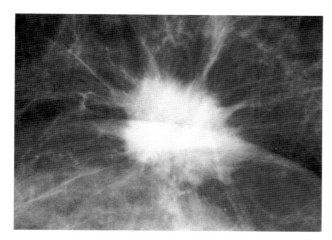

Figure 30.18 Breast cancer: mammography. There is irregular opacity with thin elongated radiating spicules. Tumour size, whether or not spicules are included, varies from 30 to 55 mm.

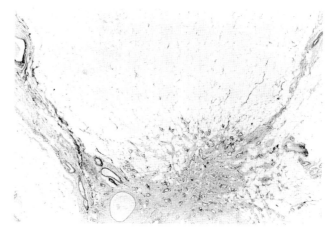

Figure 30.19 Breast cancer: histology. Spicules radiating from the lesion, without evidence of neoplastic invasion, are caused by desmoplastic reaction and fibrous tissue. (H&E, ×40.)

radiating spicules are accounted for by simple desmoplastic reaction (Figure 30.19).

It is evident that radiological measurement of tumour size may be quite different depending on how spicules are considered, and it is evident that pathological tumour size is much more reliable for clinical purposes.

The examples of radio-pathological correlation presented here confirm that in a number of instances, mammography is not completely reliable for the differential diagnosis of cancer. This limitation is intrinsic to the method: a false-negative/benign or a false-positive mammographic report in such cases is not a matter of interpretation but may be ascribed to the fact that some benign lesions simulate cancer and vice versa, as shown by the histopathological features that are consistent with and justify mammographic findings.

Such mammographic errors cannot be overcome by modifying the criteria of radiological suspicion, as this would decrease the overall accuracy of mammography to unacceptable levels. Such errors must be accepted as unavoidable, but may be corrected by adopting a multimodal diagnostic approach – that is, by using sonography, cytology and core biopsy as an adjunct to clinical and mammographic examination whenever a minimal suspicion of cancer is present.

References

1. Ciatto S, Bianchi S, Vezzosi V. Mammographic appearance of microcalcifications as a predictor of intraductal carcinoma histologic subtype. Eur Radiol1994; 4: 23–6.
2. Ciatto S, Catarzi S, Morrone D, Rosselli Del Turco M. Fine needle aspiration cytology of nonpalpable breast lesions: US versus stereotaxic guidance. Radiology 1993; 188: 195–8.
3. Linell F, Ljungberg O, Andersson I. Breast carcinoma: aspects of early stages, progression and related problems. Acta Pathol Microbiol Immunol Scand 1980; 272 (Suppl): 199–217.
4. Tabar L, Dean PB. Teaching Atlas of Mammography. New York: Thieme-Stratton, 1985: 87–136.
5. Mitnick JS, Vazquez MF, Harris MN, Roses DF. Differentiation of radial scar from scirrhous carcinoma of the breast: mammographic-pathologic correlation. Radiology 1989; 173: 697–700.
6. Ciatto S, Morrone D, Catarzi S et al Radial scars of the breast: review of 38 consecutive mammographic diagnoses. Radiology 1993; 187: 757–60.

31 The multidisciplinary team in breast cancer management

Susan O'Mahony, Judith Spencer-Knott, Anand D Purushotham

Introduction

Breast cancer is a heterogeneous disease that is diagnosed by surgical, radiological and histopathological methods and treated by a combination of surgery, radiotherapy, chemotherapy and hormone therapy. The multidisciplinary approach to the management of disease, whereby a dedicated team of health professionals with specific experience and training[1] manage patients from first presentation through diagnosis, treatment and follow-up, is particularly suited to breast cancer care. It is now accepted that the diagnosis, management and survival rates of breast cancer are superior when undertaken in specialised breast teams.[2–4] The multidisciplinary team (MDT), working to agreed protocols within these specialised units, provides quality and uniformity of care that can be audited prospectively.[5]

The multidisciplinary team

The MDT provides a broad base of expert knowledge to investigate, diagnose and treat the patient with breast cancer. It should comprise a core of essential personnel who meet regularly[6] and an extended team of health professionals active in supporting the patient or carrying out the treatment strategy.[1] The core members are a surgeon, radiologist, pathologist, clinical oncologist, medical oncologist and breast care nurse.[1] Ideally, the extended team should include a reconstructive surgeon, clinical geneticist/genetics counsellor, palliative care specialist, radiographer, primary care team, physiotherapist/lymphoedema specialist, psychiatrist/clinical psychologist and a social worker.[1] (See Figure 31.1.)

The MDT lead

The lead clinician, who must be clearly defined, takes responsibility for the work of the team as a whole, communication with patients, implementation of change and audit.[1] The primary care of breast cancer is the responsibility of the surgeon, and he or she is most likely to be the patient's first contact and therefore may be the most appropriate person to be the MDT lead.[7]

Breast care nurse

The breast care nurse (BCN) plays a pivotal part in the multidisciplinary management of breast cancer, and a detailed description of her role is merited. The psychosocial impact of breast cancer diagnosis and treatment can be significant. The incorporation of a BCN trained in counselling and communication is key to the success of the MDT. The benefits to the patient include improved understanding of her condition, enhanced involvement in decision-making, reduced anxiety, depression and somatic symptoms, increased self-esteem, and improved general health.[1]

The role of the BCN

The BCN provides a supportive and advisory service to patients who have or might have breast cancer. This support is provided to all patients diagnosed through both the symptomatic and screening services. The BCN ensures that throughout the diagnostic and treatment process, the patient receives the personal care that is required in a sensitive and

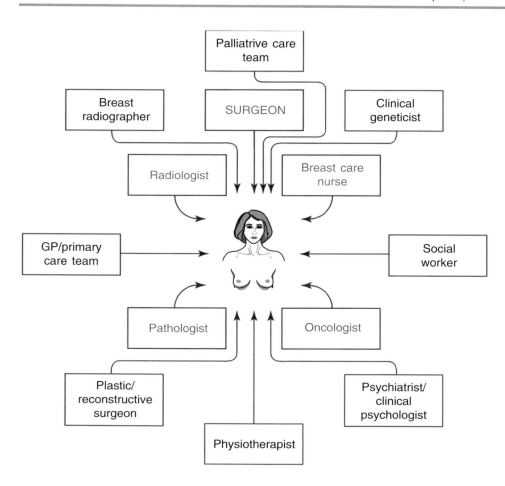

Figure 31.1 The multidisciplinary team. The core members are shown in red.

timely manner with due regard given to safety, comfort and dignity. The establishment of good communication ensures continuity of care and psychological support.

Once a diagnosis of breast cancer is given it is important that the BCN provides:

- time and privacy for confidentiality
- information and psychological support
- telephone contact
- continuity of care

Breaking 'bad news' needs to be tailored to individual needs – the process should be via stepping stones rather than an abrupt overload of information. There needs to be time to let the information sink in and explore resulting concerns. These concerns can vary enormously. The following are examples of such concerns:

- 'Everyone dies from breast cancer, don't they?'
- 'My husband had a stroke three months ago. I can't leave him alone in the house.'
- 'I felt as if an explosion had happened in my body and I was waiting for all the pieces to come down on top of me.'

- 'I fell into a black hole today. I feel as if I am drowning in the blackness.'

Patient demands and expectations have continued to change over the past few years. Access to the internet provides a wealth of information, some of which may not be relevant. Media coverage can contain alarmist messages and cause confusion. Each patient should receive relevant information about the disease and about treatment options and their effectiveness. Patients who take part in the treatment decision-making process have fewer psychological problems later on. The patient may choose to decline treatment and is entitled to support in that decision. It is important that communication continue to be open and honest. The patient needs to be aware of the possible risks of not undergoing treatment and that the opportunity remains to return and discuss the situation again.

Breast care support group

The setting up of a support group is another way of providing continuing support for any woman who has had treatment for breast cancer. The emphasis is on good health, on looking and feeling better.

Providing a network of support with monthly meetings and invited speakers allows experiences to be shared.

Requirements for a MDT

Location

The MDT should ideally be located in a suitable unit that can house outpatient clinics, clinical investigation and consultation rooms, and breast radiology services. Appropriate facilities for interdisciplinary conferences and meetings should be available. Adequate administrative support and confidentiality precautions should be in place.

Functioning

The core members of the team should hold a formal multidisciplinary meeting at least once a week to review the pathology and formulate a comprehensive management plan for each individual patient.[8] Regular communication between team members outside this formal setting should be open and encouraged. Interprofessional communication with extended members of the team is essential, and their attendance at MDT meetings should be encouraged.

Protocols

The MDT should be guided in its management decisions by written protocols based on national guidelines and interdisciplinary team consensus. These protocols must be evidence-based and updated regularly as new research is reported.[9] High-quality databases of patients should be maintained and audited regularly, to monitor and improve clinical performance and provide feedback to a cancer registry.[10]

Coordination of breast services

Each MDT works within a larger regional and national framework of breast cancer care. In the UK, breast services are localised in cancer units serving an extended local population, which in turn are aligned to larger cancer centres. The 'hub-and-spoke' model is appropriate to describe this arrangement.[11] Each cancer unit, staffed by a MDT, is a 'spoke' capable of providing an integrated breast cancer service. The 'hub' is a cancer centre that is also an academic unit. It coordinates trials, implements research-proven therapies, and provides professional, patient and public education.[11]

Advantages of the MDT

Clinical outcome

The knowledge base and treatment mix in breast cancer are too broad and labile for one person to encompass.[8] The success of the multidisciplinary model of breast cancer care is best measured by clinical outcomes. It is well documented that the survival of breast cancer patients is significantly increased with treatment by a designated and appropriately trained breast surgeon,[2–4] with a workload of more than 30 breast cancer patients per year.[12] This survival advantage is most marked when surgeons refer to oncologists and when there is increased use of adjuvant chemotherapy or hormone therapy.[11]

Of greatest significance is the reduction in mortality achieved when breast specialists within a larger, teaching hospital setting manage breast cancer.[2,13] It has been shown that care by specialist surgeons can confer 9% 5-year and 8% 10-year survival advantages to breast cancer patients.[3] Appropriateness of treatments can also be measured, with fewer mastectomies and higher rates of breast-conserving surgery in specialist units.[2,4,14] The use of adjuvant therapies such as chemotherapy and hormone treatments is also significantly higher in specialist units, resulting in a clear survival advantage.[4,6,11,15]

Continuity of care

Cancer can be seen as a medical and psychosocial diagnosis,[16] and continuity of care is of particular importance. The MDT working in a specialised breast cancer unit ensures uninterrupted, integrated and consistent medical and pyschosocial information and treatment. Location in one unit also provides convenience for the patient.[17]

Research/involvement in clinical trials

National guidelines for management of breast cancer are directly formulated from scientific evidence obtained from clinical trials. Advances in breast cancer management are ongoing, and specialist breast cancer units that treat cohorts of patients provide the ideal setting for clinical trials. It has been reported that high surgeon caseload and referral of breast cancer patients to oncologists results in an increased likelihood of entry into clinical trials.[18] While this has not been shown to confer a survival benefit per se, it is vital that the MDT be committed to the development of better care for breast cancer patients and to facilitate entry into clinical trials.[18]

Education

For the standard of breast cancer care to be maintained, junior medical staff must have experience of and training within a specialist breast team.[3] Specific protocols for the management and referral of breast disease in the community should be agreed by the MDT and clearly communicated to primary caregivers, in order to focus resources appropriately and minimize delay in diagnosis of breast cancer. Further educational opportunities can be extended to primary caregivers and to the community through educational symposia and provision of literature.

Costs

There is no doubt that provision of high-quality breast services in the multidisciplinary setting is expensive to initiate and manage. Education and training of members of the team to the exacting standards required is also costly. This is counterbalanced, however, by the more efficient and effective use of resources and improved outcomes.[1]

There is some indication that the provision of breast care services by a MDT within a specialist breast unit may reduce the volume and costs of litigation related to breast cancer management. In the USA, dissatisfaction with breast cancer diagnosis and treatment is the cause of one of the highest number of litigation claims.[19] Good communication and provision of information to patients can go a long way toward improving satisfaction.

Health professional satisfaction

It has been shown that a well-functioning MDT can improve individuals' efficiency at work, morale and work satisfaction.[20] A further reported benefit is enhanced mental health of team members as a result of working within the team environment.[21] This may be attributed to the sharing of clinical load and diagnostic responsibility. The camaraderie associated with being part of a well-functioning team may also be beneficial.

Obstacles to success

It is difficult to identify disadvantages in the multidisciplinary approach to breast cancer treatment when it is properly implemented. More appropriate is the identification of obstacles to success that can be disadvantageous to both patients and team members alike.

The MDT approach is a major departure from the traditional medical approach whereby a single, autonomous physician is responsible for the clinical decision.[8,17] This can be particularly unsettling for an individual clinician who is used to being autonomous. It can also be unsettling for the patient, who may expect to see the same clinician at each consultation. Patients are used to being under the care of one consultant, and relating to that individual as the main person responsible for their diagnosis and treatment. A perceived lack of this continuity of care may result in patients' losing confidence, with an accompanying feeling of depersonalisation of care. This problem can be largely avoided by clear definition of individual members' roles within the MDT, and good communication with the patient, providing reassurance that each team member is familiar with all aspects of their case. The BCN is of particular benefit and is very often the focal point for the patient.

Poor communication between colleagues, failure to create a flat, non-hierarchical structure within the team, clash of egos or priorities, and poor definition of the role of each team member all contribute to a dysfunctional MDT. It has been shown that 39% of senior oncology nurses and 25% of doctors cite communication with colleagues as their most stressful and challenging concerns within the multidisciplinary setting.[20] This poor communication, while stressful for team members, is disadvantageous to the optimum care of the cancer patient. One of the many benefits of a well-functioning MDT is the continuity of care and information provided to the patient. Poor interprofessional communication can result in inaccuracies or omission of information given to patients.

Despite following evidence-based protocols, a properly functioning breast cancer MDT may experience a few cases of litigation. It is unclear where ultimate responsibility lies when matters of potential litigation do arise. Failure to diagnose or delayed diagnosis of breast cancer is a good example where responsibility may lie with several members of the MDT. However, in cases where individual acts have resulted in medical negligence, all team members would not be expected to share the burden of responsibility simply by virtue of being part of the team.

Conclusions

The modern approach to breast cancer management involves the MDT working in a specialist breast unit, which in turn is aligned to a larger cancer centre. This approach has been proven to be of benefit to patients and team members, in terms of survival, appropriateness of therapy, timely provision of services, work satisfaction, and educational and research opportunities. As the management of breast cancer develops yet further with the implementation of molecular-based individualised treatment regimens, the role of the MDT will become even more important.

References

1. Cancer Guidance Sub-group of the Clinical Outcomes Group. Guidelines for purchasers: improving outcomes in breast cancer-the manual (96CC 00 21). Good Practice. London: NHS Executive, 1996: 33–7.

2. Selby P, Gillis C, Haward R. Benefits from specialised cancer care. Lancet 1996; 348: 313–18.

3. Gillis CR, Hole DJ. Survival outcome of care by specialist surgeons in breast cancer: a study of 3786 patients in the west of Scotland. BMJ 1996; 312: 145–8.

4. Sainsbury R, Rider L, Smith A, MacAdam A, on behalf of the Yorkshire Breast Cancer Group. Does it matter where you live? Treatment variation for breast cancer in Yorkshire. Br J Cancer 1995; 71: 1275–8.

5. Yarnold JR, Bliss JM, Brunt M et al. Management of breast cancer. Refer women to multidisciplinary clinics. BMJ 1994; 308: 168–71.

6. Sainsbury R. Organization of breast cancer services. Cancer Treat Rev 1997; 23: S3–11.

7. Mansel R, Blamey RW, Baildom A et al. The British Association of Surgical Oncology Guidelines for Surgeons in the Management of Symptomatic Breast Disease in the UK (1998 revision). Eur J Surg Oncol 1998; 24: 464–76.

8. Schipper H, Dick J. Herodotus and the multidisciplinary clinic. Lancet 1995; 346: 1312–13.

9. Basnett I, Gill M, Tobias JS. Variations in breast cancer management between a teaching and a non-teaching district. Eur J Cancer 1992; 28A: 1945–50.

10. Bell CMJ, Ma M, Campbell S et al. Methodological issues in the use of guidelines and audit to improve clinical effectiveness in breast cancer in one United Kingdom health region. Eur J Surg Oncol 2000; 26: 130–6.

11. Richards M, Sainsbury R, Kerr D. Inequalities in breast cancer care and outcome. Br J Cancer 1997; 76: 634–8.

12. Sainsbury R, Haward R, Rider L et al. Influence of clinician workload and patterns of treatment on survival from breast cancer. Lancet 1995; 345: 1265–70.

13. Lee-Feldstein A, Anton-Culver H, Feldstein PJ. Treatment differences and other prognostic factors related to breast cancer survival. Delivery systems and medical outcomes. JAMA 1994; 271: 1163–8.

14. Satariano ER, Swanson MG, Moll PP. Nonclinical factors associated with surgery received for treatment of early-stage breast cancer. Am J Public Health 1992; 82: 195–8.

15. Hand R, Sener S, Imperato J et al. Hospital variables associated with quality of care for breast cancer patients. JAMA 1991; 266: 3429–32.

16. Lauria MM. Continuity of cancer care. Cancer 1991; 67: 1759–66.

17. Durant JR. How to organize a multidisciplinary clinic for the management of breast cancer. Surg Clin North Am 1990; 70: 977–83.

18. Twelves CJ, Thomson CS, Young J, Gould A, for the Scottish Breast Cancer Focus Group and Scottish Cancer Therapy Network. Entry into clinical trials in breast cancer: the importance of specialist teams. Eur J Cancer 1998; 34: 1004–7.

19. Physician. Insurers Association of America. Breast Cancer Study, 1995.

20. Jenkins VA, Fallowfield LJ, Poole K. Are members of multidisciplinary teams in breast cancer aware of each other's informational roles? Qual Health Care 2001; 10: 70–5.

21. Carter AJ, West MA. Sharing the burden: teamwork in healthcare settings. In: Firth-Cozens J, Payne R, eds. Stress in Health Professionals. Chichester: Wiley, 1999: 191–202.

32 Ductal carcinoma in situ: clinical studies and controversies in treatment

Carol S Woo, Kristin A Skinner, Melvin J Silverstein

Introduction

Ductal carcinoma in situ (DCIS) is not a single disease – rather it is a heterogeneous group of lesions, presenting with a range of architectural forms, with differing growth rates, patterns, and cytological features. Patients with DCIS have a proliferation of malignant epithelial cells within the ductolobular system of the breast without evidence, by light microscopy, of invasion through the basement membrane into the surrounding stroma. Patients with this heterogeneous group of lesions have an increased risk of developing an ipsilateral invasive breast cancer, generally within the same ductal system (quadrant) as the initial DCIS. Most, but not all, experts believe that DCIS is a true malignancy, although it probably represents a range of malignant potential.

For most of the 20th century, DCIS was relatively uncommon, representing less than 1% of all newly diagnosed breast cancers.[1] With the widespread application of screening mammography, there has been a dramatic increase in the detection rate, and DCIS is now the most rapidly increasing subtype of breast cancer, with more than a fivefold increase in new cases from 1983 to 1999.[2] During 2001, there were estimated to be more than 46 000 new cases of DCIS in the USA, this now representing 19% of all cases of breast cancer diagnosed.[3]

Diagnosis of large numbers of patients with DCIS is a relatively recent phenomenon, and therefore little prospective randomised data are available to guide the complex treatment decision-making process. A range of treatments are available – from wide excision only, wide excision plus radiotherapy to mastectomy (with or without immediate reconstruc-

tion). DCIS is not a single disease entity and there is probably no correct standard treatment that is applicable to all patients. There is much controversy over the management of DCIS, but treatment should be tailored to individual patients according to the precise histopathological features of the lesion.

Clinical studies

Multi-institutional prospective randomised trials are designed to answer very specific questions, but do have their limitations. By contrast, observational and retrospective series tend not to address specific questions, but rather accumulate information on a group of patients. Well-conducted observational studies often yield results quite similar to those of prospective randomised trials.[4,5]

The first prospective, randomised trial of breast-conserving therapy for DCIS was performed by the US National Adjuvant Breast and Bowel Project (NSABP). They began a prospective randomised trial for patients with DCIS in 1985 (NSABP Protocol B-17). In this study, more than 800 patients with DCIS excised with clear surgical margins (as defined by non-transection of the tumour) were randomised into two groups: excision only versus excision plus radiotherapy. The main endpoint of the study was local recurrence, whether invasive or non-invasive disease (i.e. DCIS). The results of NSABP B-17 were published in 1993[6] and updated in 1995,[7] 1998,[8] 1999,[9] and 2001.[10]

After 12 years of follow-up, there was a statistically significant decrease of 50% in local recurrence rates for both DCIS and invasive breast cancer in patients treated with radiotherapy. The overall local recurrence rate for patients treated by excision only was 32% at 12 years. For patients treated with excision plus irradiation, it was 16%.[10] These 2001 updated data led the NSABP to continue to recommend postoperative radiotherapy for all patients with DCIS who opted for breast conservation, which was in accordance with previous updates. The NSABP acknowledged that there might be some subgroups for whom the benefits from radiotherapy were so minimal that excision alone might be adequate treatment, but these subgroups could not be consistently identified.

The early results of the B-17 trial, favouring radiotherapy for patients with DCIS, led the NSABP to perform Protocol B-24. In this trial, more than 1800 patients with DCIS were treated with excision and radiotherapy, and subsequently randomised to receive either tamoxifen or placebo. At 7 years of follow-up, 11.1% of patients treated with placebo had recurred locally, compared with only 7.7% of those treated with tamoxifen ($p = 0.02$).[10] The differences, although small, reached statistical significance for invasive disease but not for recurrence of DCIS.

The results of the European Organization for Research and Treatment of Cancer (EORTC) trial were published in 2000[11] and updated in 2001.[12] This study, EORTC Protocol 10853, was almost identical to NSABP B-17 in design and included more than 1000 patients. At 6 years of follow-up, 11% of patients treated with excision plus radiotherapy had recurred locally, compared with 20% of patients treated with excision alone. These results were similar to those obtained by the NSABP at the same stage of their trial. In contrast to the NSABP trial, half of the recurrences in each group were invasive and there was a statistically significant increase in contralateral breast cancer in patients who were randomised to receive radiotherapy.

The UK, Australia and New Zealand (the UK DCIS trial) performed a two-by-two study in which patients could be randomised into two separate arms within a trial. After excision with clear margins, patients were randomised to radiotherapy (yes or no) and/or tamoxifen versus placebo. This yielded four subgroups: excision alone, excision plus radiotherapy, excision plus tamoxifen, and finally excision plus radiotherapy plus tamoxifen. Those who received radiotherapy had a statistically significant reduction in ipsilateral breast tumour recurrence comparable to that found in the NSABP and EORTC trials. However, tamoxifen had no significant influence on rates of local recurrence.[13,14]

Despite the benefits of radiotherapy evident in the NSABP, EORTC and the UK DCIS trials, there continues to be much debate over its application in the treatment of DCIS. The US National Cancer Institute's Surveillance, Epidemiology and End Results (SEER) data suggest that approximately one-third of patients with DCIS in the USA are currently treated with excision alone.[2,15]

There are several clinical, pathological and molecular factors that might aid clinicians and patients in dealing with difficult management decisions. Research from our own group has previously shown that nuclear grade, the presence of comedo-type necrosis, tumour size and margin width are key factors in predicting local recurrence in patients with DCIS,[16,17] and analyses have shown that age is also important.[18] By using a combination of these factors, it is possible to select subgroups of patients whose absolute benefit from radiotherapy is so small that it can safely be omitted for those undergoing breast conservation. Conversely, based on these same criteria, patients can be selected whose recurrence rate is potentially high even with breast irradiation, and for whom mastectomy is therefore advisable at the outset.

Pathological classification

There is no single histopathological classification for DCIS that is universally accepted. DCIS is divided into five architectural subtypes (papillary, micropapillary, cribriform, solid, and comedo), although these are often classified as non-comedo and comedo.[19–21] Comedo DCIS is usually associated with high nuclear grade,[19–22] aneuploidy,[23] higher proliferative rates,[24] and HER2/*neu* (c-*erb*B2) gene amplification or protein overexpression,[25–31] and displays more aggressive behaviour clinically.[32–35] Non-comedo lesions tend to have the opposite features and are more indolent clinically.[36] However, such a division into comedo versus non-comedo is an oversimplification and is not appropriate for all cases of DCIS. Thus any architectural subtype may present with either high or low nuclear grade and may or may not be associated with comedo-type necrosis. It is not uncommon for high-nuclear-grade non-comedo lesions to express markers similar to those expressed by high-grade comedo lesions, and such lesions may warrant more aggressive forms of treatment. Furthermore, mixtures of different architectural subtypes within a single biopsy specimen are common, with 76% of all lesions having significant amounts of two or more architectural subtypes in our own series.

There is a lack of consensus on exactly how much comedo DCIS must be present to qualify as this subtype. The earlier work of Lagios and colleagues

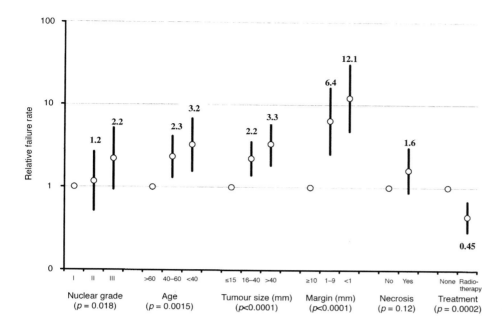

Figure 32.1 Cox multivariate analysis of factors affecting DCIS recurrence-free survival (conservatively treated patients only). Reprinted with permission from Sposto R, Epstein M, Silverstein MJ. Predicting local recurrence in patients with ductal carcinoma in situ of the breast. Error bars are 95% confidence intervals; p-values are from a Cox likelihood ratio test. In: Silverstein M, ed. Ductal Carcinoma in Situ of the Breast, 2nd edn. Philadelphia: Lippincott, Williams and Wilkins, 2002.

was qualitative rather than quantitative, with any amount of comedo DCIS (10% or 20%) being sufficient to earn the label 'comedo'. Others confirm that if any amount of comedo DCIS is present, the lesion should be classified as a comedo lesion.[20,21] However, our group consider a lesion to be comedo only if it is predominantly of this type with 50% or more of this component. Moriya and Silverberg[37,38] stipulate a figure of 70%. Poller et al[39] used comedo-type necrosis to divide DCIS into three groups. Lesions containing at least 75% comedo DCIS were called pure comedo, while those with lesser porportions of comedo DCIS (although at least 5%) were referred to as non-pure comedo DCIS. Lesions without comedo necrosis or with less than 5% were called non-comedo DCIS. Using this classification, Moriya and Silverberg were able to correlate a variety of markers (including c-*erb*B2 and S-phase fraction) with local recurrence as a measure of outcome.

For a lesion to be classified as comedo DCIS, the growth pattern should be solid and the cells should be of high nuclear grade (grade 3). However, where there is significant comedo necrosis, lesions with lower nuclear grade or of cribriform or micropapillary architecture may be designated comedo necrosis.

Moriya and Silverberg[38] classified lesions as comedo DCIS only when 70% of the lesion was high grade with solid growth and comedo-type necrosis, and a mere 8% of DCIS cases met this strict criteria. Our group used a more flexible definition, permitting inclusion of nuclear grade 2 and 3 lesions and not insisting on uniform solid growth. Moreover, only 50% of the lesion had to demonstrate these features

to be labeled comedo DCIS, resulting in 38% of lesions being classified as this subtype.

Some authors do not recognise comedo DCIS as a distinct histological subtype, but rather a feature of individual types, such as solid, papillary (including micropapillary) and cribriform.[7,40]

Therefore architectural morphology is an unsatisfactory method for classification of DCIS. Ideally, classification systems should be based on factors that reflect the biological potential of individual lesions.

Nuclear grade is a more dependable biological indicator than architecture, and has emerged as a key histopathological factor for identifying more aggressive behaviour.[19,21,32,35,41–44] In an analysis of our own series, using only DCIS patients treated with excision plus radiotherapy, nuclear grade was the only significant factor on multivariate analysis that predicted for local recurrence of both DCIS and invasive breast cancer.[17]

In a more detailed analysis, five factors were significant predictors of local recurrence by univariate analysis, namely nuclear grade, tumour size, margin width, age and treatment.[18,46,47] The presence of comedo necrosis approached multivariate significance ($p = 0.12$). Figure 32.1 depicts this multivariate analysis in graphical form.

A new system called the Van Nuys classification was introduced by our group in May 1995.[44,45] It was based upon two important predictors of local recurrence: the presence or absence of high nuclear grade

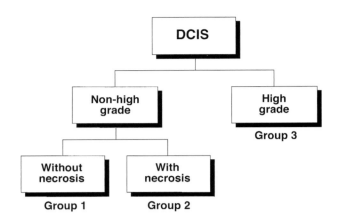

Figure 32.2 Pathological classification. DCIS patients are sorted into high nuclear grade and non-high nuclear grade. Non-high nuclear-grade cases are then sorted according to the presence or absence of comedo-type necrosis. Lesions in group 3 (high nuclear grade) may or may not show comedo-type necrosis.

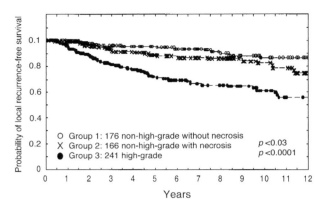

Figure 32.3 Probability of local recurrence-free survival for 583 breast conservation patients using the Van Nuys DCIS pathological classification (all $p < 0.05$). Reprinted with permission from Poller D, Silverstein MJ. Van Nuys Classification. In: Silverstein MJ, ed. Ductal Carcinoma in Situ of the Breast, 2nd edn. Philadelphia: Lippincott, Williams and Wilkins, 2002.

and comedo-type necrosis. Both factors are thought to reflect the pathobiology of tumours.

According to this classification (Figure 32.2), all high-grade lesions, irrespective of the presence or absence of comedo-type necrosis, fall within the least favourable prognostic group (group 3). The remaining non-high nuclear-grade lesions (nuclear grades 1 or 2) are subclassified by the presence (group 2) or absence (group 1) of comedo necrosis (any amount). This divides DCIS lesions into three easily identifiable groups with significantly different outcomes as measured by local tumour recurrence (Figure 32.3).

High nuclear grade was selected as the most important factor in the Van Nuys classification, based on results of our multivariate analysis showing a greater chance of recurrence after breast conservation compared with low-nuclear-grade lesions.[32,36,42–44] Similarly, comedo-type necrosis is associated with a poor prognosis[19,33–35,39,48] and is relatively easy to recognise histologically.[49]

In the Van Nuys pathological classification, there are no minimal requirements for the proportions of high nuclear grade or comedo-type necrosis. Occasional desquamated or individually necrotic cells are ignored and are not scored as comedo-type necrosis.

The most difficult aspect of nuclear grading is the intermediate-grade lesion. However, this becomes irrelevant in the Van Nuys classification system, and only nuclear grade 3 needs to be recognised, which is straightforward for most pathologists. Thus lesions have cells that are large and pleomorphic,

lack architectural differentiation and polarity, have prominent nucleoli with coarse clumped chromatin, and display mitotic figures.[19–21,39]

Diagnostic and surgical pretreatment issues

When a mammographic abnormality (microcalcifications, a non-palpable mass, a subtle architectural distortion, etc.) is found, further radiological work-up is indicated. This may include compression mammography, magnification views, ultrasonography, or magnetic resonance imaging (MRI).[50] Following this, the radiologist decides whether or not the lesion should be biopsied or the patient followed up with repeat imaging at a future date. While mammographic follow-up may be a clinically appropriate decision for many benign-appearing lesions, it often generates much anxiety, and if there is any doubt about the nature of a radiological lesion then it should probably be biopsied.

Stereotactic core biopsy is usually the procedure of choice for diagnosing DCIS. Dedicated tables with digital attachments make this a precise tool in experienced hands. For DCIS, stereotactic core biopsy using a 14-gauge needle continues to present some problems, although it remains preferable to fine-needle aspiration cytology (FNAC). Core biopsy samples are small and it may be difficult to capture the microcalcifications. In addition, the possibility of invasion in an unsampled portion of the tumour cannot be excluded. Therefore, where decisions are based on whether or not invasion is present (axillary

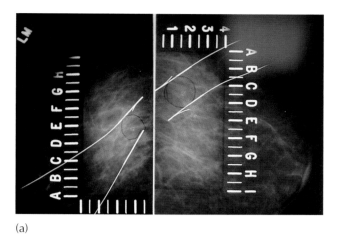
(a)

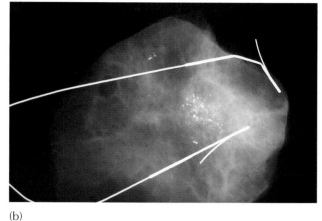
(b)

Figure 32.4   (a) Mediolateral mammogram taken after insertion of two bracketing wires around an area of microcalcification in the posterior aspect of the breast. (b) Magnification specimen radiograph of a two-wire directed breast biopsy showing a cluster of microcalcification with mammographically clear margins.

node dissection or sentinel node biopsy), a larger tissue sample may be required. The 11-gauge vacuum-assisted tools, such as the Mammotome (Ethicon Endo-surgery, Inc., Cinncinati, OH) have the capability of taking larger contiguous samples, but only about 10% of lesions are upstaged from DCIS to invasive breast cancer.[51,52]

A directed open surgical biopsy uses either a hookwire or a dye (methylene blue) to guide the surgeon to a non-palpable mammographic abnormality. Wire-guided biopsy is the preferred technique for many surgeons, as the wire can be palpated at operation. Although open wire-directed breast biopsy was the standard method for biopsy of impalpable lesions until the mid-1990s, it has since been gradually replaced by percutaneous biopsy techniques, particularly vacuum-assisted image-detected breast biopsy.[53] It is much better to establish a diagnosis preoperatively and perform a single definitive surgical procedure.

Multiple wire-directed breast biopsy remains the optimal technique for complete excision of DCIS. When excising a proven focus of DCIS, the surgeon faces two potentially conflicting aims: clear margins versus good cosmesis. From an oncological point of view, the larger the specimen excised, the greater the margins of clearance. However, optimum cosmesis is achieved when smaller amounts of tissue are removed. Much DCIS manifests as microcalcification and almost 90% of cases of DCIS undergoing surgical excision are non-palpable with no visual macroscopic correlate at operation. The use of multiple guidewires to bracket the lesion aids the surgeon greatly. DCIS lesions should be excised en bloc as a single specimen, which demands careful planning of the surgical approach and interpretation of localisa-

tion films. If involved margins mandate re-excision, the chances of achieving good cosmesis decrease. Moreover, if the specimen is removed in several pieces, it may be difficult to assess the extent of DCIS and margin status accurately.

Wire-directed excision is done using between two (Figure 32.4a,b) and four (Figure 32.5a,b) wires to bracket DCIS lesions.[54] In our practice, DCIS lesions are never removed using a single wire only. This may result in incomplete removal of the abnormality, calcifications at the edge of the specimen and positive histological margins, thus necessitating re-excision of the biopsy cavity (Figure 32.6). The bracketing wire technique maximises the chance of complete removal at the time of initial biopsy and minimises the chance of re-excision. Incomplete excisions are more likely to result when the mammographic abnormality does not correspond to the entire extent of the lesion.[55]

The excised specimen should be radiographed and the surgeon informed that the appropriate area of breast tissue has been removed. The biopsy cavity should be marked with metallic clips (Figure 32.7) which will identify the area of biopsy should radiotherapy be indicated or if local recurrence occurs. The metallic clips can also be useful should re-excision need to be performed and the specimen has been correctly orientated and marked at the time of primary surgery to identify positive margins.

If a mammographic lesion is extensive and the diagnosis unproven, complementary ultrasound examination can be performed, as approximately 10–15% of mammographically detected lesions with microcalcifications have an associated mass that can be imaged by ultrasound. This facilitates an image-guided biopsy

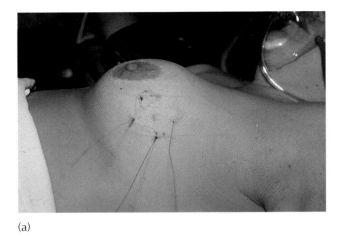

(a)

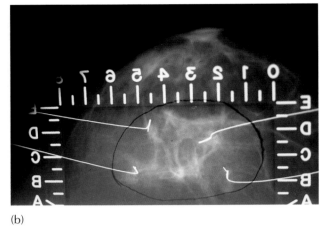

(b)

Figure 32.5 (a) Preoperative photograph of a patient with four wires in place. (b) Craniocaudal mammogram taken after insertion of four bracketing wires around an area of architectural distortion and microcalcification.

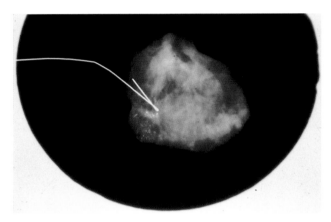

Figure 32.6 Specimen radiograph of a single-wire directed breast biopsy showing a cluster of microcalcifications at the edge of the biopsy specimen in spite of good wire placement.

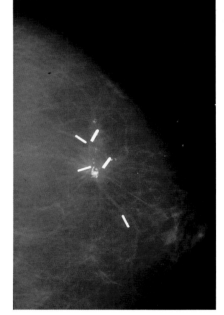

Figure 32.7 Postoperative mediolateral mammogram. Titanium clips mark the biopsy cavity.

of the mass lesion, which will help establish a diagnosis. If the patient desires breast conservation, a multiple-wire directed excision can be planned, which will optimise the chance of clear margins and good cosmesis. A large quadrant resection should not be performed unless there is cytological or histological proof of malignancy or an extremely suspicious (unequivocal) mammogram. This type of resection may lead to varying degrees of breast deformity and the definitive diagnosis may prove to be benign. Our guidelines for excision and tissue processing of a suspected DCIS are summarized in Table 32.1. After completion of the surgical procedure, the patient is wrapped with a 20–25 foot bias wrap to prevent postoperative bleeding (Figure 32.8). Using this technique, only 5 patients have been reoperated for drainage of a hematoma among more than 8000 segmental resections.

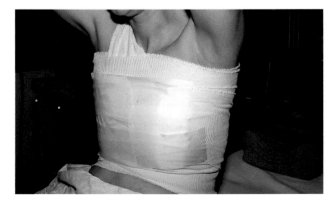

Figure 32.8 A cotton bias wrap (Fisher Imaging, Denver, CO), approximately 20–25 feet long, has been used to apply pressure to the biopsy site. This wrap is left in place for 48 hours.

Table 32.1	**Guidelines for excision of a suspected DCIS**

- Team approach (surgeon, radiologist, pathologist)
- Initial diagnosis using image-directed breast biopsy
- Use multiple hookwires to mark extent of lesion
- Remove tissue in one piece
- Multiple wire placement and magnification specimen radiography by the same radiologist
- Pathologist and radiologist communicate adequacy of excision to surgeon
- No frozen sections
- Mark margins with ink or coloured dyes
- Process all tissue sequentially

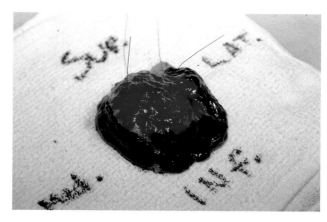

Figure 32.9 The colour-coded excision specimen with multiple wires in place oriented for the pathologist.

Handling of the biopsy specimen/tissue processing

Needle localisation, intraoperative specimen radiography and correlation with the preoperative mammogram should be performed in every case of a non-palpable lesion. Margins should be inked or dyed (Figure 32.9) and specimens should be serially sectioned at 2–3 mm intervals (Figure 32.10). The tissue sections should be arranged and processed sequentially. Pathological reporting should include a determination of nuclear grade, an assessment of the presence or absence of comedo-type necrosis, the measured size or extent of the lesion, the margin status with measurement of the closest margin, and a description of all architectural subtypes and the relative amounts of each.

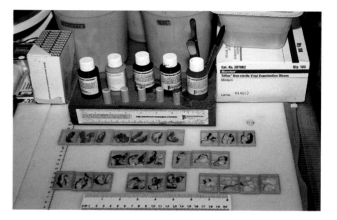

Figure 32.10 The specimen has been colour-coded with dyes and serially sectioned, and will be sequentially submitted.

For smaller lesions, tumour size should be determined by direct measurement or ocular micrometry from stained slides. For larger lesions, a combination of direct measurement and estimation, based on the distribution of the lesion in a sequential series of slides, should be used. The proximity of DCIS to an inked margin should be determined by direct measurement or ocular micrometry. The closest single distance between any involved duct containing DCIS and an inked margin should be reported.

Histological excision margins

It has previously been mentioned how tissues should be processed and the importance of inking all margins. When this has been done correctly and the pathologist reports the margins to be free of disease, what does that mean? Does it really mean that the entire lesion has been excised? There is no

clear consensus on what constitutes a clear margin, because different groups of investigators use different criteria. The Van Nuys group previously used a 1 mm margin in all directions, but this now appears to be inadequate.

Solin et al[35] have used 2 mm to define negative margins. Of interest the NSABP consider margins to be negative provided that the tumour has not been transected and tumour cells are not present at the margins; the presence of only a few connective tissue cells between the tumour and the inked margin would qualify as a clear margin.[41] Holland et al[56] require normal breast structures between the tumour and the inked margin. By contrast, the Nottingham group insists on 10 mm in all directions. The work of Faverly et al[57] suggests that 10 mm would be an appropriate criterion for clear margins. Using a serial subgross technique, they showed that only 8% of DCIS lesions have gaps (skip lesions) greater than 10 mm.

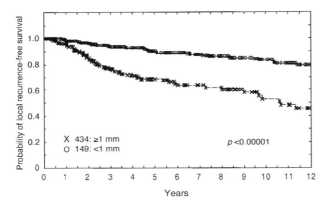

Figure 32.11 Probability of local recurrence-free survival, comparing margins of 1 mm or more with margins less than 1 mm for 583 breast conservation patients.

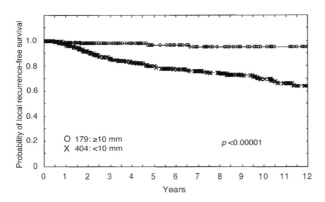

Figure 32.12 Probability of local recurrence-free survival, comparing margins of 10 mm or more with margins less than 10 mm for 583 breast conservation patients.

We have examined the importance of margins in our own series. Figure 32.11 compares the local recurrence rates when 1 mm or more is used as the definition of a clear margin. At 12 years, conservatively treated tumours with a margin of 1 mm or more had a 20% local recurrence rate and those with less than a 1 mm margin a 54% local recurrence rate. There is a significant reduction in local recurrence rates with a 10 mm margin. Tumours treated with wide excision only and a 10 mm margin of clearance had a local recurrence rate of only 5% at 12 years, compared with 36% for tumours with less than 10 mm clearance (Figure 32.12). These results are consistent with the three-dimensional work of Faverly et al[57] and with data from the Nottingham group.[58]

It may prove difficult to achieve a clearance of 10 mm at all margins when excising an impalpable lesion. Multiple hookwires will facilitate adequate

excision, but there will be cases where the pathological extent of the lesion exceeds the radiological measurements. Under these circumstances, complete excision at the first surgical attempt is less likely and re-excision of a margin(s) may be necessary.

Treatment

For most patients with DCIS, there will be no single correct treatment, and several therapeutic options will be available to a patient and her physician. These options may involve complex decision-making processes and lead to increasing frustration for both patient and physician.[59]

Counselling the patient with biopsy-proven DCIS

A patient with DCIS will be informed that she has breast cancer, but it must be emphasised that this is a special type of cancer that is potentially curable with treatment. Only a proportion of cases of DCIS will progress to invasive disease and exhibit the full cancer phenotype consisting of (a) unlimited growth, (b) genomic elasticity (resistance to treatment), (c) angiogenesis, (d) invasion and metastasis.[60,61] Pure DCIS lacks the latter two characteristics, and much current research effort is directed towards understanding why non-invasive lesions develop the ability to invade and metastasize and thus increase understanding of the neoplastic process.

When counselling a patient with DCIS, it must be emphasised that she has a borderline cancerous lesion, a 'pre-invasive' lesion, which is not a threat to her life. In our own series of patients with DCIS, the overall mortality rate is less than 0.6%, with only 5 breast cancer-related deaths among 909 patients. The 10-year Kaplan–Meier mortality rate is 1% for all patients and 1.5% for those undergoing breast conservation for DCIS lesions. The majority of other series confirm a similarly low mortality rate.[6,10,17,20,62–68]

A frequent concern expressed by patients once a diagnosis of cancer has been made is fear whether the cancer has 'spread'. Once definitive histology is available, patients with DCIS can be assured that no invasion is evident microscopically and that the likelihood of systemic spread is minimal.

Patients need to be educated that the term 'breast cancer' encompasses a wide variety of lesions with a broad range of aggressivity and malignant potential. All patients with DCIS should be reassured that they have a minimal lesion, although this may

Table 32.2   Local recurrence and death from breast cancer following mastectomy for DCIS

Authors	No. of patients	Follow-up (years)[a]	Local recurrence	Death from breast cancer
Archer et al[62]	52	11.1	0	0
Arnesson et al[63]	28	6.4	0	0
Ashikari et al[64]	110	1–10	2	1
Brown et al[69]	39	1–15	0	0
Carter and Smith[65]	38	6.2	0	1
Ciatto et al[66]	210	5.5	3	1
Farrow[67]	181	2–20	2	4
Fentiman et al[68]	76	4.8	1	1
Fisher et al[70]	28	7.1	0	1
Kinne et al[71]	101	11.5	1	1
Lagios et al[37]	53	3.7	2	1
Rosner et al[134]	182	5	–	3
Schuh et al[72]	51	5.5	0	1
Silverstein[73]	326	6.1	2	0
Simpson et al[74]	34	17.7	0	0
Sunshine et al[75]	68	10	0	3
Von Reuden and Wilson[76]	47	1–22	0	0
Westbrook and Gallagher[77]	60	5–25	1	0
Total	1684		14 (0.09%)	18 (1.1%)

[a]Mean 7.7 years.

require additional treatment involving further surgery, radiotherapy or a combination thereof. Patients should be specifically informed that they will not require chemotherapy nor will they lose their hair. Although they are unlikely to die from DCIS, patients need careful clinical follow-up.

Mastectomy

Up until the early 1980s, almost all breast cancer, including cases of DCIS, was treated with mastectomy. While breast conservation surgery has increasingly been practised for small invasive lesions, much DCIS continues to be managed with mastectomy. Thus, ironically, lesser forms of surgery have been recommended for more aggressive invasive lesions, while mastectomy has been performed for all types of DCIS presenting symptomatically. Studies on the outcome of mastectomy for DCIS relate to these symptomatic cases (often with a palpable mass) rather than screen-detected lesions, which are now much more common.

Table 32.2 lists 18 studies with a total of 1684 patients, in which mastectomy was used as the treatment for DCIS.[37,62–67,134] The local recurrence rate was 0.9% and the mortality rate was 1.1%. In our own

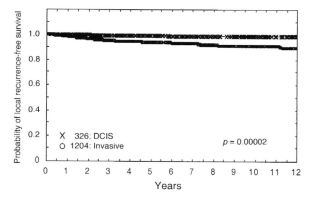

Figure 32.13   Probability of local recurrence-free survival by treatment for 1530 patients treated by mastectomy: 326 with DCIS and 1204 with invasive breast cancer. The reason why the local recurrence rate after mastectomy is so high (approximately 10% at 12 years) is that this curve includes patients with locally advanced breast cancer who received neoadjuvant chemotherapy prior to mastectomy.

series through to 2000,[73] there were 326 patients treated with mastectomy; 2 of these (1%) have recurred, but neither of them (0%) has died from breast cancer. Mastectomy is clearly a successful treatment for DCIS (Figure 32.13), but for many

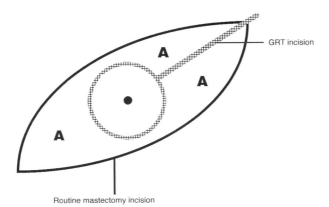

Figure 32.14   Skin incision for glandular replacement therapy (GRT: skin-sparing mastectomy and immediate reconstruction). The area marked by the letter 'A' (about 70 cm² in the average patient) represents the additional skin that would have been removed with a standard mastectomy.

patients it represents overtreatment. Mastectomy is physically deforming and may be psychologically traumatic even with optimal breast reconstruction. It remains a clinical challenge to select patients for mastectomy in order to avoid overtreatment on the one hand but to ensure that rates of local recurrence (50% of which is invasive) are minimised.

There are several indications for mastectomy, including the following:

- large diffuse lesions
- patients with documented multicentric disease (biopsy proof of DCIS in multiple quadrants)
- patients unwilling to accept even the slightest risk of death due to invasive local recurrence

- personal preference
- medical contraindications to breast conservation
- patients who are unwilling and/or unable to undergo postoperative radiotherapy and
- patients who cannot commit to long-term clinical follow-up.

When mastectomy is indicated, immediate reconstruction can be undertaken using some form of so-called 'glandular replacement therapy' (GRT).[78,79] This consists of a combination of skin-sparing mastectomy and immediate reconstruction, usually employing autologous tissue. Pure DCIS does not infiltrate the dermis and therefore this disease is particularly suited to skin-sparing mastectomy. Figure 32.14 shows the skin incision for GRT compared with standard mastectomy. With a skin-sparing technique, most of the original skin envelope is preserved and, when filled with autologous tissue, yields a breast of similar size, shape and consistency to the contralateral breast (Figure 32.15a,b). The most popular choice for autologous tissue reconstruction at our institution is a TRAM (transverse rectus abdominis myocutaneous) flap, either free or pedicled.

Breast Conservation for DCIS

Breast conservation is now routinely used for small invasive tumours, and this makes it difficult to justify the continued widespread use of mastectomy for less aggressive non-invasive disease.

There is a different approach to breast conservation treatment for DCIS compared with invasive breast cancer. Management of an invasive lesion involves (a) excision of the primary tumour with clear margins, (b) axillary node dissection or sentinel

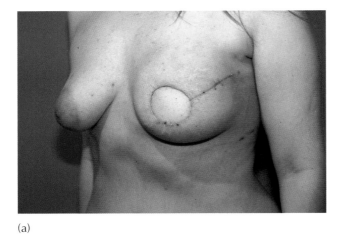

(a)

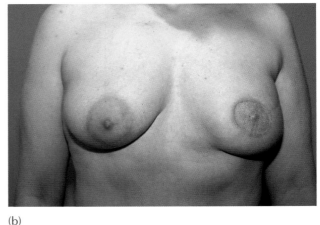

(b)

Figure 32.15   Cosmetic results of glandular replacement therapy (GRT). (a) A reconstructed breast after skin-sparing mastectomy and TRAM flap reconstruction. The island of skin that has been replaced is circular and exactly the same size as the nipple–areolar complex that has been removed. (b) The nipple–areolar complex has been reconstructed.

node biopsy, (c) whole-breast irradiation with or without a radiation boost to the area of the tumour and (d) chemotherapy for node-positive disease or a primary tumour with poor prognostic features.

Breast conservation treatment for DCIS differs in several aspects. As a minimum, the primary tumour must be excised with clear histological margins, although the optimum margin width is debatable. The issue of radiotherapy in patients with DCIS remains highly controversial, with there being no current consensus. Neither chemotherapy nor formal axillary dissection is indicated for DCIS,[80,81] although there have been reports of sentinel node positivity rates as high as 8–12% for patients with large high-grade lesions.[82]

Serial subgross studies conducted by Holland and colleagues[83,84] demonstrating that almost all DCIS lesions are unicentric suggests that many of these lesions are amenable to complete surgical excision. Nonetheless, almost one-quarter (23%) of the lesions in these studies were found to occupy more than one full quadrant of the breast. It may still be feasible to excise these more extensive lesions with wide excision and achieve an acceptable cosmetic result. High-quality mammography and an aggressive biopsy policy utilising stereotactic cores and multiple hookwires will guarantee that a higher percentage of smaller lesions will be completely excised with excellent cosmetic results.

Why is local recurrence important for conservatively treated patients with DCIS?

If all local recurrences following breast conservation surgery were non-invasive (i.e. DCIS), there would be less pressure upon surgeons to advocate mastectomy as the initial procedure for patients with DCIS. In our own series,[17,73] as in most others that have been reported,[10,20,36,85–87] approximately half of all local recurrences of DCIS were invasive disease – and herein lies the importance of local recurrence and the dilemma that it presents (Tables 32.3 and 32.4). Patients face not only further surgery (which is usually mastectomy – see below) but also a threat to their life that previously did not exist. These women initially presented with a theoretically curable lesion and by undergoing less than complete mastectomy have subsequently developed a potentially less curable form of disease. An invasive recurrence represents a biological worsening of the disease stage, which may ultimately translate into a higher mortality rate for patients initially treated with breast conservation surgery (with or without irradiation).

Local breast recurrence usually mandates mastectomy, but Solin et al[36,87–90] reported 45 local recurrences occurring in 270 breasts treated with excision and radiotherapy. The median time to local recurrence was 5.2 years. Just over half (53%) of the local recurrences were invasive and the majority of patients (42 of 45) were treated with salvage mastectomy. The breast cancer-specific survival rate at 5 years for those who recurred was 84%.

In our own series, the median time to local failure in irradiated patients was 4.8 years, which is similar to the results of Solin et al. By contrast, the median time to local failure for non-irradiated patients treated with excision only was 1.8 years. It appears that radiotherapy may prevent some local recurrences while merely delaying others.

Excision alone

For more than two decades, Lagios and colleagues[19,32,36,86] have championed breast conservation without radiotherapy. They began initially by carefully selecting patients with DCIS for excision only. There were strict criteria for eligibility and the study was confined to patients with mammographically discovered non-palpable lesions, measuring 2 mm or less in maximum extent. In addition, it was essential that the postoperative mammogram was free of microcalcifications and the margins of surgical clearance exceeded 1 mm. Lagios[86] reported an actuarial local recurrence rate of 12% at 5 years and 16% at 10 years. More recently, in his 15-year update,[91] the local recurrence rate was 20% (7% for nuclear grade 1 and 2 lesions and 36% for nuclear grade 3 lesions); there were no breast cancer-related deaths and no patients had developed distant metastases.

A number of other investigators[6,34,92] have reported similar but slightly higher rates of local recurrence for DCIS treated by excision only. The NSABP reported an actuarial local recurrence rate of 20.9% at 5 years.[6] Schwartz[34] reported a 15.3% absolute rate of recurrence at 4 years, which is approximately 20% at 5 years on an actuarial basis and is similar to the NSABP results.

Our own group has treated a total of 346 DCIS patients with excision only, and there were 61 local recurrences, of which 25 (41%) were invasive. The 5-year actuarial local recurrence rate was 19%, and there has been one breast cancer-related death in the excision-alone subgroup to date.

The average size of lesions in the series reported by Lagios was only 7 mm. This, together with the strict inclusion criteria, may account for the relatively low local recurrence rate of 12% at 5 years, which is lower than other comparable studies, some of which have shorter follow-up.

Table 32.3 Local recurrence after local excision only for DCIS

Authors	No. of patients	Follow-up (years)[a]	No. of recurrences Total	Invasive
Arnesson et al[63]	38	5	5	2
Baird et al[93]	30	3.3	4	1
Carpenter et al[94]	28	3.2	5	1
Cataliotti et al[95]	46	7.8	5	5
Eusebi et al[85]	80	17.5	16	11
Fisher et al[6]	391	3.6	64	32
Fisher et al[70]	21	7.1	9	5
Gallagher et al[96]	13	8.3	5	3
Lagios[86]	79	10	13	6
Price et al[97]	35	9	22	12
Schwartz[98]	256	6.3	71	26
Silverstein[73]	346	5.6	61	25
Total	1363		280 (21%)	129 (46%)

[a]Mean 6.0 years.

Table 32.4 Local recurrence after excision plus radiotherapy for DCIS

Authors	No. of patients	Follow-up (years)[a]	No. of recurrences Total	Invasive
Archer et al[62]	21	11.1	3	3
Baird et al[93]	8	3.3	2	1
Fisher et al[96]	399	3.6	28	8
Fisher et al[70]	27	7.1	2	1
Fourquet et al[106]	67	8.7	7	5
Haffty et al[102]	60	3.6	4	1
Hiramatsu et al[107]	76	6.2	7	4
Kurtz et al[108]	43	5.1	3	3
Kuske et al[42]	70	4.0	3	3
McCormick et al[105]	54	3.0	10	3
Ray et al[109]	58	5.1	5	1
Silverstein[73]	237	8.8	48	22
Sneige et al[110]	49	7.2	5	3
Solin et al[87]	270	10.3	45	24
Stotter et al[111]	42	7.7	4	4
White et al[112]	53	5.7	3	1
Zafrani et al[113]	55	4.6	3	1
Total	1587		182 (11%)	87 (48%)

[a]Mean 6.3 years.

Table 32.3 lists 12 studies involving a total of 1363 patients, all of whom underwent excision alone as treatment for DCIS.[6,63,70,73,85,86,93–98] The crude local recurrence rate at a mean follow-up of 6 years was 21%, and almost half (46%) of all local recurrences were invasive disease. With longer follow-up, this figure for the local recurrence rate is likely to increase, although new ipsilateral cancers will inevitably develop in some patients and cannot confidently be distinguished from true recurrences.

Therefore the figure for longer-term recurrence is an aggregate for true local recurrence and new primary tumours in the ipsilateral preserved breast. Since it is impossible to know with 100% accuracy which ipsilateral breast events are true recurrences and which are new cancers, they are generally all scored as recurrences.

Table 32.3 only lists those studies where a diagnosis of DCIS had been confirmed preoperatively and a wide excision was performed with the aim of obtaining clear margins. The series reported by Rosen et al[99] and Page et al[100,101] have therefore not been cited, as these included cases where DCIS had been missed initially. The most recent update of Page's series of patients reports a 42% local recurrence rate and a breast cancer-specific mortality rate of 22% at a median follow-up of 24 years.[101] This study offers some insight into the natural history of low- to intermediate-grade DCIS, as these patients were essentially untreated and the diagnosis was made retrospectively.

These findings and the fact that autopsy studies reveal an occult incidence of DCIS as high as 14% suggest than many DCIS lesions are not clinically significant and are unlikely to progress to invasive breast cancer.[39,102] A consensus conference on image-detected breast cancer, however, concluded that most DCIS lesions would eventually progress to invasive cancer should a patient live long enough and not die from non-breast cancer-related causes.[53]

Excision with radiotherapy

Several retrospective analyses of patients with DCIS treated with breast-conserving surgery and radiotherapy have been published.[36,42,88,103–105] Table 32.4 lists 17 studies involving a total of 1587 patients, all of whom received radiotherapy following wide excision of DCIS.[42,62,70,73,87,90,93,105–113] The local recurrence rate was 11% at a mean follow-up of 6.3 years and half (48%) of the recurrences were invasive. Solin et al[35,87–90] combined data from nine institutions in the USA and Europe into a retrospective analysis of 270 DCIS lesions treated with excision plus breast irradiation. The 15-year actuarial local recurrence rate was 19%, and recurrences were divided equally between DCIS and invasive disease. The 15-year breast cancer-specific survival rate was 96%.[87,90]

At our institution, we have treated a total of 237 DCIS patients with excision plus radiotherapy. There were a total of 48 local recurrences, of which 22 (46%) were invasive, and there have been 4 breast cancer-related deaths. The 5- and 10-year actuarial local recurrence rates for this group of DCIS patients were 12% and 20% respectively.

In 1985, the NSABP began a prospective randomised trial to evaluate postoperative breast irradiation after surgical excision of DCIS. Following wide excision with clear margins (as defined by non-transection of the tumour), patients were randomised to either ipsilateral breast irradiation or no further therapy. Axillary node dissection was undertaken until June 1987, but thereafter was optional and at the surgeon's discretion. In the event of an axillary dissection being performed, nodes had to be pathologically negative for inclusion in the trial.

The first report of this NSABP study was published in 1993.[6] A total of 790 patients were evaluable, of whom 391 were treated by excision only and 399 were treated by excision plus breast irradiation. The 5-year actuarial local recurrence rate was 10.4% for excision plus irradiation, compared with 20.9% for excision only. Thus local recurrence was halved by radiotherapy, and the difference was statistically significant. Among the 64 recurrences in the excision-only group, exactly half were invasive. By contrast, there were 28 recurrences in the excision-plus-irradiation group, only 8 of which were invasive (29%). The NSABP concluded that excision plus breast irradiation was more appropriate than excision alone for patients with localised DCIS and that in the event of local recurrence, radiotherapy significantly decreased the likelihood of invasive disease. After years of retrospective analyses, this was the first prospective randomised clinical trial for patients with DCIS, and it is of seminal importance.

The NSABP recommended radiotherapy for all patients with localised DCIS managed with breast conservation and undergoing surgical excision with clear margins. This applied to DCIS lesions of any histological architectural subtype, nuclear grade or size of the DCIS lesion. Excision alone was considered an inappropriate and inadequate treatment for DCIS.

However, the NSABP gave no analysis of local recurrence by subset. Overall, 81% of lesions were non-palpable and 85% were 20 mm or smaller in maximum extent. Almost 50% of cases showed some degree of comedo necrosis. There was no attempt to determine how these parameters affected outcome.

As stated above, the NSABP reported that radiation-treated patients had a 5-year actuarial local recurrence rate of 10.4% and non-irradiated patients a rate of 20.9%. There was no indication as to whether patients with palpable lesions had higher rates of local recurrence than impalpable ones. Moreover, it was difficult to determine how local recurrence varied with histological type, size of the lesion and margin clearance. For these and other reasons, much criticism of these results followed together with vigorous debate.[114–117]

In 1995, the NSABP published a second report, incorporating details of pathological findings from NSABP Protocol B-17.[7] Of the original 790 patients, slides were available for central pathology review on 573, and these fulfilled the criteria for diagnosis of DCIS. In this analysis, both comedo-type necrosis and margin status (close or involved) were found to be significant predictive factors for local recurrence. Some cases, originally considered to have clear margins, were reclassified as having microscopically involved margins on review. The NSABP did not change its recommendation that all patients with DCIS electing to undergo breast conservation receive radiotherapy following surgical excision with histologically clear margins.

The results of NSABP B-17 were subsequently updated in 1998,[8] 1999[9] and 2001.[10] After 12 years of follow-up, there was a statistically significant decrease in local recurrence of both DCIS and invasive breast cancer in patients treated with radiotherapy. The overall local recurrence rate for patients treated by excision only was 32% at 12 years, compared with 16% for patients treated with excision plus irradiation. Thus radiotherapy conferred a relative benefit of 50%, and the NSABP persisted with their recommendation of postoperative radiotherapy for all patients having local excision for DCIS.

The EORTC results were published in February 2000.[11] This study was almost identical to B-17 in design and included more than 1000 patients. After 6 years of follow-up, 11% of patients treated with excision plus radiotherapy had recurred locally, compared with 20% of patients treated with excision alone – results similar to those obtained by the NSABP at the same point in their trial. In contrast to the NSABP, one half of the recurrences in each group were invasive. Moreover, there was an increase in contralateral breast cancer in patients who were randomised to receive radiotherapy, which, although perhaps a chance finding, reached statistical significance ($p = 0.01$). One possible explanation for this result is the requirement for a compensatory filter or wedge during breast irradiation, which when employed on the medial tangential field can be associated with a higher scatter dose to the contralateral breast.[118–120] However, in a case–control study following over 41 000 women diagnosed with breast cancer, the relative risk of developing a second breast cancer associated with radiotherapy was only 1.19, which increased to 1.33 if the women survived at least 10 years after treatment. This suggests that radiation-induced contralateral breast cancers develop after a latent period of

approximately 10 years, and it therefore seems improbable that the increased incidence of contralateral breast cancer at 4.25 years in the EORTC trial can be attributed to the radiotherapy and is more likely a chance finding.

Should all patients with breast conservation treatment for DCIS receive radiotherapy?

There is clear evidence from published prospective randomised trials that breast irradiation reduces the local recurrence rate by approximately 50%,[10,11] and this is in accordance with our own data. However, risk–benefit analysis suggests that radiotherapy may not be appropriate for all patients and a number of issues should be considered. Radiotherapy is expensive and time-consuming, and is accompanied by significant side-effects in a small percentage of patients (cardiac, pulmonary, etc.).[121] Radiation fibrosis of the breast is a more common side-effect, particularly with the types of radiotherapy that were given in the past. Radiation fibrosis changes the texture of the breast and skin, renders mammographic follow-up more difficult, and may result in delayed diagnosis of local recurrence. The use of radiotherapy as primary treatment for DCIS precludes its use should an invasive recurrence develop at a later date. The associated changes in the skin and subcutaneous tissues can make any future skin-sparing mastectomy technically challenging. There may be some identifiable subgroups of DCIS patients in whom radiotherapy offers little improvement in local recurrence-free survival, and the statistically significant increase in contralateral breast cancer among irradiated patients (in the EORTC study) is a cause for concern.

The Early Breast Cancer Trialists' Collaborative Group (EBCTCG) has published a meta-analysis of the 10- and 20-year results from 40 unconfounded randomised trials of radiotherapy for early breast cancer.[122] Radiotherapy regimens consistently produced a reduction in local recurrence together with a reduction in 20-year breast cancer-specific mortality in the range of 2–4%. However, cardiovascular mortality was increased in those patients who received radiotherapy, and therefore the absolute survival gain with radiotherapy was only 1.2%.[123] The studies reported in the meta-analysis were conducted between 1961 and 1990. Modern radiotherapy techniques are designed to minimise cardiopulmonary exposure, but long-term cardiovascular mortality data do not as yet exist. The NSABP's 1999 update reported four breast cancer deaths among the excision-only group and seven among the excision-plus-radiotherapy group, although this difference was not statistically significant.[9] Similarly, the EORTC study also failed to show any difference in breast cancer mortality between the two treatment arms. It is important that any benefits of radiotherapy for a given subgroup of patients outweigh not only potential side-effects and complications but also inconvenience and costs.

The origins of the Van Nuys Prognostic Index

Information is now available that can aid clinicians in the selection of patients who will benefit from radiotherapy after excision versus those who do not. These same data can provide an indication of which patients may be better served by mastectomy at the outset because recurrence rates with breast conservation are unacceptably high with or without radiotherapy.

Research by ourselves[17,45] and others[7,33,34,36,37,40,48,86,92,113] has shown that various combinations of nuclear grade, the presence of comedo-type necrosis, tumour size, margin width and age are all important factors that can be used in predicting local recurrence in conservatively treated patients with DCIS. It may be possible, by using a combination of these factors, to select subgroups of patients who do not require radiotherapy in addition to complete excision or to select patients whose recurrence rate is theoretically so high, even with breast irradiation, that mastectomy is preferable.

The first two of these prognostic factors (nuclear grade and necrosis) were used to develop the Van Nuys pathological classification system for DCIS described earlier in this chapter.[45] Nuclear grade and comedo-type necrosis reflect the biology of the lesion, but neither is adequate on its own for guiding the treatment decision-making process. Tumour size and margin width together reflect extent of disease, adequacy of surgical treatment and the likelihood of residual disease. Results of multivariate analysis on our own data confirm these to be key variables in predicting behaviour and outcome of DCIS treatment (Figure 32.1).

The Van Nuys Prognostic Index (VNPI)[45–47,124,125] was derived by combining these three statistically significant predictors of local tumour recurrence in patients with DCIS, namely tumour size, margin width and pathological classification (determined by nuclear grade and necrosis). A score was given for each of the three predictors, ranging from 1 for lesions with the best prognosis to 3 for lesions with the worst prognosis. The objective with each predictor was to create three statistically distinct subgroups, using local recurrence as the marker of treatment failure. Cut-off points were determined statistically, using the log-rank test with an optimum *p*-value approach.

Research by various groups[20,33,34,37,40,48,89,90,92,113,126–128] including both our own[17,45,63,125] and the NSABP,[7] has shown that various combinations of nuclear grade, the presence of comedo-type necrosis, tumour size, margin width and age are all important factors that can be used to predict local recurrence in conservatively treated patients with DCIS.

The original Van Nuys Prognostic Index

These variables have been quantified in an attempt to make them clinically useful. The factors needed to be more than simply positive or negative results used in an anecdotal fashion. As already mentioned, the VNPI[45–47,124] combined the three statistically significant independent predictors of local tumour recurrence (tumour size, margin width, and pathological classification), and the challenge was to derive a system that would be clinically valid, therapeutically useful and user-friendly. The concept was to assign a score to each of the prognostic variables based on its relative contribution as determined by multivariate analysis. Several models were tried and thoroughly assessed.

Size score
A score of 1 was allocated for small lesions (≤15 mm), a score of 2 for intermediate sized tumours (16–40 mm) and a score of 3 for large tumours (≥41 mm).

Margin score
A score of 1 was allocated for tumour-free margins of 10 mm or more. This was most commonly achieved by re-excision with the finding of no residual DCIS or only focal residual DCIS in the wall of the biopsy cavity. A score of 2 was given for intermediate margins of 1–9 mm and a score of 3 for margins less than 1 mm (involved or close margins).

Pathological classification score[45]
A score of 3 was given for all high-grade lesions (classified as group 3), a score of 2 for non-high-grade lesions with comedo-type necrosis (group 2), and a score of 1 for non-high-grade lesions with or without comedo-type necrosis (group 1). (The classification is diagrammed in Figure 32.2.)

Tissue processing
Tissue processing is of crucial importance for a prognostic index based on pathological variables. At the time of biopsy, every effort was made to completely excise all suspect lesions. Needle localisation, intraoperative specimen radiography and

correlation with the preoperative mammogram were performed for all non-palpable cases. Margins were inked or dyed and specimens were serially sectioned at 2–3 mm intervals, with tissue sections being arranged and processed in sequence. Pathological evaluation included the subtype by pathological classification, the size or extent of the lesion, and the margin width.

Tumour size was determined by direct measurement or ocular micrometry from stained slides for smaller lesions. For larger lesions, direct measurement was used in combination with estimation, based on the distribution of the lesion in a sequential series of slides. The proximity of DCIS to an inked margin was determined by direct measurement or ocular micrometry, and the closest single distance between DCIS and an inked margin was the margin width used to calculate the margin score.

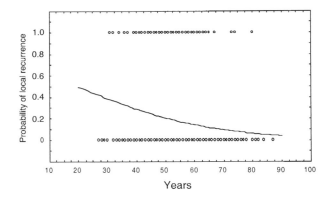

Figure 32.16 Using age as a continuous variable, the probability of local recurrence decreases as age increases. Reprinted with permission from Silverstein MJ. USC/Van Nuys Prognostic Index. In: Silverstein MJ, ed. Ductal Carcinoma in Situ of the Breast, 2nd edn. Philadelphia: Lippincott, Williams and Wilkins, 2002.

Calculating the original Van Nuys Prognostic Index

The original VNPI formula was determined by using the β-values, obtained from the initial multivariate analysis.[46,47,124] The β-values reflect the relative contribution of each factor in the estimation of the likelihood of local recurrence,[45,46,129] and were similar for all three factors. This method yielded a relatively onerous formula with 27 possible VNPI scores. The 27 subgroups fell readily into three prognostic subgroups: low, intermediate and high risk of local recurrence. As the β-values for the three factors were similar, additional analyses revealed that the formula could be simplified by omitting the β-weighting and readjusting the numerical range for each of the three subgroups. This did not compromise the clinical validity of the final formula, which was as follows:-

$$VNPI = pathological\ classification\ score +$$
$$margin\ score + size\ score$$

This formula yielded a total of seven groups, with whole-number scores ranging from 3 to 9. The most favorable (lowest) index was 3 and the worst index (highest) was 9, representing scores of 1 and 3 respectively for each of the predictors. When patients were subdivided into those with indices of 3 or 4, versus 5, 6 or 7, versus 8 or 9, the outcomes were identical when compared with the more complicated β-weighted version, and the VNPI was much easier to use.

The modified USC/Van Nuys Prognostic Index (USC/VNPI)

When age was analysed as a continuous variable, there was an inverse relationship between increas-ing age and local recurrence. Thus, in other words, with other factors being equal, the older a patient was when diagnosed with DCIS, the less likely they were to recur. Figure 32.16 is an updated version of that analysis.

Other authors have reported that age is an important factor in predicting local recurrence in patients with DCIS.[90,126–128] In a study from the Oschner Clinic, women aged under 50 had a local recurrence rate of 9.1%, compared with 2.4% in women aged over 50 ($p = 0.10$), and for women aged under 50 with a positive family history, the rate of local recurrence was as high as 20% ($p = 0.03$).[38]

The impact of age has been confirmed in other studies. Thus Vicini et al[126] reported a 10-year ipsilateral failure rate of 26.1% in women younger than 45, compared with 8.6% in older patients ($p = 0.03$). Furthermore, there was a much higher incidence of invasive local recurrence in the younger age group (19.9% vs 3.2%), which may be related to relatively smaller resection volumes and a preponderance of lesions with high nuclear grade and comedo necrosis.[126,128] On multivariate analysis, all four factors were found to be independently predictive of local recurrence in patients with DCIS: (1) young age; (2) total number of slides with DCIS; (3) the number of ducts or lobules containing malignant cells located within 5 mm of the margin; (4) the absence of pathological calcifications.[130,131] However, only the absence of pathological calcifications was an independent predictor when analysis was confined to those lesions detected by mammography.[131] The Memorial series identified young age, the presence of comedo necrosis, high nuclear grade, and close or positive margins as risk factors for local

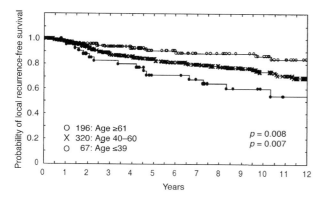

Figure 32.17 Probability of local recurrence-free survival by age for 583 breast conservation patients. Reprinted with permission from Silverstein MJ. USC/Van Nuys Prognostic Index. In: Silverstein MJ, ed. Ductal Carcinoma in Situ of the Breast, 2nd edn. Philadelphia: Lippincott, Williams and Wilkins, 2002.

Table 32.5 **The modified University of Southern California/Van Nuys Prognostic Index (USC/VNPI) scoring system**

Predictor	Score		
	1	2	3
Size (mm)	<15	16–40	>41
Margins (mm)	>10	1–9	<1
Pathological classification	Non-high-grade without necrosis	Non-high-grade with necrosis	High-grade with or without necrosis
Age (years)	≥61	40–60	≤39

1–3 points are awarded for each of four different predictors of local breast recurrence: size, margin width, pathological classification and age. Scores for each of the predictors are totalled to yield a USC/VNPI score ranging from a low of 4 to a high of 12.

recurrence, but only margin status was independently predictive.[132]

Further multivariate analysis by our group at the University of Southern California revealed that age was an independent prognostic factor (see Figure 32.1) and should be added to the VNPI with an equal weighting to other factors. An analysis of our local recurrence data by age revealed that the most appropriate breakpoints for our data were between ages 39 and 40 and between ages 60 and 61 (Figure 32.17). Based on this, a score of 3 was given to all patients aged 39 or younger, a score of 2 was given to patients aged 40–60, and a score of 1 was given to patients aged 61 or older. The new scoring system for the modified USC/VNPI is shown in Table 32.5. The final formula for the modified index is as follows:

US/VNPI = pathological classification score + margin score + size score + age score

Results using the modified USC/VNPI

Over a 12-month period through the year 2000, 583 patients with DCIS were treated with breast conservation, of whom 346 underwent excision only and 237 excision plus radiotherapy. Patients were divided into three groups with differing probabilities for local recurrence as determined by USC/VNPI scores (4, 5 or 6, versus 7, 8 or 9, versus 10, 11 or 12). Table 32.6 shows the clinical parameters for each group. The average follow-up for all patients was 83 months.

Table 32.6 **Tumour characteristics, recurrences and breast cancer deaths by USC/VNPI groups[a]**

	VNPI 4, 5 or 6	VNPI 7, 8 or 9	VNPI 10, 11 or 12	Total
No. of breast conservation patients	196	320	67	583
Average size (mm)	8.6	17.3	36.0	16.5
Average nuclear grade	1.63	2.43	2.88	2.21
No. of recurrences	4 (2%)	70 (22%)	35 (52%)	109
No. of invasive recurrences	0 (0%)	32 (46%)	15 (43%)	47 (43%)
5-/10-year local recurrence-free survival rates	99%/96%	83%/73%	54%/37%	85%/77%
Breast cancer deaths	0	4	1	5
5-/10-year breast cancer-specific survival rates	100%/100%	100%/97.7%	97.6%/97.6%	99.7%/98.5%

[a]Patients treated with mastectomy are not included in this table, since they are at limited risk for local recurrence.

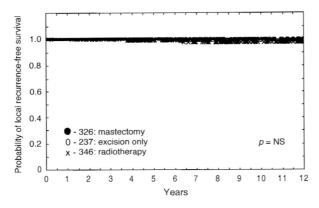

Figure 32.18 Probability of breast cancer-specific survival by treatment for 909 patients with DCIS. Reprinted with permission from Silverstein MJ. USC/Van Nuys experience by treatment. In: Silverstein MJ, ed. Ductal Carcinoma in Situ of the Breast, 2nd edn. Philadelphia: Lippincott, Williams and Wilkins, 2002.

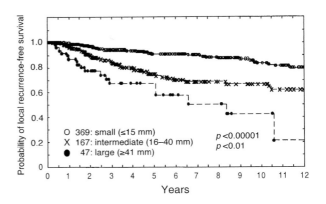

Figure 32.20 Probability of local recurrence-free survival by tumour size for 583 breast conservation patients. Reprinted with permission from Silverstein MJ. USC/Van Nuys Prognostic Index. In: Silverstein MJ, ed. Ductal Carcinoma in Situ of the Breast, 2nd edn. Philadelphia: Lippincott, Williams and Wilkins, 2002.

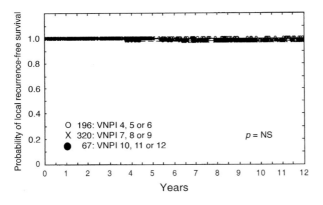

Figure 32.19 Probability of breast cancer-specific survival for 583 breast conservation patients grouped by modified USC/VNPI score (4, 5 or 6 versus 7, 8 or 9 versus 10, 11 or 12). Reprinted with permission from Silverstein MJ. USC/Van Nuys Prognostic Index. In: Silverstein MJ, ed. Ductal Carcinoma in Situ of the Breast, 2nd edn. Philadelphia: Lippincott, Williams and Wilkins, 2002.

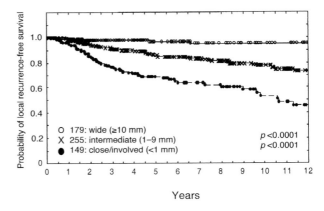

Figure 32.21 Probability of local recurrence-free survival by margin width for 583 breast conservation patients. Reprinted with permission from Silverstein MJ. USC/Van Nuys Prognostic Index. In: Silverstein MJ, ed. Ductal Carcinoma in Situ of the Breast, 2nd edn. Philadelphia: Lippincott, Williams and Wilkins, 2002.

A total of 109 patients experienced local treatment failure, of whom 48 were treated with excision plus breast irradiation and 61 with excision only. Among these 109 local recurrences, almost half (43%) were invasive (22 of 48) and there was no statistically significant difference in rates of invasive disease between patients treated with excision plus irradiation (46%) and those treated with excision alone (41%). Six patients treated with radiotherapy developed local recurrence and distant metastases, four of whom have subsequently died. One patient treated with excision only has developed fatal metastatic disease and there is no statistical difference in breast cancer-specific

survival between patients treated with excision alone and those treated with excision plus irradiation (Figure 32.18). Moreover, there is no significant difference in breast cancer-specific survival when different USC/VNPI groupings are compared (Figure 32.19). The 12-year actuarial overall survival rate, including deaths from all causes, is 90%. Rates of local recurrence-free survival for this group of 583 patients according to tumour size, margin width, pathological classification and age are shown in Figures 32.20, 32.21, 32.3 and 32.17 respectively. There is a statistically significant difference between the curves for each of the four predictors of local recurrence.

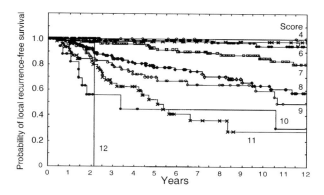

Figure 32.22 Probability of local recurrence-free survival for 583 breast conservation patients by modified USC/VNPI score 4–12. Reprinted with permission from Silverstein MJ. USC/Van Nuys Prognostic Index. In: Silverstein MJ, ed. Ductal Carcinoma in Situ of the Breast, 2nd edn. Philadelphia: Lippincott, Williams and Wilkins, 2002.

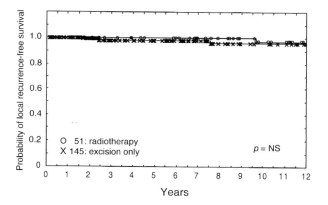

Figure 32.24 Probability of local recurrence-free survival by treatment for 196 breast conservation patients with modified USC/VNPI scores of 4, 5 or 6). Reprinted with permission from Silverstein MJ. USC/Van Nuys Prognostic Index. In: Silverstein MJ, ed. Ductal Carcinoma in Situ of the Breast, 2nd edn. Philadelphia: Lippincott, Williams and Wilkins, 2002.

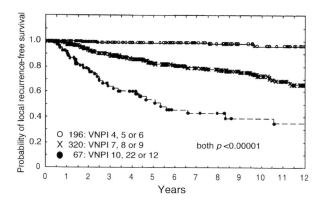

Figure 32.23 Probability of local recurrence-free survival for 583 breast conservation patients grouped by modified USC/VNPI score (4, 5 or 6 versus 7, 8 or 9 versus 10, 11 or 12). Reprinted with permission from Silverstein MJ. USC/Van Nuys Prognostic Index. In: Silverstein MJ, ed. Ductal Carcinoma in Situ of the Breast, 2nd edn. Philadelphia: Lippincott, Williams and Wilkins, 2002.

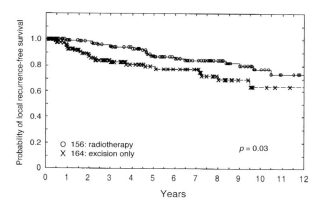

Figure 32.25 Probability of local recurrence-free survival by treatment for 320 breast conservation patients with modified USC/VNPI scores of 7, 8 or 9. Reprinted with permission from Silverstein MJ. USC/Van Nuys Prognostic Index. In: Silverstein MJ, ed. Ductal Carcinoma in Situ of the Breast, 2nd edn. Philadelphia: Lippincott, Williams and Wilkins, 2002.

Figure 32.22 shows patients by overall USC/VNPI score (4–12) while Figure 32.23 shows subgroups of patients with low (USC/VNPI score 4, 5 or 6), intermediate (USC/VNPI score 7, 8 or 9) or high (USC/VNPI score 10, 11 or 12) risk of local recurrence (statistically significant differences between subgroups).

Patients with USC/VNPI scores of 4, 5 or 6 do not show any benefit in local disease-free survival from breast irradiation (Figure 32.24) ($p > 0.05$), while patients with an intermediate risk of local recurrence (USC/VNPI score 7, 8 or 9) derive benefit from

irradiation (Figure 32.25). There is a statistically significant decrease in local recurrence rate, averaging 10–12, among patients with intermediate USC/VNPI scores who receive irradiation compared with those treated by excision alone ($p = 0.03$). Figure 32.26 divides patients with a USC/VNPI score of 10, 11 or 12 into those treated by excision plus irradiation and those treated by excision alone. Although the difference between the two groups is highly significant ($p = 0.0003$), patients with a USC/VNPI score of 10, 11 or 12 still have an extremely high risk of local recurrence even with radiotherapy and may therefore be better served by

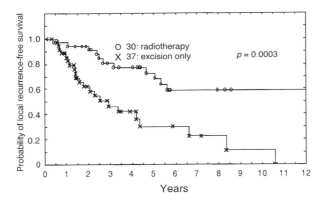

Figure 32.26 Probability of local recurrence-free survival by treatment for 67 breast conservation patients with modified USC/VNPI scores of 10, 11 or 12. Reprinted with permission from Silverstein MJ. USC/Van Nuys Prognostic Index. In: Silverstein MJ, ed. Ductal Carcinoma in Situ of the Breast, 2nd edn. Philadelphia: Lippincott, Williams and Wilkins, 2002.

Table 32.7	**Treatment guidelines based on the USC/VNPI**
USC/VNPI score	**Recommended treatment**
4, 5 or 6	Excision only
7, 8 or 9	Excision plus radiotherapy
10, 11 or 12	Mastectomy

mastectomy. Treatment recommendations based on our own practice are summarized in Table 32.7.

Discussion

DCIS is a heterogeneous group of lesions, and treatment approaches must be tailored to individual groups of patients. Some require no additional treatment following excisional biopsy, while others will benefit from radiotherapy, and for some mastectomy will be the optimum management. The most appropriate therapy must be selected for each individual patient based on available clinical and pathological data. The USC/VNPI score harnesses in a quantitative manner the evolving knowledge of prognostic factors in DCIS to define specific subsets of patients for whom the various treatment options of excision only, excision plus radiation, or mastectomy can be recommended.

Although mastectomy is curative for approximately 99% of patients with DCIS,[17,64,68,133,134] it represents overtreatment for the majority of cases currently detected by clinical and mammographic methods.

Although radiotherapy significantly decreases the risk of local recurrence by about 50% when compared with excision alone,[10,11,13] it may also represent overtreatment for a number of patients undergoing breast conservation.

The blanket recommendation by the NSABP that radiotherapy is appropriate for all patients with DCIS who are treated with breast preservation, while clearly correct based on their data, does not take account of the heterogeneity of DCIS nor of the variation in benefits from radiotherapy between different subsets that is evident from not only the NSABP data,[7,9] but also that of our own group[17,45,46] and that of others.[33,34,40,48,90,92,113]

Radiotherapy not only has significant side-effects,[121] but also changes the texture of the breast and renders subsequent mammography more difficult to interpret. Moreover, the breast cannot receive further irradiation should, at a later date, an ipsilateral invasive tumour develop that would otherwise be suitable for breast conservation treatment. Therefore radiotherapy should only be offered to those patients with DCIS who are likely to obtain a substantial benefit.

Subsets of patients who are likely to receive minimal benefit from radiotherapy can be identified using scoring systems such as the USC/VNPI (scores 4, 5 or 6), or from subset analysis of low-grade lesions,[33,37,86] small non-comedo lesions with uninvolved margins[34,98] or well-differentiated lesions.[113] This group of patients is estimated to account for approximately 30% of all cases of DCIS.

Patients with USC/VNPI scores of 10, 11 or 12 obtain the greatest absolute benefit from postexcisional radiotherapy, but rates of local recurrence remain extremely high and mastectomy should be considered for this group of patients with a very high risk of local relapse.

Patients with intermediate USC/VNPI scores of 7, 8 or 9 present the most difficult clinical challenge. For those cases with intermediate scores and margin indices of 2 or 3, local recurrence rates can be reduced by re-excision and achieving a greater margin of clearance. Radiotherapy can be considered following re-excision if the USC/VNPI score remains within the intermediate range. It should be emphasised that the USC/VNPI score is a guide to management, and for individual patients the final choice of treatment takes account not only of score value but also independent judgements made by both patient and physician.

No studies have revealed any statistically significant differences in overall mortality between the various treatment options for DCIS (wide local excision alone, wide local excision plus radiotherapy, or mastectomy). Nonetheless, there are clear differences in rates of local recurrence, and the latter is not only demoralising for patients but also represents a potential threat to life.[89,135] In our own series, as in most others,[20,34,90] approximately half of all local recurrences are invasive disease.

Discussion of management options for DCIS with patients can be very demanding, especially when no clear treatment recommendation exists. As mentioned above, the USC/VNPI provides objective guidance, and patients may wish to attempt downscoring of their lesion by choosing re-excision when margins are close or involved. This may permit adjuvant treatment with radiotherapy rather than completion mastectomy. Further excision may yield a final USC/VNPI score sufficiently low to avoid breast irradiation.

Re-excision can only result in downscoring of patients with unfavourable margin scores of 2 or 3. Occasionally, a tumour will 'upscore' when re-excision reveals a larger tumour size, higher nuclear grade, the presence of comedo necrosis or an involved margin.

The USC/VNPI score is of clinical utility because it divides patients with DCIS into three groups with statistically significant differences in risk of local recurrence following breast conservation therapy. Although a number of treatment options are available within each group (Table 32.7), the USC/VNPI score acts as a guideline – excision only for scores of 4, 5 or 6, excision plus radiotherapy for scores of 7, 8 or 9, and mastectomy for scores of 10, 11 or 12. The USC/VNPI score is an attempt to quantify the important prognostic factors for DCIS, and to translate these into clinically useful information in the treatment decision-making process.

The validity of the USC/VNPI must be independently and prospectively confirmed by other groups with access to large numbers of DCIS patients. In the future, other factors, such as molecular markers, may be integrated into the final score should they prove to be statistically important predictors of local recurrence.

Axillary lymph node dissection

Our group proposed some time ago that axillary lymph node dissection be abandoned for DCIS,[80,81] and in 1987 nodal dissection became optional for patients with DCIS entered into the NSABP B-17 trial. Subsequent reports have confirmed that axillary node dissection is not indicated for patients with DCIS.[16,17,35,136,137] Our group have found only 2 cases of nodal positivity among 363 patients undergoing axillary dissection (305 patients) or nodal sampling (58 patients). No invasive focus was found in either of these 2 patients, both of whom remain free of distant disease. Using the sentinel node biopsy technique, only 1 of 66 patients had a positive node on immunohistochemistry and all were negative on routine H & E staining. Node positivity rates as high as 10% have been found in patients with DCIS on the basis of immunohistochemical analysis.[82,138] However, the clinical significance of these immuno-histochemically detected micrometastases remains unclear, but the nature of DCIS (which has a cause-specific mortality rate of only 1%) suggests that it is a non-obligate precursor of invasive breast cancer with little or no metastatic potential.[139]

In a review of nine studies involving a total of 754 patients with DCIS, Frykberg et al[140] found the incidence of axillary lymph node metastasis to be 1.7%. Despite a low incidence of axillary nodal involvement, many authors continue to advocate axillary procedures for patients with DCIS who are deemed to be at higher risk for occult invasion.[34,141,142]

It is our current policy not to perform axillary surgery in any patient with DCIS who is undergoing breast preservation (irrespective of size, palpability, etc.) when a separate axillary incision is required. For lesions in the upper outer quadrant, a sentinel node biopsy is frequently performed via the same incision, and is always undertaken in mastectomy patients. Those patients undergoing mastectomy have larger lesions with a greater probability of occult invasion, not detected by image-guided or open biopsy techniques.[52,143] A few nodes can readily be sampled at level I, with a negative result providing additional reassurance for the patient.

Conclusions

DCIS is now a relatively common clinical diagnosis with an increasing incidence, which is partially attributable to better mammographic detection but may also reflect an underlying increase in incidence. Some cases of DCIS will progress to invasive breast cancer over a sufficiently long time period. A woman with untreated DCIS is more likely to develop an ipsilateral invasive breast cancer than someone without DCIS.

High-grade DCIS is more likely to be associated with subsequent invasive cancer than non-high-grade DCIS, and when treated conservatively is associated with higher rates of local recurrence compared with non-high-grade DCIS.

The majority of DCIS is now detected by mammography, which often shows typical patterns of microcalcifications. However, the pathological extent of DCIS is often greater than the radiological estimates and may involve more than one quadrant.

Preoperative evaluation should include magnification views and ultrasound examination, with initial biopsy under image guidance. Optimal results are obtained using larger-gauge (size 11) vacuum-assisted core biopsy techniques. The surgeon should carefully plan surgery in conjunction with the radiologist and aim to completely excise the lesion at the first attempt. Re-excision leads to inferior cosmetic results. For more extensive lesions, multiple wires can be used to bracket the lesion. If the resection margins are clear and the patient has an acceptable cosmetic result then conservation surgery is appropriate, and patients with USC/VNPI scores of 4, 5 or 6 require no further treatment. When the score is 7, 8 or 9, re-excision may be considered. Where this is not possible or re-excision fails to downscore the lesion, breast irradiation should be considered. Mastectomy with or without immediate breast reconstruction is usually recommended for scores of 10, 11 or 12. When margins are involved after initial excision, a re-excision procedure may be appropriate, although this may yield a poor cosmetic result and margins may remain positive or close. Under these circumstances, mastectomy should be discussed with the patient together with the option of immediate breast reconstruction. A skin-sparing technique can usually be employed for all types of (immediate) reconstruction, and provides an excellent cosmetic result with inconspicuous scars.

The future

Future molecular studies are likely to identify markers that will allow differentiation between those cases of DCIS that have a more aggressive potential and are likely to progress to invasive disease from cases that have no biological consequence and represent incidental radiological or pathological findings. Treatment schedules can be tailored accordingly, with more intensive therapies for the former group.

References

1. Nemoto T, Vana J, Bedwani R et al. Management and survival of female breast cancer: results of a national survey by The American College of Surgeons. Cancer 1980; 45: 2917–24.
2. Ernster V, Barclay J, Kerlikowske K et al. Incidence of and treatment for ductal carcinoma in situ of the breast. JAMA 1996; 275: 913–18.
3. Greenlee R, Hill-Harmon M, Murray T et al. Cancer Statistics 2001; CA Cancer J Clin 2001; 51: 15–36.
4. Benson K, Hartz A. A comparison of observational studies and randomised, controlled clinical trials. N Engl J Med 2000; 342: 1878–86.
5. Concato J, Shah N, Horwitz R. Randomized, controlled trials, observational studies, and the hierarchy of research designs. N Engl J Med 2000; 342: 1887–92.
6. Fisher B, Costantino J, Redmond C et al. Lumpectomy compared with lumpectomy and radiotherapy for the treatment of intraductal breast cancer. N Engl J Med 1993; 328: 1581–6.
7. Fisher E, Constantino J, Fisher B et al. Pathologic findings from the National Surgical Adjuvant Breast Project (NSABP) Protocol B-17. Cancer 1995; 75: 1310–19.
8. Fisher B, Dignam J, Wolmark N et al. Findings from National Surgical Adjuvant Breast and Bowel Project B-17. J Clin Oncol 1998; 16: 441–52.
9. Fisher E, Dignam J, Tan-Chiu E et al. Pathologic findings from the National Surgical Adjuvant Breast Project (NSABP) eight-year update of Protocol B-17: intraductal carcinoma. Cancer 1999; 86: 429–38.
10. Fisher B, Land S, Mamounas E et al. Prevention of invasive breast cancer in women with ductal carcinoma in situ: an update of the National Surgical Adjuvant Breast and Bowel Project Experience. Semin Oncol 2001; 28: 400–18.
11. Julien J, Bijker N, Fentiman I et al. Radiotherapy in breast conserving treatment for ductal carcinoma in situ: first results of EORTC randomised phase III trial 10853. Lancet 2000; 355: 528–33.
12. Bijker N, Peterse J, Duchateau L et al. Risk factors for recurrence and metastasis after breast-conserving therapy for ductal carcinoma in situ: analysis of European Organization for Research and Treatment of Cancer Trial 10853. J Clin Oncol 2001; 19: 2263–71.
13. George W, Houghton J, Cuzick J et al. Radiotherapy and tamoxifen following complete local excision (CLE) in the management of ductal carcinoma in situ (DCIS): preliminary results from the UK DCIS trial. Proc Am Soc Clin Oncol 2000; 19: 70A.
14. Houghton J, George W. Radiotherpay and tamoxifen following complete excision of ductal carcinoma in situ of the breast. In: Silverstein M, ed. Ductal Carcinoma in Situ of the Breast, 2nd edn. Philadelphia: Lippincott, Williams and Wilkins, 2002.
15. Ernster V, Barclay J, Kerlikowske K, Wilkie H, Ballard-Barbash R. Mortality among women with ductal carcinoma in situ of the breast in population-based surveillance, epidemiology and end results program. Arch Intern Med 2000; 160: 953–8.
16. Silverstein M, Barth A, Waisman J et al. Predicting local recurrence in patients with intraductal breast carcinoma (DCIS). Proc Am Soc Clin Oncol 1995; 14: 117.
17. Silverstein M, Barth A, Poller D et al. Ten-year results comparing mastectomy to excision and radiotherapy for

ductal carcinoma in situ of the breast. Eur J Cancer 1995; 31A: 1425–7.

18. Sposto R, Epstein M, Silverstein M. Predicting local recurrence in patients with ductal carcinoma in situ of the breast. In: Silverstein M, ed. Ductal Carcinoma in Situ of the Breast, 2nd edn. Philadelphia: Lippincott, Williams and Wilkins, 2002.

19. Lagios MD. Duct carcinoma in situ: pathology and treatment. Surg Clin North Am 1990; 70: 853–71.

20. Page D, Anderson T. Diagnostic Histopathology of the Breast. New York: Churchill Livingstone, 1987: 157–74.

21. Tavassoli F. Intraductal carcinoma. In: Tavassoli FA, ed. Pathology of the Breast, Ed. Norwalk, CT: Appleton and Lange, 1992: 229–61.

22. Rosen P, Oberman H. Intraepithelial (preinvasive or in situ) carcinoma. In: Rosen P, Oberman H, eds. In: Atlas of Tumor Pathology – Tumors of the Mammary Gland. Washington, DC: Armed Forces Institute of Pathology, 1993: 119–56.

23. Aasmundstad T, Haugen O. DNA ploidy in intraductal breast carcinomas. Eur J Cancer 1992; 26: 956–9.

24. Meyer J. Cell kinetics in selection and stratification of patients for adjuvant therapy of breast carcinoma. NCI Monograph 1986; 1: 25–8.

25. Allred D, Clark G, Molina R et al. Overexpression of HER-2/neu and its relationship with other prognostic factors change during the progression of in situ to invasive breast cancer. Hum Pathol 1992; 23: 974–9.

26. Barnes D, Meyer J, Gonzalez J et al. Relationship between c-erbB-2 immunoreactivity and thymidine labelling index in breast carcinoma in situ. Breast Cancer Res Treat 1991; 18: 11–17.

27. Barnes D, Bartkova J, Camplejohn R et al. Overexpression of the c-erbB-2 oncoprotein: Why does this occur more frequently in ductal carcinoma in situ than in invasive mammary carcinoma and is this of prognostic significance? Eur J Cancer 1992; 28: 644–8.

28. Bartkova J, Barnes D, Millis R et al. Immunhistochemical demonstration of c-erbB-2 protein in mammary ductal carcinoma in situ. Hum Pathol 1990; 21: 1164–7.

29. Bobrow L, Happerfield L, Gregory W et al. The classification of ductal carcinoma in situ and its association with biological markers. Semin Diagn Pathol 1994; 11: 199–207.

30. Liu E, Thor A, He M et al. The HER2 (c-erbB-2) oncogene is frequently amplified in in situ carcinomas of the breast. Oncogene 1992; 7: 1027–32.

31. van de Vijver M, Peterse J, Mooi WJ et al. Neu-protein overexpression in breast cancer: association with comedo-type ductal carcinoma in situ and limited prognostic value in stage II breast cancer. N Engl J Med 1988; 319: 1239–45.

32. Lagios M, Margolin F, Westdahl P et al. Mammographically detected duct carcinoma in situ. Frequency of local recurrence following tylectomy and prognostic effect of nuclear grade on local recurrence. Cancer 1989; 63: 619–24.

33. Schwartz G. The role of excision and surveillance alone in subclinical DCIS of the breast. Oncology 1994; 8: 21–6.

34. Silverstein M, Waisman J, Gierson E et al. Radiation therapy for intraductal carcinoma: Is it an equal alternative? Arch Surg 1991; 126: 424–8.

35. Solin L, Yeh I, Kurtz J et al. Ductal carcinoma in situ (intraductal carcinoma) of the breast treated with breast-conserving surgery and definitive irradiation. Correlation of pathologic parameters with outcome of treatment. Cancer 1993; 71: 2532–42.

36. Lagios M, Westdahl P, Margolin F et al. Duct carcinoma in situ: relationship of extent of noninvasive disease to the frequency of occult invasion, multicentricity, lymph node metastases, and short-term treatment failures. Cancer 1982; 50: 1309–14.

37. Moriya T, Silverberg S. Intraductal carcinoma (ductal carcinoma in situ) of the breast: a comparison of pure noninvasive tumors with those including different proportions of infiltrating carcinoma. Cancer 1994; 74: 2972–8.

38. Moriya T, Silverberg S. Intraductal carcinoma (ductal carcinoma in situ) of the breast: analysis of pathologic findings of 85 pure intraductal carcinomas. Int J Surg Pathol 1995; 3: 83–92.

39. Poller D, Silverstein M, Galea M et al. Ductal carcinoma in situ of the breast: a proposal for a new simplified histological classification association between cellular proliferation and c-erbB-2 protein expression. Mod Pathol 1994; 7: 257–62.

40. Fisher E, Sass R, Fisher B et al. Pathologic findings from the National surgical Adjuvant Breast Project (Protocol 6) i. Intraductal carcinoma (DCIS). Cancer 1986; 57: 197–208.

41. Kuske R, Bean J, Garcia D et al. Breast conservation therapy for intraductal carcinoma of the breast. Int J Radiat Oncol Biol Phys 1993; 26: 391–6.

42. Holland R, Peterse J, Millis R et al. Ductal carcinoma in situ: a proposal for a new classification. Semin Diagn Pathol 1994; 11: 167–80.

43. Morrow M, Schnitt S, Harris J. Ductal carcinoma in situ. In: Harris J et al, eds. Diseases of the Breast. Philadelphia: Lippincott-Raven, 1995, 355–368.

44. Silverstein M, Poller D, Waisman J et al. Prognostic classification of breast ductal carcinoma-in-situ. Lancet 1995; 345: 1154–7.

45. Silverstein M. The Van Nuys Breast Center – the first free-standing multidisciplinary breast center. Surg Oncol Clin North Am 2000; 9: 159–75.

46. Silverstein M, Poller D, Craig P et al. A prognostic index for ductal carcinoma in situ of the breast. Cancer 1996; 77: 2267–74.

47. Silverstein M, Lagios M, Craig P et al. The Van Nuys Prognostic Index for ductal carcinoma in situ. Breast J 1996; 2: 38–40.

48. Bellamy C, McDonald C, Salter D et al. Noninvasive ductal carcinoma of the breast: the relevance of histologic categorization. Hum Pathol 1993; 24: 16–23.

49. Sloane J, Ellman R, Anderson T et al. Consistency of histopathological reporting of breast lesions detected by breast screening: findings of the UK National External Quality Assessment (EQA) scheme. Eur J Cancer 1994; 10: 1414–19.

50. Tabar L, Dean P. Basic principles of mammographic diagnosis. Diagn Imag Clin Med 1985; 54: 146–57.

51. Burbank F. Stereotactic breast biopsy of atypical ductal hyperplasia and ductal carcinoma in situ lesions: improved accuracy with directional, vacuum-assisted biopsy instrument. Radiology 1997; 202: 843–7.

52. Liberman L. Clinical management issues in percutaneous core breast biopsy. Radiol Clin North Am 2000; 38: 791–807.

53. Committee CC. Image-detected breast cancer: state-of-the-art diagnosis and treatment. J Am Coll Surg 2001; 193: 297–302.

54. Silverstein M, Gamagami P, Colburn W et al. Nonpalpable breast lesions: diagnosis with slightly overpenetrated screen-film mammography and hook wire-directed breast biopsy in 1014 cases. Radiology 1989; 171: 633–8.

55. Noguchi S, Aihara T, Koyama H et al. Discrimination between multicentric and multifocal carcinomas of breast through clonal analysis. Cancer 1994; 74: 872–7.

56. Holland R, Veling S, Mravunac M et al. Histologic multifocality of Tis, T1–2 breast carcinomas. Implications for clinical trials of breast conserving surgery. Cancer 1985; 56: 979–90.

57. Faverly D, Burgers L, Bult P et al. Three dimensional imaging of mammary ductal carcinoma in situ: clinical implications. Semin Diagn Pathol 1995; 11: 193–8.

58. Blamey R, Macmilliam D, Rampaul R et al. Ductal carcinoma in situ: experience at Nottingham City Hospital 1973–2000. In: Silverstein M, ed. Ductal Carcinoma in Situ of the Breast, 2nd edn. Philadelphia: Lippincott, Williams and Wilkins, 2002.

59. Silverstein M. Intraductal breast carcinoma: two decades of progress? Am J Clin Oncol 1991; 14: 534–7.

60. Dickson R, Lippman M. Growth factors in breast cancer. Endocr Rev 1995; 16: 559–89.

61. Lippman M. The development of biological therapies for breast cancer. Science 1993; 259: 631–2.

62. Archer S, Kemp B, Gadd M et al. Ductal carcinoma in situ of the breast: comedo versus noncomedo subtype nonpredictive of recurrence of contralateral new breast primary. Breast Dis 1994; 7: 353–60.

63. Arnesson L, Smeed S, Fagerberg G et al. Follow-up of two treatment modalities for ductal carcinoma in situ of the breast. Br J Surg 1989; 76: 672–5.

64. Ashikari R, Hadju S, Robbins G. Intraductal carcinoma of the breast. Cancer 1971; 28: 1182–7.

65. Carter D, Smith R. Carcinoma in situ of the breast. Cancer 1977; 40: 1189–93.

66. Ciatto S, Bonardi R, Cataliotti L et al. Intraductal breast carcinoma. Review of a multicenter series of 350 cases. Tumori 1990; 76: 552–4.

67. Farrow J. Current concepts in the detection and treatment of the earliest of the breast cancers. Cancer 1970; 25: 468–77.

68. Fentiman I, Fagg N, Millis R et al. In situ ductal carcinoma of the breast: implications of disease pattern and treatment. Eur J Surg Oncol 1986; 12: 261–6.

69. Brown P, Silverman J, Owens P et al. Intraductal 'noninfiltrating' carcinoma of the breast. Arch Surg 1976; 111: 1063–7.

70. Fisher E, Leiming E, Anderson S et al. Conservative management of intraductal carcinoma (DCIS) of the breast. J Surg Oncol 1991; 47: 139–47.

71. Kinne D, Petrek J, Osborne M et al. Breast carcinoma in situ. Arch Surg 1989; 124: 33–6.

72. Schuh M, Nemoto T, Penetrante R et al. Intraductal carcinoma: analysis of presentation, pathologic findings, and outcome of disease. Arch Surg 1986; 121: 1303–7.

73. Silverstein M. The Van Nuys/USC experience by treatment. In: Silverstein M, ed. Ductal Carcinoma in Situ of the Breast. Philadelphia: Lippincott, Williams and Wilkins, 2002.

74. Simpson T, Thirlby R, Dail D. Surgical treatment of ductal carcinoma in situ of the breast: 10 to 20 year follow-up. Arch Surg 1992; 127: 468–72.

75. Sunshine J, Moseley H, Fletcher W et al. Breast carcinoma in situ, a retrospective review of 112 cases with a minimum 10 years follow-up. Am J Surg 1985; 150: 44–51.

76. Von Reuden D, Wilson W. Intraductal carcinoma of the breast. Surg Gynecol Obstet 1984; 158: 105–11.

77. Westbrook K, Gallager H. Intraductal carcinoma of the breast. A comparative study. Am J Surg 1975; 130: 667–70.

78. Jensen J, Handel N, Silverstein M et al. Glandular replacement therapy (GRT) for intraductal breast carcinoma (DCIS). Proc Am Soc Clin Oncol 1995; 14: 138.

79. Jensen J, Handel N, Silverstein M. Glandular replacement therapy: an argument for a combined surgical approach in the treatment of noninvasive breast cancer. Breast J 1996; 2: 121–3.

80. Silverstein M, Rosser R, Gierson E et al. Axillary lymph node dissection for intraductal carcinoma – is it indicated? Cancer 1987; 59: 1819–24.

81. Silverstein M, Rosser R, Gierson E et al. Axillary lymph node dissection for intraductal carcinoma – is it indicated? Proc Am Soc Clin Oncol 1986; 5: 265.

82. Klauber-DeMore N, Tan L, Liberman L et al. Sentinel lymph node biopsy: is it indicated in patients with high-risk ductal carcinoma in situ of ductal carcinoma in situ with microinvasion? Ann Surg Oncol 2000; 7: 636–42.

83. Holland R, Hendriks J, Verbeek A et al. Extent, distribution, and mammographic/histological correlations of breast ductal carcinoma in situ. Lancet 1990; 335: 519–22.

84. Holland R, Faverly D. Whole organ studies. In: Silverstein M, ed. Ductal Carcinoma in Situ of the Breast. Philadelphia: Lippincott, Williams and Wilkins, 2002.

85. Eusebi V, Feudale E, Foschini M et al. Long-term follow-up of in situ carcinoma of the breast. Semin Diagn Pathol 1994; 11: 223–35.

86. Lagios M. Controversies in diagnosis, biology, and treatment. Breast J 1995; 1: 68–78.

87. Solin L, McCormick B, Recht A et al. Mammographically detected, clinically occult ductal carcinoma in situ (intraductal carcinoma) treated with breast conserving surgery and definitive breast irradiation. Cancer J Sci Am 1996; 2: 158–65.

88. Solin L, Recht A, Fourquet A et al. Ten-year results of breast-conserving surgery and definitive irradiation for intraductal carcinoma of the breast. Cancer 1991; 68: 2337–44.

89. Solin L, Fourquet A, McCormick B et al. Salvage treatment for local recurrence following breast-conserving surgery and definitive irradiation for ductal carcinoma in situ (intraductal carcinoma) of the breast. Int J Radiat Oncol Biol Phys 1994; 30: 3–9.

90. Solin L, Kurtz J, Fourquet A et al. Fifteen year results of breast conserving surgery and definitive breast irradiation for treatment of ductal carcinoma in situ of the breast. J Clin Oncol 1996; 14: 754–63.

91. Lagios M. The Lagios experience. In: Silverstein M, ed. Ductal Carcinoma in Situ of the Breast. Philadelphia: Lippincott, Williams and Wilkins, 2002.

92. Ottesen G, Graversen H, Blichert-Toft M et al. Ductal carcinoma in situ of the female breast. Short-term results of a prospective nationwide study. Am J Surg Pathol 1992; 16: 1183–96.

93. Baird R, Worth A, Hislop G. Recurrence after lumpectomy for comedo-type intraductal carcinoma of the breast. Am J Surg 1990; 159: 479–81.

94. Carpenter R, Boulter P, Cooke T et al. Management of screen detected ductal carcinoma in situ of the female breast. Br J Surg 1989; 76: 564–7.

95. Cataliotti L, Distante V, Ciatto S et al. Intraductal breast cancer: review of 183 consecutive cases. Eur J Cancer 1992; 28A: 917–20.

96. Gallagher W, Koemer F, Wood WC. Treatment of intraductal carcinoma with limited surgery: long term follow-up. J Clin Oncol 1989; 7: 376–80.

97. Price P, Sinnett H, Gusterson B et al. Duct carcinoma in situ: predictors of local recurrence and progression in patients treated by surgery alone. Cancer 1990; 61: 869–72.

98. Schwartz G. Treatment of subclinical ductal carcinoma in situ of the breast by local excision and surveillance: an updated personal experience. In: Silverstein M, ed. Ductal Carcinoma in Situ of the Breast. Philadelphia: Lippincott, Williams and Wilkins, 2002.

99. Rosen P, Braun D, Kinne D. The clinical significance of pre-invasive breast carcinoma. Cancer 1980; 46: 919–25.

100. Page D, Dupont W, Roger L et al. Intraductal carcinoma of the breast: follow-up after biopsy only. Cancer 1982; 49: 751–8.

101. Page D, Dupont W, Rogers L et al. Continued local recurrence of carcinoma 15–25 years after a diagnosis of low grade ductal carcinoma in situ of the breast treated only by biopsy. Cancer 1995; 76: 1197–200.

102. Alpers C, Wellings S. The prevalence of carcinoma in situ in normal and cancer-associated breast. Hum Pathol 1985; 16: 796–807.

103. Bornstein B, Recht A, Connolly J et al. Results of treating ductal carcinoma in situ of the breast with conservative surgery and radiotherapy. Cancer 1991; 67: 7–13.

104. Haffty B, Peschel R, Papadopoulos D et al. Radiation therapy for ductal carcinoma in situ of the breast. Connecticut Med 1990; 54: 482–4.

105. McCormick B, Rosen P, Kinne D et al. Duct carcinoma in situ of the breast: an analysis of local control after conservation surgery and radiotherapy. Int J Radiat Oncol Biol Phys 1991; 21: 289–92.

106. Fourquet A, Zafrani B, Campana F et al. Breast-conserving treatment of ductal carcinoma in situ. Semin Radiat Oncol 1992; 2: 116–24.

107. Hiramatsu H, Bornstein B, Recht A et al. Local recurrence after conservative surgery and radiotherapy for ductal carcinoma in situ: possible importance of family history. Cancer J Sci Am 1995; 1: 55–61.

108. Kurtz J, Jacquemier J, Torhorst J et al. Conservation therapy for breast cancers other than infiltrating ductal carcinoma. Cancer 1989; 63: 1630–5.

109. Ray G, Adelson A, Hayhurst E et al. Ductal carcinoma in situ of the breast: results of treatment by conservative surgery and definitive radiation. Int J Radiat Oncol Biol Phys 1993; 28: 105–11.

110. Sneige N, McNeese M, Atkinson E et al. Ductal carcinoma in situ treated with lumpectomy and irradiation: histopatholocal analysis of 49 specimens with emphasis on risk factors and long term results. Hum Pathol 1995; 26: 642–9.

111. Stotter A, McNeese M, Oswald M et al. The role of limited surgery with irradiation in primary treatment of ductal carcinoma in situ breast cancer. Int J Radiat Oncol Biol Phys 1990; 18: 283–90.

112. White J, Gustafson G, Levine A et al. Outcome and prognostic factors for local recurrence in mammographically detected ductal carcinoma in-situ of the breast treated with conservative surgery and radiotherapy. Int J Radiat Oncol Biol Phys 1993; 27: 145 (abst.).

113. Zafrani B, Leroyer A, Fourquet A et al. Mammographically-detected ductal in situ carcinoma of the breast anaylyzed with a new classification. A study of 127 cases: correlation with estrogen and progesterone receptors, p53 and c-erbB-2 proteins, and proliferative activity. Semin Diagn Pathol 1994; 11: 208–14.

114. Fisher B, Redmond C, Fisher ER. Radiation therapy for in situ or localized breast cancer: the authors reply. N Engl J Med 1993; 329: 1578.

115. Lagios M, Page D. Radiation therapy for in situ or localized breast cancer. N Engl J Med 1993; 321: 1577–8.

116. Page D, Lagios M. Pathologic analysis of the NSABP-B17 Trial. Cancer 1995; 75: 1219–22.

117. Fisher E, Costantino J, Fisher B et al. Blunting the counterpoint. Cancer 1995; 75: 1223–7.

118. Fraass B, Roberson P, Lichter A. Dose to the contralateral breast due to primary breast irradiation. Int J Radiol Oncol Phys 1985; 11: 485–97.

119. Muller-Runkel R, Kalokhe G. Scatter dose from tangential breast irradiation to the uninvolved breast. Radiology 1990; 175: 873–6.

120. Boice J, Harvey E, Blettner M et al. Cancer in the contralateral breast after radiotherapy for breast cancer. New Engl J Med 1992; 326: 781–5.

121. Recht A. Side effects of radiotherapy. In: Silverstein M, ed. Ductal Carcinoma in Situ of the Breast. Baltimore: Williams and Wilkins, 1997: 347–52.

122. Early Breast Cancer Trialists' Collaborative Group. Favorable and unfavorable effects on long-term survival of radiotherapy for early breast cancer. Lancet 2000; 355: 1757–70.

123. Kurtz J. Radiotherapy for early breast cancer: Was a comprehensive overview of trials needed? Lancet 2000; 355: 1739–40.

124. Silverstein M. Van Nuys Prognostic Index for DCIS. In: Silverstein M, ed. Ductal Carcinoma in Situ of the Breast. Baltimore: Williams and Wilkins, 1997: 459–73.

125. Silverstein M, Lagios M, Groshen S et al. The influence of margin width on local control in patients with ductal carcinoma in situ (DCIS) of the breast. N Engl J Med 1999; 340: 1455–61.

126. Vicini F, Kestin L, Goldstein N et al. Impact of young age on outcome in patients with ductal carcinoma-in-situ treated with breast-conserving therapy. J Clin Oncol 2000; 18: 296–306.

127. Szelei-Stevens K, Kuske R, Yantsos VA et al. The influence of young age and positive family history of breast cancer on the prognosis of ductal carcinoma in situ treated by excision with or without radiotherapy or mastectomy. Int J Rad Oncol Biol Phys 2000; 48: 943–9.

128. Goldstein N, Vicini F, Kestin L et al. Differences in the pathologic features of ductal carcinoma in situ of the breast based on patient age. Cancer 2000; 88: 2552–60.

129. Galea M, Blamey R, Elston C et al. The Nottingham Prognostic Index in primary breast cancer. Breast Cancer Res Treat 1992; 22: 207–19.

130. Goldstein NS, Kestin L, Vicini F. Intraductal carcinoma of the breast: pathologic features associated with local recurrence in patients treated with breast-conserving therapy. Am J Surg Pathol 2000; 24: 1058–67.

131. Kestin L, Goldstein N, lacerna M et al. Factors associated with local recurrence of mammographically detected ductal carcinoma in situ in patients given breast conserving therapy. Cancer 2000; 88: 596–601.

132. van Zee K, Liberman L, Samli B et al. Long-term follow-up of women with ductal carcinoma in situ treated with breast conserving surgery: the effect of age. Cancer 1999; 86: 1757–67.

133. Bradley S, Weaver D, Bouwman D. Alternative in the surgical management of in situ breast cancer. Am Surg 1990; 56: 428–32.

134. Rosner D, Bedwani R, Vana J et al. Noninvasive breast carcinoma. Results of a national survey of The American College of Surgeons. Ann Surg 1980; 192: 139–47.

135. Silverstein M, Lagios M, Martino S et al. Outcome after local recurrence in patients with ductal carcinoma in situ of the breast. J Clin Oncol 1998; 16: 1367–73.

136. Silverstein M. Noninvasive breast cancer: the dilemma of the 1990s. Obstet Gynecol Clin North Am 1994; 21: 639–58.

137. Silverstein M, Gierson E, Colburn W et al. Can intraductal breast carcinoma be excised completely by local excision? Clinical and pathologic predictors. Cancer 1994; 73: 2985–9.

138. Dowlatshahi K, Fan M, Bloom KJ et al. Occult metastases in sentinel lymph nodes of patients with early stage breast carcinoma: a preliminary study. Cancer 1999; 86: 990–6.

139. Lagios M, Silverstein M. Sentinel node biopsy for patients with DCIS: a dangerous and unwarranted direction. Ann Surg Oncol 2001; 8: 275–7.

140. Frykberg E, Masood S, Copeland E et al. Duct carcinoma in situ of the breast. Surg Gynecol Obstet 1993; 177: 425–40.

141. Balch C, Singletary E, Bland K. Clinical decision-making in early breast cancer. Ann Surg 1993; 217: 207–22.

142. Gump F, Jicha D, Ozzello L. Ductal carcinoma in situ (DCIS): a revised concept. Surgery 1987; 102: 190–5.

143. Rosen P, Senie R, Schottenfeld D et al. Noninvasive breast carcinoma: frequency of unsuspected invasion and implications for treatment. Ann Surg 1979; 1989: 377–82.

33 Surgical treatment of early invasive breast cancer

Rache M Simmons, Michael Osborne

Introduction

The definition of 'minimal breast cancer' or 'early breast cancer' varies in the medical literature, to include ductal carcinoma in situ (DCIS), lobular carcinoma in situ (LCIS) and invasive carcinomas up to 5 mm[1] or 1 cm.[2] We define early invasive breast cancer as carcinomas less than 1 cm. This also includes DCIS with microinvasion, which is designated in the American Joint Committee on Cancer TMN system as T1*mic*,[3] defined as DCIS with an invasive component less than 1 mm.[4]

Due to the increased use of breast cancer screening through mammography and physician and patient breast self-examination, the incidence of early breast cancer has exploded in the past decade. Because of this surging incidence of early breast cancer, the clinician should be aware of the methods for diagnosis and treatment options available to these patients.

Diagnosis

As with any size of breast cancer, an early breast cancer would be detected either clinically by a palpable nodule or a change on screening mammogram or ultrasound. Due to its small size, an early breast cancer would most often be detected by breast imaging unless the lesion was located superficially in the breast.

Once the lesion has been detected, a confirmatory biopsy should be done to establish a diagnosis. This can be an image-guided needle biopsy or an excisional biopsy.

An image-guided needle biopsy can be either a fine-needle aspiration (FNA) or a core biopsy to sample the lesion. This can be done with the assistance of breast ultrasound or a mammographic stereotactic technique using a vacuum-assisted device. If the lesion is palpable, a FNA or core biopsy can also be performed without the assistance of breast imaging. Due to the limited sensitivity of FNA compared with core biopsy, and its inability to distinguish between invasive and non-invasive disease, many surgeons prefer core biopsy to FNA to establish a diagnosis. A core biopsy without evidence of invasion does not exclude the diagnosis, because of the technique's limited sampling capacity. Core biopsy samples allow additional information about the histological grade of the tumour, and the status of oestrogen and progesterone receptors (ER and PgR).

Image-guided biopsy is preferable to excision, when possible, as the oncological surgery can be planned as a one-step procedure when a pre-operative diagnosis has been established. This surgical excision can be assisted by ultrasound or mammographic localisation wire placement in non-palpable lesions.

Surgical treatment of the breast

Once a diagnosis of early breast cancer has been established, surgical treatment needs to proceed, with either breast conservation or mastectomy. The possibility of axillary metastatic involvement should also be addressed. Once the surgical treatment is complete, patients should be referred to radiation oncologists and medical oncologists to finalise planning of definitive adjuvant therapy if appropriate.

Breast conservation

The majority of small invasive breast cancers are treated by breast conservation, which includes wide local excision with negative surgical margins and radiation treatment to the breast. The studies to date, including the US National Surgical Adjuvant Breast and Bowel Project (NSABP) Protocols B-06, and the Milan Trial comparing quadratectomy with modified radical mastectomy, as well as several other clinical trials, show no statistically significant difference in overall patient survival between mastectomy and breast conservation for small invasive carcinomas.[5–11]

Several factors appear to predict the incidence of local recurrence, and would be unfavourable factors for breast conservation. Controversy exists as to what is an acceptable 'close' surgical margin, with estimates ranging from 1 cm to less than 1 mm.[12] The incidence of local failure is lower in those cases with negative final pathological margins of tumour excision than when the final pathological margins are unknown, positive, or close.[13] This emphasizes the importance of obtaining pathological tumour-free margins at the time of resection or re-excision to optimise local control.

Because of the multicentricity of breast cancer, the addition of radiation treatment to wide local excision in patients with invasive carcinoma is currently the standard of treatment. NSABP B-06 evaluated rates of local recurrence of small invasive tumours with and without radiation treatment following lumpectomy. Those patients not receiving radiotherapy, had a significantly higher rate of local recurrence.[5,8]

The radiation dose to the whole breast after lumpectomy ranges from 4500 to 5000 cGy usually given over 5 weeks.[14] Most radiation oncologists give additional treatment to the area of the tumour bed; this is referred to as a 'boost dose' and is typically in the region of 1600 cGy.[15] Surgical placement of titanium haemoclips into the biopsy cavity at the time of lumpectomy facilitates accuracy in direction of the boost dose by the radiation oncologist. These clips are also helpful in identifying the lumpectomy site on future mammography.[15]

Whether or not to boost and the appropriate dose of boost are controversial issues and may be determined by the status of the final surgical margins.[14] When patients with positive surgical margins were treated with total doses of radiation of 6600 cGy, local failure rates decreased. However, the incidence of local recurrence is still higher in patients with positive margins, with an overall failure rate of 18% at 4 years, compared to 3.7% for patients with negative margins.[16]

Mastectomy

In some patients with early breast cancer, there are contraindications to breast conservation, and the recommendation for treatment would be mastectomy with or without immediate breast reconstruc-

tion. Some of these contraindications include previous radiation to the breast area, pregnancy, extensive microcalcification, an inability to achieve tumour-free margins and multicentricity (defined as the presence of two or more separate tumour foci in different quadrants of the breast). Relative contraindications to radiotherapy include patients with connective tissue disorders, who have a higher incidence of tissue damage from radiation.[17] Another factor favouring mastectomy can be patient preference.[18] Certainly, any patient who is recommended to have a mastectomy should be offered the option of immediate reconstruction and referred to a plastic surgeon to discuss which techniques would be appropriate on an individual basis.

Surgical treatment of the axilla in early breast cancer

There are several reasons for assessing the axillary nodes for the presence of metastases in any breast cancer patient. The status of the axillary lymph nodes is important in determining the patient's stage of disease. The presence or absence of axillary lymph node metastases (ALNM) determines prognosis, which facilitates decision-making by the medical oncology team regarding adjuvant therapy. Surgical removal of metastatic nodes in the axilla significantly decreases the chance of an axillary recurrence.[17] The surgical procedure of axillary dissection may impact on overall survival, though this is debated in the medical literature.

The likelihood of axillary nodal involvement in clinically T1a,bN0M0 patients is not insignificant. In a large series of 919 patients with T1a and T1b tumours, the overall incidence of ALNM was 18.0%.[19] These data have been supported by several other series of T1a,b breast cancers, where the incidence of ALNM ranged from 10% to 27%.[20–22]

Within this group of T1a,b carcinomas, increasing tumour size has been found to increase the probability of nodal metastases.[19,23–25] When breast cancers are subdivided into T1a and T1b tumours, the incidence of ALNM for T1a tumours ranges from 0% to 10%[19,20,23,26–28] and that for T1b tumours from 10% to 23%.[19,20,23,26,28]

In addition to tumour size, the likelihood of ALNM is influenced by other factors. Favourable histological subtypes, including mucinous, medullary, papillary and tubular tumours, have been found to have fewer ALNM, which were present in 3.9% of patients with favourable tumour subtypes, compared with 13.9% of patients with a less favourable histological subtype ($p < 0.001$).[25] Histological grade of the tumour has also been found to predict ALNM in tumours smaller than 1 cm.[19,20,22,25] One study showed that T1a,b patients with tumours of histological grade 1 had a 13% chance of ALNM, compared with 16% for grade 2 tumours and 29% for grade 3 tumours.[19]

The presence of peritumoral lymphovascular invasion (LVI) has also been shown to predict the likelihood of ALNM in T1a,b tumours.[19,22] In one series, 17% of patients with ALNM had LVI, compared with 3% of patients without ($p < 0.0001$).[19]

Increasing patient age has been shown to correlate inversely with the presence of nodal metastases in early breast cancer.[19,24,25] A review of the US National Cancer Institute's Surveillance, Epidemiology and End Results (SEER) data on 12 000 women with T1a and T1b breast cancers showed that women younger than 40 had an ALNM rate of 22.6%, compared with 10.2% in women aged over 70.[25]

Even in the most favourable subgroup of early breast cancer patients – aged 50 or more, with a well-differentiated T1a tumour and without LVI – 13% had ALNM. Even among those patients aged 60 or more, 8.7% still had ALNM.[19]

Due to the incidence of ALNM in patients with early breast cancer, the status of the axilla should be assessed by sentinel lymph node biopsy or axillary dissection in all patients unless there are contraindications to axillary surgery. Evaluation of axillary metastases in patients with tumours smaller than 1 cm is particularly important because the detection of nodal metastases may significantly alter the postoperative recommendations for adjuvant therapy. The axillary nodal status may directly dictate the use of systemic therapy in a patient who would otherwise not have been offered systemic treatment. It is for these small cancers that nodal status based upon surgical staging may have the greatest impact on treatment.

Sentinel lymph node biopsy

Traditionally, axillary dissection has been performed on all patients with invasive breast cancer and is the single most important predictor of prognosis. The sentinel lymphadenectomy or 'sentinel lymph node biopsy' (SLNB) identifies the first or 'sentinel' lymph node(s) in the axillary chain to receive drainage from the tumour and is thus the most likely node to contain metastases.[29] The SLNB technique is performed by the injection of isosulfan blue or methylene blue[30] dye and/or radioactive isotope to localize the sentinel lymph node (see Figures 33.1 and 33.2).[29–38]

SLNB has been shown through several validation studies to predict axillary metastases accurately with sensitivity ranging from 93% to 98.7% and the

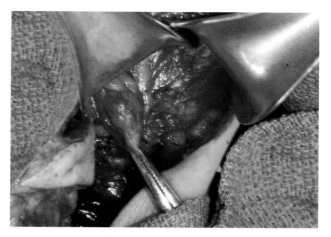

Figure 33.1 Axillary sentinel lymph node localized by methylene blue dye.

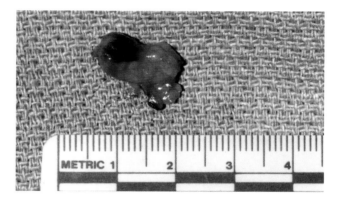

Figure 33.2 Ex vivo axillary sentinel lymph node localized by methylene dye.

false-negative rate from 0% to 6.7%.[32,34,36–39] The axillary recurrence rate for T1 tumours undergoing SLNB without axillary dissection has been shown to be 0% at 39 months.[29]

The majority of patients with early breast cancer will have negative SLNB. Positive SLNB has been documented in 8–25% of patients with T1a tumours and in 14–44% of patients with T1b tumours.[31,35,39] These numbers are slightly higher than for a traditional axillary dissection, which is probably due to the increased scrutiny with which the sentinel lymph nodes are examined.

SLNB offers a less invasive method to assess the status of the axilla, with fewer complications than a formal axillary node dissection. The potential complications of an axillary dissection include lymphoedema, infection, seroma, haematoma, neurovascular injury and arm discomfort. In patients undergoing an SLNB without an axillary dissection, the complication rate has been shown to be 3% or less.[29]

Axillary dissection

In patients who are found to have metastatic foci on SLNB, a completion axillary lymph node dissection (ALND) is typically recommended. If a patient is not a candidate for SLNB then an ALND should be performed. Contraindications to SLNB include patients with previous axillary surgery (due to axillary scar tissue and the potential inaccuracy of the technique), and pregnancy (due to a lack of data regarding fetal safety). SLNB is not being performed universally, and when a surgeon is still on a learning curve then a completion ALND may be appropriate. Several clinical trials such as the American College of Surgeons Oncology Group Z10/11 Trial and the NSABP Protocol B-32 are ongoing to evaluate the accuracy of the SLNB technique, and patients enrolled in these trials follow the protocol guidelines regarding ALND.

Bone marrow aspiration

The spread of breast cancer through the lymphatic system is measured by the status of the axillary lymph nodes, which has historically been the most important prognostic indicator for breast cancer patients. Multiple studies have suggested that the presence of bone marrow micrometastases (BMM) is equally or more predictive of distant recurrence and survival than axillary nodal status. To test for BMM, bone marrow aspirates (BMA) can be obtained at the time of surgical treatment for the primary breast cancer, as described in a number of articles[40–43] (see Figure 33.3). Samples are taken from the patient's anterior iliac crests, as described in a number of articles

Multiple studies have found a significant correlation between distant recurrence and decreased survival and the presence of BMM. One study showed the 2-year distant recurrence rate for BMM-negative patients to be 3%, versus 33% in BMM-positive patients ($p < 0.04$).[44] In a univariate analysis, Diel et al[45] showed that, at a median follow up of 36 months, the presence of BMM was associated with increased distant relapse and decreased survival ($p < 0.001$). In a multivariate analysis, the presence of BMM was found to be the strongest independent predictor of distant relapse.[45] Braun et al[42] demonstrated similar results, in which BMM was associated with the occurrence of clinical distant metastases and death from cancer-related causes ($p < 0.001$).

When prognosis is evaluated with a combination of BMM and axillary lymph node status, overall prognosis is best for those patients who are BMM-negative and lymph node-negative, conversely, those patients who are BMM-positive and lymph node-positive have the worst prognosis. Those patients who are either bone marrow-positive or lymph node-positive are intermediate in prognosis.[42]

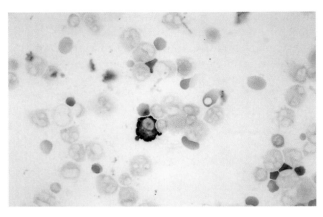

Figure 33.3 Bone marrow micrometastases in a breast cancer patient stained with cytokeratin monoclonal antibody. Courtesy of Dr Syed Hoda, The New York Presbyterian Hospital, Weill Medical School of Cornell University, Department of Pathology.

BMM have been demonstrated in 30% of T1 carcinomas[45] and may indicate a group of patients where adjuvant systemic therapy would offer a survival benefit. BMM status may serve as a complement to axillary lymph node status in assessing the likelihood of occult systemic disease in breast cancer patients. This information may be useful to clinicians in making recommendations for systemic adjuvant therapy.

Adjuvant therapy

The indication for adjuvant therapy in general is to treat those patients with substantial likelihood of having micrometastatic disease. Most medical oncologists consider this risk to be sufficiently high in node-negative patients with a tumour diameter equal to or greater than 1 cm and any patient with nodal metastases to justify adjuvant chemotherapy.[15] The indications for chemotherapy in patients with documented micrometastases in the axillary lymph nodes or the bone marrow (detected by BMA) remain debatable.

Investigational studies evaluating the impact of systemic therapy upon patients with BMM and micrometastatic disease in the sentinel lymph nodes are currently underway. The American College of Surgeons Oncology Group is exploring this question through the Z-10/Z-11 trial, in which breast cancer patients undergo lumpectomy, SLNB/axillary dissection and BMA. The treating clinicians are blinded to the immunohistochemical status of the sentinel lymph nodes and the BMA results. The patients will then all undergo breast radiotherapy and also chemotherapy/hormonal therapy as appropriate for their tumour size and nodal status. Data from this large multi-institutional trial will give insight into the clinical significance of micrometastatic disease in the sentinel node and the BMA, as well as the effectiveness of adjuvant therapy on such patients.

Tamoxifen therapy is commonly used as an adjuvant treatment in early breast cancer patients with ER-positive tumors. The recommended length of treatment for node-negative patients is 5 years.[46] Additionally, tamoxifen can be used as a chemopreventive agent to decrease the chance of an additional ipsilateral tumour in patients undergoing breast conservation or with contralateral breast cancer.[15]

The recommendations regarding tamoxifen or chemotherapy alone or a combination of both is dependent upon the clinical judgement of the treating medical oncologist. Consideration should be given to the likelihood of systemic recurrence based upon nodal status, tumour size and grade, and the status of the BMA if performed. Also, ER positivity of the tumour is predictive of the patient's response to hormonal therapy and HER2/*neu* (c-*erb*B-2) may be helpful to determine the appropriate type of chemotherapy. Another factor is the patient's age and any comorbid diseases that would reduce tolerability to a course of chemotherapy.

Prognosis

The overall prognosis for patients with early breast cancer is excellent. In one study of 218 breast cancer patients with T1a,bN0M0 tumours, the 7-year recurrence-free survival rate was 93% and the distant recurrence-free survival rate 95%.[47]

At the time of diagnosis, less than 5% of T1a,bN0 patients have clinically detectable distant metastases.[48] Due to this low incidence of systemic disease, most physicians do not initially obtain an extent-of-disease work-up including a bone scan and computed tomography (CT) scans of the lungs, brain and liver.

Surveillance

Surveillance should continue after diagnosis and treatment in early breast cancer to detect local recurrence or a new primary breast cancer in either ipsilateral or contralateral breast. According to the recommendations of the US National Comprehensive Cancer Network (NCCN version 1.2001), patients should continue diligent monthly self-examinations, and a physician should perform physical examinations at 4- to 6-month intervals to assess evidence of local recurrence and symptoms of metastatic disease. The ipsilateral arm should be evaluated to detect early signs of lymphoedema and initiate appropriate management. Mammography

should be performed every 6 months on the ipsilateral breast for 2 years and annually on the contralateral breast. Bone scans and CT scans should be performed only on patients symptomatic of systemic disease because there is no evidence of improved survival with early detection of distant metastases.[15]

References

1. Veronesi U. Clinical management of minimal breast cancer. Semin Surg Oncol 1989; 5: 145–50.
2. Simmons RM, Osborne MP. Surgical treatment of early breast cancer. In: Querci della Rovere GQ, ed. Breast Screening and Management of Early Breast Cancer. Edinburgh: Graffham Press, 1998: 205–13.
3. Hermanek P, Hutter R, Sobin LH et al. TNM Atlas: Illustrated Guide to the TNM/pTMN Classification of Malignant Tumors, 4th edn. Berlin: Springer-Verlag, 1997.
4. Fleming ID, Cooper JS, Henson DE et al. American Joint Committee on the Classification of Ductal Carcinoma in Situ, 5th edn. Philadelphia: Lippincott-Raven, 1997.
5. Fisher B, Redmond C, Poisson R et al. Eight-year results of a randomized clinical trial comparing total mastectomy and lumpectomy with or without irradiation in the treatment of breast cancer. N Engl J Med 1989; 320: 822–8.
6. Christian MC, McCabe MS, Korn EL et al. The National Cancer Institute Audit of the National Surgical Adjuvant Breast and Bowel Project Protocol B-06. N Engl J Med 1995; 333: 1469–74.
7. Fisher B, Anderson S, Redmond CK et al. Reanalysis and results after 12 years of follow-up in a randomized clinical trial comparing total mastectomy with lumpectomy with or without irradiation in the treatment of breast cancer. N Engl J Med 1995; 333: 1456–61.
8. Fisher B, Bauer M, Margolese R et al. Five year results of a randomized clinical trial comparing total mastectomy and segmental mastectomy with or without radiation in the treatment of breast cancer. N Engl J Med 1996; 312: 665–73.
9. Fisher ER, Anderson S, Tan-Chiu E et al. Fifteen year prognostic discriminates for invasive breast carcinoma. Cancer 2001; 91: 1679–87.
10. Fisher ER, Anderson S, Redmond C, Fisher B. Pathologic findings from the National Surgical Adjuvant Breast Project Protocol B-06. Cancer 1993; 71: 2507–14.
11. Veronesi U, Saccozzi R, Del Vecchio M et al. Comparing radical mastectomy with quadrantectomy, axillary dissection, and radiotherapy in patients with small cancers of the breast. N Engl J Med 1981; 305: 6–11.
12. Solin LJ, Fowble BL, Schultz DJ, Goodman RL. The significance of the pathology margins of the tumor excision on the outcome of patients treated with definitive irradiation for early stage breast cancer. Int J Radiat Oncol Biol Phys 1991; 21: 279–87.
13. Solin LJ, Fowble B, Yeh IT et al. Microinvasive ductal carcinoma of the breast treated with breast-conserving

surgery and definitive irradiation. Int J Radiat Oncol Biol Phys 1992; 23: 961–8.

14. McCormick B. Radiation and local control in early invasive breast cancer. Breast J 1999; 5: 330–4.

15. Mendenhall NP. Breast conserving therapy for early stage breast cancer. Hematol Oncol Clin North Am 2001; 15: 219–42.

16. Spivack B, Khanna MM, Tafra L et al. Margin status and local recurrence after breast-conserving surgery. Arch Surg 1994; 129: 952–7.

17. Osborne MP, Borgen PI. Role of mastectomy in breast cancer. Surg Clin North Am 1990; 70: 1023–46.

18. Frykberg ER, Bland KI. Management of in situ and minimally invasive breast carcinoma. World J Surg 1994; 18: 45–57.

19. Riveradeneira DE, Simmons RM, Christos P et al. Predictive factors associated with axillary lymph node metastases in T1a and T1b breast carcinomas: analysis in more than 900 patients. J Am Coll Surg 2000; 191: 1–8.

20. Saiz E, Toonkel R, Poppiti RJ, Robinson MJ. Infiltrating breast carcinoma smaller than 0.5 cm; Is lymph node dissection necessary? Cancer 1999; 85: 2206–11.

21. Abner A, Collins L, Peiro G et al. Correlation of tumor size and axillary lymph node involvement with prognosis in patients with T1 breast carcinoma. Cancer 1998; 83: 2502–8.

22. Chadha M, Chabon AB, Friedmann P, Vikram B. Predictors for axillary lymph node metastases in patients with T1 breast cancer. Cancer 1993; 73: 350–353.

23. Silverstein MJ, Gierson ED, Waisman JR et al. Axillary lymph node dissection for T1a breast cancer. Is it indicated? Cancer 1994; 73: 664–7.

24. Mustafa IA, Bland KI. Indication for axillary dissection in T1 breast cancer. Ann Surg Oncol 1998; 5: 4–8.

25. Maibenco DC, Weiss LK, Pawlish KS, Severson RK. Axillary lymph node metastases associated with small invasive breast carcinomas. Cancer 1999; 85: 1530–6.

26. Dowlatshahi K, Snider HC, Kim R. Axillary node status in nonpalpable breast cancer. Ann Surg Oncol 1995; 2: 424–8.

27. Chontos AJ, Maher DP, Ratzer ER, Fenoglio ME. Axillary lymph node dissection: Is it required in T1a breast cancer? J Am Coll Surg 1997; 184: 493–8.

28. Port ER, Tan LK, Borgen PI, Van Zee KJ. Incidence of axillary lymph node metastases in T1a and T1b breast carcinoma. Ann Surg Oncol 1998; 5: 23–7.

29. Giuliano AE, Haigh PI, Brennan M et al. Prospective observational study of sentinel lymphadenectomy without further axillary dissection in patients with sentinel node negative breast cancer. J Clin Oncol 2000; 18: 2553–9.

30. Simmons RM, Rosenbaum-Smith SM, Osborne M. Methylene blue dye as an alternative to isosulfan blue dye for sentinel lymph node localization. Breast J 2001; 7: 181–3.

31. McMasters KM, Tuttle TM, Carlson DJ et al. Sentinel lymph node biopsy for breast cancer: a suitable alternative to routine axillary dissection in multi-institutional practice when optimal technique is used. J Clin Oncol 2000; 18: 2560–6.

32. Smillie T, Hayasi A, Rusnak C et al. Evaluation of feasibility and accuracy of sentinel node biopsy in early breast cancer. Am J Surg 2001; 181: 427–30.

33. Cote RJ, Peterson HF, Chaiwun B et al. Role of immuno-histochemical detection of lymph node metastases in management of breast cancer. Lancet 1999; 354: 896–900.

34. Bass SS, Cox CE, Ku NN et al. The role of sentinel lymph node biopsy in breast cancer. J Am Coll Surg 1999; 189: 183–94.

35. Ollila DW, Brennan MB, Giuliano AE. Therapeutic effect of sentinel lymphadenectomy in T1 breast cancer. Arch Surg 1998; 133: 647–51.

36. Krag D, Weaver DL, Ashikaga T et al. The sentinel node in breast cancer. N Engl J Med 1998; 339: 941–6.

37. Albertini JJ, Lyman GH, Cox CE et al. Lymphatic mapping and sentinel node biopsy in the patient with breast cancer. JAMA 1996; 276: 1818–22.

38. Veronesi U, Paganelli G, Viale G et al. Sentinel lymph node biopsy and axillary dissection in breast cancer: results in a large series. J Natl Cancer Inst 1999; 91: 368–73.

39. Giuliano AE, Jones RC, Brennan M, Statman R. Sentinel lymphadenectomy in breast cancer. J Clin Oncol 1997; 15: 2345–50.

40. Simmons RM, Hoda S, Osborne M. Bone marrow micrometastases in breast cancer atients. Am J Surg 2000; 180: 309–12.

41. Janni W, Hepp F, Rjosk D et al. The fate and prognostic value of occult metastatic cells in the bone marrow of patients with breast carcinoma between primary treatment and recurrence. Cancer 2001; 92: 46–53.

42. Braun S, Pantel K, Muller P et al. Cytokeratin-positive cells in the bone marrow and survival of patients with stage I, II, or III breast cancer. N Engl J Med 2000; 342: 525–33.

43. Janni W, Gastroph S, Hepp F et al. Prognostic significance of an increased number of micrometastatic tumor cells in the bone marrow of patients with first recurrence of breast carcinoma. Cancer 2000; 88: 2252–9.

44. Cote RJ, Rosen PP, Lesser ML et al. Prediction of early relapse in patients with operable breast cancer by detection of occult bone marrow micrometastases. J Clin Oncol 1991; 9: 1749–56.

45. Diel IJ, Kaufmann M, Costa SD et al. Micrometastatic breast cancer cells in bone marrow at primary surgery: prognostic value in comparison with nodal status. J Natl Cancer Inst 1996; 88: 1652–64.

46. Fisher B, Dignam J, Bryant J. Five versus more than five years of tamoxifen therapy for breast cancer patients with negative lymph nodes and estrogen receptor positive tumors. J Natl Cancer Inst 1996; 88: 1529–1542.

47. Leitner SP, Swern AS, Weinberger D et al. Predictors of recurrence for patients with small (one centimeter or less) localized breast cancer (T1a,b N0,M0). Cancer 1995; 76: 2266–74.

48. Balch CM, Singletary SE, Bland KI. Clinical decision-making in early breast cancer. Ann Surg 1993; 217: 207–25.

34 The importance of resection margins in conservative surgery

Luigi Cataliotti, Vito Distante, Simonetta Bianchi, Lorenzo Orzalesi

Introduction

Conservative surgery is now widely accepted for small breast tumours. The introduction of more limited surgery, however, has created new challenges for both surgeons and pathologists. From an oncological point of view, a crucial consideration relates to how much surrounding breast tissue needs to be removed in order to obtain a complete resection of the tumour without compromising the cosmetic outcome. Conservative surgery is usually followed by radiotherapy with the aim of controlling both multifocal disease and residual tumour. On the basis of this rationale, surgical treatment could theoretically be restricted to simple excision of the tumour without concern for the potential presence of neoplastic foci in the residual breast. Nonetheless, the status of excision margins is the most significant determinant of local disease-free survival. Several studies have now clearly demonstrated that negative resection margins after conservative surgery are associated with the lowest rates of local recurrence.[1–7]

Schnitt et al[7] reported that surgically clear resection margins reduce local recurrence rates in patients treated with radiotherapy. The percentage of patients with local recurrence at 5 years was 0 in those patients with negative margins, compared with a rate of 21% in those with margins more than focally positive. A difference in rates of distant metastases was also observed between these two groups of patients: 14% of patients with negative margins developed distant disease, while almost one-third (32%) of those with focally positive margins did so. However, a proportion of patients in the latter group had nodal involvement. Schnitt et al[7] concluded that positive margin status may reflect tumours with a more aggressive biological behaviour.

Park et al[3] reported on rates of local recurrence at 8-year follow-up. Patients with either negative or close margins had a local recurrence rate of 7%, while those with focally positive or extensively positive margins had rates of 14% and 27% respectively. Freedman et al[8] have found that a negative resection margin, defined as more than 2 mm clearance, identifies a group of patients with a very low risk of local recurrence following breast conservation surgery and radiotherapy (7% at 10 years).

Those patients with a clearance of 2 mm or less (close margins) had similar rates of local recurrence as those with positive margins (14% at 10 years).[8] According to Sainsbury et al,[9] the presence of either invasive or in situ disease at the resection margins increases rates of local recurrence by a factor of at least 3.4 (95% confidence interval (CI) 2.6–4.6). Despite breast conservation surgery having now been practised for many years and the availability of mature data from randomised controlled trials, it remains difficult to assess which type of surgery constitutes the most effective treatment for breast cancer patients and how positive resection margins impact on rates of local recurrence when breast conservation surgery is combined with radiotherapy. These persistent uncertainties relate to several factors, including the type of surgery, technical aspects of pathological margin assessment and the lack of a universally accepted definition of margin involvement. (See Chapter 35 on local recurrence.)

Type of surgery

The term tumorectomy refers to removal of the tumour with a narrow margin of surrounding breast tissue (approximately 1 cm). Margins are grossly free of tumour at the macroscopic level but may be involved at the microscopic level. Wide local excision removes a greater volume of surrounding tissue and aims for a clearance of 1–3 cm. Quadrantectomy is a form of wide local excision in which a wide segment (a 'quadrant') of tissue is resected that includes 2–3 cm of surrounding breast tissue together with skin and pectoral fascia. The distinction between these surgical approaches is often unclear, and sometimes tumorectomy and quadrantectomy are reported as wide local excision. Several authors have reported high rates of margin positivity following tumorectomy, varying from 47% to 57%,[7,10] although Veronesi[11] found that only 16% of patients had positive margins after tumorectomy. This has created some confusion, and has led to difficulties in interpreting the results of some studies and in assessing the role of margin involvement in the local control of disease. The incidence of positive margins correlates with the type of surgical procedure, being highest for lumpectomy and lowest for quadrantectomy. Ghossein et al[12] cite positivity rates of 41% for tumorectomy, 14% for wide local excision and 7% for quadrantectomy. The surgeon should aim to carry out as wide an excision as possible that is compatible with an acceptable cosmetic result. At the same time, he or she should take account of the patient's age together with the morphology and biology of the tumour. Gage et al[13] conducted a multivariate analysis to assess the influence of various clinical and pathological factors on rates of local recurrence. For the group of patients with histologically negative margins of resection, the volume of resected breast tissue was not a significant determinant of local recurrence. The probability of attaining negative margins is related to the extent of surgical resection and consistent with the finding of Ghossein et al.[12] However, Francis et al[14] maintain that the adequacy of surgical clearance depends upon tumour aggressiveness. Using a theoretical morphological model, Faverly et al[15] concluded that tumour should be excised with a microscopically free margin of approximately 1 cm (2 cm macroscopically).

A more accurate description of the surgical procedure would facilitate interpretation of results. Moreover, correct orientation of the specimen is essential for thorough pathological assessment and in particular declaration of margin status. There are six possible resection margins: superior, inferior, medial, lateral, anterior (skin) and posterior (fascia) (Figure 34.1). It is conventional to mark superior and lateral borders for purposes of orientation. Note that when a radial quadrantic resection is performed, there are effectively four margins, two of which lie relatively close to the tumour and two further away. The former are at greater risk of neoplastic involvement. Of the two more distant margins, the more

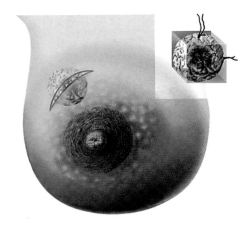

Figure 34.1 When the wide excision is more like a lump, the surgeon must mark the anterior (skin), central (nipple) and superior margins. Different-coloured or different-length stitches can be used.

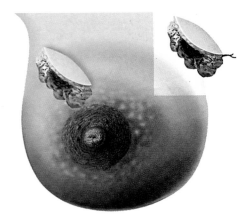

Figure 34.2 In the radial excision, the surgeon must mark only the margin close to the nipple to orientate the specimen.

proximal one, which lies close to the nipple, may exhibit intraductal spread of tumour. This type of specimen is more readily orientated by the pathologist, as it is partially covered by skin (Figure 34.2). Remodelling procedures can be integrated into breast conservation using the principles of oncoplastic surgery, which ensure both safe oncological resection and a satisfactory cosmetic outcome.[16]

Pathological assessment of margins

As stated above, close cooperation between surgeon and pathologist is mandatory, and the latter must be provided with appropriate clinical and radiological details together with the results of any previous biopsy (fine-needle aspiration cytology or core

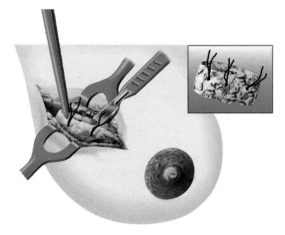

Figure 34.3 If the surgeon has to widen the excision, he or she must indicate the margin of the re-excision close to the tumour.

biopsy) and the site of the lesion in the breast. The specimen should be sent intact and correctly oriented with suture markers to the pathologist without prior sectioning by the surgeon. Where further resection is necessary, the position of this in relation to the primary specimen must be clearly indicated (and the 'outer' edge marked) (Figure 34.3). The pathologist can reconstruct the specimen if provided with adequate information, and this will help assessment of margins and strengthen confidence in the completeness of excision. For impalpable lesions, the specimen should be accompanied by a radiograph. Where the specimen X-ray reveals incomplete excision, further tissue must be resected at the time of initial surgery[17] (Figure 34.4). In addition to potential problems with surgical technique and handling of the specimen, there are also issues relating specifically to histopathological assessment. Until relatively recently, evaluation of pathological margin status was not performed routinely[7] and standardisation of techniques remains an ongoing process.

Several methods have been proposed for assessment of margins;[18,19] marking the edges of the specimen with India ink is one of the most widely used, and different coloured inks can be used to facilitate identification of individual margins. However, ink can seep into defects on the irregular surface of the specimen and track down towards the centre of the specimen. This leads to problems with definition of the true surgical (external) surface on microscopic examination.[20] Sampling errors may occur whatever method is used, and the extent of sampling is variable. There are no standardised procedures in existence at present to confirm the adequacy of excision margins, and the methods for reporting margin status to clinicians are highly variable. The

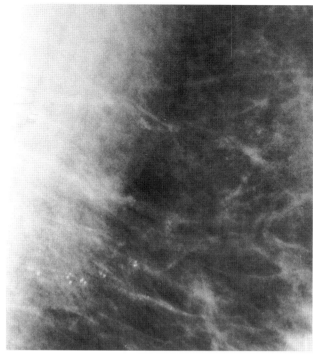

(a)

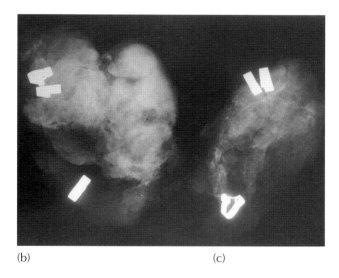

(b)　　　　　(c)

Figure 34.4 (a) Mammography shows suspect microcalcifications. (b) The X-ray of the specimen, with clockwise markers, shows the microcalcifications in the margin. (c) The X-ray of the re-excision specimen shows the residual microcalcifications with a wide clear margin.

method most commonly used is that advocated by Fisher et al.[21] This involves painting the surface of the specimen with Indian ink and obtaining sections for histopathological examination in different planes that are all perpendicular to the inked surface (Figure 34.5). The distance between the tumour and the inked margin can be accurately measured histologically. The principal disadvantage of this method is the limitation on the extent of surface sampling.

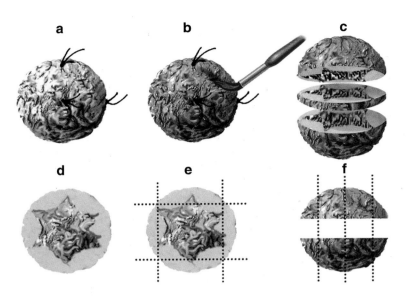

Figure 34.5 The method for reporting margin status advocated by Fisher et al.[21] (a) The superior, anterior, lateral or medial margins are marked with stitches in order to provide the proper orientation. (b) The surface of the specimen is coated with Indian ink. (c,d) The specimen is sectioned transversely to visualise the tumour. (e,f) Blocks of margins and tumour are taken in both transverse and sagittal sections.

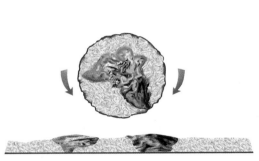

Figure 34.6 Carter's 'shaved margin method'.[22] The margin is peeled off and submitted for sectioning with the inked surface down.

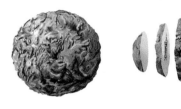

Figure 34.7 The method of Connolly and Schnitt[23] for small specimens (≤3 cm). After inking, the specimen is cut at 3–4 mm intervals and the sections are embedded to demonstrate the relationship of the tumour to the margins.

An alternative method proposed by Carter[22] consists of peeling or shaving off the surface of the specimen (in part or entirety). This 'shaved-margin method' removes tissue in a tangential manner, and a margin is considered positive if tumour is present within any areas of the histological sections of these margin shaves (Figure 34.6). This method permits the examination of a much greater proportion of the tumour surface using fewer sections than the method of Fisher et al.[21] A major disadvantage, however, is that margin width cannot be defined. Connolly and Schnitt[23] have suggested two different methods based on the size of the excised specimen. For specimens measuring 3 cm or less in maximum diameter, the margins are inked and the specimen 'bread-loafed' into 3 mm or 4 mm sections. The tissue submitted for histological examination includes the tumour with the surrounding breast tissue and its relationship to the margins of excision is clearly demonstrated (Figure 34.7). For specimens exceeding 3 cm in greatest diameter, a single incision through the centre of the tumour is made to assess the relationship between the lesion and the

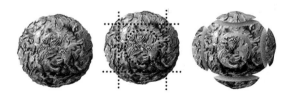

Figure 34.8 The method of Connolly and Schnitt[27] for larger specimens (>3 cm). Representative areas of margins are sampled and embedded with the inked surface down.

margins. Following this preliminary assessment, representative sections are shaved from the margins of the specimen (superior, inferior, anterior, posterior, medial and lateral) and embedded with the inked surface down (Figure 34.8).

It remains unclear whether evaluation of the shaved margin yields information of comparable utility and reliability as conventional methods in which sections are taken perpendicular to the inked surface. This is an important issue, which has been addressed in a study by Guidi et al.[24] Shaved and inked margins were examined simultaneously in a consecutive series of breast re-excision specimens. These authors found that involvement of a shaved margin was not predictive of a positive inked margin (positive predictive value 61%). By contrast, absence of tumour involvement in a shaved margin was highly predictive of a negative inked margin (negative predictive value 98%). These results suggest that the prognostic and therapeutic significance of a positive shaved margin may differ from that of a positive inked margin.[24]

Ichihara et al[25] have described a novel method for margin evaluation using an adjustable mould to prevent specimen deformation and distortion during fixation. This system has similarities to the 'shave or peeling' method and has been termed the 'pancake method'. It involves cutting a 5 mm-thick slice parallel to the margins from each side of the specimen (nipple, right side, left side and periphery). Excision is deemed adequate if no tumour is present at a depth of 5 mm. Where cancer cells are present at this depth, the corresponding blocks are examined at 10 mm depth by reprocessing and recutting the opposite side. If no tumour is present at 10 mm then excision is considered intermediate (1–5 mm). If tumour is present at this depth then excision is inadequate (<1 mm).

Veronesi et al[26] have examined the possibility of finding tumour cells in suspensions created by scraping the surface of surgical resection margins. They claim that the sensitivity of this method can exceed that of histological examination. Others have used cytological examination for margin assessment and have concluded that this can be complementary to and provide additional information than frozen section alone. Ku et al[27] reported a 97.7% correlation between histology and cytology of lumpectomy specimens.

A controversial issue relates to the use of frozen section for margin assessment, which aims to reduce rates of re-excision. Connolly and Schnitt[23] do not consider frozen section to be appropriate when margins are negative on gross examination. Under these circumstances the chance of a false-negative result is higher and these authors only undertake frozen section at the specific request of a surgical colleague. However, in a comparison of frozen and permanent histological sections, Cox et al[28] reported rates of sensitivity and specificity of 77% and 100% respectively for frozen section. Similarly, Sauter et al[29] quoted high rates of sensitivity and specificity (85% and 96% respectively) for frozen-section examination of re-excision specimens. Moreover, they concluded that the use of intraoperative frozen

section can reduce rates of re-excision in almost one-third of cases (32%).

Definition of margin involvement

There has been a lack of consensus in the literature on the definition of margin positivity. Positive margins have been interpreted to mean that tumour cells are present at the inked margins or within some arbitary distance from these. In general, a margin is considered positive when tumour exists at the surface of the specimen; when this is not the case, the exact distance between tumour cells and the closest resection margin should be stated.[30] This is particularly important in the absence of any objective definition of a negative margin.

Schnitt et al[7] consider margins to be positive when either invasive or in situ carcinoma is present at one or more margins (Figure 34.9) and close when tumour cells are present at a distance of 1 mm or less from the edge (Figure 34.10). Negativity is defined as tumour present at a distance more than 1 mm from the edge of the specimen.

For those patients with positive margins, two subdivisions are recognised: focally positive (cancer present at the margins in three low-power microscopic fields) and more than focally positive (cancer cells present at the margins in more than three low-power fields). In practice, the situation is more complex than the above scheme – some tumours are well circumscribed while others show an infiltrative

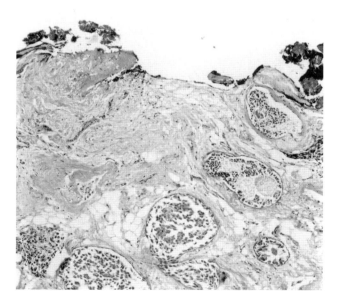

Figure 34.9 Ductal carcinoma in situ extending to the inked margin of excision.

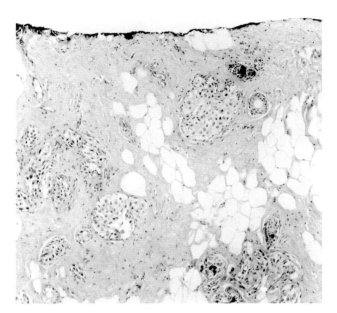

Figure 34.10 Infiltrating ductal carcinoma in which tumour cells are at a distance less than 1 mm from the inked margin of excision.

pattern of growth. Secondly, the presence of extensive involvement of peritumoral lymphatics renders determination of clearance impossible, and assessment of the adequacy of surgery is difficult even if the margins are clear.

Most breast cancers exhibit an infiltrative pattern of growth, which may be associated with the presence of an extensive intraductal component (EIC). Under these circumstances, evaluation of margins is particularly challenging for the pathologist, as is the situation with multifocality, which is present in up to 30% of cases.[31] Conversely, assessment is much more straightforward for tumours with a well-defined growth pattern without an EIC.

Gross examination of the margins at the time of surgery can provide basic information on the adequacy of surgical resection. However, misinterpretation is likely in cases of invasive lobular carcinoma, where tumour cells diffusely infiltrate the mammary stroma without any discrete mass lesion and often only subtle changes in the consistency of the breast parenchyma allude to any suspicious underlying pathology. Sauter et al[29] reported an overall sensitivity of 44% and specificity of 94% for evaluation of margins by gross inspection of the surgical specimen.

Residual tumour

It is now well recognised that the presence of tumour cells at the resection margins is not always indicative of residual tumour within the breast.[32] In the series reported by Frazier et al,[33] residual tumour was present in only about half of the cases (52.5%) of completion mastectomy or re-excision specimens when margins were positive following primary excision. Furthermore, when margins were either close or negative, residual tumour was present in 32.1% and 26.3% of cases respectively. Interestingly, Sauter et al[29] found that residual tumour was more likely when the margins of excision were unknown at the time of initial surgery compared with known margin status (42% vs 27% respectively).

The incidence of residual carcinoma following mastectomy or re-excision for DCIS appears to be higher than for invasive disease, and this may reflect the phenomenon of EIC. Silverstein et al[34] observed the presence of residual DCIS in 76% of patients with positive margins and in 43% of those with negative margins. Neuschatz et al[35] maintain that the margin status of a lumpectomy specimen containing only DCIS is the most important predictive factor for both the existence and extent of residual disease.

These data illustrate the limitations of margin evaluation in terms of adequacy of surgical resection – a significant proportion of cases with negative margins have residual disease within the breast. This accords with the results of NSABP Protocol B-06, in which local recurrence rates of 35% were observed in patients undergoing wide local excision only (no radiotherapy) with histologically negative margins.[36]

Extensive intraductal component

Wazer et al[37] investigated the influence of age and EIC on the predictive capacity of margin status for residual tumour within the conserved breast. They found that the risk of residual tumour microscopically is low irrespective of age provided that the excision margins are negative. For those tumours without an EIC, the risk of residual tumour is related to margin status and is consistently higher for young patients (aged 45 or younger) for all margin categories. When an EIC is present, the risk of residual disease is increased, irrespective of age and margin status.

An EIC and multifocality have emerged in several studies as the two most important factors predicting for both margin involvement and local recurrence.[38,39] Schnitt et al[7] found that 40% of patients with an EIC had positive margins, compared with 17% of those without an EIC. Similarly, rates of local recurrence at 5 years were significantly higher for EIC-positive tumours (20%) compared with EIC-negative tumours (7%). When an EIC is present in association with positive margins, local recurrence rates increase to 50%, but are zero when margins are clear. Therefore an EIC appears to increase local recurrence rates only when margins are involved.[9]

Dixon[6] has suggested that EIC and margin positivity are interrelated but have independent significance for prediction of local recurrence. Schnitt et al[7] recommend conservation surgery when margins are histologically negative (even if an EIC is present) and also for tumours that are focally positive in the absence of an EIC. Conversely, mastectomy or re-excision is indicated when margins are more than focally positive or are focally positive with an EIC. Most authors concur with these recommendations on treatment options for patients with margin involvement.[40]

It is clear that surgery for breast conservation should aim to excise a tumour with histologically negative margins.[1,6,11,41,42] The greater the margin of excision and hence surgical clearance, the lower is the chance of local recurrence. Some authors have proposed an adjusted radiotherapy approach in which boost doses of irradiation are tailored to margin status for maximising local control.[37] However, others have found that radiotherapy does not compensate for inadequate surgical clearance after breast conservation surgery for DCIS.[43]

References

1. DiBiase S, Komarnicky LT, Schwartz GF et al. The number of positive margins influences the outcome of women treated with breast preservation for early stage breast carcinoma. Cancer 1998; 82: 2212–20.

2. Silverstein MJ, Lagios MD, Groshen S et al. The influence of margin width on local control of ductal carcinoma in situ of the breast. N Engl J Med 1999; 340: 1455–61.

3. Park CC, Mitsumori M, Nixon A et al. Outcome at 8 years after breast-conserving surgery and radiation therapy for invasive breast cancer: influence of margin status and systemic therapy on local recurrence. J Clin Oncol 2000; 18: 1668–75.

4. Solin L, Fowble B, Schultz D, Goodman R. The significance of the pathology margins of the tumour excision on the outcome of patients treated with definitive irradiation for early stage breast cancer. Int J Radiat Oncol Biol Phys 1991; 2: 279–87.

5. Anscher MS, Jones P, Prosnitz LR et al. Local failure and margin status in early-stage breast carcinoma treated with conservation surgery and radiation therapy. Ann Surg 1993; 218: 22–8.

6. Dixon JM. Histological factors predicting breast recurrence following breast conserving therapy. Breast 1993; 2: 197.

7. Schnitt SJ, Abner A, Gelman R et al. The relationship between microscopic margins of resection and the risk of local recurrence in patients with breast cancer treated with breast-conserving surgery and radiation therapy. Cancer 1994; 74: 1746–51.

8. Freedman G, Fowble B, Hanlon A et al. Patients with early stage invasive cancer with close or positive margins treated with conservative surgery and radiation have an increased risk of breast recurrence that is delayed by adjuvant systemic therapy. Int J Radiat Oncol Biol Phys 1999; 44: 1005–15.

9. Sainsbury JRC, Anderson TJ, Morgan DAL. Breast cancer. BMJ 2000; 321: 745–50.

10. Schmidt-Ullrich RK, Wazer DE, Di Petrillo T et al. Breast conservation therapy for early stage breast carcinoma with outstanding 10-year locoregional control rates: a case for aggressive therapy to the tumour bearing quadrant. Int J Radiat Oncol Biol Phys 1993; 27: 545–52.

11. Veronesi U. How important is the assessment of resection margins in conservative surgery for breast cancer? Cancer 1994; 74: 1660–1.

12. Ghossein NA, Alpert S, Barba J et al. Importance of adequate surgical excision prior to radiotherapy in the local control of breast cancer in patients treated conservatively. Arch Surg 1992; 127: 411–15.

13. Gage I, Schnitt SJ, Nixon AJ et al. Pathologic margin involvement and the risk of recurrence in patients treated with breast-conserving therapy. Cancer 1996; 78: 1921–8.

14. Francis M, Cakir B, Ung O et al. Prognosis after breast recurrence following conservative surgery and radiotherapy in patients with node-negative breast cancer. Br J Surg 1999; 86: 1556–62.

15. Faverly DRG, Hendricks JHCL, Holland R. Breast carcinomas of limited extent. Cancer 2001; 91: 647–59.

16. Cataliotti L, Calabrese C, Orzalesi L. The response of the surgeon to changing patterns in breast cancer diagnosis. Eur J Cancer 2001; 37: S19–31.

17. Dixon JM, Ravi Sekar O, Walsh J et al. Specimen-orientated radiography helps define excision margins of malignant lesions detected by breast screening. Br J Surg 1993; 80: 1001–2.

18. Holland R, Velking SHJ, Mravunac M, Hendricks JHCL. Histologic multifocality of Tis, T1–2 breast carcinomas: implications for clinical trials of breast conserving surgery. Cancer 1985; 56: 979–90.

19. Anderson TJ. Breast cancer screening: principles and practicalities for histopathologists. Rec Adv Histopathol 1989; 14: 43–61.

20. Schnitt SJ, Connolly JL. Processing and evaluation of breast excision specimens. A clinically oriented approach. Am J Clin Pathol 1992; 98: 125–37.

21. Fisher ER, Sass R, Fisher B et al. Pathologic findings from the National Surgical Adjuvant Breast Project (Protocol 6). II. Relation of local recurrence to multicentricity. Cancer 1986; 57: 1717–24.

22. Carter D. Margins of 'lumpectomy' for breast cancer. Hum Pathol 1986; 17: 330–332.

23. Connolly JL, Schnitt SJ. Evaluation of breast biopsy specimens in patients considered for treatment by conservative surgery and radiation therapy for early breast cancer. Pathol Ann 1988; 23: 1–23.

24. Guidi AJ, Connolly JL, Harris JR, Schnitt SJ. The relationship between shaved margin and inked margin status in breast excision specimens. Cancer 1997; 79: 1568–73.

25. Ichihara S, Suzuki H, Kasami M et al. A new method of margin evaluation in breast conservation surgery using an adjastable mould during fixation. Histopathology 2001; 39: 85–92.

26. Veronesi U, Farante G, Galimberti V et al. Evaluation of resection margins after breast conservative surgery with monoclonal antibodies Eur J Surg Oncol 1991; 17: 338–41.

27. Ku NNK, Cox CE, Reintgen DS et al. Cytology of lumpectomy specimens. Acta Cytol 1991; 35: 417–21.

28. Cox CE, Ku NN, Reintgen DS et al. Touch preparation cytology of breast lumpectomy margins with histologic correlation Arch Surg 1991; 126: 490–3.

29. Sauter ER, Hoffman JP, Ottery FD et al. Is frozen section analysis of reexcision lumpectomy margins worthwhile? Cancer 1994; 73: 2607–26.

30. Fitzgibbons PL, Connolly JL, Page DL et al. Updated protocol for the examination of specimens from patients with carcinomas of the breast. A basis for checklists. Arch Pathol Lab Med 2000; 124: 1026–33.

31. Dawson PJ. What is new in our understanding of multifocal breast cancer? Pathol Res Pract 1993; 189: 111–16.

32. Singer JA. Residual breast cancer at a distance from the primary tumour. Am Surg 1993; 59: 435–7.

33. Frazier TG, Wong RWY, Rose D. Implications of accurate pathologic margins in the treatment of primary breast cancer. Arch Surg 1989; 124: 37–8.

34. Silverstein MJ, Gierson ED, Colburn WJ et al. Can intraductal breast carcinoma be excised completely by local excision? Cancer 1994; 73: 2985–9.

35. Neuschatz AC, DiPetrillo T, Steinhoff M et al. The value of breast lumpectomy margin assessment as a predictor of residual tumor burden in ductal carcinoma in situ of the breast. Cancer 2002; 94: 1917–24.

36. Fisher B, Anderson S, Redmond CK et al. Reanalysis and results after 12 years of follow-up in a randomized clinical trial comparing total mastectomy with lumpectomy with or without irradiation in the treatment of breast cancer. N Engl J Med 1995; 22: 1456–61.

37. Wazer DE, Schmidt-Ullrich RK, Ruthazer R et al. The influence of age and extensive intraductal component histology upon breast lumpectomy margin assessment as a predictor of residual tumor. Int J Radiat Oncol Biol Phys 1999; 45: 885–91.

38. Holland R, Connolly JL, Gelman R et al. The presence of an extensive intraductal component following a limited excision correlates with prominent residual disease in the remainder of the breast. J Clin Oncol 1990; 8: 113–18.

39. Campbell ID, Theaker JM, Royle GT et al. Impact of an extensive in situ component on the presence of residual disease in screening detected breast cancer. J R Soc Med 1991; 84: 652–6.

40. Peterson ME, Schueltz DJ, Reynolds C, Solin LJ. Outcomes in breast cancer patients relative to margin status after treatment with breast conserving surgery and radiation therapy: the University of Pennsylvania experience. Int J Radiat Oncol Biol Phys 1999; 43: 1029–35.

41. Fisher B, Anderson S. Conservative surgery for the management of invasive and noninvasive carcinoma of the breast: NSABP trials. World J Surg 1994; 18: 63–9.

42. Sibbering DM, Galea MH, Morgan DAL et al. Safe criteria breast conservation without radical excision. Breast 1993; 2: 198.

43. Chan KC, Knox WF, Sinha G et al. Extent of excision margin width required in breast conserving surgery for ductal carcinoma in situ. Cancer 2001; 91: 9–16.

35 Local recurrence following breast conservation treatment

Guidubaldo Querci della Rovere, Mark Kissin, Delilah Hassanally, John R Benson

Introduction

Breast conservation treatment (BCT) has become established over the past 25 years as the preferred standard of surgical management for women with early-stage breast cancer.[1] Longer-term follow-up data are now available from several prospective randomised controlled trials demonstrating survival equivalence for BCT compared with conventional mastectomy.[2–8] This introduction of conservative forms of breast surgery has coincided with the instigation of widespread mammographic screening and with smaller tumour sizes at presentation. Despite eligibility for BCT, rates of mastectomy are variable on both institutional and geographical bases. Overall rates for BCT in the USA have been cited as approximately 50%,[9,10] although a more recent estimate by Winchester[11] suggests that rates have increased to 67% for combined symptomatic and screen-detected lesions. Within the UK, rates of BCT vary from 55% to 70%, with an average of 58%.[10]

These variations in patterns of surgical management are likely to reflect differences in philosophy and education among surgeons together with an element of fear and concern among women themselves. There is a finite rate of ipsilateral breast tumour recurrence for patients undergoing BCT: approximately 5–15% at 10 years,[12–16] which translates into a lifelong risk of 1.0–1.5% per year.[17] Moreover, the psychological impact of local recurrence can be devastating and more traumatic than disclosure of the primary breast cancer diagnosis. Indeed, this event often requires a completion mastectomy and may undermine a patient's confidence in her initial treatment.[18]

Although BCT offers cosmetic benefits[19,20] with improvements in body image and sexual functioning, levels of anxiety and depression associated with breast conservation are comparable to those for mastectomy.[21] Selection of patients for BCT is of crucial importance; there is an inverse relationship between the oncological mandate of surgical radicality on the one hand and cosmesis on the other. There is a balance between the risk of local recurrence and cosmetic results, and with the advent of skin-sparing mastectomy and improvements in reconstructive techniques (including implant design), some younger patients may be better served with a mastectomy at the outset with the offer of immediate breast reconstruction.

This chapter will consider the clinicopathological risk factors and predictors of ipsilateral breast tumour recurrence (IBTR) together with its biological significance in terms of longer-term outcome, which remains a controversial issue.[22,23] Of principal concern is the relationship to distant relapse and whether local recurrence represents a determinant of distant metastases or indicates a proclivity towards development of distant disease and de facto poor prognosis. Should local recurrence have a determinant role then inadequate primary locoregional treatment may compromise survival. To quote Veronesi et al,[24] 'it is important to distinguish local recurrences linked to increased risk of distant spread from those due to inadequate local treatment'. In the latter case, patients could develop disseminated disease as a result of failure to remove residual but viable cancer cells at the time of primary treatment.

The significance of IBTR and the implications thereof for treatment strategies are perhaps better appreciated within the context of current ideas relating to the natural history of breast cancer. There are two dominant paradigms of tumour pathogenesis that have governed the management of breast cancer over the last century, but an intermediate paradigm is emerging that reflects the biological heterogeneity of this disease.

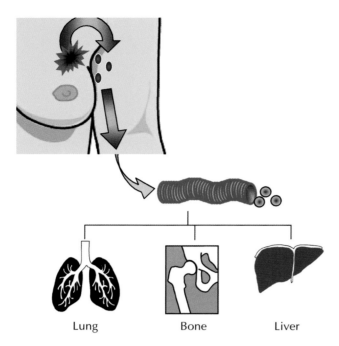

Figure 35.1 Halstedian paradigm: sequential spread of breast cancer from a single focus within the breast. Lymph node involvement precedes haematogenous dissemination, and according to this paradigm bloodstream spread cannot occur without obligate nodal disease.

Halstedian paradigm

According to the Halstedian paradigm,[25] breast cancer is a localised disease at inception that commences as a single focus and spreads in a centrifugal manner, encroaching upon ever more distant structures with progressive and sequential spread along fascial planes and lymphatics. Metastatic spread to distant organs by haematogenous dissemination is preceded by infiltration of lymph nodes, which provide a circumferential line of defence and initially serve as barriers but subsequently permit access of tumour cells into the circulation when their filtration capacity is exhausted (Figure 35.1). This hypothesis was based on the observation that local recurrence was a common antecedent to death from breast cancer following initial surgical excision. The focus of local recurrence was considered to be the cause of distant metastases, and the chances of a patient being cured were related to the extent of surgery. Thus treatments that allowed en bloc resection of tumour together with adjacent locoregional tissues offered the best chance of 'cure' and minimised the chance of local recurrence. The Halsted radical mastectomy resulted in a dramatic reduction in rates of local recurrence (from 60% to 6%), with up to three-quarters of patients remaining free of locoregional relapse at the time of death from distant disease. However, long-term survival was unaffected following radical mastectomy and the procedure incurred significant disfigurement. Nonetheless, although Halsted's radical mastectomy failed to cure most patients of breast cancer, it provided excellent local control of disease.

Forty years ago, George Crile[26] proposed that breast cancer was a systemic disease at an early stage in its natural history. This alternative hypothesis led to early forays into local tumour excision and presaged clinical trials of conservative surgery for breast cancer. Furthermore, trials of systemic therapies have demonstrated only modest absolute gains in survival of the order of 5–10%.[3–5] Rates of local relapse are inversely related to the extent of surgical resection and irradiation, but local management appears to have little, if any, impact on survival.[5] Although systemic treatment has been shown to be effective in prolonging the overall survival of breast cancer patients, other modalities of treatment such as surgery and radiotherapy have until recently had no proven benefit on long-term survival. Nonetheless, although more extensive surgery does not improve survival in patients studied hitherto, there may be a subgroup of patients with truly localised disease. For these patients, local therapy involving surgical excision (plus radiotherapy) might be curative and thus influence the natural course of the disease. There are no data to directly verify this supposition and ethical considerations would preclude any trial being conducted in which an early breast cancer remained untreated. However, analysis of long-term survival of patients treated for stage I disease prior to the widespread use of adjuvant systemic therapy suggests that breast cancer is a locoregional process in up to 75–80% of node-negative cases who may be considered statistically 'cured'.[27] In a series of patients from Memorial Sloan-Kettering Cancer Center with node-negative and node-positive tumours less than or equal to 2 cm in size (T1N0 and T1N1), comparison of observed with expected survival at a median follow-up of 18 years revealed that 89% of patients with node-negative tumours less than or equal to 1 cm were estimated to be cured, with survival curves becoming parallel or congruent during the second decade of follow-up (95% confidence interval (CI) 80–98%).[28] For tumours between 1–2 cm, the figure was slightly lower at 77% (95% CI 70–85%). Although the time taken to attain parallelism was 13 years for tumours smaller than 1 cm and 18 years for tumours between 1 cm and 2 cm, there was no statistically significant difference between the observed and expected curves after 10 years (Figure 35.2). Similar results were reported by Quiet et al[29] from the University of Chicago, although there was

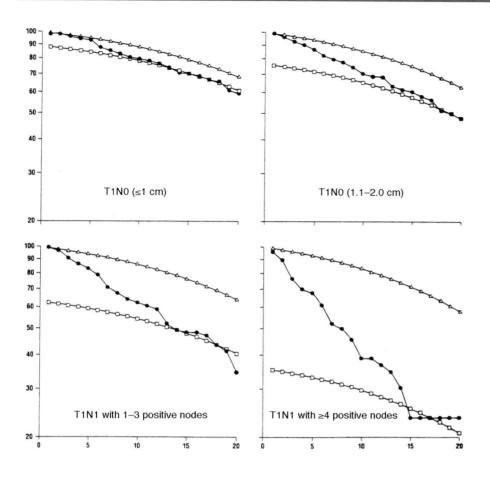

Figure 35.2 Comparison of observed (filled circles) and expected (open triangles) survival curves using a logarithmic transformation for T1N0 and T1N1 tumours. The open squares show the extrapolation to line zero of the portion of the observed curve that is approximately parallel to the normal population. The vertical intersection indicates the proportion of patients 'cured'.

no stratification of hazard ratios based on tumour size less than 2 cm. Patients with T1 tumours had an overall 20-year disease-free survival rate of 79%. Any divergence of the curves beyond 20 years is unlikely to detract from the conclusion that a substantial proportion of patients will not die of breast cancer and are likely to have achieved a 'personal cure' and to succumb to causes unrelated to breast cancer.

In a group of 100 women receiving chemotherapy for node-negative breast cancer, 67 will be successfully treated by local therapy alone, 25 will die despite chemotherapy and the remaining 8 will be 'cured' by adjuvant chemotherapy. An absolute survival benefit of 8–10% is associated with adjuvant chemo-endocrine treatment (the 5-year disease-specific survival rate increased from 67% to 75%), and complete pathological response rates of 9–10% with neoadjuvant chemotherapy are documented. Therefore in the absence of any form of local therapy, 90% of patients would theoretically die from or with breast cancer. However, following standard locoregional treatment, 50–60% of patients with breast cancer will survive for a reasonable time, implying either that local treatments are effective or that some tumours are of low innate biological aggressiveness.

Fisherian paradigm

Bernard Fisher[30] formulated an alternative hypothesis of biological predeterminism that challenged the existing paradigm based on the concept of progressive centrifugal spread according to anatomical and mechanical criteria. The fundamental tenets of this alternative paradigm are embodied in the following two statements pertaining to the clinical behaviour and pathobiology of breast cancer:[30]

- As far as survival is concerned, there is no difference between local excision, local excision plus radiotherapy and modified radical mastectomy; there is, however, a progressive decrease in local recurrence with the more aggressive treatments.
- Local recurrence is associated with worse survival, but survival is the same with the various types of treatment; local recurrence is not the cause of but simply an indicator of poor prognosis.

As mentioned in the introductory section of this chapter, clinical trials conducted by Fisher and others have demonstrated that mastectomy and breast conservation surgery are equivalent in terms

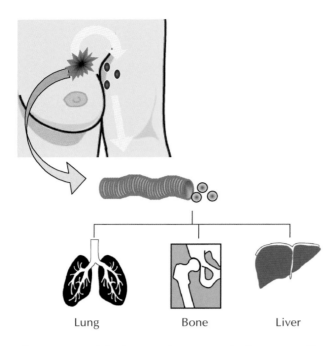

Figure 35.3 Fisherian paradigm: spread of tumour cells into the bloodstream occurs early in tumorigenesis and precedes lymph node infiltration.

Lung   Bone   Liver

of survival, [2–8] but it is the significance attributed to local recurrence that is perhaps of greater interest and has until now been underestimated. The largest breast conservation trial (NSABP B-06) confirms that postoperative irradiation improves local recurrence-free survival and in particular rates of early local recurrence at 15-year follow-up. [13] Furthermore this has been reinforced by a more recent update at 25-year follow-up. [8] Of note, distant disease-free and overall survival were similar in the three arms of the trial (wide local excision, wide local excision plus radiotherapy, and modified radical mastectomy) suggesting that residual cancer cells are a determinant of local failure but not of distant disease. These conclusions are reinforced by a meta-analysis of survival following BCT versus mastectomy, which actually reveals a non-significant survival benefit for BCT. [31]

According to the Fisherian paradigm, breast cancer is considered to be a predominantly systemic disease at the outset, with cancer cells entering the bloodstream at an early stage of tumour development via the leaky vessels of the neovasculature and lymphaticovenous communications. Initially circulating cells may be destroyed by the immune system and fail to establish viable foci of micrometastases (Figure 35.3). A corollary of Fisher's conclusions is that current forms of treatment have modest effects on reduction of mortality from breast cancer. Although a primary tumour can be excised surgically or may regress completely with chemotherapy

and/or radiotherapy, it is the existence of micrometastases at the time of presentation that will determine a patient's clinical fate. Local recurrence is viewed as an indicator of poor prognosis and reflects a host–tumour relationship that favours the development of distant disease or the activation of processes leading to a 'kick start' of micrometastases. [32] The biological potential of residual tumour cells within the breast is resonant with this more aggressive phenotype.

Factors determining local recurrence

A proportion of relapses within the ipsilateral breast following BCT represent new primary tumours. However, these are biologically unrelated to the original tumour and have independent prognostic significance. It remains uncertain what proportion of cases of IBTR are 'true' recurrences as opposed to new primaries, and most publications on IBTR have failed to distinguish between these two distinct groups. Moreover, this issue is ambiguous and some authors define a group of 'marginal miss'. In general, true local recurrences (a) occur within the index quadrant and at some arbitrary distance from the surgical scar (2–3 cm), (b) are of similar biological type and grade to the original tumour and (c) occur within 5 years from the time of primary breast cancer treatment. [24,33] Five-year survival rates are more favourable for a new primary compared with a true local recurrence (90% compared with 50–70% respectively). The distinction between these two groups can be difficult, and, with an increasing time interval to recurrence, the lesion may be situated in a different quadrant (50% probability at 5 years). Clonality studies have helped resolve some of these issues. [33]

Factors determining the risk of local recurrence following breast conservation treatment have proved difficult to define precisely for several reasons:

- Variable and indeterminate volumes of surrounding 'normal' breast tissue are excised with the primary tumour.
- More than one piece of tissue may be resected at the time of surgery, and correct identification and relative orientation of the specimens may not be possible.
- Incomplete and/or inconsistent interpretation and classification of pathological margins is common.
- Variable doses of radiotherapy have been administered to the breast with or without a boost to the tumour bed.

Notwithstanding these limitations, two factors emerge as principle determinants of local recurrence

- margin status
- the presence or absence of an extensive intra-ductal component (EIC).

Other factors have been implicated in determining the risk of local relapse, but correlations are in general much weaker than for margin status and EIC. Among these other factors, lymphatic invasion and young age (<35) have been shown to be primary predictors for increased risk of local recurrence. Consistent associations have been found for larger tumour size (>2 cm) and higher histological grade, but not for tumour subtype or nodal status.

Margin status

Gross excision of tumour is essential for acceptable rates of local control, and relapse rates may be as high as 71% in patients undergoing BCT and radiotherapy with grossly positive margins. [34] At the time of surgery, it is imperative that the surgeon examine the resected specimen to ensure that tumour does not exist in proximity to the surface of the specimen and that no macroscopic disease is detectable within the surgical cavity. For those procedures termed a 'tumorectomy' or 'lumpectomy', the surgeon aims to remove a minimum of 1 cm of normal breast tissue around the tumour. Because of the nature of breast parenchyma, this may be technically difficult to achieve with consistency and reliability, and a more practical approach is to perform a 'wide local excision', which removes 2–3 cm of surrounding breast tissue and essentially excises a column of tissue between the subcutaneous layer of the breast envelope and the pectoral fascia. With a quadrantic-style resection, although a relatively large volume of tissue is removed, the tumour does not lie equidistant from each surface and care must be taken to avoid dissecting too close to the tumour, particularly when this is positioned eccentrically in relation to the 'quadrant' of resected tissue.

Some surgeons prefer to ink the specimen in theatre and slice it into sections perpendicular to the longest axis passing through the tumour. The sections can then be inspected and further tissue resected where tumour lies close to the edge of the specimen (intraoperative frozen section can be performed prior to any re-excision).[35]

Intraoperative specimen radiography can be undertaken using a biplanar technique, and some surgeons advocate this for all cases irrespective of palpability. This can reveal additional information for palpable lesions such as calcification outside the tumour mass. However, this has not been recommended as routine practice for palpable breast tumours. [36]

As recently as 5–10 years ago, there was persistent controversy over whether surgeons should strive to remove all microscopic disease when carrying out breast conservation procedures.[13,37] This was based on inconsistent data on the predictive value of margin status and was helped to propagate by uncertainty over the biological potential of microscopic residual tumour deposits. If cancer cells remain in the tumour bed, these may subsequently form a focus for local recurrence. The capacity for adjuvant radiation or systemic therapies to eliminate such cells or modify their behaviour is debatable, although recent analyses confirm that rates of local relapse are higher in patients with close, positive or indeterminate resection margins.[38]

Some of the earlier studies examining the influence of margin status on rates of local recurrence were hampered by cases with indeterminate margins and variation in pathological methodology and criteria for designation of margin status. There is now general consensus that BCT should aim to achieve microscopically negative margins, i.e. no tumour cells present at the resection margin.[35] There has been a lack of uniformity in defining what constitutes a positive resection margin, and this in turn has compounded issues relating to microscopically negative margins and degrees of surgical clearance – how wide must a negative margin be to result in acceptable rates of local recurrence? According to the NSABP Protocol B-17,[39] a positive resection margin implies tumour cells present at the resection margin (invasive or non-invasive), and hence negative margins could be associated with tumour cells at a distance of only 1 mm from the edge of the specimen. Others consider positive margins to involve malignant cells either at the margin or within some arbitrary distance from it (e.g. 2 mm, 3 mm or 5 mm). Following inking of the specimen, random sections are usually taken perpendicular to the surface (see Chapter 34) of the specimen, which tends to be fatty and irregular in contour. A false-negative result may occur due to sampling error, and the 'shave' technique may reduce the chance of this by sampling a greater proportion of the total surface area of the specimen. Conversely, ink can track down the interstices on the surface of the specimen and yield a false-positive result due to cancer cells deep within the specimen appearing to be close to an 'inked margin'.

Historically, up to one-quarter of primary excision specimens were reported to have microscopically positive margins, but with more stringent and meticulous surgical techniques, this figure has fallen progressively. In a study involving more than 1000 patients undergoing BCT between 1970 and 1994, Mirza et al[12] reported a rate of margin positivity of approximately 10%. The NSABP and others have reported higher rates of local recurrence with microscopically positive margins, for which rates of local recurrence increase significantly with duration of follow-up compared with negative-margin tumours (regression coefficients of 0.75 ($p = 0.008$) and -0.31 ($p = 0.35$) respectively).[13,34,40–45] However, some studies have found no correlation between local recurrence and positive resection margins,[46,47] although relapse rates may have been influenced by modification of radiotherapy regimens with a proportionate increase in booster dose to 'compensate' for positive margins.

In an attempt to reconcile these conflicting reports, some authors have defined a further category of 'close' margins and found correlations between margin status and local recurrence based on strict and consistent criteria. In their seminal publication, Schnitt et al[34] defined three categories of margin:

- negative: no tumour within 1 mm of the inked margin.
- close: tumour within 1 mm of the inked margin.
- positive: tumour present at the inked margin of resection:
  - focally positive (<3 low-power fields at margins)
  - more than focally positive (>3 low-power fields at margins)

The overall local recurrence rate at 5 years was 7% (12 of 181), with rates of 0% (0 of 70), 4% (1 of 25), 6% (3 of 48) and 21% (8 of 38) respectively for each of these margin categories, and sites of first failure correlated with margin involvement ($p = 0.01$). Therefore low rates of local recurrence may obtain not only with tumour very close to the margins of resection, but also when these are focally involved with tumour. Pittinger et al[48] classified margins as negative, close or positive, with close margins having tumour 3 mm or less from the tissue edge. Local recurrence rates were similar in the negative- and close-margin groups (3%) (patients matched for tumour size, oestrogen receptor (ER) and nodal status). Among those with close margins, 49% underwent re-excision, with residual tumour being present in one-quarter of the cases. Despite this, recurrence rates were similar to those of the negative-margin group, where only 8% were re-excised, none of whom had residual tumour. Solin et al[47] defined close margins as 2 mm or less, and once again there was no difference in rates of local recurrence between negative and close groups at 5 years (approximately 14%). However, positive and close margins received higher doses of radiotherapy. Interestingly, the small numbers of cases involving positive margins in many studies preclude any robust statistical analysis. However, Smitt et al[38] found that rates of freedom from local relapse (FFLR) at 6 years were 97% for patients with negative margins versus 86% for those with close (≤2 mm), indeterminate or positive margins (there was no statistically significant difference between the latter three groups, for which rates of FFLR were 78%, 85% and 83% respectively).

Several more recent studies have examined the impact of close margins (≤2 mm) on rates of local recurrence. Although these are relatively small studies with some variability in other factors, such as age, EIC and systemic therapies, they all reveal a statistically significant increase in rates of local recurrence for 'close' compared with negative margins (Table 35.1).

Thus rates of local recurrence for close margins were approximately double those for negative margins (17–22% versus 3–8%). Therefore some inconsis-

Table 35.1 Local recurrence rates for close and negative margins

Series	No. of patients	Follow-up (years)	Rate of local recurrence (%)	
			Close[b]	Negative[c]
Peterson et al[49]	96	8 (actuarial)	17	8
Freedman et al[50]	142	0 (cumulative incidence)	14	7
Waver et al[51]	99	6 (median)	Relative risk 1.69	3
Smitt et al[38]	55	6 (actuarial)	22	3

[a]Modified from reference 38.
[b]Defined as <2 mm.
[c]Defined as >2 mm.

tency exists amongst published reports on the significance of close margins; rates of local recurrence may be equivalent to negative margins, intermediate between negative and positive margins. or similar to rates for positive margins.[35] Undoubtedly, this represents the confounding effects of other factors known to influence local recurrence together with the nuances of margin assessment.

Notwithstanding these comments, its appears that the critical factor for margin status is the absence of tumour cells at the edge of the specimen. Absolute rates of local recurrence are not influenced by the 'degree' of negativity, although intuitively it might be expected that recurrence would be less likely when the margin of clearance is greater. Several studies have confirmed that margin width per se is not a determinant of local recurrence rates.[52,53] Singletary[35] has provided a useful analysis of this issue, and points out that for patients with a 1 mm negative margin, local recurrence rates ranged from 0% to 7% (median 3%), while patients with a 2 mm negative margin had local recurrence rates of 3–10% (median 6%). However, those patients with margins that were just clear (no tumour cells within one microscopic field of the cut edge) had the lowest rates of local recurrence, ranging from 2% to 4% (median 2%). Therefore, although rates of recurrence are determined by negative margin status, no direct relationship exists between margin width and rates of local recurrence.

Extensive intraductal component (EIC)

EIC is defined as an invasive ductal carcinoma with an intraductal component representing more than 25% of the tumour together with an intraductal component in sections of adjacent breast tissue that is otherwise grossly normal. Local recurrence rates at 5 years of 21% were reported by Vicini et al[54] for EIC-positive tumours, compared with 6% for EIC-negative tumours. These clinical results are in accordance with the observational studies on mastectomy specimens undertaken by Holland et al.[55,56] The incidence of residual tumour in the surrounding breast tissue was much greater for those patients with an EIC, and this was predominantly ductal carcinoma in situ (DCIS) rather than invasive malignancy.

Several studies, including the Milan II trial, have found an EIC to be highly predictive for local recurrence following BCT.[57] In an analysis of more than 2000 women undergoing quadrantectomy as part of BCT, 119 cases of local recurrences were documented, of which 21 of 119 (18%) involved either invasive disease with an EIC (13 patients) or pure DCIS (8 patients). Furthermore, an EIC predicts for local recurrence but not distant relapse. Interest-

ingly, the NSABP trial found no association between EIC and local recurrence, and this may be related to differences in pathological criteria and personnel between institutions.[18]

The presence or absence of an EIC is correlated with margin status, and indeed an EIC is probably a predictor for positive margins. Rates of recurrence at 5 years for EIC-positive tumours with negative or close margins are 0% and 50% if margins are focally positive with an EIC.[34] Perez et al[58] reported a higher incidence of local recurrence in women aged under 40 in the presence of an EIC (17% versus 8%, $p = 0.03$). However, the relationship to margin status was unclear in this analysis of BCT for T1 and T2 tumours, and one-quarter of patients had unspecified margin status.

The significance of an EIC is that attempted breast conservation for these cases may leave further DCIS within the surrounding tumour bed and radiotherapy may not prevent subsequent proliferation and progression to invasive malignancy. Furthermore, DCIS can spread along ducts and be associated with 'skip' lesions.[35] Nonetheless, patients with an EIC but negative resection margins can be safely offered BCT. Although an EIC is a predictor for residual disease at re-excision and reflects a greater tumour burden locally,[38] it is the final margin status that determines the overall outcome.[24,45] These clinical findings are consistent with the hypothesis that an EIC relates to local disease recurrence and 'adequacy' of surgery and is not a determinant of distant disease.

Other risk factors for local recurrence

Several factors other than margin status and EIC influence rates of local recurrence, but the magnitude of correlation for each of these factors is less than for the above two principal factors.

Age
A majority of studies have confirmed that young age does correlate with an increased risk of local recurrence.[41–43,59–62] This association is particularly strong with an age cut-off of 35, but also applies to women younger than 40 or even younger than 50. Stotter et al[60] reported a significantly increased risk of local recurrence among women younger than 50 compared with those over 50, but not all studies corroborate this finding.[63] In the analysis by Mirza et al,[12] 50 years was identified as the most significant cut-off age and is a surrogate marker for the menopause. These authors and Bartelink et al[64] have speculated that breast tumours in younger women may differ biologically from those in older women.

It is recognised that there are associations between young age and multicentricity, multifocality, vascular invasion and higher tumour grade,[61,65,66] and some authors maintain that age is not an independent risk factor for local recurrence.[18] Young age has also been identified as a predictor of residual disease following re-excision. Moreover, Smitt et al[38] found that age was not a predictor of local recurrence when margins were pathologically negative.

Tumour size

Greater tumour size is a risk factor for local recurrence following BCT. For patients with tumours greater than 2 cm in maximum diameter, this association was most evident for patients not receiving radiotherapy.[37,42,67,68] Fisher et al[69] found that for patients with stage II or III node-positive disease, tumour size exceeding 5 cm was the only risk factor for local recurrence on multivariate analysis. However, it is generally more difficult to obtain pathologically negative margins for large tumours.[46] This probably accounts for the higher rates of local recurrence in the control arm of the NSABP B-06 trial compared with the corresponding group in the Milan trial (with upper size limits 4 cm and 2.5 cm respectively).

Lymphovascular invasion

There has been renewed interest in lymphovascular invasion as a risk factor for local recurrence. When tumour cells are present within lymphatic or endothelial structures beyond the confines of the main tumour, it is less likely that adequate surgical clearance will be attained, with a consequent increase in rates of local recurrence. This was confirmed in the NSABP and Milan trials, where a disproportionate number of local recurrences were observed in the groups with lymphovascular invasion. This association has been confirmed in other studies.[42,70]

Tumour type and grade

There are consistent associations between higher tumour grade and increased rates of local recurrence,[41,59,61,71] but no correlations exist for tumour type. It was a previously held view that lobular carcinoma was linked to higher rates of local recurrence due to its multicentric nature, but this has since been disproven and local recurrence rates are comparable for invasive ductal and lobular carcinomas.[72] Thus, provided that satisfactory margins of clearance are achievable, the lobular phenotype is not a contraindication to BCT.

Adjuvant therapies

With the widespread introduction of systemic treatments over the past 20 years as an integral component of breast cancer management, data have now emerged that clearly show a modulatory effect of chemo-endocrine therapies on rates of IBTR.[73–75] In the NSABP B-06 trial, node-positive patients receiving chemotherapy had a local recurrence rate of 4%, compared with 9% for node-negative patients ($p<0.05$).[73] This effect of chemotherapy on local recurrence was confirmed in a further NSABP study evaluating chemotherapy in node-negative patients.[75] In the more recent study by Mirza et al[12] on predictors of local recurrence following BCT for early breast cancer, chemotherapy resulted in a 78% reduction in rates of IBTR (hazard ratio (HR) 0.224; 95% CI 0.109–0.464; $p<0.001$). Absence of chemotherapy was an independent predictor of local relapse, and chemotherapy may compensate for 'close' surgical margins.

The NSABP B-14 trial of tamoxifen versus placebo in node-negative patients confirmed a reduction in rates of local recurrence for those receiving hormonal therapy.[73] The above-mentioned study by Mizra et al[12] revealed a 66% reduction in local recurrence attributable to adjuvant tamoxifen (HR 0.364; 95% CI 0.151–0.880; $p = 0.025$).

In an analysis of more than 1000 patients treated with BCT for T1 and T2 tumours, Perez et al[58] found that for T1 tumours, chemotherapy reduced rates of local recurrence only in women aged 40 or younger. Similarly, tamoxifen reduced rates of relapse only in women older than 40. Interestingly, there was no statistically significant impact of adjuvant systemic therapy in patients with T2 tumours.[55]

Determination of margin status

It follows from the preceding discussion that all patients should undergo re-excision if either invasive or non-invasive tumour is present at the resection margins. It is the final margin status that is critical to outcome. and failure to achieve a 'negative' margin is an indication for mastectomy. Interestingly, there are limited data suggesting that patients with positive margins and an associated IBTR rate in excess of 30% may risk impairment of long-term survival,[44] which is most likely attributable to an increased chance of distant metastases.[34,44]

What constitutes a satisfactory margin of clearance? According to the above studies, close margins with tumour cells present within 3 mm or even 1 mm of the inked margin are associated with acceptable rates of local recurrence (<5% at 5 years, or 1% per year). Many American surgeons consider a margin clearance of 2–3 mm to be appropriate,[76] and this echoes the view of the British Association of Surgical Oncologists. Nonetheless, some breast units stipulate that patients undergoing wide local excision should have a radial margin of clearance of 5 mm. This pathological mandate has led to re-excision rates of up to 50% in the personal experience of one of the authors (MK) and others.[77] A re-excision rate of 39% based on a policy of a final radial margin clearance of 5 mm was cited by Mirza et al.[12] A further excision compromises the ultimate cosmetic result, which is inversely related to the volume of tissue excised. The amount of tissue removed at re-excision is rather imprecise and a matter of surgical judgement. Moreover, it is unusual to find residual tumour when re-excision is performed to achieve a wider margin of clearance rather than a 'negative' margin per se. By contrast, further disease will be found in approximately 40–50% of cases undergoing re-excision for positive margins.

Re-excision not only involves an additional period of hospitalisation, with concomitant costs, but may also delay commencement of adjuvant therapies. Various innovative methods are being developed and evaluated that permit more accurate assessment of margin status, which in turn is the most important predictor of residual cancer cells in the tissue adjacent to the surgical cavity.

Multicoloured inking system

Differential inking can be applied to the six surfaces of the resection specimen. This allows the pathologist to better define the individual margins than when the more familiar Indian ink and orientation sutures are used (which can become displaced/avulsed during processing of the specimen). This may necessitate re-excision of the entire cavity in the event of margin positivity, whereas multicoloured inks permit a re-excision of the appropriate part of the cavity. Such selective re-excision reduces the total volume of tissue re-excised but does not increase rates of local recurrence.[78]

Intraoperative specimen analysis

With the increasing use of percutaneous biopsy techniques and definitive preoperative diagnosis, the indications for intraoperative frozen-section examination have changed in recent years. The technique currently has value in assessing margin status at the time of primary surgery in an attempt to ascertain completeness of tumour excision and to reduce rates of re-excision. Using an 'orange peel' method, Noguchi et al[79] reported an overall accuracy of 86%,

with rates of sensitivity and specificity of 83% and 86% respectively. However, there are concerns about using intraoperative frozen-section examination for small tumours, where sacrifice of tissue may jeopardise definitive permanent sections and render interpretation of borderline lesions such as atypical ductal hyperplasia more difficult. Furthermore, the cost–benefit advantages of frozen section may be thwarted by the need to defer mastectomy pending discussion of results (and possible immediate breast reconstruction) with the patient.

An alternative method for assessing the completeness of excision is to sample the surgical cavity following lumpectomy, wide local excision or quadrantectomy. Biopsies can be taken randomly from the walls of the cavity or a thin shaving of the entire wall can be performed. The pathological status of the cavity or shave biopsy is considered to be concordant with that of the resected specimen. Frozen-section analysis under these circumstances yields a sensitivity of 91% and a specificity of 100%.[80] Moreover, residual tumour is found in approximately 25% of cases[81] with random biopsies and more than one-third of cases when cavity wall shaving is undertaken.[82] However, these methods are labour-intensive and unsuited to routine surgical practice.[18]

A promising and relatively simple method for sampling surgical margins is touch preparation cytology. This method relies on the selective adherence of tumour cells to a glass surface, which can be subsequently fixed and stained with H&E. Proponents of this technique claim that it is cost-effective and can accurately assess resection margins (sensitivity and specificity 100%).[83]

Intraoperative imaging for margin assessment

Intraoperative ultrasound (IOUS) is currently being evaluated as a method for guiding excision of both palpable and impalpable lesions with the aim of achieving negative margins at the time of primary surgery. Harlow et al[84] successfully employed this technique for the resection of 65 non-palpable carcinomas, and obtained pathologically negative margins in 63 cases (97%). Others have used IOUS to enhance surgical accuracy during resection of palpable lesions.[85,86] This technique can also help to estimate the macroscopic margin of surrounding normal breast tissue and to direct re-excision at the time of first surgery. Newer imaging modalities such as magnetic resonance imaging (MRI) and positron emission tomography (PET) have high sensitivity and specificity, and may permit the detection of residual disease following conservation surgery.[87–89]

With widespread adoption of stricter and more standardised criteria for pathological margin assessment, coupled with attention to surgical technique, the majority of patients nowadays have a final margin status that is microscopically negative for tumour foci. Although increased rates of local recurrence associated with positive margins and an EIC suggest that incomplete removal of tumour may contribute to local recurrence, patients with negative margins have a finite rate of local recurrence despite 'adequate' surgical excision.

Attention has recently focused on determining risk factors for local recurrence among patients with negative margins of excision.[17] As discussed earlier in this chapter, the width of the negative margin is not directly correlated with rates of local recurrence.[35] Nonetheless, trials of BCT have confirmed that wider resections of tissue are associated with lower rates of local recurrence. Thus, in the surgery-only arms of the NSABP and Milan trials, rates of local recurrence were approximately 53% (at 10 years) and 8.8% (at 3 years) respectively. The former group of patients underwent 'lumpectomy' (a 1 cm macroscopic margin of surrounding breast tissue), while the latter group had a quadrantic resection, which removes 2–3 cm of adjacent breast tissue. Rates of local recurrence are therefore more than threefold greater for lumpectomy compared with quadrantectomy. Rather than assessing the width of the resection margin, Goldstein et al[90] have suggested that an assessment of the amount of carcinoma in the vicinity of the inked margin (and not the distance from it) may be a better predictor of local recurrence in patients with 'negative' margins.

Conventional histopathological parameters have not proved to be useful for stratifying risk in this 'negative'-margin group. However, expression profiles for some of the newer biological and molecular markers may be predictive of local recurrence patterns for this particular group of patients. Thus higher levels of expression of the HER2/*neu* (c-ErbB-2) oncoprotein, p53 and the mitogenic growth factor IGF-I (insulin-like growth factor I) have been reported to be associated with increased rates of local recurrence following BCT.[91,92] Until more data are available, HER2/*neu* overexpression should not be considered a contraindication to BCT.[93] Another approach for predicting relapse in patients with negative margins is 'molecular margin assessment'. Grossly normal adjacent breast tissue can be analysed for genetic changes such as loss of heterozygosity (LOH) at defined chromosomal loci.[94,95] Such changes may confer an increased risk of local relapse in patients with margins deemed 'negative' on conventional pathological assessment.

Molecular profiling with DNA microarrays is beginning to yield patterns of tumour expression that correlate with disease-free and overall survival. It is possible in the future that a particular 'signature' may be associated with an increased risk of local recurrence, and corresponding treatment recommendations could be modified accordingly.[22]

The significance of local recurrence

The surgical dogma that mandates a finite degree of surgical excision in order to minimise local recurrence may be misguided – if local recurrence does not affect survival then why strive to prevent local recurrence and in so doing risk overtreating patients? In the NSABP B-06 trial, 43% of patients undergoing wide local excision only had developed local recurrence at 9 years of follow-up, compared with only 12.2% for those receiving radiotherapy post lumpectomy. Despite the great variation in the incidence of IBTR, this does not translate into survival differences, and Fisher et al[68] concluded that no causal relationship exists between IBTR and distant disease. Fisher subsequently examined differences in distant disease-free survival between patients with and without IBTR using a Cox regression model based on the fixed covariates of age, nodal status, tumour size and grade, together with the time-varying covariate of IBTR.[68] IBTR was found to be the strongest predictor for distant disease and was considered to be a marker for increased risk but not a cause of distant metastases (3.41-fold increased risk; 95% CI 2.70–4.30). Early local recurrence was associated with a shorter disease-free interval and IBTR was better correlated with distant disease than tumour size, which has been reported to be highly predictive for the development of distant metastases. Others have also concurred that local recurrence following BCT is an indicator of poor prognosis.[96,97] Moreover, the timing of IBTR has prognostic significance, with an interval of less than 2 years being associated with a 5-year survival rate of 38%, compared with 90% when IBTR occurred beyond a 2-year interval ($p = 0.026$).[15] IBTR is an independent predictor of distant disease and a marker of risk, but not an instigator of distant metastases. Although locoregional treatment in the form of surgery or radiotherapy may prevent or reduce the chance of expression of the marker, such therapy does not alter the intrinsic risk of developing distant disease. Fisherian precepts would dictate that breast cancer be managed by simple surgical excision of the primary lesion in conjunction with systemic therapy. Although rates of local recurrence would be greater, overall survival would be unaffected. Moreover, such a strategy is less likely to eliminate a marker of risk for the development of distant disease, and IBTR under these circumstances would indicate the need for systemic therapy to maximise survival. It is a matter of judgement as to what constitutes an 'acceptable' rate of local recurrence. Rates of almost 40% were witnessed in the control arm of the NSABP B-06 trial. Although rates of this magnitude are not acceptable by current standards of care, it may be inappropriate to employ treatment schedules whose primary purpose is to minimise absolute rates of local recurrence in the absence of any longer-term survival gain. Indeed, it might be argued that were this the prime objective of locoregional therapies then all patients should undergo mastectomy!

Can locoregional treatment influence survival?

There is limited evidence that not all cases of breast cancer are systemic at the outset and that a subgroup of patients with early breast cancer exist for whom micrometastatic spread has not occurred prior to clinical (or mammographic) detection. Firstly, some of Halsted's patients survived for several decades following surgery and among a group of untreated patients at the Middlesex Hospital, survival rates of 20–30 years were documented. These observations suggest that some patients may never have developed micrometastatic disease.[98] Secondly, analysis of data from the Guy's trial reveals that survival may be compromised by inadequate locoregional treatment. Patients with T1 tumours randomised to wide local excision (and suboptimal doses of radiotherapy) had higher rates of local recurrence, and reduced survival was noted for stage II patients.[99] However, longer-term follow-up of the Guy's data by Hayward[100] suggests that some patients with stage I and II disease treated by mastectomy have achieved hazard ratios similar to those of an aged-matched population, with the observed/expected deaths ratio approaching but not attaining unity. Finally, two randomised studies of postmastectomy radiotherapy have shown a survival benefit (approximately 10%) in a subgroup of premenopausal node-positive patients receiving chemotherapy, suggesting that persistence of local or regional disease can lead to distant metastases and impaired survival.[101,102] Furthermore, the most recent overview from the Early Breast Cancer Trialists' Collaborative Group (EBCTCG) suggests an overall survival benefit from local radiation to either the breast following BCT or the chest wall following mastectomy.[103] Survival percentages at 20 years yield a ratio of 0.911 in favour of radiotherapy (Figure 35.4). These results support the Halstedian paradigm, as does the reduction in mortality from breast cancer screening,

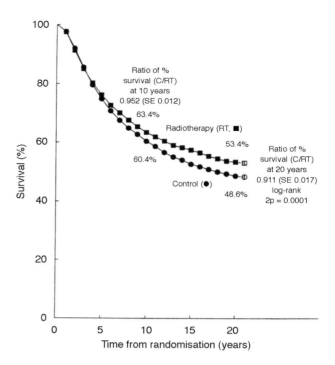

Figure 35.4 Absolute effects of radiotherapy on cause-specific survival: breast cancer death rates calculated by subtraction of the non-breast-cancer mortality rate from the all-cause mortality rate.

which aims to detect cancers during the preclinical phase when they remain localised without micrometastatic dissemination.[104,105] Breast cancer is a heterogeneous disease for which 'small' if rapid may mean 'late', while 'large' if slow may still be early.[106] Some tumours behave in a relatively indolent, 'benign' manner, while others are inherently more biologically aggressive and lethal despite intensive therapies at both a local and a systemic level. As micrometastases can never be excluded, any irrefutable declaration that a tumour remains genuinely localised at the time of diagnosis is impossible. The propensity to metastasise can be estimated using prognostic indices, and current attempts at genetic fingerprinting may increase predictive capacity.

Local recurrence as a determinant or indicator of metastasis

Locoregional treatments such as surgery or radiotherapy are potentially curative in the absence of micrometastases when disease is confined to the breast and lymph nodes. Under these circumstances, when local management is incomplete, viable cells persist within locoregional tissues and can develop into distant metastases at a later date. Therefore, where micrometastases either are absent at presentation or have been obliterated by systemic therapy, local recurrence is a determinant of distant disease and assumes a different significance from Fisher's postulate of local recurrence being a marker for distant disease. By contrast, where micrometastases exist and have not been ablated with systemic therapy, local recurrence would be an indicator of poor prognosis, with foci of residual tumour and distant occult disease maintained in a state of dynamic equilibrium until some event triggers recurrence. Local recurrence predicts for and is a marker for distant disease whether BCT precedes[107] or follows[15,68] systemic therapy, and timing of recurrence is important (the earlier the recurrence, the greater the chance of distant disease). Both events are manifestations of the same biological process, which reflects the intrinsic behaviour of any particular breast tumour. However, studies have revealed partial independence amongst prognostic factors in determining the potential for local and distant relapse. In their study of IBTR in more than 2000 patients undergoing BCT with quadrantic resection, Veronesi et al[24] found that tumour size and nodal status are correlated with distant but not local disease recurrence, while young age and peritumoral invasion predict for both local and, to a lesser extent, distant disease relapse. Local recurrence conferred an overall increased risk of distant relapse of 4.62-fold (95% CI 3.34–6.39). There was actually evidence of an inverse relationship between nodal status and local recurrence, which may be due to confounding effects of concomitant chemotherapy. Furthermore, EIC predicts for local recurrence only, which under these circumstances represents inadequate local treatment and is not a marker for an inherently increased risk of distant metastases. Of interest, the benefits of chemotherapy may be compromised when locoregional control is inadequate, due to the reduced efficacy of chemotherapy in the presence of a greater tumour cell burden in locoregional tissues. Any persistent locoregional disease could become a source of distant metastases.[108] Indeed, this phenomenon may account for the notable survival benefit for node-positive patients receiving a combination of chemotherapy with postmastectomy radiotherapy compared with chemotherapy alone. Nodal retrieval in the Danish trial was modest, which poses doubts regarding the adequacy of locoregional surgery. This may have led to an apparent survival benefit from radiotherapy due to a relative lack of efficacy of chemotherapy secondary to inadequate locoregional management and the presence of 'oligometastases'.[109] Within the trials of BCT, most of the cases of local recurrence occur against a background of micrometastatic disease and therefore represent a marker of distant relapse. Those patients without micrometastases at

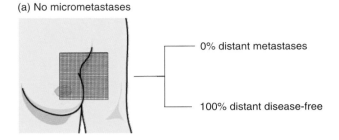

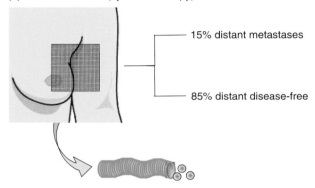

Figure 35.5 (a) Adequate locoregional treatment is potentially curative in the absence of micrometastases. (b) In the presence of micrometastases, about 15% of patients will relapse at distant sites, despite therapy. Local recurrence in this situation is an indicator of poor prognosis.

presentation and who undergo adequate locoregional treatment have the same outcome irrespective of the type of surgery. However, where there is inadequate or incomplete locoregional therapy, survival differences may emerge because local recurrence is a determinant of distant disease and may render systemic therapy less effective. It is perhaps not surprising that no survival difference is detectable in BCT trials, because the majority of patients have received adequate primary locoregional treatment and local recurrence is not a cause of distant disease. Those cases where local recurrence is a determinant of distant failure are probably too few and follow-up too short to have any statistical impact. Thus adequate locoregional treatment is potentially curative in the absence of micrometastases, but in their presence relapse will occur at distant sites in approximately 15% of patients and local recurrence is an indicator of poor prognosis (Figure 35.5). When locoregional treatment is inadequate, residual tumour cells will cause local recurrence and possibly distant disease in a proportion of patients despite the absence of micrometastases at presentation. In the presence of micrometastases, inadequate locoregional treatment can reduce the efficacy of systemic therapy, leading

(a) No micrometastases

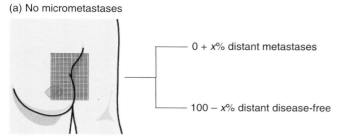

0 + *x*% distant metastases

100 – *x*% distant disease-free

(*x* = distant disease determined by local recurrence)

(b) Micrometastases (systemic therapy)

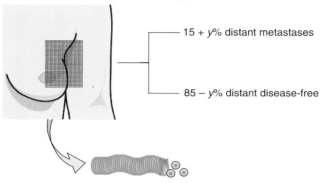

15 + *y*% distant metastases

85 – *y*% distant disease-free

(*y* = reduction in efficacy of systemic therapy due to inadequate locoregional control)

Figure 35.6   (a) When locoregional control is inadequate, residual tumour cells will cause local recurrence and possibly distant disease in a proportion (*x*) of patients. Despite the absence of micrometastases, survival is reduced because of poor locoregional management. (b) Even with micrometastases, inadequate locoregional treatment will reduce the efficacy of systemic therapy, leading to a reduction (*y*) in the number of patients remaining free of distant disease.

to a reduction in the number of patients remaining free of distant disease (Figure 35.6).

Implications for management

In attempts to improve outcomes for all patients, overtreatment becomes a contentious and unavoidable consequence – consider women with T1N0 breast cancer:

- 70% do not benefit from axillary dissection
- 60% do not require radiotherapy
- 95% fail to obtain statistical benefit from chemotherapy (approximately 65% of patients will be treated for a 5% absolute gain in survival).

There are important medical and financial implications from these figures. It would be provocative to suggest that all patients are managed in accordance with Fisherian principles. Thus cases of early breast cancers amenable to conservative surgery would undergo lumpectomy only, without axillary dissection or postoperative radiotherapy. Those tumours with an innate risk of dissemination would subsequently declare themselves with the manifestation of local recurrence, which would be an indicator and not an instigator of distant relapse and poor prognosis. A higher rate of local recurrence would be the price for avoiding unnecessary adjuvant treatment in those patients (40–50%) who do not relapse either locally or systemically after simple lumpectomy. Radiotherapy and systemic (chemohormonal) therapy would be administered at the time of local relapse (unless this mandated mastectomy).

However, local relapse can be psychologically devastating for a patient, even when she is informed that long-term survival is unaffected. Although most studies to date have revealed a 65% reduction in rates of IBTR following radiotherapy,[58] the absolute benefits from adjuvant radiotherapy may become even less in the future with increased attention to surgical resection margins. It is the surgical resection that has the predominant impact on local recurrence, and Holmberg[110] has reiterated our own contention that most women do not develop local recurrence at 5–10 years. He also estimates that the cost of preventing local recurrence at 5 years exceeds the cost of a life-year saved by screening.

There is potential for the application of a more selective policy for radiotherapy in patients undergoing BCT. This seems more likely as patients present with smaller tumours and better surgical clearance is achieved. Indeed, in the Milan trial, women aged 55 or older derived minimal benefit from the addition of radiotherapy to quadrantic resection.[111,112] Furthermore, in the Uppsala–Örebro study, although radiotherapy improved locoregional control, the absolute rates of local recurrence were acceptable even without radiotherapy, particularly for women aged over 55 with invasive ductal carcinoma (7.7% versus 2.3%).[113] Perez[58] has reported that patients with T1 and T2 tumours undergoing BCT do not benefit from a boost dose when surgical excision margins are negative, in contrast to patients with close or positive margins. Intraoperative radiotherapy (IORT) and partial breast irradiation[114–116] are innovative techniques that may permit a more selective and tailored approach to radiotherapy with cost savings. In those circumstances where radiotherapy can be omitted as primary treatment, it can be employed as part of the salvage strategy.

Although randomised clinical trials have previously failed to identify any group of patients for whom local recurrence produces a decrement in survival,[5,117] these may not have possessed the power to detect any effect of attenuated locoregional treatment on overall survival.[118] The numbers of events are relatively small and some cases of distant recurrence may not yet have occurred at the time of analysis. The overview by the EBCTCG previously referred to has revealed that prevention of four isolated locoregional recurrences by radiotherapy at 10 years prevents one breast cancer death at 20 years (a 5% absolute mortality reduction).[103] Vicini et al[23] have undertaken a retrospective study to assess the influence of IBTR on distant disease, and in particular to clarify whether this is a determinant or marker of increased risk for relapse at distant sites. They employed a matched-pair analysis comparing distant metastases in patients with and without local recurrence in order to overcome confounding effects and competing risks that could potentially contribute to distant failure. A distinction was also made between true recurrences/marginal misses within the index quadrant and recurrence elsewhere in the breast, which is more likely to be a new primary. Vicini et al[23] found that only the former had an impact on overall survival and that distant metastases usually followed local recurrence in time sequence. Furthermore, a secondary delayed peak was observed, suggesting that local recurrence could be a cause of distant disease by secondary dissemination from a recurrent focus within the breast.

These clinical results accord with the intuitive assumption that viable cancer cells remaining in the peritumoral tissue of the breast following BCT will ultimately proliferate and metastasise to distant sites. The biological consequence of these residual foci of tumour cells depends upon whether they represent a 'determinant' or an 'indicator' of distant disease. As mentioned above, in the absence of micrometastases, adequate locoregional management can theoretically cure patients, and local recurrence in this group represents persistent disease and a failure to eradicate all tumour cells with primary treatment. It is a determinant of distant disease, the probability of which depends upon both temporal and innate biological factors.

locoregional treatment. For the former group, it is important to administer maximal locoregional therapy at the time of initial diagnosis with curative intent. For the latter group, minimal early locoregional treatment would suffice, as any local recurrence developing secondary to 'inadequate' locoregional treatment would not have an impact on survival, but would be an indicator of a relationship between tumour and host that favoured distant relapse. It would be an indication for maximal treatment at the time of local recurrence, including systemic therapy. Clearly, distinction between these two groups is difficult, but may be aided in the future by microarray techniques that better characterise the biology of individual tumours and provide a molecular 'portrait'. Interestingly, it may be surmised that as tumour size has fallen progressively in recent years, a lower proportion of patients will have micrometastases at the time of diagnosis and therefore disease confined to the locoregional tissues. For these patients, inadequate locoregional treatment at the outset will lead to higher rates of local recurrence, which represent a determinant of distant disease and can directly affect overall survival.

This proposal could be tested in a prospective randomised trial comparing minimal treatment at presentation (and maximal treatment at the time of relapse) with conventional treatment in patients aged 50–70 with T1N0 and non-invasive cancers. Such a trial may reveal a reduction in overall survival as a consequence of suboptimal primary treatment (wide local excision with or without sentinel lymph node biopsy) and hence poorer local control. Moreover, a study of this nature would generate much controversy and would probably be deemed both unethical and unacceptable to many clinicians and patient advocacy groups. Notwithstanding such reservations, a trial of this design may help to resolve some of the uncertainties and contradictions in management of breast cancer patients and establish whether persistent cancer cells in locoregional tissues constitute a source of distant metastases.

Maximal treatment at initial diagnosis versus relapse

Where local recurrence is a determinant of distant disease, treatment at relapse may prevent distant dissemination, and the timing of diagnosis and initiation of treatment are critical. However, where local recurrence develops against a background of pre-existing micrometastatic disease, local recurrence represents a marker for distant disease that would have developed whatever the extent of primary

Management of local recurrence

In contrast to local recurrence following BCT, locoregional failure after mastectomy is more closely correlated with the conventional histological parameters of tumour size, histological grade and nodal status. Chest wall recurrence is also increased when lymphovascular invasion is prominent. It is impossible to formulate a single management strategy for locally recurrent breast cancer that is applicable to all patients. Each patient should be assessed individually with a precise and tailored treatment plan.

The management of locally recurrent breast cancer is dependent on several key factors:

- site of recurrence
- previous treatment modalities
- concomitant systemic disease
- tumour marker measurements
- patient preference

The various treatment options for recurrent disease mirror those for the treatment of primary breast cancer, and include surgery, radiotherapy and systemic therapies (chemotherapy and hormonal therapy). The choice of treatment must reflect the previous therapies that have been followed by failure of local disease control. A crucial determinant of management strategy is the presence or absence of concomitant systemic disease. Patients presenting with locally recurrent breast cancer should always undergo restaging with the following investigations:

- routine blood tests (full blood count, liver function tests, bone profile and calcium)
- bone scan
- liver ultrasound or computed tomography (CT) scan of abdomen
- CT scan of the chest

Ipsilateral breast tumour recurrence without systemic disease

BCT without radiotherapy is associated with a local recurrence rate in excess of 30% overall.[5] However, for smaller grade 1 or special-type tumours in older women, acceptable rates of local recurrence with surgery only may be feasible. In principle, under these circumstances, local recurrence could be treated with further wider excision followed by radiotherapy, provided that satisfactory cosmesis could be maintained. When both surgical resection (wide local excision/quadrantectomy) and radiotherapy have already been employed as treatment for the primary tumour, recurrence in the breast should be treated by mastectomy. This yields a 10-year disease-free survival rate of 50–60% and the rates of complications for salvage mastectomy are comparable to those for primary mastectomy despite surgery within an irradiated field.[60,72,119–122] In those cases where the axilla has not previously been treated, a formal axillary dissection should be carried out at the time of salvage mastectomy. In a study by Kurtz et al[120] involving 118 patients, approximately half were treated with salvage mastectomy and the other half with further BCT.

Rates of subsequent local recurrence were higher in patients treated with an additional conservation procedure. Kurtz et al[120] advocate the selective use of further BCT, which should be restricted to local recurrences that are isolated mobile lesions of 2 cm diameter or smaller occurring in an originally node-negative patient. However, larger recurrences can be successfully managed initially with induction chemotherapy, either to render them operable or to permit further BCT.

Local recurrence in the axilla without systemic disease

Isolated axillary recurrences when operable should be treated by a formal level II/III axillary clearance when this has not been undertaken as part of the primary treatment, i.e. after sentinel node biopsy or axillary sampling with or without radiotherapy. Recurrences following axillary dissection can sometimes be treated by local excision, but this can be technically challenging when tumour is adherent to vital structures such as the axillary vein. Radiotherapy to the axilla and supraclavicular area can be considered as an alternative option and is necessary for cases of inoperable axillary recurrence (if it has not been used previously). This can be employed in conjunction with chemo-endocrine therapies to maximize response and obtain local control of disease.

Local recurrence in the chest wall without systemic disease

Chest wall recurrence following mastectomy can be classified according to the extent of recurrent disease (Table 35.2).

Table 35.2	Treatment of chest wall recurrence following mastectomy
Type of recurrence	**Treatment**
Single spot	Wide excision + radiotherapy (if not used previously)
Multiple spots	Radiotherapy (not previously used) or wide excision (± flap)
Widespread disease	Radiotherapy (not previously used) and/or chemotherapy
Ulcerating/fungating tumour	Excision of necrotic tissue for palliation/control of bleeding sites; topical charcoal for odour control/antibiotics

Local recurrence in the presence of systemic disease

Where local recurrence occurs in the setting of metastatic disease, local and systemic therapies are of palliative value only, but can provide useful relief of symptoms. The development of local recurrence simultaneously with distant metastases accounts for approximately 10% of all patients with local failure after BCT. Furthermore, this dual manifestation of local and distant disease is the strongest argument for IBTR being a marker rather than a determinant of distant disease. Clearly, a proportion of patients with local recurrence apparently in the absence of systemic disease will have micrometastases and are at higher risk for subsequent overt metastatic disease at distant sites.

Prognosis of local recurrence

In the majority of cases, local recurrence is a marker of a poor-prognosis disease and therefore portends a worse outcome in general. Furthermore, not only does local recurrence per se reflect a poorer prognosis, but the time interval between primary treatment and recurrence is of relevance: when this interval is less than 2 years, the chance of distant disease is significantly greater. Overall and disease-free survival rates following treatment for IBTR range from 50% to 80% and 50% to 60% respectively.[119,121,123]

Conclusions

Until recently, the concept of biological predeterminism appeared pre-eminent and a worthy successor to the Halstedian doctrine of centrifugal spread of cancer. However, evidence has now emerged from clinical trials that casts doubt on the universal application of this concept to breast tumours. The most recent overview by the EBCTCG suggests that prevention of local recurrence can save lives. Although this evidence pertains to reductions in local relapse resulting from adjuvant radiotherapy, the principle must also apply to surgical modalities. Mastectomy in both radical and modified forms was rejected as standard treatment for all breast cancers, not for failure to reduce local recurrence, but rather for its lack of impact on overall survival.

There are implications for treatment. On the one hand, can we justify continuing to follow Fisherian principles on the basis that the current evidence is premature and inadequate to modify practice? Alternatively, should we revert to Halstedian principles of more thorough locoregional management at the time of presentation? An 'intermediate' (or 'spectrum') paradigm may be relevant, encompassing elements of both Fisher and Halsted but less restrictive than either of these paradigms in pure form. However, this is difficult to translate into practice, as differentiation between the basic groupings is difficult. There are a group of patients in whom failure to perform mastectomy (with or without chest wall radiotherapy) at the outset will risk compromise of longer-term outcome due to local recurrence acting as a determinant of distant disease. This contention is supported by a recent analysis of rates of local recurrence and survival in breast cancer patients undergoing various intensities of locoregional treatments. Higher-risk patients receiving lesser surgery without radiotherapy exhibited higher rates of local recurrence, with evidence of impaired survival after the first 5 years (4% difference), suggesting that local recurrence as an event can have an impact on longer-term survival in some patients.[124] Newer molecular markers and gene expression profiles may help to identify this group in the future,[125] but what about the present?

A compromise solution and pragmatic approach may be to select those patients for whom more aggressive locoregional treatment at the outset may confer a survival advantage. This is likely to include younger patients, who should be informed that lesser treatments may be associated with local recurrence and in turn a small but significant decrement in survival. For those patients aged under 35 who develop early local recurrence (within 2 years of diagnosis), the administration of systemic therapy would be appropriate. Furthermore, where patients have received prior systemic treatment at presentation, local recurrence should prompt consideration of additional systemic intervention. The absolute benefits of adjuvant chemo-endocrine treatment are greater the higher the risk of systemic relapse. It could therefore be argued that as local recurrence is a highly significant prognostic marker for distant disease recurrence, chemo-endocrine treatment should be prescribed for all cases of local recurrence. However, it must be acknowledged that this hypothesis has not been tested in a randomized trial and is not evidenced-based.

It seems likely that large multicentre and multinational trials will be necessary in the future to define more precisely the factors influencing local recurrence in margin-negative cases and for identification of the subgroup of patients for whom local recurrence represents a determinant of distant disease. Such studies will possess the appropriate power to detect modest differences in outcome based on relatively small numbers of events.[17]

References

1. NIH Consensus Conference. Treatment of early stage breast cancer. JAMA 1991; 265: 391–5.

2. Atkins H, Hayward JL, Klugman DJ et al. Treatment of early breast cancer: a report after 10 years of a clinical trial. BMJ 1972; ii: 423–9.

3. Veronesi U, Saccozzi R, Del Vecchio M et al. Comparing radical mastectomy with quadrantectomy, axillary dissection and radiotherapy in patients with small cancers of the breast. N Engl J Med 1981; 305: 6–11.

4. Sarrazin D, Dewar JA, Arriagada R et al. Conservative management of breast cancer. Br J Surg 1986; 73: 604–6.

5. Fisher B, Redmond C, Poisson R et al. Eight year results of a randomised clinical trial comparing total mastectomy and lumpectomy with or without irradiation in the treatment of breast cancer. N Engl J Med 1989; 320: 822–7.

6. Blichert-Toft M, Rose C, Andersen JA et al. Danish randomised trial comparing breast-conserving therapy with mastectomy: six years of life-table analysis. J Natl Cancer Inst Monogr 1992; 11: 19–25.

7. van Dongen JA, Voogd AC, Fentiman IS et al. Long-term results of a randomised trial comparing breast-conserving therapy with mastectomy: European Organisation for Research and Treatment of Cancer 10801 trial. J Natl Cancer Inst 2000; 92: 1143–50.

8. Fisher B, Joeng J-H, Anderson S et al. Twenty-five year follow-up of a randomised trial comparing radical mastectomy, total mastectomy and total mastectomy followed by irradiation. N Engl J Med 2002; 347: 567–75.

9. Margolese RG. Surgical considerations for invasive breast cancer. Surg Clin North Am 1999; 79: 1031–46.

10. Locker G, Sainsbury R, Cuzick J. Breast surgery in the ATAC trial: women from the United States are more likely to have mastectomy. Breast Cancer Res Treat 2002; 76: S35.

11. Winchester DL. Data-based breast management. Presented at the 85th Annual Meeting of the American Radium Society, Houston, TX, April 2003.

12. Mirza NQ, Vlastos G, Meric F et al. Predictors of locoregional recurrence amongst patients with early-stage breast cancer treated with breast-conserving therapy. Ann Surg Oncol 2002; 9: 256–65.

13. Fisher B, Anderson S, Redmond CK et al. Reanalysis and results after 12 years of follow up in a randomized clinical trial comparing total mastectomy with lumpectomy with or without irradiation in the treatment of breast cancer. N Engl J Med 1995; 333: 1456–61.

14. Jacobsen JA, Danforth DN, Cowan KH et al. Ten year results of a comparison of conservation with mastectomy in the treatment of stage I and II breast cancer. N Engl J Med 1995; 332: 907–11.

15. Touboul E, Buffat L, Belkacemi Y et al. Local recurrence and distant metastases after breast-conserving surgery and radiation for early breast cancer. Int J Radiat Oncol Biol Phys 1999; 43: 25–38.

16. Haffty BG, Reiss M, Beinfield M et al. Ipsilateral breast tumour recurrence as a predictor of distant disease: implications for systemic therapy at the time of relapse. J Clin Oncol 1996; 14: 52–7.

17. Schnitt SJ. Risk factors for local recurrence in patients with invasive breast cancer and negative surgical margins of excision. Am J Clin Pathol 2003; 120: 485–8.

18. MacMillan RD, Purushotham AD, George WD. Local recurrence after breast-conserving surgery for breast cancer. Br J Surg 1996; 83: 149–55.

19. Beadle GF, Silver B, Botnick L et al. Cosmetic results following primary radiation therapy for early breast cancer. Cancer 1984; 54: 2911–18.

20. Rose MA, Olivotto I, Cady B et al. Conservative surgery and radiation therapy for early breast cancer: long-term cosmetic results. Ann Surg 1989; 124: 153–7.

21. Fallowfield LJ. Psychosocial adjustment after treatment for early breast cancer. Oncology 1990; 4: 89–100.

22. Querci della Rovere G, Benson JR. Ipsilateral local recurrence of breast cancer: determinant or indicator of poor prognosis. Lancet Oncol 2002; 3: 183–7.

23. Vicini FA, Kestin L, Huang R et al. Does local recurrence affect the rate of distance metastases and survival in patients with early-stage breast carcinoma treated with breast conserving therapy? Cancer 2003; 97: 901–19.

24. Veronesi U, Marubini E, Del Vecchio M et al. Local recurrences and distant metastases after conservative breast cancer treatments: partly independent events. J Natl Cancer Inst 1995; 87: 19–27.

25. Halsted WS. The results of operation for the cure of cancer of the breast performed at the Johns Hopkins Hospital form June 1889 to January 1894. Johns Hopkins Hosp Rep 1894-95; 4: 297.

26. Crile G. Treatment of breast cancer by local excision. Am J Surg 1965; 109: 400–3.

27. Hellman S. Natural history of small breast cancers. J Clin Oncol 1994; 12: 2229–34.

28. Rosen PP, Groshen S, Saigo PE et al. A long term follow up study of survival in stage I (T1N1M0 and stage II (T1N1M0 breast carcinoma. J Clin Oncol 1989; 7: 355–66.

29. Quiet CA, Ferguson DJ, Weichselbaum RR, Hellman S. Natural history of node-negative breast cancer: a study of 826 patients with long term follow up. J Clin Oncol 1995; 13: 1144–51.

30. Fisher B. The evolution of paradigms for the management of breast cancer. Persp Cancer Res 1992; 52: 2371–83.

31. Abrams J, Chen T, Giusti R. Survival after breast-sparing surgery versus mastectomy. J Natl Cancer Inst 1994; 86: 1672–3.

32. Baum M, Benson JR. Current and future roles of adjuvant endocrine therapy in management of early carcinoma of the breast. In: Senn H-J, Goldhirsch RD, Gelber RD, Thurlimaan B, eds. Recent Results in Cancer Research 140 – Adjuvant Therapy of Breast Cancer V. Berlin: Springer–Verlag, 1996: 215–26.

33. Haffty BG, Carter D, Flynn SD et al. Local recurrence

versus new primary: clinical analysis of 82 breast relapses and potential applications for genetic fingerprinting. Int J Radiat Oncol Biol Phys 1993; 27: 575–83.

34. Schnitt SJ, Abner A, Gelman R et al. The relationship between microscopic margins of resection and the risk of local recurrence in patients with breast cancer treated with breast-conserving surgery and radiation therapy. Cancer 1994; 74: 1746–51.

35. Singletary SE. Surgical margins in patients with early-stage breast cancer treated with breast conservation therapy. Am J Surg 2002; 184: 383–93.

36. National Coordinating Group for Breast Screening Pathology. Pathology Reporting in Breast Cancer Screening, 2nd edn. Sheffield: NHS Breast Screening Programme, 1995.

37. van Dongen JA, Bartelink H, Fentimen I et al. Factors influencing local relapse and survival and results of salvage treatment after breast conserving treatment in operable breast cancer. EORTC trial 10801. Breast conservation compared with mastectomy in TNM stage I and II breast cancer. Eur J Cancer 1992; 28A: 808–15.

38. Smitt MC, Nowels K, Carlson RW et al. Predictors of re-excision findings and recurrence after breast conservation. Int J Radiat Oncol Biol Phys 2003; 57: 979–85.

39. Fisher ER, Costantino J, Fisher B et al. Pathologic findings from the National Surgical Adjuvant Breast and Bowel Project (NSABP) Protocol B-17. Cancer 1995; 75: 1310–19.

40. Ryoo MC, Kagan AT, Wollin M et al. Prognostic factors for recurrence and cosmesis in 393 patients after radiation therapy for early mammary carcinoma. Radiology 1989; 172: 555–9.

41. Kurtz JM, Jacquemir J, Amalric R et al. Risk factors for breast recurrence in premenopausal and postmenopausal patients with ductal cancers treated by conservation therapy. Cancer 1990; 65; 1867–78.

42. Borger JH. The impact of surgical and pathological findings on radiotherapy of early breast cancer. Radiother Oncol 1991; 22: 230–6.

43. Borger J, Kemperman H, Hart A et al. Risk factors in breast conservation therapy. J Clin Oncol 1994; 12: 653–60.

44. Di Biase S, Komarnicky LT, Schwartz GF et al. The number of positive margins influences the outcome of women treated with breast preservation for early stage breast carcinoma. Cancer 1998; 82: 2212–20.

45. Smitt MC, Nowels KW, Zdeblick MJ et al. The importance of the lumpectomy surgical margin status in long term results of breast conservation. Cancer 1995; 76: 259–67.

46. Schmidt-Ulrich R, Wazer D, Tercilla O et al. Tumour margin assessment as a guide to optimal conservation surgery and irradiation in early-stage breast carcinoma. Int J Radiat Oncol Biol Phys 1989; 17: 733–8.

47. Solin LJ, Fowble BL, Schultz DJ, Goodman RL. The significance of the pathology margins of the tumor excision on the outcome of patients treated with definitive irradiation for early stage breast cancer. Int J Radiat Oncol Biol Phys 1991; 21: 279–87.

48. Pittinger TP, Maronian NC, Poulter CA, Peacock JL. Importance of margin status in outcome of breast conserving surgery for carcinoma. Surgery 1994; 116: 605.

49. Petersen ME, Schultz DJ, Reynolds C et al. Outcomes in breast cancer patients relative to margin status after treatment with breast-conserving surgery and radiation therapy: the University of Pennsylvania experience. Int J Radiat Oncol Biol Phys 1999; 43: 1029–35.

50. Freedman G, Fowble B, Hanlon A et al. Patients with early stage invasive cancer with close or positive margins treated with conservative sugery and radiation have an increased risk of breast recurrence that is delayed by adjuvant systemic therapy. Int J Radiat Oncol Biol Phys 1999; 44: 1005–15.

51. Wazer DE, Schmidt-Ulrich RK, Ruthazer R et al. Factors determining outcome for breast-conserving irradiation with margin-directed dose escalation to the tumor bed. Int J Radiat Oncol Biol Phys 1998; 40: 851–8.

52. Assersohn L, Powles TJ, Ashley S et al. Local relapse in primary breast cancer patients with unexcised positive surgical margins after lumpectomy, radiotherapy and chemoendocrine therapy. Ann Oncol 1999; 10: 1451–5.

53. Gage I, Schnitt SJ, Nixon AJ et al. Pathologic margin involvement and the risk of recurrence in patients treated with breast conserving therapy. Cancer 1996; 78: 1921–8.

54. Vicini FA, Recht A, Abner A et al. Recurrence in the breast following conservative surgery and radiation therapy for early-stage breast cancer. J Natl Cancer Inst Monogr 1992; 11: 33–9.

55. Holland R, Veling SHJ, Mravunac M, Hendricks JHCL. Histologic multifocality of Tis, T1-2 breast carcinomas: implications for clinical trials of breast-conserving surgery. Cancer 1985; 56: 979–90.

56. Holland R, Connolly JL, Gelman R et al. The presence of an extensive intraductal component following a limited excision correlates with prominent residual disease in the remainder of the breast. J Clin Oncol 1990; 8: 113–18.

57. Veronesi U, Volterrani F, Luini A et al. Quadrantectomy versus lumpectomy for small size breast cancer. Eur J Cancer 1990; 26: 671–3.

58. Perez CA. Conservation therapy in T1–T2 breast cancer: past, current issues and future challenges and opportunities. Cancer J Sci Am 2003; 9: 442–53.

59. Recht A, Connolly JL, Schnitt SJ et al. The effect of young age on tumor recurrence in the treated breast after conservative surgery and radiotherapy. Int J Radiat Oncol Biol Phys 1987; 14: 3–10.

60. Stotter AT, McNeese MD, Ames FC et al. Predicting the rate and extent of locoregional failure after breast conservation therapy for early breast cancer. Cancer 1989; 64: 2217–25.

61. Kurtz JM, Jacquemir J, Amalric R et al. Why are local recurrences after breast-conserving therapy more frequent in younger patients? J Clin Oncol 1990; 8: 591–8.

62. Kurtz JM, Spitalier JM, Amalric R et al. Mammary recurrences in women younger than forty. Int J Radiat Oncol Biol Phys 1988; 15: 271–6.

63. Nolber MP, Venet L. Prognostic factors in patients undergoing curative irradiation for breast cancer. Int J Radiat Oncol Biol Phys 1985; 11: 1323–31.

64. Bartelink H, Borger J, van Dongen J et al. The impact of tumour size and histology on local control after breast conserving therapy. Radiother Oncol 1988; 11: 297–303.

65. Sismondi P, Bordon R, Arisio R et al. Local recurrences after breast conserving surgery and radiotherapy: correlation of histopathological risk factors with age. Breast 1994; 3: 8–13.

66. de la Rochefordiere A, Asselain B, Campana F et al. Age as a prognostic factor in pre-menopausal breast carcinoma. Lancet 1993; 341: 1039–43.

67. Fisher B, Anderson S. Conservative surgery for the management of invasive and non-invasive carcinoma of the breast: NSABP trials. National Surgical Adjuvant Breast and Bowel Project. World J Surg 1994; 18: 63–9.

68. Fisher B, Anderson S, Fisher ER et al. Significance of ipsilateral breast tumour recurrence after lumpectomy. Lancet 1991; 338: 327–331.

69. Fisher BJ, Perera FE, Cooke AL et al. Long term follow-up of axillary node-positive breast cancer patients receiving adjuvant systemic therapy alone: patterns of recurrence. Int J Radiat Oncol Biol Phys 1997; 38: 541–50.

70. Locker AP, Ellis IO, Morgan DAL et al. Factors influencing local recurrence after excision and radiotherapy for primary breast cancer. Br J Surg 1989; 17: 890–4.

71. Clark RM, McCulloch PB, Levine MN et al. Randomised clinical trial to assess the effectiveness of breast irradiation following lumpectomy and axillary dissection for node-negative breast cancer. J Natl Cancer Inst 1992; 84: 683–9.

72. Kurtz JM, Jacquemier J, Torhorst J et al. Conservation therapy for breast cancers other than infiltrating ductal carcinoma. Cancer 1989; 63: 1630–5.

73. Fisher B, Costantino J, Redmond C et al. A randomised clinical trial evaluating tamoxifen in the treatment of patients with node-negative breast cancer who have estrogen-receptor positive tumours. N Engl J Med 1989; 320: 479–84.

74. Fisher B, Redmond C, Dimitrov NV et al. A randomised clinical trial evaluating sequential methotrexate and fluorouracil in the treatment of patients with node-negative breast cancer who have estrogen-receptor negative tumours. N Engl J Med 1989; 320: 473–8.

75. Fisher B, Dignam J, Wolmark N et al. Tamoxifen in treatment of intraductal breast cancer: National Surgical Adjuvant Breast and Bowel Project B-24 randomised controlled trial. Lancet 1999; 353: 1993–2000.

76. Balch GC, Mithani SK, Kelly MC. Intraoperative evaluation of surgical margins in breast conserving therapy. In: Bland KI, Copeland EM, eds. The Breast, 3rd edn. Philadelphia: WB Saunders, 2004.

77. Abraham SC, Fox K, Fraker D et al. Sampling of grossly grossly benign breast re-excisions: a multidisciplinary approach to assessing adequacy. Am J Surg Pathol 1999; 23: 316.

78. Gibson GR, Lesnikoski B-A, Yoo J et al. A comparison of ink-directed and traditional whole cavity re-excision for breast lumpectomy specimens with positive margins. Ann Surg Oncol 2001; 8: 693–704.

79. Noguchi M, Minami M, Earshi M et al. Pathologic assessment of surgical margins on frozen and permanent sections in breast conserving surgery. Breast Cancer 1995; 2: 27–33.

80. Weber S, Storm FK, Stitt J, Mahvi DM. The role of frozen section analysis of margins during breast conservation surgery. Cancer J Sci Am 1997; 3: 273–7.

81. Umpleby HC, Herbert A, Royle G and Taylor I. Wide excision of primary breast cancer: the incidence of residual carcinoma at the site of excision. Ann R Coll Surg Engl 1988; 70: 246–8.

82. Macmillan RD, Purushotham AD, Mallon E et al. Breast conserving surgery and tumour bed positivity in patients with breast cancer. Br J Surg 1994; 81: 56–8.

83. Klimberg VS, Westbrook KC, Korourian S. Use of touch preps for diagnosis and evaluation of surgical margins in breast cancer. Ann Surg Oncol 1998; 5: 220–6.

84. Harlow SP, Krag DN, Ames SE et al. Intra-operative ultrasound localisation to guide surgical excision of non-palpable breast carcinoma. J Am Coll Surg 1999; 189: 241–6.

85. Moore MM, Whitney LA, Cerilla L et al. Intra-operative ultrasound is associated with clear lumpectomy margins palpable infiltrating ductal breast carcinoma. Ann Surg 2001; 233: 761–8.

86. Smith LF, Rubio IT, Henry-Tillman R et al. Intraoperative ultrasound-guided breast biopsy. Am J Surg 2001; 180: 419–23.

87. Adler DD, Wahl RL. New methods for imaging the breast: techniques, findings and potential. AJR Am J Roentgenol 1995; 164: 19–30.

88. Tillman GF, Orel SG, Schnall MD et al. Effect of breast magnetic resonance imaging on the clinical management of women with early-stage breast carcinoma. J Clin Oncol 2002; 20: 3413–23.

89. Greco M, Crippa F, Agresti R et al. Axillary lymph node staging in breast cancer by 2-fluoro-2-deoxy-D-glucose positron emission tomography: clinical evaluation and alternative management. J Natl Cancer Inst 2001; 93: 630–5.

90. Goldstein N, Kestin L, Vicini F. Factors associated with ipsilateral breast failure and distant metastases in patients with invasive breast carcinoma treated with breast-conserving therapy: a clinicopathological study of 607 neoplasms from 583 patients. Am J Clin Pathol 2003; 120: 500–27.

91. Haffty BG, Brown F, Carter D et al. Evaluation of HER-2/neu oncoprotein expression as a prognostic indicator of local recurrence in conservatively treated breast cancer: a case–control study. Int J Radiat Oncol Biol Phys 1996; 35: 751–7.

92. Turner BC, Haffty BG, Narayanan L et al. Insulin-like growth factor-I receptor over-expression mediates cellular radioresistance and local breast cancer recurrence after lumpectomy and radiation. Cancer Res 1997; 57: 3079–83.

93. Freedman G, Haulou AL, Fowble BL et al. Recursive partitioning and the risk of ipsilateral breast tumour recurrence in early stage breast cancer. J Clin Oncol 2002; 20: 4015–21.

94. Deng G, Lu Y, Zlotnikov G et al. Loss of heterozygosity in normal tissue adjacent to breast carcinomas. Science 1996; 274: 2057–9.

95. Li Z, Moore DH, Meng ZH et al. Increased risk of local recurrence is associated with allele loss in normal lobules of breast cancer patients. Cancer Res 2002; 62: 1000–3.

96. Chauvet B, Reynaud-Bougnoux A, Calais G et al. Prognostic significance of breast relapse after conservative treatment in node-negative early breast cancer. Int J Radiat Oncol Biol Phys 1990; 19: 1125–30.

97. Whelan T, Clark R, Roberts R et al. Ipsilateral breast tumour recurrence post-lumpectomy is predictive of subsequent mortality: results from a randomized trial. Int J Radiat Oncol Biol Phys 1994; 30: 11–16.

98. Bloom HJG, Richardson WW, Harries EJ. Natural history of untreated breast cancer (1805–1933). Comparison of untreated and treated cases according to histological grade of malignancy. BMJ 1962; i: 213–21.

99. Hayward J, Caleffi M. The significance of local control in the primary treatment of breast cancer. Arch Surg 1987; 122: 1244.

100. Hayward J. Controversies in breast cancer management. Presented at the 8th International Congress on Senology, Rio de Janiero, Brazil, May 1994.

101. Ragaz J, Jackson SM, Le N et al. Adjuvant radiotherapy and chemotherapy in node-positive pre-menopausal women with breast cancer. N Engl J Med 1997; 337: 956–62.

102. Overgaard M, Hansen PS, Overgaard J et al. Post-operative radiotherapy in high risk pre-menopausal women with breast cancer who receive adjuvant chemotherapy. N Engl J Med 1997; 337: 949–55.

103. Early Breast Cancer Trialists' Collaborative Group. Favourable and unfavourable efects on long term survival of radiotherapy for early breast cancer: an overview of the randomised trials. Lancet 2000; 355: 1757–70.

104. Forrest P. Breast Cancer – The Decision to Screen. London: The Nuffield Provincial Hospitals Trust Publications, 1990.

105. Wald N, Frost C, Cuckle H. Breast cancer screening: the current position. BMJ 1991; 302: 845–6.

106. Thornton H. The voice of the breast cancer patient – a lonely cry in the wilderness. Eur J Cancer 1997; 33: 825–8.

107. Rouzier R, Extra J-M, Carton M et al. Primary chemotherapy for operable breast cancer: Incidence and prognostic significance of ipsilateral breast tumour recurrence after breast-conserving surgery. J Clin Oncol 2001; 19: 3828–35.

108. Hellman S. Stopping metastases at their source. N Engl J Med 1997; 337: 996–7.

109. Querci della Rovere G, Daniels I. Local treatment for breast cancer. Breast 1998; 7: 174–5.

110. Holmberg L. Breast conserving surgery without radiotherapy. Acta Oncol 1995; 34: 681–3.

111. Veronesi U, Luini A, Del Vecchio M et al. Radiotherapy after breast-preserving surgery in women with localised cancer of the breast. N Engl J Med 1993; 328: 1587–91.

112. Veronesi U, Cascinelli N, Mariani L et al. Twenty year follow up of a randomized study comparing breast conserving surgery with radical mastectomy for early breast cancer. N Engl J Med 2002; 347: 1227–31.

113. Liljegren G, Holmberg L, Bergh J et al. 10 year results after sector resection with or without postoperative radiotherapy for stage I breast cancer: a randomized trial. J Clin Oncol 1999; 17: 2326–33.

114. Veronesi U, Orecchia R, Luini A et al. A preliminary report of intraoperative radiotherapy (IORT. in limited-stage breast cancers that are conservatively treated. Eur J Cancer 2001; 37: 2178–83.

115. Vaidya JS, Joseph D, Hilaris B et al. Targetted intra-operative radiotherapy (TARGIT) for breast cancer. Breast Cancer Res Treat 2002; Suppl 1: S18 (abst).

116. Vaidya JS, Tobias J, Baum M et al. Intraoperative radiotherapy for breast cancer. Lancet Oncol 2004; 5: 165–73.

117. Veronesi U, Volterrani F, Luini A et al. Quadrantectomy versus lumpectomy for small size breast cancer. Eur J Cancer 1990; 26: 671–3.

118. Lippman M. How should we manage breast cancer in the breast, or 'Buddy, can you paradigm?' J Natl Cancer Inst 1995; 87: 3–4.

119. Osborne MP, Simmons RM. Salvage surgery for recurrence after breast conservation surgery. World J Surg 1994; 18: 93–7.

120. Kurtz JM, Amalric R, Brandone H et al. Results of salvage surgery for mammary recurrence following breast conserving therapy. 1988; 207: 347–51.

121. Osteen RT. Risk factors and management of local recurrence following breast conservation surgery. World J Surg 1994; 18: 76–80.

122. Barr LC, Brunt AM, Goodman AG et al. Uncontrolled local recurrence after treatment of breast cancer with breast conservation. Cancer 1989; 64: 1203–7.

123. Ames FC, Balch CM. Management of local and regional recurrence after mastectomy or breast conservation treatment. Surg Clin North Am 1990; 70: 1115–23.

124. Grey R. BCRM, Manchester, 2004.

125. Ramaswamy S, Golub TR. New methods for imaging the breast: techniques, findings and potential. AJR Am J Roentgenol 1995; 164: 19–30.

36 Management of the axilla I

Marco Greco, Massimiliano Gennaro

Introduction

It was Halsted[1] who first clearly recognised that breast cancer often spreads early, via the lymphatic ducts, to the axillary lymph nodes. He reasoned that the resulting axillary metastases were a potential source of tertiary spread. Axillary dissection thus came to be viewed as an essential part of the curative approach to breast cancer, in which it was considered important to remove all possible disease sites by en bloc removal of the breast, lymphatic vessels and lymph nodes. The theoretical underpinning of this approach was the belief that breast cancer spreads progressively and sequentially from a single focus to the axillary lymph nodes, followed by haematogenous dissemination.

Later, after even more radical surgery failed to improve breast cancer survival, the disease came to be considered as a systemic one from its earliest phases. In this scheme, dissemination via the lymphatic ducts was stochastic in nature and did not necessarily precede haematogenous spread. Nevertheless, the role of axillary dissection remained clear, although the emphasis shifted from treatment to staging. The aim of axillary dissection was to obtain prognostic information to stratify patients in terms of risk of recurrence, to obtain regional control and to serve as a guide for adjuvant therapy. This concept is embodied in the current TNM (tumour, node, metastasis) staging of breast cancer.

For more than a century, axillary dissection has been routinely applied to most women with the disease, with the following specific objectives:

- to remove local disease
- to prevent recurrence
- to stage breast cancer
- to plan adjuvant treatment

Now, however, the indication for axillary dissection has changed radically as a result of progress on several fronts. It has become clear that aggressive surgery is not always necessary for oncological radicality, while quality of life and avoidance of excessive morbidity have become much more important than formerly; screening and increased public awareness have resulted in earlier diagnosis; at the same time there have been major advances in treatment and diagnosis (preoperative, intraoperative and postoperative).

Axillary involvement

Studies to understand the dynamics of spread of cancer cells to regional lymph nodes were conducted from the middle of the 20th century and concentrated on the axilla. If cancer cells travelled in the lymphatic ducts to be taken up by the axillary lymph nodes then the first, second and third echelons should be involved in orderly succession. The Netherlands Cancer Institute was one of the first centres to investigate this issue. In a study published in 1958,[2] they found a clear correlation between disease stage and subclavian node involvement (third axillary level), as assessed by intraoperative biopsy of the axillary apex. This result corroborated the prognostic role of third-level axillary involvement; however, the significance of the finding (Table 36.1) that 4% of stage I cases had third-level axillary involvement was less clear.

Table 36.1	**Netherlands Cancer Institute study: relation between tumour stage and involvement of the axillary apex (AB)**
Stage	**AB-positive (%)**
I	4
II	17
IIIa	40

A retrospective study from the National Cancer Institute, Milan shed further light on the issue. Axillary nodal metastases by level were analysed in 1446 consecutive breast cancer patients who had received complete axillary dissection and were found to have axillary involvement.[3]

The main conclusions were as follows:

- The spread of breast cancer to the axilla was regular: skip metastases (higher-level involvement without lower-level involvement) were observed in only 1.3% of cases.
- The probability of second- or third-level disease was related to the number of lymph nodes involved at the first level (Table 36.2); furthermore, in a large proportion (54%) of cases with first-level involvement, there was also higher-level involvement.
- In cases with first- and second-level involvement, the risk of third-level involvement was related to tumour size.
- Complete axillary dissection gave much more accurate and reliable prognostic information than partial dissection. In particular third-level involvement has grave prognostic implications and can change treatment plans.

The recent advent of sentinel node biopsy has further contributed to our understanding of the development and distribution of metastatic lymph nodes from breast cancer. As first shown by Cabanas[4] in penile cancer and then by Morton et al[5] in early-stage melanoma, injection of suitable tracer material peritumorally results in it being taken up by, and travelling in, the lymphatic ducts to reach the lymph node or nodes that first drain the tumour area. Such nodes are sentinel nodes, and a wealth of accumulated evidence has shown that these are almost always the first lymph nodes to be colonised by cancer cells arriving from the primary tumour via the lymphatic ducts.

The technique of identifying the sentinel node using blue dye or a radiopharmaceutical as tracer is known as lymph node mapping. Lymph node mapping in breast cancer does not always lead to the identification of a sentinel node in the first level of the axilla. Intramammary, interpectoral, subclavian and internal mammary chain sentinel nodes have been well documented. In theory, therefore, histological analysis of the sentinel node provides more reliable prognostic information than axillary dissection, since the sentinel node is the one that first receives lymph from the tumour area.

The usual policy when the sentinel node is positive is to perform axillary dissection. However, in women with early breast cancer, it has been found that 40–50% of those with a positive sentinel node have no other regional lymph nodes involved. Furthermore the risk of involvement of non-sentinel nodes is proportional to the volume of metastases of the sentinel node.[6–8] These findings have led to second-generation trials both in Europe and the USA, to determine if it is safe to omit axillary dissection in those cases with minimal sentinel node involvement (namely where only micrometastases are present).

Indications for axillary surgery

The traditional surgical approaches to the axilla are:

- axillary sampling
- low axillary dissection (first and second levels)
- full axillary clearance (first, second and third levels)

The choice of the most appropriate option involves balancing the requirement for information against the risk of complications and sequelae. Full clearance in particular can be associated with significant postoperative rates of morbidity including arm lymphoedema, shoulder stiffness in addition to arm hypoesthesia or paresthesia arising from damage to the intercostobrachial nerve. Rarely, surgical damage to the long thoracic nerve or the thoracodorsal pedicle can lead to winged scapula or atrophy of the latissimus dorsi muscle.[9] The more aggressive is the axillary intervention, the greater is the risk of such sequelae. Conversely, less aggressive approaches are likely to provide incomplete prognostic information and can compromise local control.

The advent of sentinel node biopsy seems to have partially resolved this dilemma; it is a minimally

Table 36.2	**National Cancer Institute, Milan study (1990): metastatic involvement of axillary levels II and III in relation to the number of metastatic nodes at level I**

No. of involved nodes at level I	Percentage with involvement at levels II or III
1	12.1
2	19.5
3	37.5
4	40.3
>4	83.9

invasive procedure that provides accurate information about locoregional involvement. Two types of tracer are in use: blue dye (methylene blue, patent blue, isosulfan blue, etc.) and technetium-99m (^{99m}Tc)-labelled radiocolloids (albumin microaggregate, colloidal sulfur, etc.). Blue dye is injected in the operating room and requires a relatively large incision to enable the surgeon to follow the blue lymph ducts to the blue lymph node; it is a cheap and relatively simple procedure and does not require special equipment. When radiotracer is used, it is usually injected 12–24 hours prior to surgery in a nuclear medicine setting. Routine precautions against radioactive contamination must be adhered to. Lymphoscintigraphy can be performed to ensure that a sentinel node is detected. During surgery itself, a gamma-detecting probe is used to locate the node, which can be removed via a small incision placed directly over the node.

Appropriate training is required for both methods. Use of the radioactive tracer method alone identifies an axillary sentinel more often than the blue dye method alone; the use of dual localization methods is reported to provide the highest rate of sentinel node identification (>95%).

The method is 100% specific (no false positives) and failure to find cancer cells in the sentinel nodes (false negative) is influenced by two factors:

- the number of sentinel nodes identified per patient.
- the thoroughness and intensity of histological examination of the excised nodes.

If a node is extensively involved by metastasis, the lymphatic flow may be diverted to other lymph nodes. In such cases, the node, which takes up tracer is not the sentinel node, and if this node turns out to be negative, there is false negative result. For this reason, many surgeons insist that all nodes taking up tracer should be considered sentinel nodes and be removed and examined. Furthermore, any nodes that are palpable intraoperatively should also be removed and examined.[10]

Sentinel node involvement may be minimal and difficult to identify by conventional hematoxylin and eosin (H&E) staining of a limited number of sections. To overcome this, multiple step sections per node may be examined and immunohistochemical or polymerase chain reaction (PCR) techniques employed. This may reduce the number of false negatives and increase the negative predictive value of the method.[11,12] These exhaustive procedures greatly increase the pathologist's workload and result in significantly higher proportions of node-positive cases than historical reports on series examined by traditional methods. More common too is the finding of micrometastases only, or even the presence of just a few isolated cancer cells. The prognostic significance of these micrometastases is unlikely to be the same as for more substantial lymph node deposits. It should be noted, however, that second-look studies after standard pathological examinations reveal up to 4–8% of false negative cases (a negative predictive value for the original examination of 90–95%).

Notwithstanding these considerations, it may be estimated that about 30% of patients with T1 tumours without clinical evidence of axillary disease have pathological axillary lymph node involvement. The converse argument is that in 70% of these patients, axillary dissection serves no purpose. Minimally invasive sentinel node biopsy makes it possible to identify these cases, so that axillary dissection may be avoided. As noted above, some authors initially considered that only the node taking up the greatest quantity of tracer was the sentinel node. Subsequently, all nodes taking up tracer were recognized as potential sentinel nodes and removed in order to increase diagnostic accuracy. For this reason many surgeons in the UK consider that sentinel node biopsy is analogous to their 'axillary sampling' or 'blind biopsy'. One study has shown that four-node sampling, in which four nodes are removed at random from the first axillary level, included the sentinel node in a high proportion of cases (80%). Moreover, these blindly sampled lymph nodes were able to predict the state of the axilla with an accuracy similar to that of sentinel node biopsy.[13–15]

Although the sentinel node technique usually focuses on the axilla, past experience with extended radical mastectomy showed that about 20% of patients had involvement of the internal mammary chain and about 9% had involvement at this site only.[16] The use of a radiotracer and lymphoscintigraphy not uncommonly reveals uptake to this and other nodal areas (the subclavian region, interpectorally or within the breast itself). This has rekindled interest in alternative drainage pathways from the breast parenchyma and the possibility of obtaining prognostic information from them. According to this reasoning, sentinel nodes should be removed and examined from whichever site they are revealed.

Several, multicentre, trials have validated the sentinel node concept in women with relatively small unifocal breast cancer and a clinically uninvolved axilla, and it has rapidly become established as a standard treatment for such women. The method is also being evaluated (i) in women with more advanced tumours treated with neoadjuvant chemotherapy, who might safely forego axillary dissection if the sentinel node

Table 36.3	Negative predictive value of PET as a method of identifying involved axillary lymph nodes in relation to the size of the primary breast cancer

Tumour size	Negative predictive value (%)
T1a–b	97.3
T1c	93.5
T2	94.4

is negative, (ii) in cases of multifocal and multicentric primaries, and (iii) in local relapse after breast-conserving surgery. However, opinion is divided on the appropriateness of sentinel node biopsy in these situations.

Positron emission tomography (PET) is also being evaluated as a method of identifying lymph nodes which warrant biopsy and is complementary to established sentinel node procedures. It is also being evaluated as a method in its own right for identifying metastatic lymph nodes and hence for selecting patients who need not undergo axillary dissection. A prospective study at the National Cancer Institute, Milan assessed the use of 2-fluoro-2-deoxy-D-glucose as a selection tool. Cells with a high rate of glucose metabolism (such as cancer cells) preferentially take up this substance, and nodes containing malignant cells can be identified with good spatial resolution if PET is used in association with computed tomography (CT–PET). This method has been found to have a high negative predictive value when used to identify lymph node metastases (Table 36.3).[17] This functional imaging methodology has several advantages:

- It is non-invasive.
- It provides whole-body staging.
- Its diagnostic accuracy does not depend on the size or site of the cancer or whether it is unifocal or multifocal.
- It can be repeated.
- Results are reproducible and independent of the operator.

The aforementioned objectives of axillary surgery have not changed with current approaches to breast cancer management. What has changed, though, is the surgical treatment, and methods of selecting those patients who will benefit the most from invasive axillary procedures. Complete axillary dissection is no longer indicated or justified when the sentinel nodes, or other appropriately sampled lymph nodes, are free of tumour.

What future for axillary staging?

Many attempts have been made to reduce the extent of locoregional treatment for breast cancer in the past few years, in line with universal trends to employ less aggressive surgical treatments for all types of cancer. The most notable of the modified radical innovation in this area was the replacement of mastectomy by conservative surgery and breast radiotherapy.[18] With regard to axillary dissection, seminal trials have provided some evidence justifying omission of this procedure in selected patients.

The randomised prospective B-04 trial of the National Surgical Adjuvant Breast and Bowel Project (NSABP), first published in 1977 and more recently updated, found that survival was identical in clinically node-negative patients irrespective of whether they received prophylactic axillary dissection, axillary irradiation, or no axillary treatment (unless and until relapse occurred in which case they received axillary dissection).[19,20] The authors concluded that lymph node metastasis was an indicator but not a governor of survival.

Preliminary results of a UK multicentre randomised prospective trial conducted by the Cancer Research Campaign were also published in 1977. This trial recruited patients with both clinically positive and clinically negative axillae, and randomised patients to mastectomy alone or mastectomy plus radiotherapy to the regional lymphatic field.[21] The trial concluded that untreated axillary nodes did not appear to act as a source of tertiary spread and that delayed (therapeutic) radiotherapy can achieve the same objective as immediate radiotherapy to the axilla.

Thus, it seems that, from a strictly therapeutic point of view, axillary treatment can be safely avoided in clinically node-negative patients, particularly if staging information is considered to be of secondary importance.

Management of nodes in the internal mammary chain provides further information on the safety of leaving locoregional nodes untreated. Patients at the National Cancer Institute, Milan were randomly allocated to internal mammary chain dissection or no such treatment. Among those whose internal mammary nodes were removed, pathological involvement of nodes carried a worse prognosis than negativity, particularly when the axillary nodes were positive as well. Nevertheless, there was no difference in overall survival between these two groups, and local failure was rare among the non-treated patients.

Another aspect to be considered is local control. This was highlighted by a prospective observational study on 401 breast cancer patients with no clinical involvement of the axilla. None received axillary treatment, and unexpectedly low rates of axillary relapse were observed at 5 years follow up (2%, 1.7% and 10% for T1a, b and c respectively) in comparison to the expected percentage of nodal involvement.[22] The implication of these findings is that only a fraction of lymph node metastases will give rise to progressive disease.

Another aspect to consider is that the role of nodal involvement in determining adjuvant treatment has become much less important than formerly. In accordance with widely accepted guidelines, most node-negative patients now receive chemotherapy, hormone therapy or both, depending on age, hormone receptor status, tumour grade and other features of the primary tumour.[23,24] As a consequence, it can be argued that only a limited number of patients who receive no axillary assessment will be undertreated.[25] In addition, various biological characteristics of the primary tumour have emerged as potential prognostic factors able to identify breast cancer patients at high risk of recurrence, irrespective of whether axillary status is known. A promising study in this area came from the National Cancer Institute, Milan, which examined the use of a prognostic score, based on four established prognostic factors, to identify four subgroups with different prognoses. It was found that node-positive patients with a good prognostic score had better survival than node-negative patients, and that node-negative patients with a bad score had similar survival to node-positive patients.[26] Another study, from the Netherlands Cancer Institute, used microarray technology to evaluate a 70-gene prognostic profile in consecutive patients with primary breast cancer. The method was reported to be a more powerful predictor of outcome than established determinants, and was independent of nodal status.[27] These findings suggest that pathological axillary nodal status may soon become irrelevant as a guide to decision making in breast cancer management. They have also rendered the TNM staging system outdated, since it is based solely on clinical and anatomical considerations. A revised system incorporating not only pathological and biological criteria, but also gene profiling, is likely to emerge in the near future.

Conclusion

Outside a clinical trial setting, axillary dissection should perhaps be considered an unnecessary procedure if adjuvant systemic treatment is already indicated on the basis of other criteria. It is unclear whether such patients should receive axillary radiotherapy to forestall the risk of local axillary recurrence. Clinical trials and retrospective analyses have shown that radiation to the entire or lower part of the axilla can reduce the number of such recurrences. The alternative policy of no initial axillary treatment, with full axillary clearance (or radiotherapy) for recurrent axillary disease, has no adverse effect on outcome. Full axillary dissection may have advantages over radiotherapy in such cases, and it is more likely to be definitive.

References

1. Halsted WS. The results of operation for the cure of cancer of the breast performed at the John Hopkins Hospital from June 1889 to January 1894. Johns Hopkins Hosp Rep 1894–5; 4: 297.
2. Van Slooten EA, Hampe JF. Indicatiestelling voor de behandeling van mammacarcinoom; bepaling van de operabiliteit door proefexcisie van de subclaviculaire klieren. Jaarbeok van kankeronderzoek Kankerbestrijding 1958; 8: 64.
3. Veronesi U, Luini A, Galimberti V et al. Extent of metastatic axillary involvement in 1446 cases of breast cancer. Eur J Surg Oncol 1990; 16: 127–33.
4. Cabans RM. An approach for the treatment of penile cancer. Cancer 1997; 39: 456–66.
5. Morton DL, Wen DR, Wong JH et al. Technical details of intraoperative lymphatic mapping for early stage melanoma. Arch Surg 1992; 127: 392–9.
6. Veronesi U, Paganelli G, Viale G et al. A randomized comparison of sentinel-node biopsy with routine axillary dissection in breast cancer. N Engl J Med 2003; 349: 546–53.
7. Krag DN, Julian TB, Harlow SP et al. NSABP-32: phase III, randomized trial comparing axillary resection with sentinel lymph node dissection: a description of the trial. Ann Surg Oncol 2004; 11(3 Suppl): 208S-10S.
8. Viale G, Sonzogni A, Pruneri G et al. Histopathologic examination of axillary sentinel lymph nodes in breast carcinoma patients. J Surg Oncol 2004; 85: 123–8.
9. Ernst MF, Voogd AC, Balder W, et al. Early and late morbidity associated with axillary levels I–III dissection in breast cancer. J Surg Oncol 2002; 79: 151–5.
10. McCarter MD, Yeung H, Fey J et al. The breast cancer patient with multiple sentinel nodes: when to stop? J Am Coll Surg 2001; 192: 692–7.
11. Krag DN, Weaver DL. Pathological and molecular assessment of sentinel lymph nodes in solid tumors. Semin Oncol 2002; 29: 274–9.
12. Viale G, Maiorano E, Mazzarol G et al. Histologic detection and clinical implications of micrometastases in axillary sentinel lymph nodes for patients with breast carcinoma. Cancer 2001; 92: 1378–84.
13. Macmillan RD, Barbera D, Hadjiminas DJ et al. Sentinel

node biopsy for breast cancer may have little to offer four-node-samplers. Results of a prospective comparison study. Eur J Cancer 2001; 37: 1076–80.

14. Sato K, Tamaki K, Takeuchi H et al. Management of the axilla in breast cancer: a comparative study between sentinel lymph node biopsy and four-node sampling procedure. Jpn J Clin Oncol 2001; 31: 318–21.

15. Ahlgren J, Holmberg L, Bergh J, Liljegren G. Five-node biopsy of the axilla: an alternative to axillary dissection of levels I–II in operable breast cancer. Eur J Surg Oncol 2002; 28: 97–102.

16. Veronesi U, Cascinelli N, Greco M et al. Prognosis of breast cancer patients after mastectomy and dissection of internal mammary nodes. Ann Surg 1985; 202: 702–7.

17. Greco M, Crippa F, Agresti R et al. Axillary lymph node staging in breast cancer by 2-fluoro-2-deoxy-D-glucose-positron emission tomography: clinical evaluation and alternative management. J Natl Cancer Inst 2001; 93: 630–5.

18. Veronesi U, Cascinelli N, Mariani L et al. Twenty-year follow-up of a randomized study comparing breast-conserving surgery with radical mastectomy for early breast cancer. N Engl J Med 2002; 347: 1227–32.

19. Fisher B, Montague E, Redmond C et al. Comparison of radical mastectomy with alternative treatments for primary breast cancer. A first report of results from a prospective randomized clinical trial. Cancer 1977; 39(6 Suppl): 2827–39.

20. Fisher B, Anderson S, Bryant J et al. Twenty-year follow-up of a randomized trial comparing total mastectomy, lumpectomy, and lumpectomy plus irradiation for the treatment of invasive breast cancer. N Engl J Med 2002; 347: 1233–41.

21. Baum M, Coyle PJ. Simple mastectomy for early breast cancer and the behaviour of the untreated axillary nodes. Bull Cancer 1977; 64: 603–10.

22. Greco M, Agresti R, Cascinelli N et al. Breast cancer patients treated without axillary surgery: clinical implications and biologic analysis. Ann Surg 2000; 232: 1–7.

23. National Institutes of Health Consensus Development Panel. National Institutes of Health Consensus Development Conference Statement: Adjuvant Therapy for Breast Cancer, November 1–3, 2000. J Natl Cancer Inst 2001; 93: 979–89.

24. Goldhirsch A, Wood WC, Gelber RD, et al. Meeting highlights: Updated International Expert Consensus on the Primary Therapy of Early Breast Cancer. Seventh International Conference on Adjuvant Therapy of Primary Breast Cancer. J Clin Oncol 2003; 21: 3357–65.

25. Greco M, Gennaro M, Valagussa P et al. Impact of nodal status on indication for adjuvant treatment in clinically node negative breast cancer. Ann Oncol 2000; 11: 1137–40.

26. Menard S, Bufalino R, Rilke F et al. Prognosis based on primary breast carcinoma instead of pathological nodal status. Br J Cancer 1994; 70: 709–12.

27. Van De Vijver MJ, He YD, Van't Veer LJ et al. A gene expression signature as a predictor of survival in breast cancer. N Engl J Med 2002; 347: 1999–2009.

37 Management of the axilla II*

Guidubaldo Querci della Rovere, John R Benson

Introduction

Some form of axillary surgery is an integral component of the locoregional management of early breast cancer. Despite the widespread introduction of techniques for breast conservation over the past 30 years, the procedure of choice has been a formal axillary dissection (level II). Alternative options such as axillary sampling have been championed by a surgical minority and are the subject of continuing controversy.[1] Increasing rates of lymph node negativity have spurred the investigation of non-invasive methods for imaging the axillary nodes, but these are questionable as a staging modality due to limitations of resolution at the microscopic tumour level. The advent of sentinel node biopsy has generated much enthusiasm as a method that permits pathological evaluation of nodal tissue yet potentially avoids unnecessary surgical dissection and minimises morbidity. In some countries, sentinel node biopsy has been adopted as the standard of care in the absence of trial data evaluating not only rates of morbidity but also regional recurrence and overall survival. Techniques of sentinel node biopsy appear promising as a staging procedure, but in this era of the 'sentinel rush' it is important to ensure that this nascent method be incorporated into the surgical management of breast cancer in an appropriate manner that does not ultimately compromise patient care and outcome. A selective and flexible approach to axillary surgery is most likely to prove 'ideal'.[2] Three basic issues will be considered in this chapter:

- Is there a group of patients with such a low probability of nodal involvement that an axillary procedure can be omitted?
- Is the concept and technique of sentinel node biopsy sufficiently accurate and robust that rates of axillary recurrence and possibly long-term survival are not impaired as a consequence of either withholding systemic therapies or failing to remove non-sentinel nodes
- Are some patients better served by formal axillary dissection at the outset due to a relatively high probability of nodal metastases (based on host and primary tumour characteristics).

Indications for axillary dissection

Halsted's radical mastectomy encompassed axillary dissection as part of the 'en bloc' removal of local and regional tissue in continuity.[3] This surgical approach was underpinned by the paradigm of progressive and sequential spread of breast cancer from a single focus within the breast to axillary nodes, with subsequent haematogenous dissemination[4]. The operation was carried out with therapeutic intent and, although successful at controlling local disease, did not have any impact on long-term survival. However, this early cohort of patients presented with larger tumours and the incidence of axillary metastases was relatively high. The failure

---

*This chapter was originally published as 'The case for axillary dissection' in Advances in Breast Cancer 2004; 1(2): 3–8.

of radical surgery to improve survival led to the hypothesis that breast cancer is a systemic disease at or near inception and distant disease could exist without obligate nodal involvement. Although it was acknowledged that axillary dissection provided no survival benefit (consonant with the Fisherian paradigm), the status of the axillary nodes was and remains the single most powerful prognostic indicator, and until recently was a crucial factor in the selection of patients for chemotherapy.[5] Furthermore, removal of involved nodes provides locoregional control, with rates of axillary recurrence being sixfold higher (18% vs 3%) for untreated axillae.[6] With heightened public awareness and mammographic screening programmes, breast cancers are increasingly being diagnosed at an earlier stage. Historically, almost half of symptomatic patients (46%) had positive axillary nodes,[7] but with the introduction of screening programmes 25–30% of all patients currently have nodal involvement at presentation. Those patients with negative axillae do not benefit from surgical clearance, and this stage shift has prompted the investigation of less intrusive methods for surgical management of the axilla.

Although the majority of studies (e.g. the US National Surgical Adjuvant Breast and Bowel Project (NSABP) Protocol B-04)[6,8] have failed to demonstrate any survival advantage from axillary dissection, others have suggested that some benefit may be derived from more thorough node dissection.[9–11] A recent analysis from a study in Cardiff comparing modified radical mastectomy with simple mastectomy revealed an overall survival difference of 15% at 11 years (personal communication). Of interest, the NSABP B-04 trial was confounded by salvage dissection for regional recurrence and did not possess the power to detect a small survival difference (<7%), which may have been masked by a type II error. A meta-analysis of all data involving 3000 cases suggests a survival benefit of 5.4%.[12] Nonetheless, a problem with such meta-analyses is distinguishing between the effects of removing nodal tissue per se, and the influence of adjuvant systemic treatment on overall survival. In that study, however, adjustments were made for the benefit of adjuvant chemotherapy. Thus it is conceded that a small survival benefit may result from axillary dissection, which has an established role as a staging procedure and for achieving regional control.

Current status of axillary management

The recognition that axillary dissection was principally a staging procedure with concomitant morbid-ity led to the investigation of alternative methods for staging the axilla. These included axillary sampling and more recently sentinel lymph node biopsy. The former consists of the removal of a minimum of four nodes at level I, which are assessed histologically with routine paraffin sections. If one or more nodes contain metastatic tumour then either a delayed axillary dissection is undertaken or the axilla is irradiated. This has been validated as a staging procedure[13] but is still associated with significant morbidity and rates of local recurrence of up to 10%. The principle of the sentinel node hypothesis was first proposed by Cabanas[14] in 1977 in the context of inguinal lymphatic drainage from penile cancer. The concept was applied to melanoma by Morton et al[15] at the beginning of the 1990s and subsequently pioneered in breast cancer patients by Guiliano et al.[16] The technique is a diagnostic test for assessing the histological status of nodes in the axillary basin. According to the sentinel node hypothesis, there is a single node that first receives drainage of lymph from the primary breast tumour and acts as the 'first port of call'. The concept is Halstedian and presupposes a sequential and orderly spread of cancer cells to the sentinel node, from whence passage to higher-echelon nodes occurs. If the sentinel node does not contain metastasis then the remaining non-sentinel nodes are likewise presumed to be tumour-free. Conversely, if tumour deposits are found in the sentinel node then it is implicit that there is non-sentinel node involvement and completion axillary dissection is undertaken. With increasing experience with the technique, the concept has turned out to be slightly imperfect. Usually, more than a single node is identified as being 'sentinel' or the true sentinel node is inapparent, leading to the removal of several nodes – which in effect constitutes a targeted sampling. Nevertheless, the incidence of skip metastases is low (2%)[17] and the negative predictive value of the technique high (97%).[18] A crucial parameter is the false-negative rate, which is the proportion of patients incorrectly diagnosed as node-negative. False-negative rates are usually quoted as approximately 5%, which is only slightly higher than those for conventional axillary dissection and is considered acceptable. However, in the conventional dissection, nodal tissue is excised and the consequences of false negativity and potential under staging are less consequential. By contrast, with sentinel node biopsy, inappropriate management decisions may ensue and undetected tumour deposits in non-sentinel nodes may become a source of distant metastases, with impairment of both locoregional control and overall survival. Many studies quote false-negative rates above 5%, and rates as high as 17% have been cited. Calculation of the rate may yield a misleadingly low figure in some papers (the denominator should be the number of patients with positive nodes and not the total number of patients).[19,20]

Problems and limitations of axillary sampling and sentinel node biopsy

Axillary sampling

A frequent predicament when undertaking axillary sampling is lack of certainty that four nodes have been retrieved. It is often difficult to confidently identify nodes among the fibrofatty tissue of the axilla. To overcome this problem, some surgeons have evolved the technique by preoperative injection of blue dye, which permits a guided sampling. As discussed above, in the event of nodal metastases, further axillary treatment is required.

Sentinel node biopsy

Technique

The technique of sentinel node biopsy was initially assessed in peer-reviewed pilot studies using blue dye only (patent blue-V, isosulfan blue and methylene blue). These identified the sentinel node in only 65.5% of cases, and a learning curve for the technique was evident as further experience was accrued. Krag et al[21] introduced radioactive tracers (technetium-99m (^{99m}Tc) colloid) as an alternative method for identification of the sentinel node, while other groups have used a dual localisation method with detection of 'blue' and 'hot' nodes. This combined approach allows the successful identification of the sentinel node in more than 95% of cases and is associated with the shortest learning curve.[22–24] Morrow et al[25] randomised patients to identification of the sentinel node using either dye or isotope alone and showed these to be of comparable efficacy. There is an international consensus that a combination of dye and isotope is optimal, but other aspects of methodology, such as site of injection and lymphoscintigraphy, remain contentious. The dye/isotope can be introduced by intratumoral, peritumoral, subcutaneous, intradermal or subareolar injection. There has been a trend recently toward subareolar injection, which is associated with less 'shine through', although it may give poorer visualisation of the internal mammary chain.[26] Interestingly, a subareolar site may require a greater massage effect which could encourage the migration of tumour cells to the sentinel node and these could be a potential source of micrometastases (particularly those detected only on immunohistochemistry). These have been termed 'traumatic metastases' or 'traumets'.[27]

Definition

The original definition of the sentinel node was strict – the first node draining the tumour. Not only is there usually more than one sentinel node in the axillary basin, but lymphoscintigraphy may reveal nodes in the internal mammary chain or supraclavicular zones. The existence of multiple candidate sentinel nodes is a potential flaw in the pathophysiology of the sentinel node hypothesis; the number of nodes detected is to some extent a time-dependent phenomenon. Dye or isotope will be retained for an indeterminate period of time in the 'sentinel' node(s) before proceeding to higher-echelon nodes. Methodological issues such as the time interval between injection and node harvesting, together with colloid particle size, are critical determinants of sensitivity and specificity. If hypothetically there were a range of different coloured dyes (blue, yellow, green, etc.), would there be a cognate sentinel node for each colour? On average, there are two or three axillary sentinel nodes; and McCarter et al[28] reported that three nodes were required to identify 99% of positive patients and more than four sentinel nodes were found in 15% of patients. Removal of three or four sentinel nodes from the axilla really represents a sophisticated form of axillary sampling. Nodes that are judged palpable at operation (clinically node-negative) are always removed, irrespective of whether they are blue or hot. Where several nodes are blue, the presence of a blue afferent lymphatic does not necessarily indicate sentinel status. Some surgeons now choose to remove all blue-stained nodes and sometimes adjacent nodal tissue as a 'limited orientated axillary dissection' in an effort to avoid delayed axillary surgery.[29] It is not understood why some blue nodes are 'cold' and some hot nodes are not blue (approximately 10%). Clearly, there is a risk of a false-negative result if an insufficient number of sentinel nodes are removed, yet there is pressure not to resect non-sentinel nodes, in order to minimise morbidity and validate the procedure.

Location of the sentinel node

The sentinel node is usually found in the lower part of the axilla among level I nodes. Identification and removal is relatively straightforward and morbidity low. Occasionally, the sentinel node is located at level II[30] and rarely at level III, when removal can incur significant surgical insult. A delayed axillary dissection is technically challenging, and it might be argued that when the sentinel node is encountered at higher levels, a formal dissection should be undertaken at the time. Extra-axillary sites may harbour the sentinel node when radioactive tracers are employed. Significant surgical morbidity can result from removal of internal mammary nodes, and no survival benefit has been demonstrated from these more aggressive surgical procedures.[31] Moreover, it is uncommon for the internal mammary nodes to be involved in the absence of metastases in the axillary nodes (9%), which undermines its value as additional staging information.

Pathological assessment

The sentinel node has been subjected to much more intensive pathological scrutiny than nodal tissue from a conventional axillary dissection, where nodes are usually bisected only. The sentinel node undergoes multiple step sections, which greatly increases the chance of finding tumour cells (diameter 15 μm).[32] In order to validate the hypothesis, it has been essential to exhaustively examine the sentinel node to confidently declare it free of tumour. Less intensive protocols would increase false-negative rates and undermine the premise upon which the sentinel node biopsy technique is based. Using both H & E and immunohistochemical methods, the probability of non-sentinel lymph node involvement when the sentinel node is free of tumour has been estimated at less than 0.1%.[33] The absolute incidence of node positivity is higher when the sentinel node biopsy technique is used. Much of this upstaging is attributable to the detection of micrometastases (often by immunohistochemical methods only), and the clinical significance of these and isolated clusters of tumour cells (submicroscopic deposits) remains controversial.[34,35] Circulating tumour cells must undergo both arrest and proliferation to form viable metastatic foci.[36] Furthermore, the phenomenon of isolated sentinel node positivity (approximately 50% of node-positive cases) has led some authors to suggest that completion axillary dissection could be omitted in some patients with micrometastases in the sentinel node detected only with immunohistochemistry. Others maintain that at present the prediction of non-sentinel node involvement is not sufficiently accurate to avoid completion axillary dissection in selected cases of sentinel node positivity. In particular, tumour grade does not appear to predict for non-sentinel node metastases. Interestingly, most validation studies have not examined non-sentinel nodes as intensively as the sentinel node. Conceivably, some of these nodes may have contained tumour cells, implying that some false-negative rates are deceptive.[35]

Complications

Although there are reports of reduced morbidity of sentinel node biopsy compared with axillary dissection,[37] the only randomised trial assessing short-term treatment-related morbidity concluded there was no significant difference between the two techniques.[38] It is imperative to await data on longer-term morbidity, together with rates of local recurrence and overall survival. Unfortunately, many cases of sentinel node biopsy are now undertaken outside a trial setting, and therefore much potentially valuable follow-up information is likely to be unavailable for future analysis. Similarly, will sentinel node biopsy cases be an exception to the UK National Institute for Clinical Excellence (NICE) recommendation that routine follow-up of breast cancer patients be limited to 3 years?

Training

There is a learning curve associated with the sentinel node biopsy technique and surgeons must be appropriately trained and validation undertaken with approximately 30–40 consecutive cases (20 cases in the USA).[39] A high rate of successful identification of the sentinel node and a correspondingly low false-negative rate (5–10%) must be confirmed before an individual surgeon or institution can employ this method for staging the axilla in routine practice. However, higher false-negative rates do not necessarily imply that the technique is being improperly conducted. Blue/hot nodes may be successfully identified and removed, but subsequent correlation pathologically with non-sentinel nodes is partially dependent on the nuances of histological assessment.

There will be a continued stream of new trainees for instruction in the technique; validation will have to be carried out on selected patients who will undergo mandatory completion axillary dissection. This raises ethical issues and such a discriminatory demand may invoke problems with patient consent and even medicolegal action.

The need for and the benefit of axillary surgery

If it is acknowledged that axillary dissection does not confer any survival gain then its benefits must be assessed indirectly on the basis of improved survival from adjuvant systemic therapies administered according to nodal status. The most recent overview by the Early Breast Cancer Trialists' Collaborative Group (EBCTCG) concludes that axillary nodal status remains the strongest prognostic factor on multivariate analysis but that the proportional benefits of chemotherapy are similar in node-negative and node-positive patients.[40] Moreover, the absolute benefits in postmenopausal women are similar for the two nodal groups. Thus axillary staging is now less important in the selection of patients for adjuvant chemotherapy, while is based on size and other characteristics of the primary tumour. For smaller tumours (<2 cm), axillary dissection is a dominant selection criterion for chemotherapy. However, the absolute benefits of chemotherapy for node-positive patients with small tumours is of the order of 1–2%.

In a review of 355 cases of breast cancers up to 20 mm in diameter from the Royal Marsden Hospital, the incidence of nodal metastases in women above age 55, with oestrogen receptor-positive tumours up to 10 mm without lymphovascular invasion, was 2.7% for grade 1 and 11% for grade 2 tumours. In over 90% of node-positive cases, only one node is positive. With an incidence of nodal metastases of between 2% and 11%, 5000 to 500 patients will need to receive axillary surgery and 98 to 89 patients adjuvant chemotherapy in order for just 1 or 2 patients to have a benefit. The average cost of an axillary staging procedure is approximately £3000.[41] The cost of these 1–2 patients benefitting from chemotherapy is therefore estimated between £1.5 and £15 million. It is likely that for older women (aged over 55) with smaller tumours, the risk to benefit ratio of finding the small number of node-positive cases and the modest gains from chemotherapy do not justify any form of axillary surgery – staging (sentinel node biopsy) or therapeutic (axillary lymph node dissection) – at the primary operation. An acceptable option in women aged over 55 with small tumours is to advocate a two-stage procedure: excision of the primary tumour, with a deferred decision on the need for axillary surgery (staging or therapeutic).

Analyses of axillary nodal metastases in smaller tumours have yielded variable results. When tumour type in addition to size is taken into account, a subgroup emerges with a probability of nodal involvement of less than 5%. In a review of almost 13 000 patients, Maibenco et al[42] found a frequency of nodal metastases of only 3.9% in T1a tumours of favourable histological types (tubular, mucinous and papillary). They concluded that axillary lymph node dissection could be reasonably avoided in T1a (grade 1, papillary, mucinous, tubular) and T1b (mucinous and tubular) tumours, and others have suggested this this may apply to all patients aged over 40 with grade 1 tumours and no adverse prognosticators.[43] With the advent of sentinel node biopsy, many have advocated its use in these smaller tumours with a low probability of nodal involvement (including ductal carcinoma in situ (DCIS) with micro-invasion[44]). Nonetheless, we believe that there remains a strong argument for omission of any axillary surgery in these prognostically favourable groups and possibly certain older patients for whom the cost-to-benefit ratio justifies the avoidance of axillary surgery (typically fewer than 5 patients per 100 would have their management altered on the basis of information derived from nodal pathology).

There may, however, be a subgroup of patients with a small survival advantage from axillary dissection. This is likely to include younger women, for whom gains in survival may not be apparent for many years. Improved longer-term outcome following postmastectomy radiotherapy is evident after more prolonged follow-up (the prevention of four isolated local recurrences at 10 years prevents one breast cancer death at 20 years).[45] Younger women also represent a group among whom there is a higher probability of lymph node involvement and for whom axillary lymph node dissection at the outset may be more appropriate than sentinel node biopsy. For example, women aged under 40 with grade 3 tumours exceeding 2 cm in size have a 40% chance of positive axillary nodes. Is this figure too high to justify sentinel node biopsy, which may necessitate further axillary surgery and delays in chemotherapy?

Alternatives to axillary node dissection

It is our view that axillary dissection (level II) should remain the standard of care for management of the axilla in early breast cancer patients until longer-term results of randomised controlled trials comparing this with sentinel node biopsy are available. Axillary sampling and sentinel node biopsy are acceptable methods for staging the axilla.

A promising technique for the detection of metastatic lymph nodes is positron emission tomography (PET) scanning.[46] This technique does not detect the 'first' draining node but 'metastatic' nodes, and could potentially render redundant any surgical diagnostic procedure. It has relatively good sensitivity and specificity but remains inferior to histopathological assessment for the detection of micrometastases.

Conclusions

The question of a possible survival benefit remains a critical issue in assessing the role of axillary dissection in the management of breast cancer. If a survival benefit is confirmed then axillary lymph node dissection should be the standard of care. In the absence of any survival benefit, axillary sampling and sentinel node biopsy are acceptable alternatives to axillary dissection, but the results of longer-term evaluation and follow-up are essential.

Sampling may be more biologically appropriate, and the cost-to-benefit ratio may favour sampling over sentinel node biopsy when resources are limited.

As increasing numbers of breast cancer patients are presenting with earlier-stage disease where the probability of lymph node involvement is low, it is reasonable to consider a two-stage surgical procedure, with any final decision on axillary surgery being made after complete histopathological assessment of the primary tumour. This may permit avoidance of axillary surgery altogether in some patients. However, we would support the recommendation that routine axillary dissection be undertaken in all patients with tumours larger than 2 cm with or without lymphovascular invasion and in all patients with sentinel node positivity.[20] The frequency of multiple sentinel nodes is higher in this group, although the chance of nodal involvement may be modest and axillary sampling could be an appropriate alternative (dye-guided).[47]

As any survival advantage from axillary lymph node dissection may only emerge with longer follow-up, this procedure should be discussed with younger women, who have a proportionately greater life-expectancy.

References

1. MacMillan RD, Rampaul RS, Blamey RW. Sentinel node biopsy in breast cancer. Lancet 2001; 358: 1815.

2. Gemignani ML, Borgen PI. Is there a role for selective axillary dissection in breast cancer? World J Surg 2001; 25: 809–818.

3. Halsted WS. The results of operation for the cure of cancer of the breast performed at the John Hopkins Hospital from June 1889 to January 1894. Johns Hopkins Hosp Rep 1894–5; 4: 297.

4. Benson JR, Baum M. Changing philosophical perspectives in breasts cancer. In: Tobias J, Henderson C, Houghton J, eds. Breast Cancer – New Horizons in Research and Treatment. London: Arnold, 2001: 12–29.

5. Fisher B, Bauer M, Wickerham DL et al. Relation of number of positive nodes to the prognosis of patients with primary breast cancer: an NSABP update. Cancer 1983; 52: 1551.

6. Fisher B, Montague E, Redmond C et al. Ten-years results of a randomised clinical trial comparing radical mastectomy and total mastectomy with or without irradiation. N Engl J Med 1985; 312: 674.

7. Carter CL, Allen C, Henderson DE. Relation of tumour size, lymph node status and survival in 24,740 breast cancer cases. Cancer 1989; 73: 505–8.

8. Fisher B, Montague E, Redmond C et al. Comparison of radical mastectomy with alternative treatments for primary breast cancer. Cancer 1977; 39: 2827.

9. Harris JR, Osteen RT. Patients with early breast cancer benefit from effective axillary treatment. Breast Cancer Res Treat 1985; 5: 17–21.

10. Gardner B, Feldman J. Are positive axillary nodes in breast cancer markers for incurable disease? Ann Surg 1993; 218: 270–8.

11. Moffat FL, Sewofsky GM, Davis K et al. Axillary node dissection for early breast cancer: some is good but all is better. J Surg Oncol 1992; 51: 8.

12. Orr RK. The impact of prophylactic axillary node dissection on breast cancer survival – a Bayesian meta-analysis. Ann Surg Oncol 1999; 6: 109–16.

13. Steel RJ, Forrest APM, Chetty U. The efficacy of axillary sampling in obtaining lymph node status in breast cancer. Br J Surg 1985; 72: 368–9.

14. Cabanas RM. An approach for the treatment of penile carcinoma. Cancer 1997; 39: 456–66.

15. Morton DL, Wen DR, Wong JH et al. Technical details of intra-operative lymphatic mapping for early stage melanoma. Arch Sur 1992; 127: 392–9.

16. Guiliano AE, Kirgan DM, Guenther JM, Morton DL. Lymphatic mapping and sentinel lymphadenectomy for breast cancer. Ann Surg 1994; 220: 391–401.

17. Veronesi U, Luini A, Galimberti V, Marchini S et al. Extent of metastatic involvement in 1446 cases of breast cancer. Eur J Surg Oncol 1990; 16: 127–33.

18. Veronesi U, Paganelli G, Galimberti et al. Sentinel node biopsy to avoid axillary dissection in breast cancer with clinically negative lymph nodes. Lancet 1997; 349: 1864–7.

19. McMasters KM, Giuliano AE, Ross MI et al. Sentinel lymph node biopsy for breast cancer – not yet standard of care. N Engl J Med 1998; 339: 990–5.

20. Sachdev U, Murphy K, Derzie A et al. Predictions of non-sentinel lymph node metastasis in breast cancer patients. Am J Surg 2002; 183: 213–17.

21. Krag D, Weaver D, Ashikaga T et al. The sentinel node in breast cancer. A multicentre validation study. N Engl J Med 1998; 339: 941–6.

22. Albertini JJ, Lyman GH, Cox C et al. Lymphatic mapping and sentinel node biopsy in the patient with breast cancer. JAMA 1996; 276: 1818.

23. Cody HS. Management of the axilla in early stage breast cancer: will sentinel node biopsy end the debate? J Surg Oncol 1999; 71: 137–9.

24. Veronesi U, Paganelli G, Galimberti V et al. Sentinel node biopsy to avoid axillary dissection in breast cancer with clinically negative lymph nodes. Lancet 1997; 349: 1864.

25. Morrow M, Rademaker AW, Bethke KP et al. Learning sentinel node biopsy: results of a prospective randomised trial of two techniques. Surgery 1999; 126: 714–20.

26. Smith LF, Cross MJ, Klimberg VS. Sub-areolar injection is a better technique for sentinel lymph node biopsy. Am J Surg 2000; 180: 434–7.

27. Rosser RJ. Safety of sentinel lymph node dissection and significance of cytokeratin micromatastases. J Clin Oncol 2001; 19: 1882.

28. McCarter MD, Yeung H, Fey J et al. The breast cancer patients with multiple sentinel nodes: when to stop? J Am Coll Surg 2001; 192: 692–7.

29. Salmon RJ, Marcolet A, Vieira M, Languille O. Sentinel node biopsy or limited orientated axillary dissection (L.O.A.D.) in early breast cancer. Eur J Surg Oncol (in press).

30. Roumen RMH, Valkenburg JGM, Geuskens LM. Lymphoscintigraphy and feasibility of sentinel node biopsy in 83 patients with primary breast cancer. Eur J Surg Oncol 1997; 23: 495–502.

31. Veronesi U, Cascinelli N, Greco M et al. Prognosis of breast cancer patients after mastectomy and dissection of internal mammary nodes. Ann Surg 1985; 202: 702.

32. Viale G, Bosari S, Mazzarol G et al. Intra-operative examination of axillary sentinel lymph nodes in breast carcinoma patients. Cancer 1999; 85: 2433–9.

33. Turner RR, Ollila DW, Krasne DL. Histopathological validation of the sentinel lymph node hypothesis for breast carcinoma. Ann Surg 1997; 226: 271.

34. International (Ludwig) Breast Cancer Study Group. Prognostic importance of occult axillary lymph node micrometastases from breast cancers. Lancet 1990; 335: 1565–8.

35. Millis RR, Springall R, Lee AH et al. Occult axillary lymph node metastases are of no prognostic significance in breast cancer. Cancer 2002; 86: 396–401.

36. den Bakker MA, Van Weeszenberg A, de Kanter AY et al. Non-sentinel lymph node involvement in patients with breast cancer and sentinel node micrometastasis; too early to abandon axillary clearance. J Clin Pathol 2002; 55: 932–5.

37. Schrenk P, Rieger P, Shamiyeh A, Wayand W. Morbidity following sentinel node biopsy versus axillary lymph node dissection for patients with breast carcinoma. Cancer 2000; 88: 608–14.

38. Rietman JS, Dijkastra PU, Geertzen JH et al. Short-term morbidity of the upper limb after sentinel lymph node biopsy or axillary lymph node dissection for stage 1 or 2 breast carcinoma. Cancer 2003; 98: 690–6.

39. Schwartz GF, Giuliano AE, Veronesi U. Proceedings of the Consensus Conference on the Role of Sentinel Lymph Node Biopsy in Carcinoma of the Breast, April 19–22, 2001, Philadelphia, Pennsylvania. Cancer 2002; 94: 2542–53.

40. Early Breast Cancer Trialists' Collaborative Group. Polychemotherapy for early breast cancer: an overview of the randomised trials. Lancet 1998; 352: 930–42.

41. Ronka R, Smitten KV, Sintonen H et al. The impact of sentinel node biopsy and axillary staging strategy on hospital costs. Ann Oncol 2004; 15: 88–94.

42. Maibenco DC, Weiss LK, Pawlish KS et al. Axillary lymph node metastases associated with small invasive breast carcinomas. Cancer 1999; 85: 1530.

43. Mustafa IA, Bland KI. Indications for axillary dissection in T1 breast cancer. Ann Surg Oncol 1998; 5: 4–8.

44. Keshgar MRS, Ell PJ. Clinical role of sentinel lymph node biopsy in breast cancer. Lancet Oncol 2002; 3: 105–10.

45. Early Breast Cancer Trialists' Collaborative Group. Favourable and unfavourable effects on long term survival of radiotherapy for early breast cancer: an overview of randomised trials. Lancet 2000; 355: 1757–70.

46. Greco M, Crippa F, Agresti R et al. Axillary lymph node staging in breast cancer by 2-fluoro-2-deoxy-D-glucose-positron emission tomography: clinical evaluation and alternative management. J Natl Cancer Inst 2001; 93: 630–5.

47. Benson JR, Querci della Rovere G. Sentinel node biopsy in breast cancer. Lancet 2001; 358: 1815.

38 The role of intraoperative radiotherapy (IORT) in the conservative management of early-stage breast cancer

Roberto Orecchia, Alberto Luini, Giovanna Gatti, Mattia Intra, Mario Ciocca, Umberto Veronesi

Introduction

Intraoperative radiotherapy (IORT) is a technique that permits the administration of a high dose of radiation as a single fraction at the time of surgery. It can be employed either alone or in combination with conventional external-beam therapy as an irradiation boost. The technique allows precise application of radiation dosage to the target area with minimal exposure of surrounding tissues, which are retracted and shielded during delivery of the radiation. IORT facilitates an integrated approach to the multidisciplinary treatment of cancer[1] and emphasises the interaction between surgery and radiotherapy in three principal aspects:

- It reduces the chance of residual disease at the site of surgery by eliminating microscopic tumour foci.
- It maximises the radiobiological effect of a single high dose of irradiation, with attainment of total dosage levels locally within the breast that exceed those of external-beam therapy.
- It optimises combined surgical and radiotherapy treatment with early irradiation, reducing the risk of tumour recurrence secondary to growth of residual disease at the site of surgery.

IORT therefore potentially intensifies the tumour-kill effect of surgery and radiotherapy and minimises the chance of local failure. For patients with disease confined to locoregional tissues, this may increase the chance of definitive cure. Its use does not preclude the administration of chemotherapy or other systemic adjuvant therapies.

Initial experience with IORT dates back to the 1920s, but poor technical facilities restricted its use to the palliative treatment of locally unresectable tumours. With the development of orthovoltage equipment in the 1940s, the potential role of IORT in conjunction with external-beam radiation became better defined. During the 1960s, generation of electron beams from linear accelerators replaced low-energy radiation,[2] with the advantages of more homogeneous dose distribution, sparing of underlying tissue due to lower exit dose, and reduction in total duration of treatment. When applied with external electron beams, IORT involves transferring the patient from the operating theatre (with an open surgical wound) to the treatment room where the linear accelerator is located. Following administration of radiotherapy, the patient must be returned to the operating theatre for completion of the surgical procedure. This constitutes a major limitation of the technique and precludes its widespread application due to logistical problems of patient transfer and significant lengthening of anaesthesia time.

Over the past 25 years, the indications for high-dose-rate intraoperative brachytherapy (HDR-IORT) have been increasing.[3] Although brachytherapy yields a less homogeneous dose distribution than electron beams, different applications can adapt to the irregular configurations of the surgical bed, which is impractical for electron collimators. Moreover, HDR-IORT is amenable to dose fractionation, with further treatment sessions being carried out using catheters positioned during surgery and remaining in situ for a few days (perioperative treatment). This permits a higher total dosage to be delivered than with a single fraction.

An important advance for IORT occurred in the mid-1990s with the development of miniaturised mobile linear accelerator prototypes.[4] These devices can be readily positioned in proximity to the operating table and possess an arm that can be manipulated into the required position for irradiation. These accelerators have a variable spectrum of electron energy and have the particular advantage of being accommodated in any operating theatre without major structural modifications. Mobile shields can be positioned appropriately in relation to the operating field to provide maximum radioprotection. This avoids any transfer of the patient, and surgical time is prolonged by approximately 20 minutes only. Other devices that are sources of low energy X-rays (approximately 50 kV) have been developed for intraoperative irradiation (and can similarly be placed in any operating room).[5] They can be secured to a stereotactic support for precise placement within any body cavity.

During the past two decades, several IORT applications have been evaluated,[6] with improvements in local control for intermediate or locally advanced cancers, including rectal, gastric and gynaecological malignancies in addition to bone and soft tissue sarcomas.[7–10] Local control rates of over 90% have been recorded for many primary tumours, with lower rates of between 40% and 80% for malignant gliomas, stage III lung cancer and inoperable pancreatic carcinomas. More recently, IORT has been employed as sole treatment for some tumours, including breast cancer, with promising results.[11–13]

Different IORT system configurations

For most institutions using IORT, patients must be transported to the radiotherapy department and back to the operating theatre while still under general anaesthesia. This presents logistical problems and hampers the development of an integrated approach to IORT. An alternative arrangement is the use of a satellite operating room within the radiotherapy department that is adjacent to the linear accelerator or brachytherapy suite. This reduces the hazards associated with transfer of an anaesthetised patient between departments. Further developments that aim to integrate IORT into the operative schedule and minimise the risk of infection and disruption of other schedules include the following.

Dedicated IORT suite

A dedicated IORT facility involves multidisciplinary input to construct a specialised electron accelerator for exclusive use within the operating theatre. Although this represents the ideal set-up, it is expensive and the dual-function (surgery and radiotherapy) suite must be located close to surgical services, pathology, radiology and other facilities.[4] An important aspect of the IORT suite is a modified operating table that has the versatility of movement to permit accurate geometric alignment of the electron beam. A popular method of achieving this docking exercise is the 'hard-dock system' whereby the applicator is directly connected to the linear accelerator and alignment is dependent upon movements of the operating table. By contrast with a 'soft-dock system', the applicator is fixed in relation to the patient, with no physical connection between linear accelerator and applicator. A laser system ensures that correct geometric alignment is achieved by the combined movements of the operating table and the linear accelerator gantry.

Mobile accelerator with electrons at a maximum energy of 9–12 MeV

This is a limited-energy device that permits use of an accelerating 'in-axis' structure directly inserted into the warhead. It characteristically emits low levels of environmental irradiation over a wide dosage range,[14] although some stray radiation comes from both patient and bed-generated 'bremsstrahlung'. These stray rays, which constitute no more than 0.5% of the total electron dose, are absorbed by additional lead barriers placed around the operating table and a lead shield (15 cm thick) beneath the surgical bed corresponding to the axis of the electron field (a beam-stopper). A principal feature of this apparatus is the high dose per impulse, with values of 2.5–12 cGy per impulse (compared with 0.06 cGy per impulse for traditional accelerators). Ionisation cameras for low-dose dosimetry cannot therefore be used and chemical dosimeters containing an iron sulfate solution (Fricke's method) are preferred. Radiochromic film can also be used to calibrate monitor cameras. Electron-beam collimation is achieved through lightweight cylindrical applicators with a diameter varying between 4 cm and 12 cm and terminal angles of between 0° and 45°. The diameter of the applicator determines its length, since uniformity of distribution in the treatment field is due to scattering from the applicator walls (no scatter filters). This scattering effect also impacts upon dose rate: smaller applicator diameters are associated with higher dose output because more electrons are scattered from the walls to reach the beam field. Dosimetric procedures must be performed in a water puppet at maximal dose depth for flat applicators and a depth corresponding to the beam axis for angular applicators.

Low-energy X-ray (<50 keV) stereotactic system

This is a miniaturised source composed of a probe approximately 10 cm long and 1 mm thick.[5] The source is connected to a structure that can be positioned according to stereotactic coordinates and a predetermined point. This distribution around the source is approximately spheroidal, thus ensuring that the dose distribution is isotropic when the source is placed at the centre of a spheroidal applicator. There is a very steep dose gradient, with rapid attenuation of dose with increasing distance from the source (15–20%/mm) and the dose rate is 2 Gy/min for a spheroidal applicator 2 cm in diameter. The principal disadvantages of this system (in common with other orthovoltage devices) are limited penetration at depth (20 Gy at 0.2 cm and 5 Gy at 1 cm), a relatively long period for delivery of a therapeutic dose (20–30 min) and a greater volume of irradiated normal tissue. Moreover, in the case of breast irradiation, the spherical dose distribution does not allow sparing of skin overlying the tumour bed. Solid spherical applicators of various diameters are available to provide peritumoral irradiation following lumpectomy. An ionisation camera with flat parallel electrodes used in a water puppet allows evaluation of basal and applicator-specific dosimetry. These measurements can be integrated with data from radiochromic films analysed through a microdensitometer.

HDR brachytherapy source projectors

A source projector is a device that can transfer a small sealed radioactive source from a shielded container to the particular anatomical zone to be treated.[3] Besides the container, the equipment consists of a system for source transfer, a guidance tube, catheters, applicators, and a control board and alarm devices. The whole device is operated through a computerised control system and compatible systems are used to calculate dose distribution and treatment planning. Each punctiform radioactive source is characterised by high activity (approximately 10 Ci) that can yield a dose rate in excess of 2 Gy/min. The radioactive element (iridium-192, ^{192}Ir) is contained in a cylinder just over 1 mm in diameter, and the source position can be programmed for each of the 18–20 catheters available, with stationing time varying from 0 to 1000 s per position/impulse. Computerisation allows the source to move in a series of positions within the catheters at preset space and time intervals, yielding a series of impulses that allow the administration of a therapeutic radiation dose over a short time interval. The most important performance parameters for this equipment include linearity, accuracy, reproducibility of the timing system, and validation of source activity through an ionisation camera and specific electrometer. Where a dedicated HDR-IORT suite is not available, the HDR-brachytherapy afterloader can be easily transferred from the radiotherapy department to a modified operating room containing a shielding system. A range of surface and interstitial applicators ensure optimum treatment of different target positions and size.[15] Moreover, there is a specific device designed for intracavity breast irradiation (an intralumpectomy cavity), which is an inflatable spheroidal balloon catheter with a central lumen that can be used in conjunction with an HDR source. Following treatment, the balloon is deflated with recovery of approximately 2 ml of saline introduced at the time of catheter insertion.[16]

Irrespective of the location and systems used to deliver IORT treatment, the technique demands a high level of multidisciplinary collaboration to optimise procedures and guarantee adherence to quality assurance protocols.[17] The following aspects require specific attention:

- equipment
- procedures
- personnel
- clinical images and evaluation of outcome

Rationale for the use of IORT in breast conservation treatment

Standard conservation treatment for early-stage breast cancer consists of excision of the primary tumour with histologically clear resection margins, axillary surgery (level II dissection or sentinel node biopsy) and radiotherapy to the remaining breast.[18,19] External-beam radiotherapy is conventionally delivered with tangential fields in 25–30 daily fractions over a 5- to 6-week period. The total dosage to the breast is usually 40–50 Gy, with an optional booster dose to the tumour bed of 10–15 Gy (for positive resection margins).[20,21] When applying an external boost, the field is usually enlarged so as to encompass an adequate volume of breast tissue in order to avoid geographical error. This enlarged field can lead to a higher rate of late complications such as fibrosis and telangiectasia.[22] The boost can be delivered either with an electron field or with attenuated tangential photon fields. Alternatively, ^{192}Ir implants can be used with a brachytherapy technique. IORT has recently been investigated as a means for booster delivery followed 2–3 weeks later by conventional external-beam irradiation.[23–25] There is some controversy over the impact of ipsilateral breast tumour recurrence on overall survival when the risk of local recurrence is relatively high. All trials of breast conservation treatment have confirmed benefits of radiotherapy in terms of local control; rates of local recurrence at 5 years varied from 2% to 20% and from 27% or 42% with and without radiotherapy respectively.[26] The improvement in rates of local control ranged from 10% to 36% with the application of radiotherapy. Although studies have identified subgroups of women at lower risk of recurrence (e.g. the older age group), a uniform and reliable risk factor profile has not yet been defined.[27,28] Furthermore, controversy persists over the minimum radiation treatment required for adequate local control without compromise of therapeutic effect.[29] Appropriate clinical endpoints are avoidance of troublesome side-effects and shortening of treatment duration, which can indirectly improve quality of life (QoL). A patient's fear of local recurrence may adversely affect QoL even when she is cognisant that overall survival outcome is unaffected by ipsilateral breast tumour recurrence and subsequent salvage mastectomy. Hayman et al[30] described a 'trade-off' between fear and consequence of local recurrence on the one hand and toxicity and inconvenience of radiotherapy on the other.

Researchers at the Christie Hospital and Holt Radium Institute in Manchester, UK have investigated the use of more restricted forms of external breast irradiation; in a randomised study involving more than 700 patients, electron-beam radiotherapy of the tumour-bearing quadrant alone has been compared with whole-breast irradiation following lumpectomy. All patients had tumours measuring less than 4 cm and were node-negative.[31] At a median follow-up of 8 years, the crude rate of ipsilateral breast tumour recurrence was 19.5% in the limited-field irradiation group and 10% in those receiving whole-breast irradiation. This trial employed a rather unusual radiation schedule and no patients were offered adjuvant systemic chemotherapy. There was also a higher prevalence of lobular carcinoma and a higher risk of local failure in the localised-field arm of the trial.[32]

Brachytherapy has been routinely employed in some centres for provision of a boost at the surgical site. More recently, this technique has been investigated as sole radiation treatment for a selected group of patients. Fentiman et al[33] treated patients undergoing breast conservation treatment with ^{192}Ir implants alone to the primary tumour bed. Using an after-loading technique, 55 Gy were delivered on a continuous basis for 5 days. After a median follow-up of 6 years, tumour recurrence occurred in 37% of patients. The observed rate of in-breast recurrence was significantly higher than rates of local recurrence in patients receiving both external radiation (50 Gy) and a boost to the tumour bed with ^{192}Ir implants (25 Gy). Dale et al[34] have pointed out that

the biologically effective dose (BED) in patients treated with ^{192}Ir implants alone was around 15–20% lower than in patients treated with the combined modality. This was considered to account almost completely for the difference in local recurrence rate.[34] By contrast, in a series of 50 consecutive patients with infiltrating ductal carcinoma (≤30 mm maximum diameter with no extensive intraductal component (EIC)) and excised with clear margins, treatment with brachytherapy of the tumour bed only was associated with no cases of locoregional or distant failures at a median follow-up of 47 months. Moreover, good or excellent results have been achieved in almost all (98%) patients.[35] Evidence is emerging from other studies to suggest that, in appropriately selected patients, brachytherapy alone with accelerated treatment schedules may be a safe treatment option with no increase in distant metastases or impairment of overall survival compared with combined radiation schedules.[36]

Long-term results of the Milan III trial comparing quadrantectomy, axillary dissection and radiotherapy (QUART) with quadrantectomy and axillary dissection without radiotherapy reveal that 86% of ipsilateral breast tumour recurrences occur in the index quadrant.[27] These findings support the employment of more limited radiotherapy aimed at elimination of residual cancer cells in the vicinity of the primary tumour. This concept accords with the observations of Holland et al[37] on the incidence of residual tumour in mastectomy specimens, and suggest that whole-breast irradiation can be avoided.

The technique of IORT offers the potential to deliver a relatively high intensity of radiation safely as a single dose to the tumour bed at the time of surgery while sparing adjacent normal surrounding breast tissue.[1,6] IORT has yielded small but statistically significant benefits in terms of local control for a variety of cancers, including pancreatic, colorectal, gastric, gynaecological and soft tissue malignancies. However, experience with IORT in breast cancer patients is limited, with only a few small published studies to date. Initial studies examined the use of IORT as a boost to the tumour bed in conjunction with external-beam radiation (delivered following IORT). In 1989, Dobelbower et al[25] published the first interim analysis of a retrospective study involving 21 breast cancer patients. Longer-term follow-up of this trial was published in 1997 at the same time as a study from a French group involving 51 patients.[23,24] The rationale for using IORT in these pilot studies was a reduction of the boost volume together with an improvement in side-effect profile. A total of 72 patients with stage I and II breast cancer were treated between 1984 and 1996 with IORT to the tumour bed following lumpectomy. The study protocol stipulated that all tumours be excised with histologically free margins and all underwent axillary dissection. Doses of radiation varied from 10 Gy (69 patients) to 15 Gy (3 patients) and were delivered with electron beams (6–20 MeV) adjusted to the amount of tissue to be irradiated. All patients subsequently received postoperative external irradiation of 45–50 Gy. No significant side-effects were observed when IORT was administered at a dosage of 10 Gy (<10% of patients with mild fibrosis) and all patients had an excellent cosmetic result. Furthermore, at follow-up ranging from 2 years to 12 years, no cases of ipsilateral breast tumour recurrence have been observed.

IORT as the sole mode of irradiation has the potential for accurately treating the tumour bed in a selected group of patients with early-stage breast cancer. The applicator can be applied under direct vision at the tumour bed within the open surgical field. Skin and subcutaneous tissues are not irradiated, thus reducing potential side-effects and improving cosmetic outcome. In particular, for patients with a relatively low risk of ipsilateral breast tumour recurrence, it may be possible to replace conventional radiotherapy with a single intraoperative dose that is equivalent to a full course of fractionated external-beam radiotherapy. There are obvious advantages of such an approach in terms of overall treatment time, logistics, patient comfort, cost and QoL. The relative biological effect of a single IORT dose is estimated to be 1.5–2.5 times higher than that of the dose delivered with external-beam radiotherapy. More specifically, the equivalence of IORT to standard 2 Gy fractionation can be calculated using the linear–quadratic model and computing the survival fraction of clonogenic units with different (α/β) ratios. For example, a total dose of 60 Gy given with 2 Gy fractionation is equivalent biologically to a single dose of IORT of 22.3 Gy (with an α/β ratio at 10 Gy acceptable for mammary tumours).[38,39] We have chosen a level of 21 Gy as corresponding to a full treatment dose. The potential incidence and extent of IORT effects on healthy tissues in the longer term remain unknown. Previous studies lack certifiable data and have limited follow-up. More recent studies involve patients with better prognosis and adequate duration of follow-up such that complication rates and adverse sequelae can be more accurately documented.[40] Formulae for radio-biological equivalence (linear–quadratic model, biological equivalent dose (BED), etc.) cannot fully predict the possible late effects of a single dose of high-intensity IORT.

Animal testing with canine models has provided information on short-term complications of IORT and data on maximum tolerated doses (MTD) for various organs and tissues such as peripheral nerves (15 Gy) cardiac atrium (20 Gy), lung (20 Gy) and skeletal muscle (23 Gy).[41] For these reasons, it is mandatory that comprehensive follow-up policies be incorporated into future clinical programmes of IORT. Precise follow-up schedules will be dictated by the specific disease together with IORT intensity (low-dose adjuvant treatment, combined treatment with pre- or postoperative external-beam irradiation, and combination with further systemic treatments). Evaluation of side-effects should distinguish between toxicities specific to IORT and multidisciplinary treatment toxicity. It is preferable to use an internationally accepted scale for event quantification.

ELIOT: electron intraoperative treatment

A period of 4 months of intensive testing together with personnel training was undertaken prior to activation of the ELIOT (electron intraoperative treatment) programme at the European Institute of Oncology, Milan. Between July 1999 and February 2002, more than 250 patients with a mean age of 59 (range 33–80) were treated. All patients had histologically confirmed invasive carcinoma with a maximum diameter not exceeding 2.5 cm and unifocality evident on imaging with mammography and/or ultrasound examination. Additional information on tumour extent was obtained in selected patients by magnetic resonance imaging (MRI) or breast scintigraphy with technetium-99m (^{99m}Tc)-MDP. Exclusion criteria included previous biopsy performed at another institution, systemic diseases (systemic lupus erythematosus, scleroderma, dermatomyositis, polyarteritis, etc.) and tumour location (lesions in the tail of the breast or close to the skin). A clinical programme was planned and developed in three phases:

1. A dose-escalation study was undertaken to define the maximum tolerated dose (single fraction) and establish relative efficacy between a single IORT dose and a conventional fractionated schedule of external beam radiotherapy.
2. A phase II study was undertaken using the MTD level reached (21 Gy) to assess acute and immediate toxicity in a larger cohort of patients.
3. An ongoing prospective randomised study compared standard external-beam irradiation (50 Gy to the whole breast and a 10 Gy boost to the tumour bed) with a single dose of intraoperative limited-field irradiation to evaluate the effectiveness of this approach in terms of local control, regional control, distant disease-free and overall survivals, cosmetic outcome, and cost.

Surgical procedure of ELIOT

Surgical techniques for ELIOT have been standardised at every stage.

Tumour removal

A wide excision of tumour is performed via either a radial incision or a periareolar incision for tumours relatively close to the areola (for which mastectomy is not mandated). For cases of impalpable lesions, a guided resection of the lesion is performed after radioisotopic localisation with ^{99m}Tc. A surgical margin of at least 1 cm around the tumour is aimed for, according to the volume of the breast. The specimen is examined and the tumour characterised in terms of size, histological type, focality and resection margins. A specimen X-ray is obtained to verify the presence of the lesion and to estimate its eccentricity and closeness to resection margins. Patients with a unifocal invasive carcinoma and clinically negative axillary nodes undergo sentinel node biopsy, but otherwise complete axillary dissection is performed. For lesions in the upper outer quadrant, it is usually possible to undertake the axillary procedure through the breast incision, while for other topographies, a counterincision is made in the axillary region (radial or transverse). Drains are placed in both the breast and axilla.

Preparation of the breast for ELIOT

Following tumour resection, the deep surface of the remaining breast parenchyma is mobilised off the fascia of the pectoralis major muscle for a distance of 5–10 cm around the tumour bed. This will permit approximation of tissue in the centre of the tumour bed and place breast parenchyma directly in the line of the radiation beam. The superficial surface of the parenchyma is separated from the subcutaneous tissue for approximately 4–5 cm in each direction, taking care not to disturb the blood supply of the skin flaps created during this procedure. The portion of the breast tissue that is treated with ELIOT is henceforth referred to as the 'target'. In order to minimise radiation exposure of the chest wall and ensure that maximal doses of radiation are delivered to the breast parenchyma, protective plates are positioned between the breast and the pectoral muscle. A dedicated lead disc (5 mm thickness) and an aluminium disc (4 mm thickness) are commonly used for this purpose to collectively shield and protect the chest wall (Figure 38.1). It is important to reconstruct the breast parenchyma in order to expose the appropriate portion of the gland to the radiation beam and avoid excessive inhomogeneity in the target volume. The electron-beam energy is selected on the basis of the thickness of the target volume, and the optimum dose distribution within the gland is attained if the thickness of the irradiated target remains as uniform as possible. Following mobilisation and undermining of the breast parenchyma, the gland is sutured in accordance with the defect resulting from surgical extirpation of the tumour (Figure 38.2). The anatomy and

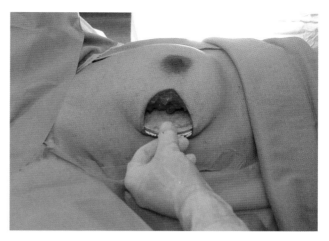

Figure 38.1 After wide excision of the cancer, a lead disc is positioned underneath the breast over the pectoral muscle.

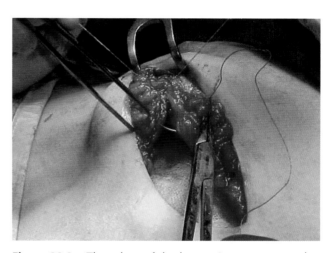

Figure 38.2 The edges of the breast tissue are sutured.

thickness of the breast are partially restored, with protection of the underlying thoracic wall. The precise thickness of the breast tissue is measured with a special device and the biologically effective electron energy is selected. The skin must be held away from the collimator to avoid inadvertent irradiation of the skin in the vicinity of the surgical breach (Figure 38.3). If the skin lies in contiguity with the Perspex collimator, its margin will receive approximately 5% of the total dose. A special piece of equipment has been developed that completely spares the skin from radiation exposure during delivery of ELIOT. This consists of a metallic ring with a variable diameter that is adjusted according to an individual patient's anatomy (Figure 38.4). This ring is connected to fine non-traumatic metallic hooks, which anchor the skin margins and gently retract the skin away from the radiation field. A wet sterile gauze can also be placed between the skin and the collimator to create a further tissue-equiva-

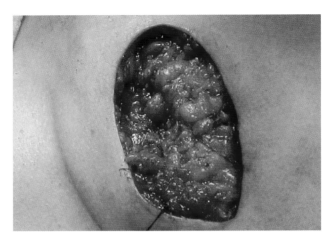

Figure 38.3 The suturing is completed and the breast tissue is exposed for the radiotherapy treatment.

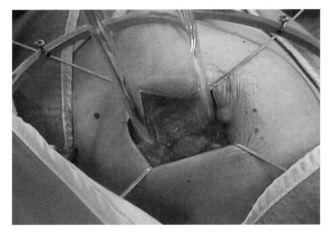

Figure 38.4 The radiotherapy applicator is positioned inside the wound.

lent barrier that can absorb low-energy electrons scattered around the edge of the collimator. Once the breast tissue has been sutured and the skin edges securely fixed, the sterile collimator can be positioned to ensure that the entire target volume is included within the radiation field. The portion of breast tissue that is to be irradiated (the clinical target volume) corresponds to a zone of 4–5 cm around the surgical resection site. However, depending on breast size, tumour location and glandular transposition, up to 10 cm of breast parenchyma may be irradiated. The collimator diameter is selected on the basis of the area to be treated and should cover both the tumour bed and a safe margin. The thickness of the target tissue will determine the energy of the electron beam.

The applicator is placed in direct contact with the breast tissue, and the linear accelerator can be manipulated under remote control to allow position-

ing of the collimator within the operating field. Care should be taken to avoid any herniation of breast tissue into the collimator, which would expose the superficial part of the gland to excessive radiation. The remote control of the linear accelerator facilitates accurate positioning of the collimator by the radiation technologist, and the connection to the distal part of the applicator is made in exactly the desired position.

Radiation treatment

Once the applicator is in position, a series of mobile shields are placed around the operating table to protect against scattering of X-rays. All personnel leave the operating room and the radiation equipment is switched on via the control panel. Radiation is delivered in two consecutive phases, each of which represents half of the prescribed dose. Using this method, the dose delivered in the first phase can be controlled and the dose in the second phase adjusted if necessary. In practice, any difference between planned and delivered dosage is rarely more than ±1.5%. The whole procedure is completed in 2–4 minutes.

Removal of ELIOT device and wound closure

After radiation treatment has been completed, the applicator is removed immediately from the surgical wound and the linear accelerator withdrawn from the area of the operating table. The sutures within the breast parenchyma are cut in order to allow removal of the lead and aluminium discs. The breast tissue is then reconstructed once more and the skin and subcutaneous tissues closed using absorbable monofilament material. The postoperative course is usually uneventful.

Results

The first two studies have been concluded to date. A total of 105 patients have been enrolled into the dose-escalation trial (55 patients) and the phase II study (50 patients) at a dose level of 21 Gy. All patients underwent a quadrantic resection and just under half (45 patients) had a complete axillary dissection, with 55 patients undergoing sentinel node biopsy, while 5 patients had untreated axillae. The majority of patients had small tumours measuring 20 mm or less (83%) located in the upper outer quadrant (65%). Three-quarters (74%) of the tumours were invasive ductal carcinomas, most commonly grade 1 or 2 and oestrogen receptor-positive (84%). Only 33% of tumours were progesterone receptor-positive and 58% had a low index of proliferation as measured with the Ki67 monoclonal antibody.

Dose-escalation study

The first 10 patients in this study received a single intraoperative dose of 10 Gy as an anticipated boost followed by conventional fractionated external-beam irradiation at a total of 44 Gy (22 fractions). Seven patients received 15 Gy followed by external irradiation at a total dose of 40 Gy (20 fractions). All other patients were treated with ELIOT alone, with three different dose levels: 17 Gy (8 patients), 19 Gy (6 patients) and 21 Gy (24 patients). A dose level of 21 Gy was administered to all planned patients, and no major acute or intermediate side-effects were observed at a follow-up of between 10 and 20 months. A few patients experienced mild pain in the irradiated area, and other complications included haematoma (3 patients), fibrosis of breast tissue (3 patients) and transient oedema of the breast (3 patients). One patient developed an in-breast recurrence at 6 months, but in a different quadrant, suggesting multifocal carcinoma not recognised at the time of surgery. One patient developed distant metastases without local recurrence. The cosmetic outcome was good in all patients, and in particular no erythema of the skin was observed, because of its retraction away from the radiation beam.

Phase II study

A total of 50 patients have been treated in this study with radiation administered at the 90% isodose and not at D_{max}. This adjustment to the dosage schedule corresponds to a D_{max} of 23.2 Gy. It was observed in the first study that 20% of patients had a slight underdosage of the target when tumours were deeply situated, with a tissue thickness of 25 mm or more. This modification has permitted better homogeneity of dose distribution, with less than 5% of cases receiving slightly less than 80% of the prescribed dose on limited areas of the target. Although follow-up remains rather short, the observed rate of acute toxicity is similar to that of the previous group of patients.

Phase III randomised study

This is an ongoing study and accrual is expected to be complete in 3 years' time. A total of 235 patients were recruited in the first 14 months of the study.

Discussion

The results of the Milan III trial at 12-year follow-up reveal that approximately 85% of recurrence in the ipsilateral breast occurs in the previously involved quadrant, thus supporting the use of a more restricted radiation schedule aimed at eliminating potential residual cancer cells in the index quadrant.[27]

As an alternative to a prolonged course of external irradiation, some clinicians have treated patients with low- or high-dose-intensity ^{192}Ir implants placed in the tumour bed and constituting the sole source of radiation treatment in patients undergoing breast conservation therapy.[33–36] Rates of local control were high (92–100%) in all studies except one.[33] Moreover, cosmetic outcomes and distant disease-free and overall survival were comparable to those in patients treated with a combined schedule. External-beam irradiation of the index quadrant alone has been compared with whole-breast irradiation in patients who are clinically node-negative with tumours measuring less than 4 cm.[31,32] Following tumour excision, patients were randomised into two groups. One group received radiation of the whole breast and regional lymph nodes while the other group were irradiated with an electron field confined to the tumour bed. A clear advantage emerged in terms of local control for whole-breast irradiation. At a median follow-up of 8 years, the crude in-breast recurrence rate was 19.5% in the limited-irradiation group and 10% for those who had whole-breast irradiation. It should be noted, however, that there were proportionately more patients with invasive lobular carcinoma in the limited-field arm and none of the patients received systemic therapy.

The technique of IORT is compatible with the basic oncological tenets of breast conservation surgery. The extent of breast tissue resection is the same and the need to position an applicator does not modify the skin incision. Radial or periareolar incisions are acceptable as for standard treatment modalities, and these will be determined by tumour size and location within the breast. In order to ensure good coverage of the clinical target volume by radiation and concomitant protection of healthy tissues within the operative field, the portion of breast tissue to be irradiated must be adequately prepared. The surgeon has an important role to play in this respect, and close cooperation between surgeon and radiation physics personnel is crucial for maximal success with this technique. ELIOT is relatively easy to perform and only marginally prolongs the duration of the surgical procedure. Indeed, the actual episode of irradiation is completed within 2–4 minutes and the overall duration of the radio-surgical procedure is less than 30 minutes. In the case of sentinel node biopsy, this will also include the time taken for intraoperative assessment of the sentinel node. Interestingly, sentinel node biopsy is likely to be more frequently practised in the future, and ELIOT could be undertaken while awaiting results of sentinel node examination.

Subsequent mobilisation of breast tissue after surgical excision to expose the 'target' for radiation does prolong operating time, but facilitates post-resection reconstruction and improves the final cosmetic result.

There have been no signs of ischaemia or necrosis of the skin flaps secondary to this mobilisation procedure, which should spare subcutaneous blood vessels. The rate of postoperative complications (pain, seroma, haematoma or infection) observed for ELIOT patients was not increased compared with a matched group of non-ELIOT patients, and the length of hospital stay was similar for the two groups. Precautions for protecting healthy tissue such as placement of lead and aluminium shields and the use of a special device to retract the skin edges dramatically reduced the exposure of these tissues to radiation and resulted in a low incidence of radiation-induced sequelae. Furthermore, the cosmetic outcome was favourable for all patients.

Additional clinical investigation and evaluation is mandatory to determine the optimum role and indications for the use of IORT. These studies should be undertaken only in highly specialised cancer centres and both the economic and social costs should be assessed alongside clinical efficacy. Standardised international models are perhaps the most suitable system for the development and evaluation of these technically complex treatment methods, where personnel training and specificity of equipment and apparatus are critical determinants of outcome.

Acknowledgements

The authors are very grateful to AICF (American Italian Cancer Foundation) and IRC (Associazione Italiana Ricerca sul Cancro) for their important support for this research. Appreciation is also expressed to Dr SE Franzetti for her editorial assistance.

References

1. Calvo FA, Micaily B, Brady LW. Intraoperative radiotherapy: a positive view. Am J Clin Oncol 1993; 16: 418–23.
2. Abe M. History of intraoperative radiation therapy. In: Dobelbower RR Jr, Abe M, eds. Intraoperative Radiation Therapy. Boca Raton, FL: CRC Press, 1989: 2–9.
3. Hu KS, Enker WE, Harrison LB. High-dose-rate intraoperative irradiation: current status and future directions. Semin Radiat Oncol 2002; 12: 62–80.
4. Willet CG, Gunderson LL, Busse PM et al. IOERT treatment factors. Technique, equipment. In: Gunderson LL et al, eds. Current Clinical Oncology: Intraoperative Irradiation: Techniques and Results. Totowa, NJ: Humana Press, 1999: 65–85.
5. Briggs DS, Thomson ET. Radiation properties of a miniature X-ray device for radiosurgery. Br J Radiol 1996; 69: 544–7.
6. Vaeth JM. Intraoperative Radiation Therapy in the Treatment of Cancer. Basel: Karger, 1997.
7. Gunderson LL, Nelson H, Martenson JA et al. Locally advanced primary colorectal cancer: intraoperative electron and external-beam irradiation ± 5-FU. Int J Radiat Oncol Biol Phys 1997; 37: 601–14.
8. Sindelar WF, Kinsella TJ, Tepper JE et al. Randomized trial of intraoperative radiotherapy in carcinoma of the stomach. Am J Surg 1993; 165: 178–87.
9. Garton GR, Gunderson LL, Webb MJ et al. Intraoperative radiation therapy in gynecologic cancer: update of the experience at a single institution. Int J Radiat Oncol Biol Phys 1997; 37: 839–43.
10. Eble MJ, Lehnert TH, Schwarzbach M et al. IORT for extremity sarcomas. Front Radiat Ther Oncol 1997; 31: 146–51.
11. Veronesi U, Orecchia R, Luini A et al. Focalised intraoperative irradiation after conservative surgery for early stage breast cancer. Breast 2001; 10: 84–9.
12. Veronesi U, Orecchia R, Luini A et al. A preliminary report of intraoperative radiotherapy (IORT) in limited-stage breast cancers that are conservatively treated. Eur J Cancer 2001; 37: 2178–83.
13. Gatzmeier W, Orecchia R, Gatti G et al. Intraoperative radiation therapy in the treatment of cancer of breast cancer. A new therapeutic alternative in the conservative treatment of breast cancer? Its potential role and future perspectives. Experience from the European Institute of Oncology (EIO), Milan. Strahlenther Onkol 2001; 177: 330–7.
14. Piermattei A, Delle Canne S, Azario L et al. Linac Novac7 electron beam calibration using GAF-Chromic film. Physica Medica 1999; 15: 277–83.
15. Nag S, Martinez-Monge R, Gupta N. Intraoperative radiation therapy using electron-beam and high dose rate brachytherapy. Cancer J Sci Am 1997; 10: 94–101.
16. Herbert M, Alecu R, Alecu M. Initial experience with novel brachytherapy device for early stage breast cancer treatment. Radiother Oncol 2001; 60: S19 (abst).
17. Palta JR, Biggs P, Hazle JD et al. Intraoperative electron beam radiation therapy: technique, dosimetry, and dose specification: report of Task Force 48 of the Radiation Therapy Committee, American Association of Physicists in Medicine. Int J Radiat Oncol Biol Phys 1995; 33: 725–46.
18. Veronesi U, Saccozzi R, Del Vecchio M et al. Comparing radical mastectomy with quadrantectomy, axillary dissection, and radiotherapy in patients with small cancers of the breast. N Engl J Med 1981; 305: 6–11.
19. Veronesi U, Paganelli G, Viale G et al. Sentinel lymph node biopsy and axillary dissection in breast cancer: results in a large series. J Natl Cancer Inst 1999; 91: 368–73.

20. Bartelink H, Horiot JC, Poortmans P et al. Recurrence rate after treatment of breast cancer with standard radiotherapy with or without additional irradiation. N Engl J Med 2001; 345: 1378–87.

21. Romestaing P, Lehingue Y, Carrie C et al. Role of a 10 Gy boost in the conservative treatment of early breast cancer: results of a randomized clinical trial in Lyon, France. J Clin Oncol 1997; 15: 963–8.

22. Vrieling C, Collette L, Fourquet A et al. The influence of the boost in breast-conserving therapy on cosmetic outcome in the EORTC 'Boost Versus No Boost' trial. EORTC Radiotherapy and Breast Cancer Cooperative Groups. European Organization for Research and Treatment of Cancer. Int J Radiat Oncol Biol Phys 1999; 45: 677–85.

23. Merrick HW, Battle JA, Padgett BJ et al. IORT for early breast cancer: a report on long-term results. Front Radiat Ther Oncol 1997; 31: 126–30.

24. DuBois JB, Hay M, Gely S et al. IORT in breast carcinomas. Front Radiat Ther Oncol 1997; 31: 131–7.

25. Dobelbower RR, Merrick HW, Eltaki A et al. Intra-operative electron beam therapy and external photon beam therapy with lumpectomy as primary treatment for early breast cancer. Ann Radiol 1989; 6: 497–501.

26. Early Breast Cancer Trialists' Collaborative Group (EBCTCG). Favourable and unfavourable effects on long-term survival of radiotherapy for early breast cancer: an overview of the randomised trials. Lancet 2000; 355: 1757–70.

27. Veronesi U, Marubini E, Mariani L et al. Radiotherapy after breast-conserving surgery in small breast carcinoma: long term results of a randomized trial. Ann Oncol 2001; 12: 997–1003.

28. Schnitt SJ, Hayman J, Gelman R et al. A prospective study of conservative surgery alone in the treatment of selected patients with stage I breast cancer. Cancer 1996; 77: 1094–100.

29. Kurtz JM, Kinkel K. Breast conservation in the 21st century. Eur J Cancer 2000; 36: 1919–24.

30. Hayman JA, Fairclough DL, Harris JR et al. Patient preferences concerning the trade-off between the risks and benefits of routine radiation therapy after conservative surgery for early-stage breast cancer. J Clin Oncol 1997; 15: 1252–60.

31. Ribeiro GG, Magee B, Swindell R et al. The Christie Hospital Breast Conservation Trial: an update at 8 years from inception. Clin Oncol 1993; 5: 278–83.

32. Magee B, Swindell R, Harris M et al. Prognostic factors for breast recurrence after surgery and radiotherapy: results from a randomized trial. Radiother Oncol 1996; 39: 223–7.

33. Fentiman IS, Poole C, Tong D et al. Inadequacy of iridium implant as sole radiation treatment for operable breast cancer. Eur J Cancer 1996; 32: 608–11.

34. Dale RG, Jones B, Price P. Comments on 'Inadequacy of iridium implant as sole radiation treatment for operable breast cancer, Fentiman et al., Eur J Cancer 1996, 32: 608–611.' Eur J Cancer 1997; 33: 1707–8.

35. Vicini F, Kini VR, Chen P et al. Irradiation of the tumor bed alone after lumpectomy in selected patients with early stage cancer treated with breast conserving therapy. J Surg Oncol 1999; 70: 33–40.

36. Vicini F, Baglan K, Kestin L et al. The emerging role of brachytherapy in the management of patients with breast cancer. Semin Oncol 2002; 12: 31–9.

37. Holland R, Connoly JL, Gelman R et al. The presence of an extensive intraductal component (EIC) following a limited excision correlates with prominent residual disease in the remainder of the breast. J Clin Oncol 1990; 8: 113–18.

38. Okunieff P, Sundaraman S, Chen Y. Biology of large dose per fraction radiation therapy. In: Gunderson LL et al, eds. Current Clinical Oncology: Intraoperative Irradiation: Techniques and Results. Totowa, NJ: Humana Press, 1999: 25–46.

39. Strandqvist M. Time–dose relationship. Acta Radiol 1994; 55: 1–30.

40. Azinovic I, Calvo FA, Puebla F et al. Long-term normal tissue effects of intraoperative electron radiation therapy (IOERT): late sequelae, tumor recurrence, and second malignancies. Int J Radiat Oncol Biol Phys 2001; 49: 597–604.

41. Sindelar WF, Johnstone PA, Hoekstra HJ, Kinsella TJ. Normal tissue tolerance to intraoperative irradiation. In: Gunderson LL et al, eds. Current Clinical Oncology: Intraoperative Irradiation: Techniques and Results. Totowa, NJ: Humana Press, 1999: 131–73.

39 Radiotherapy in early breast cancer

Simon G Russell, Charlotte E Coles, Assem Rostom

Introduction

Breast cancer is the most common malignancy in women, with about 180 000 new cases a year in Europe. Despite this increasing incidence, documented mortality rates for the period 1990–2000 have declined in the UK and USA, which is most likely attributable to a combination of screening and adjuvant systemic therapies.[1] The UK NHS Breast Screening Programme (NHSBSP) was introduced in the late 1980s and has resulted in a stage migration, with an increased proportion of T1 tumours ($\leq$2 cm). This could translate into reduced mortality rates and is an issue that is elaborated upon by Benson in Chapter 5. Similarly, tamoxifen has been widely used as adjuvant hormonal treatment over a similar period, with confirmed reductions in breast cancer deaths. Mortality figures may also have improved following the introduction of multidisciplinary team working, whereby newly diagnosed and suspected breast cancers are managed in the context of a multidisciplinary setting with collective management input from surgeons, radiologists, pathologists, radiation/medical oncologists and breast care nurses. Many cases of breast cancer are detected at an early stage, and can be managed with breast-conserving surgery, postoperative radiotherapy and, increasingly, systemic treatment. Breast irradiation constitutes a significant component of radiotherapy workload, and currently consumes 30% of radiotherapy resources in the UK.

Radiotherapy of the breast presents special challenges, as the anatomy and surrounding structures render this an inherently difficult site to irradiate in a homogeneous manner. It has a complex three-dimensional (3D) shape, which may have been modified further by surgery, and it is located at the body–air interface. There are also vital organs in close proximity, such as the lungs and heart (in the case of left-sided tumours), which are at risk from radiation damage. Single-plane 2D radiotherapy breast plans can lead to substantial dose inhomogeneities, particularly in women with larger breasts. An inhomogenous dose may lead to increased normal-tissue side-effects and poor cosmetic results in the longer term, which can cause significant psychological morbidity for patients.

Radiotherapy following breast-conserving surgery

Since the pioneering work of Sir Geoffrey Keynes[2] in the 1920s and 30s on the use of conservative surgery and definitive radiotherapy, this form of management gained in popularity throughout Europe and the USA in the second half of the 20th century and has become the standard of care for many cases of early breast cancer. Patients must be appropriately selected for breast-conserving surgery based on factors such as tumour size ($\leq$3 cm), proximity to or involvement of the nipple, and multifocality. Breast size, tumour grade and age of the patient are other factors that may need to be taken into account when considering suitability for breast conservation. Prospective randomised controlled trials have shown that breast-conserving surgery and radiotherapy is as effective as mastectomy in terms of overall survival.[3] Several seminal trials have demonstrated that radiotherapy following breast-conserving surgery decreases rates of local recurrence when compared with surgery alone.[4–7] It is yet to be established if there is a group of patients with favourable features who could be spared breast irradiation, and this question remains the subject of ongoing trials. Four randomised controlled trials have addressed whether, in selected groups of patients, radiotherapy could be avoided following breast-conserving surgery. All of these studies showed a consistently higher rate of local recurrence when radiotherapy was omitted. Furthermore, no subgroup could be identified that did not benefit from radiotherapy.[4–7] However, the benefits of radiotherapy in patients aged over 55 with small (<1 cm) tumours of favourable histology are likely to be marginal, and omission of radiotherapy in this subgroup could be considered.

Radiotherapy following breast-conserving surgery is delivered to the entire remaining breast tissue, and in most centres around the world, the commonest dose used is 46–50 Gy administered in daily fractions of 2 Gy. However, in the UK, experience suggests that 40 Gy given in 15 fractions over 3 weeks (2.67 Gy per fraction) provides similar rates of local control and late normal-tissue effects as 2 Gy per fraction regimens. This issue of dosage should be clearer when the results of the UK START trial are published. A further radiation boost to the tumour bed using an electron field is frequently administered to further decrease local recurrence.[8,9] Radiation fields to the breast or chest wall extend from the midline to the midaxillary line laterally (or 1 cm beyond palpable breast tissue), to the suprasternal notch superiorly and 1 cm below the inframammary fold inferiorly. Surgical incisions and drains should remain within these boundaries to avoid excessive irradiation of lung tissue. At the time of surgery, it is essential to ensure adequate haemostasis to prevent haematoma formation. Clips can be deployed at the surgical site and tumours should be excised with an 'adequate' margin of clearance (see Chapter 35).

Nodal irradiation

The role of regional nodal irradiation following breast-conserving surgery is controversial and has not yet been addressed in a clinical trial. Recommendations are therefore based on extrapolating the data from postmastectomy trials. Following any form of axillary surgery, clinical indications for irradiation of the axilla represent a balance between the risk of regional recurrence and potential morbidity. Axillary irradiation following surgical clearance has not been shown to improve either local control or survival, but does increase the incidence of lymphoedema (up to 40%) and is generally contraindicated. If, however, there is suspicion of residual disease in the axilla following clearance then radiotherapy should be considered. The practice of internal mammary nodal irradiation remains one of the most controversial areas of breast radiotherapy. Isolated nodal recurrence is rare and the lack of data currently precludes its routine use.

Contraindications to breast-conserving surgery and radiotherapy include large or multicentric breast tumours, previous irradiation, extensive ductal carcinoma in situ (DCIS) and pregnancy.

Timing of radiotherapy following breast-conserving surgery and chemotherapy

When chemotherapy is prescribed, it can delay radiotherapy by up to 6 months. Concerns have been expressed that delaying radiotherapy until after chemotherapy is potentially unsafe and might increase rates of local recurrence. The optimal sequencing of these modalities was studied by Recht et al,[10] who randomised patients to four cycles of an anthracycline-containing chemotherapy regimen followed by breast radiotherapy or to radiotherapy followed by the same chemotherapy schedule. With a median follow-up of 5 years, the overall survival rate was 81% in the chemotherapy-first group and 73% in the radiation-first group ($p = 0.11$). The local relapse rate was higher in the chemotherapy-first group (14% compared with 5%), but the distant recurrence rate was less (20% compared with 32%). It is therefore recommended that patients who are at a greater risk of local relapse should undergo radiotherapy first, while those at a greater risk of distant failure receive chemotherapy first. Any resultant delay in radiotherapy is unlikely to have an impact on local control.

Postmastectomy radiotherapy

For more than 50 years, radiotherapy has been combined with mastectomy, but the indications for chest wall and regional nodal irradiation continue to evolve. All trials have shown that postmastectomy radiotherapy reduces the proportional risk of local failure by two-thirds to three-quarters. The effects on relapse-free and overall survival have been variable between trials, but those involving more than 200 patients have generally shown trends in favour of improvements in recurrence-free and overall survival.[11] The first meta-analysis of postmastectomy radiotherapy trials was published in 1987, and showed a poorer overall survival in the radiation group.[12] These data have since been updated,[13] and reveal a decrease in deaths from breast cancer but an increase in the non-breast-cancer death rate, yielding overall equality of survival. An initial meta-analysis by the Early Breast Cancer Trialists' Collaborative Group (EBCTCG) failed to reveal any overall survival advantage at 10 years for patients receiving postmastectomy radiotherapy.[14] Patients undergoing breast irradiation following breast-conserving surgery were included and there was no subset analysis based on the use of systemic adjuvant therapy. A meta-analysis by Whelan et al[15] of 11 trials in which all patients received systemic treatment concluded that locoregional irradiation reduced mortality from breast cancer (hazard ratio (HR) 0.80; 95% confidence interval (CI) 0.71–0.89; $p = 0.0001$). The EBCTCG published a more comprehensive meta-analysis in 2000.[16] A total of 40 unconfounded randomised trials of radiotherapy for early breast cancer were analysed. It involved central review of individual patients' data on recurrence and cause-specific mortality from 20 000 women, half of whom had 'node-positive' disease. Radiotherapy fields included not only chest wall (or breast) but also axillary, supraclavicular and internal mammary nodal areas. For patients receiving radiation, there was a decrease in the rate of local recurrence from 27.2% to 8.8% at 10 years. Although breast cancer mortality was reduced ($2p = 0.0001$), other causes of death (particularly cardiovascular) were increased ($2p = 0.0003$). The overall survival rate at 20 years was 37.1% with radiotherapy versus 35.9% for the group control ($2p = 0.06$), with a survival percentage of 0.967 in favour of radiotherapy.[12] As reported by Cuzick et al,[13] postmastectomy radiation significantly improved breast-cancer-specific survival, but overall survival was unaffected, due to an increase in non-cancer deaths. Many of these data relate to outdated modes of radiotherapy, and newer radiation techniques employ tangential fields (particularly avoiding the heart and vasculature) that minimise toxicity and could improve overall survival. Van de Steene et al[17] reanalysed the EBCTCG data, excluding trials that began before 1970, small trials, trials with poor survival rates and trials using radiation fractions that are no longer employed. A significant survival benefit for the radiotherapy arm was found for recent trials ($2p<0.05$), large trials ($2p<0.03$), trials using standard fractionation ($2p<0.02$) and trials with a favourable crude survival ($2p<0.03$). Van de Steene et al[17] concluded that adjuvant radiotherapy significantly improves overall survival of breast cancer patients provided that current techniques are used and treatment is given with standard fractionation. The results of this study stress the importance of reducing cardiovascular and other late toxicities in adjuvant radiotherapy schedules for breast cancer.

Perhaps the two most important recent studies addressing postmastectomy radiotherapy are those of the British Columbia group[18] and the Danish Breast Cancer Cooperative Group.[19] The former randomised 318 premenopausal women with node-positive breast cancer to mastectomy and chemotherapy with or without irradiation. Radiotherapy was given to the chest wall and locoregional lymph nodes between the fourth and fifth cycles of cyclophosphamide, methotrexate and fluorouracil (CMF). After 15 years of follow-up, the women assigned to chemotherapy plus radiotherapy had a 33% reduction in the rate of recurrence (relative risk (RR) 0.67; 95% CI 0.50–0.90) and a 29% reduction in mortality from breast cancer (RR 0.71; 95% CI 0.51–0.99). The overall survival rate was 54% for patients receiving postmastectomy radiotherapy, compared with 46% for women treated with systemic chemotherapy alone.[18] The Danish study was much larger, randomising 1708 premenopausal women with stage II or III breast cancer to mastectomy and chemotherapy (CMF) alone or to mastectomy, CMF, and irradiation of the chest wall and regional lymph nodes. The local recurrence rate was reduced from 32% to 9% ($p<0.001$), while the relapse-free and overall survival rates at 10 years improved from 34% to 48% and 45% to 54% respectively ($p<0.001$). An important aspect of this study was that the use of modern radiotherapy techniques minimised cardiac irradiation and there was no increase in reported non-breast-cancer deaths. The relative risk of death from any cause was reduced by 29%.[20]

It remains unclear whether patients with 1–3 positive lymph nodes benefit from postmastectomy radiotherapy. In the Danish study, this category represented a large proportion of patients, but many did not undergo formal axillary dissection, which may have underestimated the number of positive nodes and increased the risk of local recurrence due to residual microscopic disease in the axillae. This may have resulted in an apparent survival benefit from postmastectomy irradiation due to inadequate locoregional surgical treatment. Interestingly, postmastectomy radiotherapy in both the British Columbia and Danish trials yielded the same proportional benefits in patients with 1–3 positive nodes as for those with 4 or more involved nodes. However, with more prolonged follow-up, benefits are statistically more robust in the group with 4 or more nodes. Table 39.1 summarises the American Society of Clinical Oncology (ASCO) guidelines regarding postmastectomy radiation.[21] There is general consensus that patients with 4 or more involved nodes should receive postmastectomy radiotherapy. Curiously, the proportional reduction in locoregional failure was greater for patients with 1–3 positive nodes.[22,23] The role of radiation in postmastectomy patients with small tumours and 1–3 positive lymph nodes is the subject of an ongoing national Intergroup trial and the proposed UK SUPREMO study.

Table 39.1 Summary of ASCO postmastectomy radiotherapy (PMRT) guidelines

1. **Patients with ≥4 positive axillary lymph nodes** PMRT is recommended.

2. **Patients with 1–3 positive axillary lymph nodes** There is insufficient evidence to make recommendations or suggestions for the routine use of PMRT in patients with T1/2 tumours with 1–3 positive nodes.

3. **Patients with T3 or stage III tumours** PMRT is suggested for patients with T3 tumours with positive axillary nodes and patients with operable stage III tumours.

4. **Patients undergoing preoperative systemic therapy** There is insufficient evidence to make recommendations or suggestions as to whether all patients initially treated with preoperative systemic therapy should be given PMRT.

5. **Modifications of these guidelines for special patient subgroups** There is insufficient evidence to make recommendations or suggestions for modifying guidelines regarding the routine use of PMRT based on other tumour-related, patient-related or treatment-related factors.

6. **Chest wall irradiation** In patients given PMRT, adequate treatment of the chest wall should be mandatory.

7. **Details of chest wall irradiation** There is insufficient evidence to make recommendations or suggestions regarding such aspects of chest wall irradiation as total dose, fraction size, the use of bolus and the use of scar boosts.

8. **Axillary nodal irradiation** Full axillary radiotherapy should not be given routinely to patients undergoing complete or level I/II axillary dissection. There is insufficient evidence to make suggestions or recommendations as to whether some patient subgroups might benefit from axillary irradiation.

9. **Supraclavicular nodal irradiation for patients with ≤4 positive axillary lymph nodes** The incidence of clinical supraclavicular failure is sufficiently great in these patients that a supraclavicular field should be irradiated.

10. **Supraclavicular nodal irradiation for patients with 1–3 positive axillary lymph nodes** There is insufficient evidence to make recommendations as to whether or not a supraclavicular field should be used for these patients.

11. **Internal mammary nodal irradiation** There is insufficient evidence to make suggestions or recommendations as to whether or not deliberate internal mammary nodal irradiation should be used in any patient subgroup.

12. **Sequencing of PMRT and systemic therapy** There is insufficient evidence to recommend the optimal sequencing of chemotherapy, tamoxifen and PMRT. It is suggested, on the basis of the available evidence regarding toxicities, that doxorubicin not be administered concurrently with PMRT.

13. **Integration of PMRT and reconstructive surgery** There is insufficient evidence to make recommendations or suggestions with regard to the integration of PMRT and reconstructive surgery.

14. **Long-term toxicities** The potential long-term risks of PMRT include lymphoedema, brachial plexopathy, radiation pneumonitis, rib fractures, cardiac toxicity and radiation-induced second neoplasms. Data suggest that the incidence of many of these toxicities is lower when modern radiotherapy techniques are used, although follow-up in patients treated with current radiotherapy is insufficient to rule out the possibility of very late cardiac toxicities. From the available evidence, with its limitations, however, it appears that, in general, the risk of serious toxicity from PMRT (when performed using modern techniques) is low enough that toxicity considerations should not limit its use in most circumstances when otherwise indicated.

15. **Toxicity considerations for special patient subgroups** There is insufficient evidence to make recommendations or suggestions that PMRT should not be used for some subgroups of patients because of increased rates of toxicity (such as radiation carcinogenesis) compared with the rest of the population.

Radiotherapy following neoadjuvant chemotherapy and mastectomy

The issue of radiotherapy following mastectomy in the setting of neoadjuvant chemotherapy poses diffi-cult problems and there are significantly fewer trial data upon which to base decisions. Because of the histological changes consequent to chemotherapy, pathological parameters that are normally used to guide radiotherapy become distorted. Buchholz et al[24] at the MD Anderson Cancer Centre, compared local recurrence rates in neoadjuvant chemotherapy patients with those previously reported after mastectomy and adjuvant chemotherapy. As might be anticipated, there was a higher risk of local recurrence in the neoadjuvant group than the adjuvant group when compared stage for stage. When considering radiotherapy after induction chemotherapy and surgery, both the pretreatment clinical stage and the postmastectomy pathological stage must be taken into account. In a retrospective series of inflammatory carcinomas, those treated with chemotherapy and mastectomy alone had a 59% local recurrence rate, compared with 15% if additionally treated with radiotherapy.[25] Currently, there are no data available for outcomes of clinical stage I and II disease treated with neoadjuvant chemotherapy. In general, patients requiring mastectomy following neoadjuvant chemotherapy should receive radiotherapy.

Radiotherapy following reconstruction

Many younger women undergoing mastectomy opt for breast reconstruction, as either an immediate or a delayed procedure. Although immediate reconstruction has a number of advantages for the patient, the need for postmastectomy radiation must be considered when selecting the optimum form of reconstruction (with respect to both timing and technique). Aside from any effects of radiotherapy on long-term cosmetic outcome, reconstructive surgery may impair the efficacy of postmastectomy radiotherapy and increase cardiac and lung irradiation. These outstanding questions remain to be answered in appropriate clinical trials.

The late toxicity of breast radiotherapy

Serious long-term side-effects from radiotherapy are rare, and with modern radiotherapy techniques these risks can be minimised.

Lymphoedema is a recognised complication of breast cancer patients undergoing treatment, occurring in 5–10% of patients undergoing standard level II axillary dissection. In addition to discomfort and impaired function, it can also lead to depression and anxiety. Lymphoedema occurs most commonly in those who have both axillary surgery and radiotherapy (40%). Modern surgical and radiotherapy techniques can reduce the incidence of this complication, as can prompt treatment of soft tissue infection and weight loss in the obese.[26] Radiation pneumonitis affects approximately 1% of irradiated breast cancer patients and presents with cough,

fever and dyspnoea. The incidence of pneumonitis is higher if nodal irradiation is added or if concurrent chemotherapy is given. The risk of pneumonitis may be decreased by limiting the volume of irradiated lung; modern radiotherapy techniques make this feasible.[27] Nonetheless, pneumonitis is usually clinically insignificant, with few long-term sequelae. Certain types of postoperative radiotherapy to the chest wall and lymph nodes are associated with an increase in cardiac mortality due to exposure of the heart; this only applies to left-sided tumours using standard tangential beam arrangements. An analysis of over 200 000 women in the US National Cancer Institute (NCI) Surveillance, Epidemiology and End-Results (SEER) database[28] showed that the overall relative risk for cardiac mortality in women receiving radiotherapy to the left side was 1.17 (95% CI 1.01–1.36), although other studies have not confirmed this finding. With modern radiotherapy techniques, cardiac radiation dosimetry can be further improved, with a potential decrease in cardiac mortality, which may become evident in future clinical studies.

The incidence of radiation-induced brachial plexus injury following nodal irradiation is less than 1%.[29] This figure may be lower with modern radiation techniques, and historically higher rates of brachial plexopathy may have been due in part to inadvertent patient movement between radiotherapy dosages to the breast and supraclavicular lymph nodes. When brachial plexus injury is suspected, cross-sectional imaging is essential to exclude tumour recurrence. Secondary malignancy is a rare complication of any radiation treatment, and the incidence of sarcoma in the irradiated breast field is 0.2% at 10 years.[30] Smokers have a slightly increased risk of lung cancer on the ipsilateral side, which is not apparent in non-smokers.[31]

Intensity-modulated radiotherapy

Intensity-modulated radiotherapy (IMRT) refers to variation of radiation fluence across the beam. The major value of IMRT for breast radiotherapy is the reduction of dose inhomogeneity within the target volume. A secondary advantage is the reduction of high-dose irradiation to normal tissues. 3D radiotherapy planning and IMRT techniques have been developed with the aim of improving dose homogeneity to the breast and reducing normal-tissue side-effects.

IMRT has evolved very rapidly over the last few years and the majority of publications on this subject report dosimetric analysis as opposed to clinical outcome. Initial clinical experience with

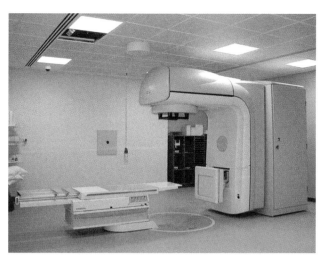

Figure 39.1   Simens Primus Dual Energy 6/15 MeV Linear Accelerator with electron facility installed in the Oncology Centre at Addenbrooke's Foundation NHS Trust, June 2003.

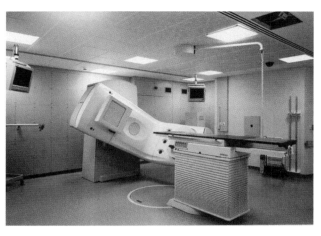

Figure 39.2   Siemens Primus Linear Accelerator with Multileaf collimators, Auto-field sequencing and Electronic Portal Imaging facilities.

IMRT using multiple static fields reported on the treatment of 10 patients with breast cancer who showed minimal or no acute skin reactions.[32] A further report from the same institution later commented on cosmetic results at 12 months in 95 patients treated with IMRT.[33] The cosmetic outcome was rated as excellent/good in 94 of these patients (99%), none of whom experienced persistent breast pain or developed telangiectasia or significant fibrosis.

To date, there has been only one randomised controlled trial designed to investigate late normal-tissue side-effects.[34] This was carried out at the Royal Marsden Hospital and involved 305 patients with early breast cancer. Women with larger breasts were specifically selected for the trial on the premise that these patients would be more susceptible to dose inhomogeneities. They were randomised to either standard radiotherapy or forward-planned IMRT using either a metal compensator or multiple static fields. The primary endpoint was breast appearance following radiotherapy, which was assessed with serial photographs. Interim analysis was completed in September 2002 and favoured IMRT; a change in breast appearance was scored in 60 of 116 (52%) patients allocated standard 2D treatment and 42 of 117 (36%) patients allocated IMRT (p = 0.05). A further randomised controlled trial investigating the clinical relevance of IMRT irrespective of breast size is underway at Addenbrooke's Oncology Centre, Cambridge. At least two confirmatory trials would provide sufficient impetus to adopt IMRT as standard practice for breast cancer patients within the UK with potential benefits for many women.

Intraoperative radiotherapy techniques (see Chapter 38)

The technique of intraoperative radiotherapy (IORT) using a portable electron-beam-driven device has the advantage of delivering partial breast irradiation at the time of surgery and avoiding outpatient visits for external-beam or high-dose-rate (HDR) brachytherapy. However, the biologically equivalent dose remains uncertain and definitive histological resection margins are unknown at the time of irradiation. Veronesi's group at the European Institute of Oncology in Milan have considerable experience of using ELIOT (electron intraoperative treatment), which consists of a mobile linear accelerator with a robotic arm. A single fraction of radiotherapy is given with a Perspex applicator using 3–9 MeV electrons. The chest wall is shielded with an aluminium–lead disc and the skin is stretched out of the radiation field. The target volume consists of the surgical bed and a 1–3 cm margin of surrounding breast tissue. A pilot study on 86 women treated with a single fraction of 17–21 Gy showed the technique to be well tolerated by patients. With a reported mean follow-up of 8 months, it is not, however, possible to comment on issues of late normal-tissue side-effects and local tumour control.[35] There is an ongoing trial in Milan that randomises patients to either whole-breast radiotherapy (60 Gy) or ELIOT (21 Gy) following quadrantectomy. The ELIOT programme is discussed in detail in Chapter 38.

An alternative IORT device is the Intra-beam, a portable device that delivers low-voltage (50 kV) photons.[36] Pilot studies of intraoperative targeted radiotherapy (Targit) in the UK, USA, Europe and Australia have treated a total of 185 patients. In the majority of patients included in these studies, whole-breast external-beam radiotherapy was administered, but Targit replaced the boost dose to the tumour bed. At a median follow-up of 22 months, there have been two recurrences and satisfactory cosmetic results. A multicentre randomised trial is currently underway that allocates breast conservation patients to whole-breast radiotherapy or Targit. This yields a dosage of 20 Gy to the surface of the applicator, with attenuation to 5 Gy at a distance of 1 cm.[37] Individual participating centres have the option of adding external-beam radiotherapy to those patients deemed as 'high-risk' for ipsilateral breast tumour recurrence.

Perhaps IORT will replace the use of a booster dose and can be administered at the time of primary surgery – this could potentially save up to 2 weeks of machine time per patient.

Partial breast irradiation

It is estimated that the majority of ipsilateral breast tumour recurrences following breast conservation surgery will be in the vicinity of the tumour site, i.e. the index quadrant. It might therefore be argued that irradiation of the entire breast is unnecessary and will add little to local control. For quadrantectomy, Veronesi et al[38] reported that the incidence of ipsilateral new primary tumours was the same as for new primary lesions in the contralateral breast.

Several groups are now exploring the use of partial breast irradiation, which has become feasible with recent developments in computer technology and software equipment. However, there are potential problems associated with these techniques of partial breast irradiation. Physicists and radiographers must undergo specific training in what are fairly sophisticated techniques and the relevant hardware and software packages are relatively expensive. Movement of the breast during respiration can result in geographical mistargetting. Furthermore, identification of the precise boundaries of the tumour bed post surgery can be difficult. The NCI Division of Cancer Treatment and Diagnosis has recently hosted a workshop to address these issues as part of its radiation research programme. This meeting served to highlight some of the difficulties of this approach, including appropriate selection of patients (based on clinical and pathological parameters), radiation dose/fractionation and localisation of the target volume.[39] Several ongoing trials will attempt to answer these questions.

Conclusions

Radiotherapy has a proven role in the management of early breast cancer and been shown not only to decrease ipsilateral local recurrence but also to improve survival in certain categories of patients following both breast-conserving surgery and mastectomy. Despite recent advances in radiation technology, the majority of centres worldwide use basic radiotherapy techniques based on 2D breast data. The incorporation of new approaches to breast radiotherapy, such as IMRT and partial breast irradiation, may lead to a reduction in longer-term morbidity without compromise of local control. These more complex radiotherapy methods will demand precise delineation of the tumour bed and application of appropriate margins. Ongoing and proposed randomised trials will evaluate these concepts, and will determine the levels of safety and efficacy associated with the new techniques.

References

1. Benson JR, Purushotham A. Trends in breast cancer incidence, survival and mortality. Lancet 2000; 356: 590–3.

2. Keynes G. Conservative treatment of cancer of the breast. BMJ 1937; ii: 643–9.

3. Fisher B, Anderson S, Bryant J et al. Twenty-year follow-up of a randomized trial comparing total mastectomy, lumpectomy, and lumpectomy plus irradiation for the treatment of invasive breast cancer. N Engl J Med 2002; 347: 1233–41.

4. Veronesi U, Salvadori B, Luini A et al. Breast conservation is a safe method in patients with small cancer of the breast. Long-term results of three randomised trials on 1,973 patients. Eur J Cancer 1995; 31A: 1574–9.

5. Veronesi U, Luini A, Del Vecchio M et al. Radiotherapy after breast-preserving surgery in women with localized cancer of the breast. N Engl J Med 1993; 328: 1587–91.

6. Liljegren G, Holmberg L, Bergh J et al. 10-year results after sector resection with or without postoperative radiotherapy for stage I breast cancer: a randomized trial. J Clin Oncol 1999; 17: 2326–33.

7. Clark RM, McCulloch PB, Levine MN et al. Randomized clinical trial to assess the effectiveness of breast irradiation following lumpectomy and axillary dissection for node-negative breast cancer. J Natl Cancer Inst 1992; 84: 683–9.

8. Romestaing P, Lehingue Y, Carrie C et al. Role of a 10–Gy boost in the conservative treatment of early breast cancer: results of a randomized clinical trial in Lyon, France. J Clin Oncol 1997; 15: 963–8.

9. Bartelink H, Horiot JC, Poortmans P et al. Recurrence rates after treatment of breast cancer with standard

radiotherapy with or without additional radiation. N Engl J Med 2001; 345: 1378–87.

10. Recht A, Come SE, Henderson IC et al. The sequencing of chemotherapy and radiation therapy after conservative surgery for early-stage breast cancer. N Engl J Med 1996; 334: 1356–61.

11. Recht A. Postmastectomy radiotherapy. In: Gradishar WJ, Wood WC, eds. Advances in Breast Cancer Management. Amsterdam: Kluwer, 2000: 39–51.

12. Cuzick J, Stewart H, Peto R et al. Overview of randomised trials of postoperative adjuvant radiotherapy in breast cancer. Cancer Treat Rep 1987; 71: 15–29.

13. Cuzick J, Stewart H, Rutqvist L et al. Cause-specific mortality in long-term survivors of breast cancer who participated in trials of radiotherapy. J Clin Oncol 1994; 12: 447–53.

14. Early Breast Cancer Trialists' Collaborative Group: effects of radiotherapy and surgery in early breast cancer: an overview of the randomized trials. N Engl J Med 1995; 333: 1444–55.

15. Whelan TJ, Julian J, Wright J et al. Does locoregional radiation therapy improve survival in breast cancer? A meta-analysis. J Clin Oncol 2000; 18: 1220–9.

16. The Early Breast Cancer Trialists' Collaborative Group. Favourable and unfavourable effects on long term survival of radiotherapy for early breast cancer: an overview of the randomised trials. Lancet 2000; 355: 1757–70.

17. Van de Steene J, Soete G, Storme G. Adjuvant radiotherapy for breast cancer significantly improves overall survival. Radiother Oncol 2000; 55: 263–72.

18. Ragaz J, Jackson SM, Le N et al. Adjuvant radiotherapy and chemotherapy in node-positive premenopausal women with breast cancer. N Engl J Med 1997; 337: 956–62.

19. Overgaard M, Hansen PS, Overgaard J et al. Postoperative radiotherapy in high-risk premenopausal women with breast cancer who receive adjuvant chemotherapy. Danish Breast Cancer Cooperative Group 82b trial. N Engl J Med 1997; 337: 949–55.

20. Hojris I, Overgaard M, Christensen J et al. morbidity and mortality of ischaemic heart disease in high risk breast cancer patients after adjuvant post-mastectomy systemic treatment with or without radiotherapy. Lancet 1999; 354: 1425–30.

21. Recht A, Edge SB, Solin LJ et al. Post-mastectomy radiotherapy: clinical practice guidelines of the American Society of Clinical Oncology. J Clin Oncol 2001; 19: 1539–69.

22. Overgaard M, Jensen MB, Overgaard J et al. Operative radiotherapy in high risk post menopausal breast cancer patients given adjuvant tamoxifen: Danish Breast Cancer Cooperative Group DBCG 82c randomized trial. Lancet 1999, 353: 1641–8

23. Kuske RR. Adjuvant chest wall and nodal irradiation: maximize cure, minimize late cardiac toxicity. J Clin Oncol 1998; 16: 2579–82.

24. Buchholz TA, Katz A, Strom EA et al. Pathological factors that predict for local-regional recurrences after mastectomy are different for breast cancer patients

25. Fleming RYD, Asmar L, Buzdar AU et al. Effectiveness of mastectomy by response to induction chemotherapy for control in inflammatory breast cancer. Ann Surg Oncol 1997; 4: 452–61.

26. Kisin MW, Querci della Rovere G, Easton D, Westbury G. Risk of lymphoedema following the treatment of breast cancer. Br J Surg 1986; 73: 580–4.

27. Lingos TI, Recht A, Vicini F et al. Radiation pneumonitis in breast cancer patients treated with conservative surgery and radiation therapy. Int J Radiat Oncol Biol Phys 1991; 21: 355–60.

28. Paszat LF, Mackillop WJ, Groome PA et al. Mortality from myocardial infarction after adjuvant radiotherapy for breast cancer in the Surveillance, Epidemiology, and End-Results cancer registries. J Clin Oncol 1998; 16: 2625–31.

29. Powell S, Cooke J, Parsons C. Radiation-induced brachial plexus injury: follow-up of two different fractionation schedules. Radiother Oncol 1990; 18: 213–20.

30. Taghian A, de Vathaire F, Terrier P et al. Long-term risk of sarcoma following radiation treatment for breast cancer. Int J Radiat Oncol Biol Phys 1991; 21: 361–7.

31. Inskip PD, Stovall M, Flannery JT. Lung cancer risk and radiation dose among women treated for breast cancer. J Natl Cancer Inst 1994; 86: 983–8.

32. Kestin LL, Sharpe MB, Frazier RC et al. Intensity modulation to improve dose uniformity with tangential breast radiotherapy: initial clinical experience. Int J Radiat Oncol Biol Phys 2000; 48: 1559–68.

33. Vicini FA, Sharpe M, Kestin et al. Optimizing breast cancer treatment efficacy with intensity-modulated radiotherapy. Int J Radiat Oncol Biol Phys 2002; 54: 1336–44.

34. Yarnold J, Donovan E, Bleackley N et al. Randomised trial of standard 2D radiotherapy (RT) versus 3D intensity modulated radiotherapy (IMRT) in patients prescribed breast radiotherapy. Clin Oncol 2002; 14: S40.

35. Veronesi U, Orecchia R, Luini A et al. A preliminary report of intraoperative radiotherapy (IORT) in limited-stage breast cancers that are conservatively treated. Eur J Cancer 2001; 37: 2178–83.

36. Vaidya JS, Baum M, Tobias JS et al. Targeted intra-operative radiotherapy (Targit): an innovative method of treatment for early breast cancer. Ann Oncol 2001; 12: 1075–80.

37. Vaidya JS, Tobias JS, Houghton J et al. Intra-operative breast radiation: the targeted intra-operative radiotherapy (Targit) trial. Breast Cancer Res Treat 2003; 82: S2.

38. Veronesi U, Cascinelle N, Mariani L et al. Twenty year follow up of a randomized study comparing breast conserving surgery with radical mastectomy for early breast cancer. N Eng J Med 2002; 347: 1227–32.

39. Walker P, Arthur D, Bartlink H et al. Workshop on partial breast irradiation: state of the art or science. Bethesda, MD. 8–10 December 2002. JNCI 2004; 96: 175–84.

40 Systemic adjuvant therapies for early breast cancer

Jean Abraham,* Cheryl Palmer,* Bristi Basu, Helena Earl

Introduction

In the Western world, breast cancer is the commonest cancer occurring in women and the second commonest cause of cancer-related death. Mortality rates in breast cancer have shown a decline since 1995.[1] This is thought to be due to ongoing changes in the treatments available and the delivery of these treatments to all women with breast cancer. The wider implementation of breast screening programmes is also beginning to impact on population mortality from breast cancer, as shown in the Scandinavian study reported in the Lancet.[2] Screening has changed the stage distribution at diagnosis, with more women now presenting with smaller cancers and a better prognosis.

As an introduction to this chapter on systemic therapy in early breast cancer, we will summarize two consensus statements and then discuss the evidence to support the conclusions made.

2000 NIH Consensus Conference[3,4]

The summary consensus from the above conference published in 2001 was as follows:

1. Accepted prognostic and predictive factors include age, tumour size, lymph node status, histological tumour type, grade, mitotic rate and hormone receptor status.
2. Novel technologies, including tissue and expression microarrays and proteomics, have great potential.

3. Adjuvant hormonal therapy should be offered only to women whose tumours express hormone receptor protein. Currently, 5 years of tamoxifen is standard adjuvant hormonal therapy, although ovarian ablation is an alternative for selected premenopausal women.
4. Adjuvant polychemotherapy improves survival and should be recommended to the majority of women with localized breast cancer, regardless of lymph node, menopausal or hormone receptor status.
5. Anthracycline-containing regimens confer a small but statistically significant improvement in survival when compared with non-anthracycline-containing regimens.
6. The role of taxanes in the adjuvant treatment of lymph node-positive breast cancer remains unclear.
7. Adjuvant dose-intensive chemotherapy regimens in high-risk breast cancer and the use of taxanes in node-negative breast cancer should be confined to randomized trials.
8. There is a need for trials to evaluate the role of adjuvant chemotherapy in women older than 70.
9. The effects of adjuvant treatments on a patient's quality of life need to be evaluated in randomized clinical trials, particularly premature menopause, weight gain, cognitive impairment and fatigue.

2003 St Gallen Consensus Conference[5]

The 2001 St Gallen Consensus Conference[6] had agreed that the treatment of node-positive breast cancer should be defined by age and biological

---

*Joint first authors – made equal contributions to the manuscript.

Table 40.1   Risk categories of node-negative breast cancer[a]

Risk group	Endocrine-responsive	Endocrine-unresponsive
Minimal-risk	ER and/or PgR expressed AND *all* the following features: pT ≤2 cm AND Grade 1 AND age ≥35	NA
Average-risk	ER and/or PgR expressed AND *at least one* of the following features: pT >2 cm OR grade 2–3 OR age <35	ER and PgR absent

ER, oestrogen receptor; PgR, progesterone receptor; NA, not applicable.
[a]Modified from the St Gallen 2001 Consensus.

---

characteristics. Risk categories in this group were eliminated. However, in women aged under 35 with hormone receptor-positive disease, it was felt that a combination of chemotherapy and endocrine treatment should be offered, and that chemotherapy alone was inadequate. In 2003, the consensus panel again concurred that nodal status is the principal determinant of baseline prognosis, with node-positive disease forming a separate risk group.

In these recommendations, there are two risk categories for node-negative disease (Table 40.1). Hormone responsiveness remains the primary determinant when deciding on adjuvant therapy (Table 40.2). If 10% or more of cells stain positively for either the oestrogen or progesterone receptor (ER or PgR), then this is considered a satisfactory threshold for endocrine responsiveness. If ER is absent then node-negative disease, which would otherwise be regarded as low-risk, becomes average-risk.

Hormonal treatments and related trials

Tamoxifen is a partial ER agonist and selective ER modulator (SERM). Approximately 75% of invasive

---

Table 40.2   Adjuvant systemic treatment recommendations for patients with operable breast cancer

Risk group	Endocrine-responsive		Endocrine-unresponsive	
	Premenopausal	Postmenopausal	Premenopausal	Postmenopausal
Node-negative minimal-risk	Tamoxifen *or* no treatment	Tamoxifen *or* no treatment	NA	NA
Node-negative average-risk	OA/GnRH analogue + tamoxifen [± chemotherapy] *or* Chemotherapy → tamoxifen [± GnRH analogue/OA] *or* GnRH analogue/OA	Tamoxifen *or* Chemotherapy → tamoxifen	Chemotherapy	Chemotherapy
Node-positive	Chemotherapy → tamoxifen [± GnRH analogue/OA] *or* OA/GnRH analogue + tamoxifen [± chemotherapy]	Chemotherapy → tamoxifen *or* Tamoxifen	Chemotherapy	Chemotherapy

NA, not applicable; OA, ovarian ablation; GnRH, gonadotrophin-releasing hormone.

breast cancer tumours express ER or PgR. Tamoxifen is the most commonly prescribed cancer drug, and until recently had an almost unimpeachable role in the treatment of hormone receptor-positive breast cancer for both pre- and postmenopausal women. Over the last 30 years, many studies have looked at the roles of tamoxifen in cancer therapy. The Early Breast Cancer Trialists' Collaborative Group (EBCTCG)[7] was set up to evaluate the large amount of statistically variable data produced by a multitude of trials. They published an overview in 1998, which looked at trials started prior to 1990, of tamoxifen versus no tamoxifen, mostly with 10 years of follow-up. Data were available on 37 000 women from 55 trials, of whom 18 000 had ER-positive tumours and 12 000 had unknown ER status. It was concluded that 5 years of tamoxifen was better than less than 5 years, with the proportional reductions in mortality risk at 1, 2 and 5 years being 14%, 18% and 28% respectively. This reduction is seen regardless of age and prior chemotherapy. With 15 years of follow-up, the 2000 Oxford Overview backed the survival benefit from tamoxifen.[8] Importantly, this review led to the concept of there being a gradation of benefit dependent upon the strength of ER-positivity. For patients with a strongly ER-positive tumour, the reduction in 10-year mortality is 36%. This concept has led to a greater emphasis on ER-positivity scoring from a pathological viewpoint (e.g. the Allred Score).

The 1998 EBCTCG overview also found that tamoxifen given following chemotherapy provides additional benefit. Again, 5 years of tamoxifen produced the best outcomes, whereby further proportional reductions in recurrence and mortality of 52% and 47% occurred, when compared with chemotherapy alone. Trials have now been performed comparing concurrent and sequential chemo-endocrine treatment, and early results reported at the 2002 meeting of the American Society of Clinical Oncology (ASCO) showed that sequential chemo-endocrine therapy with tamoxifen following chemotherapy results in improvements in survival.[9,10] Neither age nor menopausal status significantly altered the benefits produced by tamoxifen. No benefit was seen in women with ER-poor tumours. However, two trials analysed in the overview found tamoxifen to be of benefit in the small number of ER-negative/PgR-positive tumours. Tamoxifen was also shown to produce a relative risk reduction for cancer of around 30% in the contralateral breast. In premenopausal, node-negative, hormone receptor-positive, low-risk patients, chemotherapy is not standard treatment, and some might consider tamoxifen unnecessary, but its benefits in terms of secondary prevention deserve consideration.[11] Although tamoxifen has no impact on disease-free or overall survival in hormone recep-

tor-negative patients, it is likely to offer protection against a second primary cancer.

Trials such as aTTom (adjuvant Tamoxifen Treatment offer more) and ATLAS (Adjuvant Tamoxifen Longer Against Shorter) are looking at the value of extending tamoxifen treatment to beyond 5 years. These trials randomise ER-positive women to receive either 5 more years of tamoxifen or no further treatment. Some trials, including the National Surgical Adjuvant Breast and Bowel Project (NSABP) B14 trial, have, however, shown no survival advantage in those taking tamoxifen for more than 5 years.

In addition to an improvement in long-term survival from breast cancer, tamoxifen also helps to preserve bone and lipid metabolism.[6,12–14] However, tamoxifen carries risks of thromboembolism, endometrial cancer and visual disturbances, as well as less serious but potentially debilitating toxicities due to oestrogen withdrawal, including hot flushes and urogenital symptoms. There has been a need, therefore, for the development of both more effective and less toxic adjuvant hormonal treatments.

Aromatase inhibitors block the production of oestrone peripherally from androstenedione and the production of oestradiol from testosterone, both in the ovary and peripherally in the sites of hormone aromatization. In premenopausal women, their use may cause a reflex ovarian hyperstimulation syndrome and they are not recommended. Third-generation non-steroidal (triazole) aromatase inhibitors, such as anastrozole and letrozole (which suppress aromatase activity by 98%),[15] and the steroidal aromatase inhibitor exemestane, are being evaluated in clinical trials.

The role of tamoxifen as first-choice endocrine therapy is currently under review as the data regarding aromatase inhibitors begin to mature from some of the large randomized controlled trials. In January 2005, the ASCO Technology Assessment Panel reviewed the recent data from these trials and their implications for clinical practice.[16]

Three different designs of adjuvant trials with aromatase inhibitors in postmenopausal women are being or have been tested.[17] Some, but by no means all, of these trials are described below.

Direct comparison trials

The ATAC ('Arimidex' and Tamoxifen Alone or in Combination) trial was a phase III, multinational, multicentre, double-blind, randomized controlled trial.[18–20] It included 9366 postmenopausal women with early breast cancer and compared the tolerability and efficacy of anastrozole alone versus tamoxifen alone versus anastrozole plus tamoxifen. Where chemotherapy was used, it was completed prior to randomization. Initial analyses at 33 and 47 months led to the combination treatment arm being closed due to low efficacy. The reasons for this are not currently clear. After a median follow up of 68 months, anastrozole significantly increased disease-free survival (hazard ratio (HR) 0.87; 95% confidence interval (CI) 0.78–0.97; $p = 0.01$) and time to recurrence. Anastrozole also significantly reduced distant metastases and contralateral breast cancers. Although both tamoxifen and anastrozole were relatively well tolerated, anastrozole was superior in terms of a lower incidence of hot flushes, urogenital symptoms, weight gain, thromboembolism, ischaemic cerebrovascular events and endometrial cancer. However, tamoxifen afforded greater protection against musculo- skeletal disorders and fractures. It may be that the aromatase inhibitors will need to be combined routinely with a bisphosphonate, and the ASCO panel recommend routine bone density monitoring with appropriate treatment implementation for osteoporosis in women on aromatase inhibitors.

Sequential trials

The IES (Intergroup Exemestane Study)[21] randomized 4742 women between treatment with 2 or 3 years of tamoxifen either to continue for a total of 5 years or to receive exemestane to complete 5 years of hormonal therapy. At a median follow-up of 30.6 months, significant reductions were found in recurrences, contralateral breast cancer and deaths in the exemestane arm.

As a consequence of the results of IES, the TEAM trial, which originally involved a 5-year direct comparison between tamoxifen and exemestane, was stopped. It has restarted with a new sequential design of exemestane for 5 years versus tamoxifen for 2–3 years switching to exemestane for completion of 5 years of treatment.

The Italian Study (ITA)[22] was designed similarly to IES, but using anastrozole instead of exemestane. It only enrolled 426 patients and has not yet reported definitive effects.

The Breast International Group (BIG) 01-98 trial was a randomised four-arm study using letrozole 2.5 mg and tamoxifen 20 mg. It randomized 8028 patients between (1) 5 years of tamoxifen, (2) 5 years of letrozole, (3) 2 years of tamoxifen followed by 3 years of letrozole or (4) 2 years of letrozole followed by 3 years of tamoxifen, each arm having 5 years of follow-up. At 3 years, the results, presented at St

Gallen in 2005, indicate that letrozole prolongs disease-free survival (HR 0.81) in comparison with tamoxifen. Letrozole was associated with an increased risk of bone fractures but a reduced risk of venous thrombosis.

Additive trials

In the National Cancer Institute of Canada (NCIC) Intergroup trial MA-17, 5187 postmenopausal women who were ER-positive or ER-unknown, and disease-free following 5 years of adjuvant tamoxifen, were randomized either to 5 years of further treatment with letrozole or to placebo.[23] After a median follow-up of 28.8 months, the data safety monitoring board stopped the study as a result of a significant reduction in breast cancer events within the letrozole arm of the trial. The study showed an overall benefit in distant disease-free survival and a statistically significant survival advantage for women who had node-positive disease.

In a similar study using exemestane, the NSABP B-33 trial randomized patients between further treatment with 2 years of exemestane or observation upon completion of 5 years of tamoxifen.

The outcomes of these aromatase inhibitor trials pose a number of questions relating to the use and indications for both tamoxifen and aromatase inhibitors, for which some answers and guidance have been given by the ASCO Technology Panel.

1. *Is there sufficient new evidence to recommend that aromatase inhibitors be used as initial adjuvant therapy in postmenopausal women with ER-positive breast cancer?* It is apparent from the above studies that aromatase inhibitors are the optimal treatment for any post-menopausal women with ER-positive breast cancer for whom tamoxifen is contraindicated. However, for postmenopausal women with ER-positive breast cancer with no contraindication to tamoxifen, the answer is still not entirely clear. The ASCO panel decision was that the optimal adjuvant hormonal therapy for postmenopausal women with ER-positive breast cancer should include an aromatase inhibitor either as initial therapy or after treatment with tamoxifen.

2. *Are there particular patient groups who should receive initial aromatase inhibitor therapy rather than tamoxifen?* The ASCO panel had previously stipulated that any postmenopausal women who develop breast cancer while receiving tamoxifen or other SERMs should be treated with an aromatase inhibitor. Some members of

the panel felt that data from the ATAC trial indicated that postmenopausal women with ER-positive, PgR-negative breast cancer might receive greater benefit from initial aromatase inhibitor therapy. Postmenopausal women with HER2-overexpressing breast cancers had exhibited higher response rates with aromatase inhibitors. However, the number of women with HER2-overexpressing tumours in the ATAC trial was small, and so currently there is no clear answer to this question.

3. *Do the MA-17 results indicate that aromatase inhibitors should be used in postmenopausal women with ER-positive breast cancer who have completed 5 years of therapy with tamoxifen?* MA-17 is the only trial to produce a statistically significant overall survival advantage ($p = 0.04$). This was seen in the node-positive subgroup. The median follow-up from MA-17 is only 2.5 years, and so it is reasonable to recommend a minimum of 2.5 years of an aromatase inhibitor after completion of tamoxifen treatment, especially in those with node-positive disease.

4. *Do the IES and ITA results indicate that aromatase inhibitors should be used in postmenopausal women with ER-positive breast cancer who have had 2–3 years of tamoxifen therapy?* The optimum timing of any switch from tamoxifen to aromatase inhibitors is uncertain. Changing treatment after 2–3 years in the IES trial produced a 4.7% projected absolute difference in disease-free survival at 3 years. It cannot be concluded that switching treatment after 2–3 years is advantageous for most patients, since the trials did not investigate treatment after extended years.

5. *What is the optimal duration of adjuvant treatment with aromatase inhibitors?* Current trials have not yet addressed the issue of whether more than 5 years of treatment with an aromatase inhibitor would confer additional benefit. It is now planned to extend NSABP B-33 and MA-17 beyond 10 years in order to answer this question. Those women who received an aromatase inhibitor in years 6–10 will now have the option to be re-randomised and to either continue with their aromatase inhibitor or receive a placebo for years 11–15.

Other issues are also still outstanding. It is not known whether initial use of an aromatase inhibitor followed by tamoxifen would be more effective. In women who are rendered amenorrhoeic by chemotherapy, the use of aromatase inhibitors may be unwise. These women are not necessarily biochemically postmenopausal. Trials are currently running to assess whether an aromatase inhibitor in combination with ovarian ablation might be efficacious in premenopausal women. Until results are available, the ASCO panel do not recommend such treatment unless patients are enrolled in a relevant trial. These include (i) the Austrian Breast Cancer Study Group (ABCSG) trial 12 comparing 3 years of tamoxifen plus goserelin with 3 years of anastrozole plus goserelin; (ii) SOFT (Suppression of Ovarian Function Trial: International Breast Cancer Study group (IBCSG) 24-02) looking at 5 years of tamoxifen versus ovarian ablation plus tamoxifen versus ovarian ablation plus exemestane (where ovarian ablation can be achieved with bilateral oophorectomy, radiation or triptorelin); and (iii) TEXT (Tamoxifen and EXemestane Trial: IBCSG 25-02), using 5 years of tamoxifen plus triptorelin or 5 years of exemestane plus triptorelin. It is also as yet uncertain whether the third-generation aromatase inhibitors can be used interchangeably.

The technology assessment by the ASCO panel has produced guidelines only, and the ultimate decision regarding treatment choice will rest with the clinician and the patient. Other areas will also need to be looked at, such as mechanisms of hormone resistance, the potential role of other SERMs, and combinations of treatments including cytokines and other new biological agents. Within all of these adjuvant trials, the primary endpoint is disease-free survival. However, it is imperative that the impact of hormonal manipulation on quality of life, organ toxicities, bone and lipid metabolism, and cognitive function also be taken into account. Emerging results indicate that aromatase inhibitors in ER-positive postmenopausal women in the adjuvant setting *may* become the hormonal treatment of choice.

Ovarian suppression and related trials

Ovarian ablation has long been known to improve outcomes in premenopausal women. The EBCTG performed a meta-analysis of at least 12 trials in 1996.[24] Patients had had either surgical or radiation-induced ovarian suppression. From these data, it was clear that ovarian ablation improves both disease-free and overall survival, but the significance of ER status and whether ablation provided additional benefits on top of chemotherapy were not apparent. This meta-analysis also showed that the benefits of ovarian ablation might be reduced in patients who have had prior chemotherapy (because of chemotherapy-induced amenorrhoea). The proportional improvement in overall survival is 24% in the absence of chemotherapy but only 8% in those who have received chemotherapy. For women aged less than 50 ovarian ablation produced a 20% proportional reduction in 15-year mortality. However, in women who continue to menstruate, ovarian ablation is of greater benefit. Women who develop chemotherapy-induced amenorrhoea tend to have a better prognosis.[25–27] The IBCSG trials I, II, V and VI showed that women aged under 35 have a particularly poor prognosis despite adjuvant chemotherapy, which is worse if they are ER-positive and did not achieve chemotherapy-induced amenorrhoea. Chemotherapy alone is not adequate in this group of patients.[28]

Goserelin (Zoladex) is a luteinizing hormone releasing hormone (LHRH) receptor agonist. The LHRH receptor agonists produce medical castration, suppressing ovarian function in pre- and perimenopausal women after initial stimulation. They have some obvious advantages over surgical or radiation-induced ovarian suppression. They are potentially reversible on cessation of treatment, so allowing preservation of fertility. In the ZEBRA (Zoladex Early Breast Cancer Research Association) trial, following 2 years of goserelin treatment, menses returned in 90% of women aged 40 or less and in 70% of women over 40.[29–31] There have also been some recent reports of the use of LHRH agonists concurrently with chemotherapy, in women younger than 40 in an attempt to preserve fertility following adjuvant systemic chemotherapy.[32] Premature menopause that is irreversible carries with it increased risks of heart disease and osteoporosis, and, in addition, surgical procedures require an anaesthetic. Ovarian radiation also suppresses ovarian function more slowly than LHRH agonists.[33]

Trials with goserelin have been set up to answer two major questions:

1. Does goserelin with or without tamoxifen provide an alternative to chemotherapy in patients with ER-positive disease?
2. Does goserelin confer any additional benefit when combined with standard treatment (surgery ± radiotherapy ± tamoxifen ± chemotherapy)?

The optimum duration of LHRH agonists is not yet known and has not been properly addressed. Two years of goserelin is generally recommended; this recommendation originates from the ZEBRA trial, where, at the time, 2 years of adjuvant tamoxifen together with goserelin was given. It is also not clear whether there are subsets of premenopausal hormone receptor-positive women (depending, for example, on age, grade of tumour, or other newer molecular classifiers) who would derive most benefit from ovarian ablation. All premenopausal women have been eligible to enter the various ovarian ablation trials, and it is well established that those achieving chemotherapy-induced amenorrhoea probably gain little from this additional intervention. Thus, trials involving only women who do

not achieve chemotherapy-induced amenorrhoea are proposed in order to compare ovarian ablation with no ovarian ablation.

Trials looking into goserelin with or without tamoxifen as an alternative to chemotherapy include the ZEBRA trial, ABCSG AC05[34,35] and the Italian Breast Cancer Adjuvant Study Group (GROCTA) 02 trials.[36,37]

The ZEBRA trial was a large (1640 patients) randomised, multicentre, international trial. Node-positive pre- and perimenopausal women, following surgery, were randomized between monthly goserelin for 2 years versus 6 cycles of CMF (cyclophosphamide, methotrexate and 5-fluorouracil (5-FU)) chemotherapy. The mean follow-up was 7.3 years. In ER-positive patients, goserelin and CMF were equivalent in terms of overall, disease-free and distant disease-free survival, whilst in ER-negative patients, CMF was superior. Amenorrhoea occurred in both groups, but more rapidly and more often reversibly in those who received goserelin. In a subgroup analysis, there was no difference in bone mineral density, although initially there was greater loss in the goserelin group with some recovery on cessation of treatment. Quality of life, not surprisingly, was better in those on goserelin.

The ABCSG AC05 study involved 1034 hormone receptor-positive premenopausal women. Following surgery, they were randomized between monthly goserelin for 3 years with tamoxifen for 5 years and 6 cycles of CMF. At a median follow-up of 60 months, disease-free survival was in favour of the goserelin and tamoxifen arm and there was a non-statistically significant trend in favour of goserelin and tamoxifen in terms of overall survival.

A smaller number of patients were involved in the GROCTA 02 study, where 244 ER-positive pre- or perimenopausal women were allocated either 6 cycles of CMF chemotherapy or ovarian suppression (goserelin for 2 years, ovarian irradiation or oophorectomy), together with tamoxifen for 5 years. The mean follow-up was 89 months, and no significant differences in disease-free or overall survival were found.

It is probably safe to conclude from these trials that in ER-positive pre- and perimenopausal women, goserelin has equivalent efficacy (disease-free survival) to that of CMF, and that goserelin plus tamoxifen is at least as effective as CMF chemotherapy without the cytotoxic side-effects. However, as new chemotherapy regimens emerge, especially with anthracyclines being standard treatment, it is not known whether ovarian ablation will still be of equal efficacy.

Trials examining the role of goserelin in addition to standard treatment include the ZIPP (Zoladex In Premenopausal Patients) trial,[38,39] an Intergroup trial, INT-0101[40] and the IBCSG VIII trial.[41,42]

The ZIPP trial enrolled 2710 women, of any ER status, and initially had four arms: (1) goserelin for 2 years, (2) tamoxifen for 2 years, (3) goserelin and tamoxifen for 2 years; or (4) no treatment following standard adjuvant therapy. However, as preliminary results were emerging in favour of tamoxifen, many centres decided to give this agent routinely. Initial results from this trial are available for a median of 5 years of follow-up. Goserelin produced a significant improvement in disease-free and overall survival. The greatest benefit was seen in women with ER-positive tumours who had not received prior chemotherapy.[43]

INT-0101 involved 1504 women with ER-positive, node-positive tumours. Following surgery, all patients received CAF (cyclophosphamide, doxorubicin and 5-FU) chemotherapy. The three arms of the trial then involved (1) no further treatment; (2) goserelin for 5 years or (3) goserelin and tamoxifen for 5 years. The median follow-up was 6.2 years. A significant improvement in 5-year disease-free survival was apparent for the arm with goserelin and tamoxifen (77%) as compared with goserelin alone (70%), which in turn was better than chemotherapy alone (67%). No difference was seen in overall survival.

The IBCSG VIII trial recruited 1063 pre- or perimenopausal node-negative breast cancer patients. It used four arms initially, but the no-treatment arm was dropped. The remaining three arms were: (1) six cycles of CMF followed by goserelin for 2 years, (2) six cycles of CMF or (3) goserelin for 2 years. Results have been reported at a median follow-up of 7 years, the primary endpoint being disease-free survival. For women with ER-positive disease, chemotherapy alone was equivalent to goserelin alone, with a 5-year disease-free survival rate of 81%, whereas sequential treatment provided a non-significant improvement in DFS of 86%. In women whose disease was ER-negative, CMF produced a 5-year disease-free survival rate of 88% and goserelin only 73%. It was concluded from this study that in this subset of women, those who are ER-negative should receive chemotherapy and those who are ER-positive should be considered either for chemotherapy and ovarian ablation or ovarian ablation alone. However, it should be remembered that ovarian ablation was equivalent to CMF and has not been compared with newer chemotherapy regimes.

The SOFT study is ascertaining whether the addition of ovarian ablation offers any benefit.

Current practice generally recommends that ovarian suppression by whatever means should be a key feature of adjuvant treatment in high-risk premenopausal women with early breast cancer. LHRH analogues may prove to be the best way of achieving this. Along with the NIH 2000 Consensus and the 2001 St Gallen Consensus, the European Society of Mastology (EUSOMA) drew up guidelines for the endocrine therapy of breast cancer in March 2002.[44] It was agreed and proposed that premenopausal women should be offered an LHRH agonist for 2 years, with or without 5 years of tamoxifen or chemotherapy. LHRH agonists should also be offered to premenopausal women who fail to become amenorrhoeic with chemotherapy, in whom menses return after completion of chemotherapy, or whose levels of oestrogens or follicle-stimulating hormone fail to fall adequately.

Adjuvant chemotherapy

The benefits of adjuvant chemotherapy derive from a direct cytotoxic effect on the tumour cells and/or an indirect effect mediated by suppression of oestrogen function in premenopausal women. Evidence supporting the role of adjuvant chemotherapy in early breast cancer is presented in the overview by the EBCTCG.[45] This report was the result of over a decade of collection and analysis of individual patient data from 18 000 women enrolled into 47 trials beginning before 1990. This analysis looked at the effect of prolonged polychemotherapy versus no chemotherapy. The overview also analysed data from 6000 women in 11 trials involving shorter versus longer durations of chemotherapy and data from 6000 women in 11 trials of anthracycline-containing regimens versus CMF. The results showed the following:

- Polychemotherapy produced a significant proportional reduction in recurrence of 35% in women younger than 50 and 20% in women aged 50–69. Unfortunately, few women aged over 70 had been included.
- Polychemotherapy produced proportional reductions in mortality of 27% in women younger than 50 and 11% in women aged 50–69.
- The reduction in recurrence was mainly observed in the first 5 years of follow-up. However, the difference in survival was seen in the first 10 years.
- Proportional reductions in risk were similar for women with lymph node-positive or node-negative disease.
- In women younger than 50 with node-negative disease, the 10-year survival rate increases from

71% increases to 78% (an absolute benefit of 7%) and in those with node-positive disease, the 10-year survival rate increases from 42% to 53% (an absolute benefit of 11%).

- In women aged 50–69 with node-negative disease, the 10-year survival rate increases from 67% to 69% (an absolute benefit of 2%) and in those with node-positive disease, the 10-year survival rate increases from 46% to 49% (an absolute benefit of 3%).
- The benefits of polychemotherapy seemed to occur irrespective of hormone receptor status, menopausal status at presentation and use of tamoxifen.
- Comparisons of shorter versus longer durations of chemotherapy did not show any survival advantage for treatment lengths longer than 3–6 months.

Overall, combination chemotherapy is a more effective adjuvant therapy than single-agent chemotherapy, reducing the annual risk of death by about 20%.[46] The effects of combination chemotherapy are most marked in women younger than 60 and those who were premenopausal when commencing treatment.

Evidence for use of anthracycline-containing regimens versus CMF

Deciding which combination chemotherapy to use is dependent upon recurrence risk, patient preference, performance status and comorbidities. The EBCTCG 1998 overview analysed data from 6000 women in 11 trials of anthracycline-containing regimens versus CMF. Anthracycline regimens demonstrated reduced recurrence and mortality rates, although at the time the available data were not complete. In September 2000, this overview was updated.[7] There were then 14 000 women in 15 trials. The data confirmed that anthracycline regimens continued to yield greater benefit in terms of reduction in recurrence and mortality rates in comparison with CMF. This benefit lasted for 10 years, with an absolute gain of about 4% in recurrence and survival in node-positive women. For node-negative women, there is an absolute survival gain of 1.7% at 5 years. In the individual trials, treatment benefit was almost exclusively found where anthracyclines were given in an intensive schedule with other chemotherapy agents.

The two main anthracyclines used in Europe and North America are epirubicin and doxorubicin. There are no trials directly comparing the efficacy of these two drugs in the adjuvant setting. However, a meta-analysis of 13 randomized trials comparing epirubicin and doxorubicin in metastatic breast cancer showed that epirubicin was equally efficacious and had fewer toxicities at equivalent doses.[47]

Optimal treatment length, dose and schedule of chemotherapy

The EBCTCG overview analysed data from 6000 women in 11 trials involving shorter versus longer durations of chemotherapy. No significant improvements in recurrence or mortality rates were gained by use of chemotherapy for longer than 6 months. The NSABP B-15 trial compared six cycles of CMF versus four cycles of AC (doxorubicin and cyclophosphamide) versus four cycles of AC followed by three cycles of CMF.[48] The results of this trial showed that four cycles of AC were equivalent to six cycles of CMF.

A number of trials have examined the issue of dose escalation and optimal dose. The NSABP B-22 trial[49] involved 2305 node-positive women randomized to receive AC chemotherapy. In each arm the dose and intensity of doxorubicin remained the same but the dose and intensity of cyclophosphamide were varied. No difference in overall survival or disease-free survival was seen in either the dose-intensified or dose-escalated arms compared with the standard arm (600 mg/m²). In the Cancer and Leukemia Group B (CALGB) 9344 study, dose escalation of doxorubicin in 3170 node-positive women randomized to 60 (standard), 70 or 90 mg/m² showed no improvement in overall or disease-free survival with higher dosage.[50]

However, in the recently reported CALGB 9741 taxane-containing study, which randomized patients between arms examining dose-dense (chemotherapy given 2-weekly with granulocyte colony-stimulating factor (G-CSF) support) and scheduling issues, there was a clear advantage in terms of disease-free and overall survival for women receiving dose-dense therapy.[51] Quality of life was also improved with G-CSF, and this study showed that not only was treatment completed more quickly, but it was on the whole more tolerable. We will not review high-dose chemotherapy studies in this chapter but given the negative results of all such studies, the results of randomized studies such as CALGB 9741 are of considerable interest. There is a strong hint that more intensive therapy does provide an advantage for moderate- and high-risk women with breast cancer, and that there is indeed an important dose-intensity/response relationship for adjuvant chemotherapy.

Following the successful CALGB 9741 adjuvant study, showing a strongly positive result for dose-dense therapy, it is of interest to consider early reports of piloted adjuvant treatments from this group. There has been a report of a pilot adjuvant phase II study of dose-dense FEC (5-FU, epirubicin and cyclophosphamide) followed by weekly paclitaxel and docetaxel.[52] This phase II study looked at both feasibility and efficacy. FEC (500:100:500 mg/m^2) was given in a dose-dense schedule every 2 weeks for six cycles with G-CSF support, followed by weekly paclitaxel (80 mg/m^2) and docetaxel (35 mg/m^2) for 18 weeks (a total of 30 weeks of treatment). Unfortunately, this dose-dense schedule produced significant toxicity, with grade 3/4 pneumonitis in 4 of 44 (9%) patients with symptoms severe enough to require prolonged hospitalization. This complication seemed wholly attributable to the dose-dense FEC. Seventeen patients proceeded with the second phase of weekly taxanes for 18 weeks, and, after completion of this, 2 of 17 (11%) patients developed severe pleural and pericardial effusions, again requiring hospitalization. This protocol is not being developed further for high-risk patients, and may set an upper limit to the degree of intensification achievable with G-CSF support alone rather than stem cell haematological support.

One study reported at ASCO 2003 addresses both an anthracycline and a scheduling question.[53] NEAT (National Epirubicin Adjuvant Trial) and McNEAT (BR9601 Scottish Cancer Therapy Network Trial) were presented as a prospectively agreed meta-analysis. The trial shows a very significant advantage for ECMF (epirubicin four cycles then CMF four cycles) chemotherapy in terms of both disease-free survival (HR 0.69; 95% CI 0.57–0.83; p<0.0001) and overall survival (HR 0.65; 95% CI 0.52–0.80; p<0.0001) when compared with standard classical CMF for six cycles. This is the first large adjuvant chemotherapy study (2391 patients) to be carried out in the UK and is a seminal result for the UK breast cancer research community. The study is the most strongly positive amongst the few individual trials that demonstrate an advantage for anthracycline-based chemotherapy.[54,55] This advantage is demonstrated across all stratification groups and, although there are some differences between subgroups, there is no statistically significant interaction. The study has been reported as a preplanned meta-analysis with a smaller trial run by the Scottish Cancer Therapy Network, which asked broadly similar questions. The analysis was event-driven and the fact that it was carried out 18 months after the predicted date suggests another important observation. The results for patients treated in the standard CMF arm were considerably better than those that had been predicted before the trial started. The trial has shown an advantage for the Bonadonna block-scheduling anthracycline approach,[56] and has also improved outcomes for breast cancer patients by insisting on adherence to the two classical CMF

schedules (oral or intravenous cyclophosphamide). Direct comparisons in the metastatic setting had already shown 3-weekly CMF to be inferior, and Bonadonna's analysis of his original CMF study showed that less than 85% dose delivery of classical CMF resulted in inferior outcomes.[57] The group reported at ASCO 2002 that the ECMF regimen is tolerable.[58] Quality-of-life data have been collected longitudinally over 24 months, and again set a standard for adjuvant chemotherapy trials in breast cancer. This study confirms the benefit of anthracyclines and shows that, unlike four cycles of AC, which was shown to be equivalent to the ECMF block scheduling is definitely superior to classical CMF. The emergence of myelodysplastic syndromes (MDS) and acute myeloid leukaemia (AML) in the FEC D1 and 8 studies (the only other studies to show in a 'stand-alone way' the superiority of anthracyclines) is of concern.[59] To date, no cases of MDS or AML have been reported in either the NEAT or the Scottish studies, although follow-up in this study is shorter (median duration 37 months). However, with longer follow-up, epirubicin 400 mg/m^2 given in this schedule will hopefully prove not only effective but also safer than the more intensive FEC schedules.

Taxanes

Taxanes (paclitaxel and docetaxel) are a new class of chemotherapeutic agents, for which there is emerging evidence to support their use in the adjuvant setting in moderate- and high-risk younger patients.

The CALGB 9344 trial, involved 3121 node-positive women who were randomized to receive either four cycles of AC alone or four cycles of AC followed by four cycles of paclitaxel.[50] At a median follow-up of 69 months, there is no effect of doxorubicin dose escalation on disease-free or overall survival. However, the addition of paclitaxel given sequentially provides hazard ratios for disease-free survival of 0.83 (95% CI 0.73–0.94; p = 0.0023) and for overall survival of 0.82 (95% CI 0.71–0.95; p = 0.0064) for all 3121 patients randomized. In an unplanned subset analysis, the hazard ratio for disease-free survival of additional paclitaxel was 0.72 (95% CI 0.59–0.86) for ER-negative tumours (1279 patients), whereas ER-positive tumours (94% treated with tamoxifen sequentially) showed a hazard ratio of 0.92 (95% CI 0.79–1.08). This paper therefore suggests a significant interaction between additional paclitaxel and ER status (with or without tamoxifen). However, this is not confirmed in other trials (see below), and although ER status is balanced in the two arms of the study, it is important to remember that this was neither a stratification factor nor was there a preplanned subgroup analysis on the basis of ER status.

Other trials include the NSABP B-28 in which node-positive women were randomized to receive either four cycles of AC alone or four cycles of AC followed by four cycles of paclitaxel. At ASCO 2003, Mamounas et al[60] presented the updated results of this study, which examined the additional treatment of four cycles of paclitaxel 225 mg/m^2 to the standard of four cycles of AC. In this study, 3060 patients were randomized, and there is now a median follow-up of 64 months. Disease-free survival shows a relative risk of relapse of 0.83 ($p = 0.008$) in favour of the addition of paclitaxel, although overall survival does not show the same advantage (relative risk 0.94; $p = 0.46$). There appears to be no interaction of taxanes with ER-positivity, although a confounding factor may be the concomitant treatment of ER-positive patients with tamoxifen. If there was an interaction with ER-positivity (i.e. less effect of taxanes in ER-positive patients) then the effect might be exaggerated by the early addition of tamoxifen. The interaction of chemotherapy and tamoxifen appears to be a negative one, presumably because of the reduction in mitotic rate from tamoxifen acting as a cytotoxic agent in ER-positive tumours.

In terms of number deaths in this study, there are no significant differences between the standard and experimental arms. This is perhaps because the prognosis of patients is very good and it is too early to detect differences in survival (median of 64 months follow-up). This study now supports the earlier results of CALGB 9344,[50] which show a benefit from the addition of taxanes. However, in this earlier study, there was a clear interaction between ER status and benefit of taxanes, although there are now rather more studies showing lack of any interaction than studies showing any positive interaction for ER-negative disease.[61]

This report again reiterates the difference in biology between hormone receptor-positive and -negative disease. Analysis of relapse and survival in the first 5 years is more informative for the hormone receptor-negative group, for whom the majority of events have already occurred. This contrasts with the hormone receptor-positive population, for whom many more events occur after the 5-year time point.[62] Similarly, the interaction of chemotherapy treatments seems to have more effect in the hormone receptor-negative population within the first 5 years, and in the hormone receptor-positive population after this time.[63] This makes some sense when tumour biology is taken into account, and it should be remembered when analysing these adjuvant studies – this particular study includes 66% hormone receptor-positive women.

The NSABP B-27 trial compared neoadjuvant (i.e. preoperative) AC four cycles alone versus neoadjuvant AC four cycles followed by postoperative docetaxel four cycles versus neoadjuvant AC four cycles followed by neoadjuvant docetaxel four cycles. A 65% clinical response rate was seen in the AC–docetaxel neoadjuvant arm compared with a 40% response in the other two arms. Similarly, the pathological complete response rate was significantly increased in the same arm: 25.6% versus 13.7%.[64] However, at the 2004 San Antonio Breast Cancer Symposium, it was reported that there was no survival advantage with taxane use in this trial.[64]

Two trials, BCIRG-01 and PACS-01, have looked at docetaxel efficacy in node-positive breast cancer, purportedly using more intensive anthracycline-based control arms. BCIRG was reported at a median follow-up of 55 months at the 2003 San Antonio Breast Cancer Symposium and has been recently published.[65] It compared six cycles of FAC (5-FU, doxorubicin and cyclophosphamide) with six cycles of TAC (docetaxel, doxorubicin and cyclophosphamide), with overall survival rates of 81% and 87% respectively ($p = 0.01$). This led to widespread use of TAC as standard chemotherapy in the USA. However, there has been one study showing that FAC is equivalent to CMF administered 3–weekly,[66] and hence there is less enthusiasm to adopt TAC in Europe.

PACS-01 compared six cycles of FEC was compared with three of FEC followed by three of docetaxel. At a median follow-up of 60 months, the overall survival rates were 87% and 91% respectively. The use of an anthracycline regimen known to be more effective than CMF may prove to be practice-changing, and Europe may switch to a standard adjuvant regimen containing taxanes.

There are a number of ongoing trials involving over 22 000 women and as yet unreported, that will help to clarify the role of taxanes in the adjuvant setting in early breast cancer. In particular, the UK trial (TACT) has just completed recruiting over 4000 women. This study examines the addition of docetaxel four cycles to anthracycline-based chemotherapy. Standard treatment in the trial was either the ECMF experimental arm from the recently reported NEAT study[53] or eight cycles of day 1-only FEC. The recently initiated adjuvant studies across the world will incorporate detailed analysis of molecular markers (assessing candidate genes and microarrays) to define new predictive and prognostic markers.

HER2/*neu*

A greater understanding of the biology of cancer is leading to more specifically targeted therapies.

Predicting which cases of early breast cancer will benefit from certain treatments will avoid unnecessary toxicity. Human epidermal growth factor receptor 2 (HER2) is a 185 kDa transmembrane tyrosine kinase that is expressed by normal and malignant breast epithelial cells and is overexpressed in 25–30% of all breast cancers.[67] Women with HER2-positive breast cancer have a poorer prognosis.[67–70] HER2/neu gene overexpression is often associated with other adverse prognostic factors, including ER and PgR negativity,[71] higher tumour stage,[69] higher tumour grade,[72] increased number of positive axillary lymph nodes[68] and DNA ploidy.[73] Both visceral and osseous metastases are more common in breast cancers that overexpress HER2/neu. It may be that increased epidermal growth factor receptor (EGFR) levels increase metastatic spread.[74,75] HER2 positivity may also increase resistance to CMF chemotherapy and hormonal manipulation;[76] however, the evidence for this is not conclusive.

Trastuzumab (Herceptin) is a humanized recombinant monoclonal IgG that targets HER2. In March 2002, the National Institute of Clinical Excellence (NICE) in the UK issued guidelines on the use of trastuzumab in advanced breast cancer. Its role in the adjuvant setting has yet to be determined and clinical trials are ongoing. These include (1) NSABP B-31 looking at AC four cycles followed by either paclitaxel alone or paclitaxel and trastuzumab; (2) the Intergroup study, which involves AC four cycles followed by paclitaxel alone, or paclitaxel and trastuzumab together, or paclitaxel then trastuzumab; and (3) HERA, in which women receiving any chemotherapy and/or radiotherapy are randomized to 3-weekly trastuzumab for 12 months or 24 months or to observation only. The choice of taxanes is based on results from metastatic breast cancer trials where trastuzumab has been found to increase the effectiveness of chemotherapy with doxorubicin or paclitaxel.[77] There are potential limitations to the use of trastuzumab in early breast cancer due to cardiotoxicity in patients treated concurrently or previously with anthracyclines, which at present are accepted standard chemotherapy in this setting.

Controversial issues

1. *What is the optimal treatment for elderly (>70) women with average- to high-risk hormone receptor-negative tumours?* The answer to this question is uncertain because chemotherapy trials to date have excluded this age group. In fit elderly women who have a good quality of life and performance status, it may be reasonable to treat them in a similar manner to postmenopausal hormone receptor-negative women aged under 70. Many trials addressing

this issue are underway worldwide.

2. *What is the optimal treatment for women with small (<1 cm) hormone receptor-negative tumours?* The problems associated with answering this question include small, underpowered trials without data on hormone receptor status and difficulties with amounts of tissue available for analysis of hormone receptor status.[78] Analysis of published data shows that a favourable histological grade is associated with a good prognosis and that blood or lymphatic vessel invasion is a poor prognostic indicator. In clinical practice, nodal status, together with tumour size and tumour grade, are used to assess risk of recurrence. In the UK, the Nottingham Prognostic Index (NPI)[79] is used to help determine the relative risk of recurrence: NPI = tumour size (cm) × 0.2 + nodal stage + tumour grade) (where nodal stage is determined as follows: no nodes involved = 1; 1–3 nodes involved = 2; ≥4 nodes involved = 3). On the basis of this index and individual patient characteristics and choice, a decision is made regarding treatment options.[80] The NPI has never been popular in the USA where a combination of staging with the AJCC TNM scoring system together with prognostic information derived from SEER (Surveillance, Epidemiology and End-Results) tends to be used. Histological grade is not routinely factored into the decision-making process in the USA. Lately, the web-based programme Adjuvant! (www.adjuvantonline.com) has become widely accepted in both Europe and the USA. It was developed to incorporate grade and TNM/SEER and has been independently validated.[81] The answer to the above question may be clarified in the future by using microarray technology to establish an expression signature, which may predict high-risk patients and early onset of metastatic disease.[82–84]

Summary

We have presented here evidence for the use of hormonal treatment and chemotherapy as adjuvant therapy in early breast cancer for both pre- and postmenopausal women. To date, the majority of information is available from large randomized trials looking at combinations of hormone manipulation and chemotherapy. New agents, combinations and schedules are being tested as these emerge from development programmes of academic institutions and the pharmaceutical industry. Human genome and breast cancer genome research heralds a new era in which we may be able to answer some outstanding fundamental questions in this field. Which women really need treatment? And what treatment do they need? At present, our clinical decisions at an individual patient level are far from accurate. As clinicians, we are aware of the inadequacy of our clinical decision-making and the failure of our present-day prognostic and predictive scores to individualize therapy for our patients. On the one hand, the desire to provide treatments that curativere may result only in overtreatment of women without 'significant' micrometastatic disease. But, on the other hand, our desire to lessen the burden of adjuvant treatments may result in relapse and death of our patients. These dilemmas and difficulties are apparent to clinicians on a daily basis during their interactions with early breast cancer patients. Decision-making at present seems to be more of an 'art-form' and needs to become more of a 'science'. The molecular age will yield tests that will identify patients with 'significant' micrometastatic disease at the outset, and will eventually deliver tests which predict response to current hormonal agents and chemotherapy and to a range of newer agents that will become available to our patients in the near future.

We hope that this chapter is helpful for clinicians facing the difficult problem of advising women with early breast cancer on optimal forms of systemic therapy.

References

1. Beral V, Hermon C, Reeves, Peto R. Sudden fall in breast cancer death rates in England and Wales. Lancet 1995; 345: 1642–43.

2. Tabar L, Yen MF, Vitak B et al. Mammography service screening and mortality in breast cancer patients: 20-year follow-up before and after introduction of screening. Lancet 2003; 361: 1405–10.

3. National Institutes of Health Consensus Development Conference. J Natl Cancer Inst Monogr 2001; 30: 1–152.

4. National Institutes of Health Consensus Development Conference Statement. Adjuvant Therapy for Breast Cancer, November 1–3, 2000. J Clin Oncol 2001; 93: 979–89.

5. Senn H-J, Thürlimann B, Goldhirsch A et al. Comments on the St. Gallen Consensus 2003 on the Primary Therapy of Early Breast Cancer. Breast 2003; 12: 569–82.

6. Goldhirsch A, Glick JH, Gelber RD et al. Meeting Highlights: International Consensus Panel on the Treatment of Primary Breast Cancer. J Clin Oncol 2001; 19: 3817–27.

7. Early Breast Cancer Trialists' Collaborative Group. Tamoxifen for early breast cancer: an overview of the randomised trials. Lancet 1998; 351: 1451–67.

8. Early Breast Cancer Trialists' Collaborative Group. 2000 analysis overview results. Fifth Meeting of the Early Breast Cancer Trialists' Collaborative Group. Oxford, UK, 21–23 September 2000.

9. Albain KS, Green SJ, Ravdin PM et al, for SWOG, ECOG, CALGB, NCCTG, and NCIC-CTG. Adjuvant chemohormonal therapy for primary breast cancer should be sequential instead of concurrent: initial results from Intergroup trial 0100 (SWOG-8814). Proc Am Soc Clin Oncol 2002; 21: Abst 143.

10. Pico C, Martin M, Jara C et al. Epirubicin–cyclophosphamide (EC) chemotherapy plus tamoxifen (T) administered concurrently (Con) versus sequential (Sec): randomised phase III trial in postmenopausal node-positive breast cancer (BC) patients. GEICAM 9401 study. Proc Am Soc Clin Oncol 2002; 21: Abst 144.

11. Fisher B, Constantino JP, Wickerham DL et al. Tamoxifen for prevention of breast cancer: report of the National Surgical Adjuvant Breast and Bowel Project P-1 study. J Natl Cancer Inst 1998; 90: 1371–88.

12. Bilimoria MM, Assikis VJ, Jordan VC. Should adjuvant tamoxifen be stopped at 5 years? Cancer J Sci Am 1996; 2: 140–50.

13. McDonald CC, Alexander FE, Whyte BW et al. Cardiac and vascular morbidity in women receiving adjuvant tamoxifen for breast cancer in a randomised trial. BMJ 1995; 311: 977–80.

14. Love RR, Mazess RB, Barden HS et al. Effects of tamoxifen on bone mineral density in postmenopausal women with breast cancer. N Engl J Med 1992; 326: 852–6.

15. Lonning PE. Pharmacology of the new aromatase inhibitors. Breast 1996; 5: 202.

16. Winer EP, Hudis C, Burstein HJ et al. American Society of Clinical Oncology Technology Assessment on the Use of Aromatase Inhibitors As Adjuvant Therapy for Postmenopausal Women With Hormone Receptor-Positive Breast Cancer: Status Report 2004. J Clin Oncol 2005; 23: 1–11.

17. Ragaz J. Adjuvant trials of aromatase inhibitors: determining the future landscape of adjuvant endocrine therapy. J Steroid Mol Biol 2001; 79: 133–41.

18. Baum M. The ATAC (Arimidex, Tamoxifen, Alone or in Combination) adjuvant breast cancer trial in postmenopausal (PM) women. Breast Cancer Res Treat 2001; 69: 210 (Abst 218).

19. Baum M, Budzar AU, Cuzick J et al. ATAC Trialists' Group. Anastrozole alone or in combination with tamoxifen versus tamoxifen alone for adjuvant treatment of postmenopausal women with early breast cancer: first results of the ATAC randomised trial. Lancet 2002; 359: 2131–9.

20. ATAC Trialists' Group. Results of the ATAC (Arimidex, Tamoxifen, Alone or in Combination) trial after completion of 5 years' adjuvant treatment for breast cancer. Lancet 2005; 365: 60–2.

21. Coombes RC, Hall E, Gibson LJ et al. A randomized trial of exemestane after two to three years of tamoxifen therapy in postmenopausal women with primary breast cancer. N Engl J Med 2004; 350: 1081–92.

22. Boccardo F, Rubagotti A, Amoroso D et al. Anastrazole appears to be superior to tamoxifen in women already

receiving adjuvant tamoxifen treatment. Breast Cancer Res Treat 2003; 82: Abst 3.

23. Goss PE, Ingle JN, Martino S et al. A randomized trial of letrozole in postmenopausal women after five years of tamoxifen therapy for early-stage breast cancer. N Engl J Med 2003; 349: 1793–802.

24. Early Breast Cancer Trialists' Collaborative Group. Ovarian ablation in early breast cancer: overview of the randomised trials. Lancet 1996; 348: 1189–96.

25. Poikonen P, Saarto T, Elomaa I et al. Prognostic effect of amenorrhoea and elevated serum gonadotrophin levels induced by adjuvant chemotherapy in premenopausal node-positive breast cancer patients. Eur J Cancer 2000; 36: 43–8.

26. Del Mastro L, Venturini M, Sertoli MR et al. Amenorrhoea induced by adjuvant chemotherapy in early breast cancer patients: prognostic role and clinical implications. Breast Cancer Res Treat 1997; 43: 183–90.

27. Pagani O, O'Neill A, Castiglione M. Prognostic impact of amenorrhoea after adjuvant chemotherapy in premenopausal breast cancer patients with axillary node involvement: results of the International Breast Cancer Study Group (IBCSG) trial VI. Eur J Cancer 1998; 34: 632–40.

28. Aebi S, Gelber S, Castiglione-Gersch M et al. Is chemotherapy alone adequate for young women with oestrogen receptor-positive breast cancer? Lancet 2000; 355: 1869–74.

29. Kaufmann M, on behalf of the ZEBRA Trialists' group. Zoladex™ (goserelin) vs CMF as adjuvant therapy in pre/perimenopausal, node-positive, early breast cancer: preliminary efficacy results from the ZEBRA study. Breast 2001; 10 (Suppl 1): S30 (Abst P53).

30. Kaufmann M, Jonat W, Blamey R et al. Zoladex Early Breast Cancer Research Association (ZEBRA) Trialists' Group. Survival analyses from the ZEBRA study. Goserelin (Zoladex) versus CMF in premenopausal women with node-positive breast cancer. Eur J Cancer 2003; 39: 1711–17.

31. Jonal W. Zoladex™ (goserelin) vs CMF as adjuvant therapy in pre-/perimenopausal, node-positive, breast cancer: first efficacy results from the ZEBRA study. Eur J Cancer 2000; 36: S67.

32. Recchia F, Sica G, De Filippis S et al. Ovarian protection with goserelin (G) during chemotherapy for early breast cancer: long term results of a phase II study. Proc Am Soc Clin Oncol 2002; 21: Abst 162.

33. Boccardo F, Rubagotti A, Perrotta A et al. Ovarian ablation versus goserelin with or without tamoxifen in pre-perimenopausal patients with advanced breast cancer; results of a multicentric Italian study. Ann Oncol 1994; 5: 337–42.

34. Jakesz R, Hausmaninger H, Samonigg E et al. Comparison of adjuvant therapy with tamoxifen and goserelin versus CMF in premenopausal stage I and II hormone-responsive breast cancer patients: four-year results of Austrian Breast Cancer Study Group (ABCSG) Trial 5. Proc Am Soc Clin Oncol 1999; 18: 67a (Abst 250).

35. Jakesz R, Hausmaninger H, Samonigg E et al. Complete endocrine blockade with tamoxifen and goserelin is superior to CMF in the adjuvant treatment of premenopausal, lymph node-positive and -negative patients with hormone-responsive breast cancer. Breast 2001; 10 (Suppl 1): S10 (Abst S26).

36. Boccardo F, Rubagotti A, Amoroso D et al. Cyclophosphamide, methotrexate and fluorouracil versus tamoxifen plus ovarian suppression as adjuvant treatment of oestrogen receptor-positive pre-/perimenopausal breast cancer patients: results of the Italian Breast Cancer Adjuvant Study Group 02 randomised trial. J Clin Oncol 2000; 18: 2718–27.

37. Boccardo F, Rubagotti A, Amoroso D et al. CMF vs tamoxifen (TAM) plus ovarian suppression (OS) as adjuvant treatment of ER positive (ER+) per-/perimenopausal breast cancer (BCA) patients (pts). Breast 2001; 10 (Suppl 1): S32 (Abst P62).

38. Rutqvist LE. Zoladex® and tamoxifen as adjuvant therapy in premenopausal breast cancer: a randomised trial by the Cancer Research Campaign (CRC) Breast Cancer Trials Group, the Stockholm Breast Cancer Study Group, the South-East Sweden Breast Cancer Group & the Gruppo Interdisciplinare Valutazione Interventi in Oncologia (GIVIO). Proc Am Soc Clin Oncol 1999; 18: 67a (Abstr 251).

39. Baum M, Houghton J, Odling-Smee W et al. Adjuvant 'Zoladex' in premenopausal patients with early breast cancer: results from the ZIPP trial. Breast 2001; 10 (Suppl 1): S32–3 (Abst RP64).

40. Davidson N, O'Neill A, Vukov A et al. Effect of chemohormonal therapy in premenopausal, node-positive, receptor-positive breast cancer: an Eastern Cooperative Oncology Group phase III Intergroup trial (E5188 INT-0101). Breast 1999; 8: 232–3 (Abst 069).

41. Castiglione-Gersch M, Gelbert RD, O'Neill A et al, for the International Breast Cancer Study Group. Systemic adjuvant treatment for premenopausal node-negative breast cancer. Eur J Cancer 2000; 36: 549–50.

42. International Breast Cancer Study Group (IBSCG). Adjuvant chemotherapy followed by goserelin versus either modality alone for premenopausal lymph node-negative breast cancer: a randomized trial. J Natl Cancer Inst 2003; 95: 1833–46.

43. Baum M, Houghton J, Sawyer W et al. Management of premenopausal women with early breast cancer: Is there a role for goserelin? Proc Am Soc Clin Oncol 2001; 20: 27a (Abst 103).

44. Blamey RW. Guidelines on endocrine therapy of breast cancer. EUSOMA. Eur J Cancer 2002; 38: 615–34.

45. Early Breast Cancer Trialists' Collaborative Group. Polychemotherapy for early breast cancer: an overview of the randomised studies. Lancet 1998; 352: 930–42.

46. Hortobagyi GN. Treatment of breast cancer. N Engl J Med 1998; 339: 974–84.

47. Findlay BP, Walker-Dilks C. Epirubicin alone or in combination chemotherapy, for metastatic breast cancer: Provincial Breast Cancer Disease Site Group and the Provincial Systemic Treatment Disease Site Group. Cancer Prev Control 1998; 2: 140–6.

48. Fisher B, Brown AM, Dimitrov NV et al. Two months of doxorubicin–cyclophosphamide with and without interval reinduction therapy compared with six months of cyclophosphamide, methotrexate and 5-fluorouracil in positive node breast cancer patients with tamoxifen non-responsive tumours, results from NSABP-B15. J Clin Oncol 1990; 8: 1483–96.

49. Fisher B, Anderson S, Wicerham DL et al. Increased intensification and total dose of cyclophosphamide in a doxorubicin–cyclophosphamide regimen for the treatment of primary breast cancer: findings from NSABP-B22. J Clin Oncol 1997; 15: 1858–69.

50. Henderson IC, Berry DA, Demetri GD et al. Improved outcomes from adding sequential paclitaxel but not from escalating doxorubicin dose in an adjuvant chemotherapy regimen for patients with node-positive primary breast cancer. J Clin Oncol 2003; 21: 976–83.

51. Citron ML, Berry DA, Cirrincione C et al. Randomized trial of dose-dense versus conventionally scheduled and sequential versus concurrent combination chemotherapy as postoperative adjuvant treatment of node-positive primary breast cancer: first report of Intergroup trial C9741/Cancer and Leukemia Group B trial 9741. J Clin Oncol 2003; 21: 1431–9.

52. Dang CT, Moynahan ME, Dickler MN, et al. Phase II study of dose-dense (DD) 5-fluorouracil, epirubicin, and cyclophosphamide followed by alternating weekly paclitaxel (P) and docetaxel (D) in high-risk node-positive (N+) breast cancer (BCA): feasibility and efficacy. Proc Am Soc Clin Oncol 2003; 22: Abst 46.

53. Poole CJ, Earl HM, Dunn JA, et al for the NEAT and SCTBG Investigators. NEAT (National Epirubicin Adjuvant Trial) and SCTBG BR9601 (Scottish Cancer Trials Breast Group) phase III adjuvant breast trials show significant relapse-free and overall survival advantage for sequential ECMF. Proc Am Soc Clin Oncol 2003; 22: Abst 13.

54. Levine MN, Bramwell VH, Pritchard KI et al. Randomised trial of intensive cyclophosphamide, epirubicin, and fluorouracil chemotherapy compared with cyclophosphamide, methotrexate, and fluorouracil in premenopausal women with node-positive breast cancer. J Clin Oncol 1998; 16: 2651–8.

55. Coombes RC, Bliss JM, Wils J et al. Adjuvant cyclophosphamide, methotrexate and fluorouracil versus fluorouracil, epirubicin and cyclophosphamide chemotherapy in premenopausal women with axillary node-positive operable breast cancer: results of a randomised trial. J Clin Oncol 1996; 14: 35–45.

56. Bonadonna G, Zambetti M, Valagussa P. Sequential or alternating doxorubicin and CMF regimens in breast cancer with more than three positive nodes. JAMA 1995; 273: 542–7.

57. Bonadonna G, Valagussa P, Moliterni A et al. Adjuvant cyclophosphamide, methotrexate, and fluorouracil in node-positive breast cancer, the results of 20 years of follow-up. N Engl J Med 1995; 332: 901–6.

58. Earl HM, Poole CJ, Dunn J et al, on behalf of the NEAT Steering Committee: NEAT – National Epirubicin Adjuvant Trial, a multi-centre phase III randomised trial of epirubicin × 4 and classical CMF × 4 (ECMF) versus CMF × 6 (CMF). Proc Am Soc Clin Oncol 2002; 21: Abst 2050.

59. Crump M, Tu D, Shepherd L et al. Risk of acute leukaemia following epirubicin-based adjuvant chemotherapy: a report from the National Cancer Institute of Canada Clinical Trials Group. J Clin Oncol 2003; 21: 3066–71.

60. Mamounas EP, Bryant J, Lembersky BC et al. Paclitaxel (T) following doxorubicin/cyclophosphamide (AC) as adjuvant chemotherapy for node-positive breast cancer: results from NSABP B-28. Proc Am Soc Clin Oncol 2003; 22: Abst 12.

61. Nabholtz J, Pienkowski T, Mackey J et al. Phase III trial comparing TAC (docetaxel, doxorubicin, cyclophospha-mide) in the adjuvant treatment of node positive breast cancer (BC) patients: interim analysis of the BCIRG 001 study. Proc Am Soc Clin Oncol 2002; 21: Abst 141.

62. Ravdin P, Olivotto A, Speers C et al. Should estrogen receptor (ER) negativity alone be an indication for chemotherapy in T1N0 breast cancer? Proc Am Soc Clin Oncol 2003; 22: Abst 55.

63. Valero V, Buzdar AU, McNeese M et al. Primary chemotherapy in the treatment of breast cancer: the University of Texas MD Anderson Cancer Center experience. Clin Breast Cancer 2002; 3: S63–8.

64. NSABP. The effect on primary tumour response of adding sequential taxotere to adriamycin and cyclophosphamide: preliminary results from NSABP protocol B27. Breast Cancer Res Treat 2001; 69: Abst 5.

65. Martin M, Pienkowski T, Mackey J et al. Adjuvant docetaxel for node-positive breast cancer. N Engl J Med 2005; 352: 2302–13.

66. Martin M, Villar A, Sole-Calvo A et al, on behalf of the GEICAM group (Spanish Breast Cancer Research Group), Spain. Doxorubicin in combination with fluorouracil and cyclophosphamide (iv FAC regimen day 1, 21) versus methotrexate in combination with fluorouracil and cyclophosphamide (iv CMF regimen day 1, 21) as adjuvant chemotherapy for operable breast cancer: a study by the GEICAM group. Ann Oncol 2003; 14: 833–42.

67. Slamon DJ, Clark GM, Wong SG et al. Human breast cancer: correlation of relapse and survival with amplification of the HER2/neu proto-oncogene. Science 1987; 235: 117–82.

68. Slamon DJ, Godolphin W, Jones LA et al. Studies of the HER2/neu proto-oncogene in human breast and ovarian cancer. Science 1989; 244: 707–12.

69. Press MF, Pike MC, Chazin VR et al. HER-2/neu expression in node-negative breast cancer: direct tissue quantification by computerised image analysis and association of overexpression with increased risk of recurrent disease. Cancer Res 1993; 53: 4960–70.

70. Seshadri R, Figaira FA, Horsfall DJ et al. Clinical significance of HER-2/neu oncogene amplification in primary breast cancer. The South Australia Breast Cancer Study Group. J Clin Oncol 1993; 11: 1936–42.

71. Quenel N, Wafflart J, Bonichon F et al. The prognostic value of c-*erb*B-2 in primary breast carcinomas: a study of 942 cases. Breast Cancer Res Treat 1995; 35: 283–91.

72. Berger MS, Locher GW, Saurer S et al. Correlation of c-*erb*B-2 gene amplification and protein expression in human breast carcinoma with nodal status and nuclear grading. Cancer Res 1988; 48: 1238–43.

73. Sal O, Sullivan S, Sun XF et al. Simultaneous analysis of c-*erb*B-2 expression and DNA content in breast cancer using flow cytometry. Cytometry 1994; 16: 160–8.

74. Kallioniemi OP, Holli K, Visakorpi T et al. Association of c-*erb*B-2 protein overexpression with high rate of cell proliferation, increased risk of visceral metastasis and poor long-term survival in breast cancer. Int J Cancer 1991; 49: 650–5.

75. Pantel K, Schlimok G, Braun S et al. Differential expression of proliferation-associated molecules in individual micrometastatic carcinoma cells. J Natl Cancer Inst 1993; 85: 1419–24.

76. Ravan PM, Chamness GC. The c-*erb*B2 proto-oncogene as a prognostic and predictive marker in breast cancer. A paradigm for the development of other macro-molecular markers – a review. Gene 1995; 159: 336.

77. Slamon DJ, Leyland-Jones B, Shak S et al. Use of chemotherapy plus a monoclonal antibody against HER2 for metastatic breast cancer that overexpresses HER2. N Engl J Med 2001; 344: 783–92.

78. Fisher B, Dignam J, Tan-Chiu E et al. Prognosis and treatment of patients with breast tumours of one centimetre or less and negative axillary lymph nodes. J Natl Cancer Inst 2001; 93: 112–20.

79. Galea MH, Blamey RW, Elston CE et al. The Nottingham Prognostic Index in primary breast cancer. Breast Cancer Res Treat 1992; 22: 207–19.

80. D'Erediat G, Giardina C, Martellotta M et al. Prognostic factors in breast cancer: the predictive value of the Nottingham Prognostic Index in patients with a long-term follow-up that were treated in a single institution. Eur J Cancer 2001; 37: 591–6.

81. Olivotto IA, Bajdik C, Ravdin PM et al. An independent population-based validation of the decision-aid for stage I–II breast cancer. Proc Am Soc Clin Oncol 2004; 23: 522 (Abst 14S).

82. Sorlie T, Perou CM, Tibshirani R et al. Gene expression patterns of breast carcinomas distinguish tumour subclasses with clinical implications. Proc Natl Acad Sci USA 2001; 98: 10869–74.

83. West M, Blanchette C, Dressman H et al. Predicting the clinical status of breast cancer by using gene expression profiles. Proc Natl Acad Sci USA 2001; 98: 11462–7.

84. van't Veer LJ, Dai H, van de Vijver MJ et al. Gene expression profiling predicts clinical outcome of breast cancer. Nature 2002; 415: 530–6.

41 Medicolegal aspects

Simon Levene

Preliminary

Breast screening and the subsequent management of patients have medicolegal implications that are worth considering against a background of the law of negligence generally.

First, some statistics that may give comfort. It was estimated that in 1978 less than 1% of patients were injured by negligent care in the United States, and only 10% of those patients sought the advice of a lawyer.[1] No comparable study has been carried out in the UK, but there is no reason to suppose that patients in the UK are more litigious than those in America. Thus the proportion of injured patients seeking legal advice in the UK is likely to be well below 10%. In seeking to understand the legal process, it is important to bear in mind the following points:

- The majority of potential claimants never get as far as issuing proceedings.
- Where negligence results in litigation, an overwhelming majority of claims result in negotiated settlements rather than in court action.
- Most contested trials find in favour of the defendant.
- Most of the typical medical costs are spent on administrative and legal fees.

To illustrate, the following is a summary of one English firm's experience out of the first 50 cases of clinical negligence concluded in 2002:

- 26 were discontinued following investigation either before or after the issue of protective proceedings;
- 15 were concluded successfully after the issue of proceedings and before trial;
- 6 were discontinued after the issue of proceedings;

- 3 were taken to trial: in one case the Claimant lost, in one case the Claimant won, and in one case the parties reached a settlement in the middle of the case for about a third of the value the Claimant had put on it.

Following the creation of the National Health Service Litigation Authority (NHSLA), it was predicted that cases would settle more readily and at an earlier stage in the litigation process. Many doctors feared that the NHSLA (in consultation with Health Trusts and Health Authorities) would take litigation decisions on purely commercial grounds: they felt that the Defence Unions had been more protective. It is certainly true that cases now settle faster, and Defendants admit liability sooner: recent procedural changes have put pressure on Defendants to admit liability at an early stage, by penalising them financially if they do not. Statistics are not readily available, and it is not clear to what extent the NHSLA and these procedural changes are responsible.

Negligence

The aim of this chapter is to give the legal background against which the law scrutinises the practice of medicine.

By 'negligence' is meant a breach in the duty of care that one person owes to another. This is not laid down by statute: the test is one that has evolved from judgements over the years. In the case of a motorist, the duty of care is obvious: a car is a dangerous object, and a motorist owes a duty to other road users to drive it carefully. The case of a doctor is more complex, but in essence the doctor owes the patient *a duty to provide the standard of care that the patient is reasonably entitled to expect*. Negligence is treatment that falls below this standard.

It must always be remembered that although the test is a legal one, it has evolved (and it is still applied) in the light of evidence given to the courts by medical experts: except in the most flagrant of cases (e.g. the removal of the wrong breast or leaving a swab in a patient after an operation), the Court will not be competent to judge the issue of negligence without help from expert practitioners.

The principles of negligence are the same whatever medical discipline is being considered, although a court will take into account the fact that different disciplines (e.g. general surgeons and gynaecologists) might have different approaches to medical problems. However, it is important to remember that the clinician under scrutiny is to be judged by his own speciality. So, a casualty officer who treats a neurological case on an emergency admission is to be judged by the standard of a casualty officer, not a consultant neurologist. On the other hand, an A&E consultant should realise when it is appropriate to refer a patient to a neurologist: he cannot simply rely on the fact that as an A&E consultant he would not be expected to provide expert neurological care. This is recognised in the medical profession, and the courts took note of it in *Sidaway* v. *Board of Governors of the Bethlem Royal and Maudsley Hospital* :[2] the law clearly requires a different degree of skill from a specialist in his own special field than from a general practitioner. In the field of neurosurgery, it would be necessary to substitute for the phrase 'no doctor of ordinary skill', the phrase 'no neurosurgeon of ordinary skill'. All this is elementary, and firmly established law.

A medical practitioner is not obliged to achieve success: his duty is to exercise reasonable skill and care. The classic formulation of the test is found in *Lanphier* v. *Phipos*:[3]

> 'Every person who enters into a learned profession undertakes to bring to the exercise of it a reasonable degree of care and skill. He does not undertake, if he is an attorney, that at all events you shall gain your case, nor does a surgeon undertake that he will perform a cure; nor does he undertake to use the highest possible degree of skill. There may be persons who have higher education and greater advantages than he has, but undertakes to bring a fair, reasonable and competent degree of skill...'

The test is now known as the 'Bolam' test, from MCNAIR J's famous jury direction in *Bolam* v. *Friern Hospital Management Committee*:[4]

> 'A doctor is not guilty of negligence if he has acted in accordance with a practice accepted as proper by a responsible body of medical

men skilled in that particular art... Putting it the other way round, a doctor is not negligent, if he is acting in accordance with such practice, merely because there is a body of opinion which takes a contrary view.'

The Bolam test works by looking for broad consensus in the medical profession, and allows practitioners to make advances in treatment and techniques without making every advance a bandwagon onto which they must all leap. It is also important to look at the doctor's specialisation or lack of it. In *Hucks* v. *Cole*,[5] the Court pointed out that the defendant was to be judged as a general practitioner with a diploma in obstetrics, although part of a doctor's ability lies in knowing when he is getting out of his depth and when to refer a patient for more specialised advice. In the case of a junior hospital doctor, there are two possible tests, both taken from *Wilsher* v. *Essex Health Authority*.[6] In the higher test, which comes from MUSTILL LJ's judgment:

> 'The standard is not just that of the averagely competent and well-informed junior houseman (or whatever the position of the doctor) but of such a person who fills a post in a unit offering a highly specialised service.'

In the lower test, which comes from Sir Nicholas Browne-Wilkinson's judgment:

> 'If the standard of care required of such a doctor is that he should have the skill required of the post he occupies, the young houseman or the doctor seeking to acquire specialist skill in a special unit would be held liable for short-comings in the treatment without any personal fault on his part at all.'

The former test is the one generally used, and was confirmed by the Court of Appeal in *Wilsher* v. *Essex Area Health Authority*.[7] In other words, the standard to be expected of a consultant who heads a team sets the standard for the work of the team as a whole. If it were otherwise, the experience of the treating doctor would become a relevant factor, and an inexperienced doctor, while more likely to make mistakes, would be less likely to be successfully sued. If a procedure is beyond the capacity of a junior doctor, it should not be entrusted to him, and if he finds himself out of his depth in the course of a procedure, he should seek the help of a more senior colleague. (This is one of the commonest criticisms in 'birth trauma' cases.)

Errors of judgement

In *Whitehouse* v. *Jordan*,[8] Lord Denning sought to redefine medical negligence as something other than an error of judgement. He proposed putting this question to the average competent and careful practitioner:

> 'Is this the sort of mistake that you yourself might have made? If he answers 'Yes, even doing the best I could, it might have happened to me', then it is not negligent.'

When *Whitehouse* v. *Jordan* went to the House of Lords, however, the judgment reaffirmed the Bolam test and deprecated the use of the term 'error of judgement':

> 'It is high time that the unacceptability of such an answer be finally exposed. To say that a surgeon committed an error of clinical judgement is wholly ambiguous, for, while some such errors may be completely consistent with the due exercise of professional skill, other acts of omission in the course of exercising clinical judgement may be so glaringly below proper standards as to make a finding of negligence inevitable. I would have it accepted that the true doctrine was enunciated in *Bolam* v. *Friern Hospital Management Committee*!'

In the light of all this, it is clear that a great deal of medical treatment, even if administered with all due skill and care, involves some degree of risk. It is inevitable that mishaps will occur for which the patient has no remedy.[9] In *Mahon* v. *Osborne*,[10] SCOTT LJ discussed the position of the surgeon in a context which has universal application to the law of negligence as follows:

> 'It is not every slip or mistake which imports negligence and, in applying the duty of care to the case of the surgeon, it is peculiarly necessary to have regard to the different kinds of circumstances that may present themselves for urgent attention....'

Causation

It is not enough to prove that a practitioner was negligent. The Claimant also has to prove that she was injured by this negligence. Here, the issue of medical consensus has no part. This was considered in the case of *Loveday* v. *Renton*,[11] in which the Court had to decide whether pertussis vaccine could cause permanent brain damage in young children. The question was purely one of causation, and the Claimant argued that the court was only concerned to ascertain the general state of medical opinion on the question, not whether that opinion was well founded. STUART-SMITH LJ disposed of the argument thus:

> 'It is fundamental to the Bolam test, which is concerned only with the issue of breach of duty, that if a doctor acts in accordance with the practice and opinion of a respectable and responsible body of medical opinion he is not guilty of negligence, even if another respectable and responsible body holds different views ... It is obvious that the court is not concerned to decide the merits of one practice as opposed to others, but only to determine if a respectable and responsible body of medical practitioners would have acted as the Defendant acted. But it is equally obvious that such a test cannot apply to the issue of causation, where the question is: Did the treatment, in this case vaccination, cause brain damage?'

> 'Since by a parity of reasoning if there is a respectable and responsible body of medical opinion which holds the view that it is not proved that the vaccine causes brain damage, a Plaintiff must fail on causation ... the court has to determine the factual issue by weighing and evaluating all the evidence in the case and seeing whether at the end of the day the Plaintiff has discharged the onus of proof on all the evidence. That is the approach I propose to adopt.'

The majority of claims arising out of the management of breast cancer founder on the issue of causation. The onus is on the Claimant to establish that a failure to diagnose, or a late diagnosis, made a significant difference to the patient's prognosis. Suppose that a Unit has a policy of screening patients every 3 years, and negligently fails to call a woman for 5 years, or fails to detect a cancer on mammography. Then any of the following might be the case: (i) the screening would not have picked up any abnormality (in which case there is no loss), or (ii) the screening would have picked up an abnormality, but the delay makes no difference to the prognosis (in which case there is again no loss), or (iii) the woman's life, or breast, could have been saved if the diagnosis had been made earlier.

Only (iii) would give rise to a claim for substantial damages, but even then the Claimant would have to prove that no reasonable doctor would have delayed a screening for so long. Thus it would not be enough for a Claimant to show that a clinic was in breach of its own protocols (although this would help her): she must show that the delay was unreasonable by any standards.

There may be tension between the protocol of a screening clinic and the circumstances of an individual patient. Although it would be exceedingly difficult for a patient to establish that the protocol was one that no clinic could reasonably operate, it might well be easier to prove that the protocol was applied so rigidly that significant factors were ignored in her particular case. Where a clinic decides that it is inappropriate to screen a woman who is asking to be screened, the issue will be whether, given all the patient's circumstances, it was reasonable to refuse.

Innovative practice

Having ascertained the standard of care that a patient was entitled to expect, a Court then goes on to consider how the care provided to the Claimant measured up to that standard. Professional practice may change over time so that what was once accepted as the correct procedure is no longer considered to be respectable or responsible. In Bolam, MCNAIR J pointed out that a medical practitioner cannot obstinately and pigheadedly carry on with some old technique if it has been proved to be contrary to what is really substantially the whole of informed medical opinion.[12]

Thus there is an obligation on doctors to keep up to date with developments otherwise you might get surgeons today saying: 'I don't believe in anaesthetics. I don't believe in antiseptics. I am going to continue to do my surgery in the way it was done in the eighteenth century.' That would clearly be wrong.[13]

In his book 'Professional Negligence',[14] Professor Michael A Jones says of the doctor's duty to keep up to date:

'There is an inevitable tension between the doctor's obligation to keep up to date, and the trite observation that doctors should not adopt any and every new idea until it has been proved to be both effective and safe. Doctors should not subject patients to untried methods of treatment unless the traditional approach has proved ineffective and the anticipated benefits are justified by the risks. On the other hand, despite the emphasis within many malpractice actions on complying with common practice, the Courts are careful to avoid the suggestion that findings of negligence may stifle innovation. A new technique may carry an unforeseen danger, not withstanding the reasonable efforts of the profession to identify risks in advance, and this will not be held negligent.'

It goes without saying that a doctor is only to be criticised by the medical standards at the time of his criticised act: he cannot be expected to apply techniques or standards not then current. See *Roe* v.

Minister of Health.[15] Contemporary literature is often of crucial importance, although it is possible to construct an excessively flimsy case for either the Claimant or the Defendant out of too extensive a literature search: it is often easy to find support somewhere in the literature for a particular course, but it can be more difficult to prove that such literature represents mainstream practice. Literature must be mainstream: doctors (even specialists) are too busy to read everything. It is always helpful to take standard textbooks as the starting point: if the criticised doctor departed from approved practice and cannot give a satisfactory reason why he did so, a wise Health Authority will not contest the claim:

'One must be careful when considering documents culled for the purpose of a trial, and studied by reference to a single isolated issue, not to forget that they once formed part of a flood of print on numerous aspects of industrial life, in which many items were bound to be overlooked. However conscientious the employer, he cannot read every textbook and periodical, attend every exhibition and conference, on every technical issue which might arise in the course of his business: nor can he necessarily be expected to grasp the importance of every single item which he might come across. Thus, if a works doctor regularly read *The Lancet* from cover to cover he would have seen the modest announcement of the V-51R ear plug in the edition of 28 April 1951 but it would be unrealistic to hold that all shipbuilders and repairers were thereafter on notice of the existence of plastic ear plugs whose manufacturers claimed an attenuation of 30 db.'[16]

The fact that a procedure was standard is not necessarily the end of the matter, however. In *Clarke* v. *Adams*,[17] the Claimant was severely burned during a course of heat treatment administered by a physiotherapist. Before the treatment, he had been given warning in the form approved by the Chartered Society of Physiotherapists, but the Court held that this warning was not enough to safeguard him.

Defensive medicine

What effect does the definition of negligence have on treatment? Does it stifle innovation, or penalise conservatism? In one sense, it is bound to favour defensive medicine, because a doctor is likely to feel that if a pioneering procedure, never before performed, goes wrong, he will be unable to call up a body of medical opinion in support. The Courts are aware of this problem, however, and are prepared not only to reject an established practice shown to be manifestly wrong, but also to approve a practice that had never been tried before:

'I think that, in an appropriate case, a judge would be entitled to reject a unanimous medical view if he were satisfied that it was manifestly wrong and that the doctors would have been misdirecting themselves as to their duty in law.'[18]

Nor is innovation precluded by the test. Because the burden is on the Claimant to prove that there has been negligence, he cannot simply point to his treatment and say that 'innovation = not approved by a reputable body of medical opinion'. See *Hunter* v. *Hanley*:[19]

'It follows from what I have said that in regard to allegations of deviation from ordinary professional practice ... such deviation is not necessarily evidence of negligence. Indeed, it would be disastrous if this were so, for all inducement to progress in medical science would then be destroyed. Even a substantial deviation from normal practice may be warranted by the particular circumstances. To establish liability by a doctor where deviation from normal practice is alleged, three facts require to be established. First of all it must be proved that there is a usual and normal practice; secondly it must be proved that the defender has not adopted that practice; and thirdly (and this is of crucial importance) it must be established that the course the doctor adopted is one which no professional man of ordinary skill would have taken if he had been acting with ordinary care.'

Landau v. *Werner*[20] sounds a warning:

'A doctor might not be negligent if he tried a new technique, but if he did he must justify it before the Court. If his novel or exceptional treatment had failed disastrously he could not complain if it was held that he went beyond the bounds of due care and skill as recognised generally.'

In *Roe* v. *Minister of Health*,[21], Lord Denning made specific mention of the need for the law not to stifle innovation:

'It is so easy to be wise after the event and to condemn as negligence that which was only a misadventure. We ought always to be on our guard against it, especially in cases against hospitals and doctors. Medical science has conferred great benefits on mankind but these benefits are attended by considerable risks. We cannot take the benefits without taking the risks. Every advance in technique is also attended by risks. Doctors, like the rest of us have to learn by experience; and experience often teaches in a hard way. Something goes wrong and shows up a weakness, and then it is put right ....

'We should be doing a disservice to the community at large if we were to impose liability on hospitals and doctors for everything that happens to go wrong. Doctors would be led to think more of their own safety than of the good of their patients. Initiative would be stifled and confidence shaken. A proper sense of proportion requires us to have regard to the conditions in which hospitals and doctors have to work. We must insist on due care for the patient at every point, but we must not condemn as negligence that which is only a misadventure.'

Where a practitioner is embarking on a novel treatment, he is under a greater duty than usual to inform and warn the patient.

Disclosure of risks

The Bolam test governs all aspects of the practitioner–patient relationship, from initial information, through diagnosis and advice, to treatment and after-care. In Sidaway,[22] the House of Lords considered the duty of disclosure to a patient of the advantages and disadvantages or risks and benefits of a proposed course of treatment. The opinion was held that the issue of whether non-disclosure of a particular risk should be condemned as a breach of the doctor's duty of care is one to be decided primarily on the basis of expert medical evidence. However, a Judge might in certain circumstances come to the conclusion that disclosure of a particular risk was so obviously necessary to an informed choice on the part of the patient that no reasonably prudent medical man would fail to make it. The House of Lords rejected the alternative view that different standards should apply to the disclosure of risks, as pertained with the law in Canada. In upholding the Bolam test, Lord Bridge specifically referred to the following passage in the Canadian case of *Reibl* v. *Hughes*:[23]

'To allow expert medical evidence to determine what risks are material and, hence, should be disclosed and, correlatively, what risks are not material is to hand over to the medical profession the entire question of the scope of the duty of disclosure, including the question whether there had been a breach of that duty. Expert medical evidence is, of course relevant to a finding of risks that reside in or are a result of recommended surgery or other treatment. It should also have a bearing on their materiality but this is not a question that is to be concluded on the basis of the expert medical evidence alone. The issue under consideration is a different issue from that involved where the question is whether the doctor carried out his professional activities by applicable professional standards. What is under consideration here is the patient's right to know what risks are involved in undergoing or foregoing certain surgery or other treatment.'

It is not enough for a court to determine that a doctor did not give the patient appropriate warnings about a procedure or treatment. If the warning was inappropriate, what would the patient have done when given an appropriate warning? The Court applies a subjective test in determining what the patient would have chosen if properly informed: see *Ellis* v. *Wallsend District Hospital*.[24] This raises a difficulty, because a doctor's opinion that a course of treatment is desirable may lead him to soft-pedal the warnings, and the patient may well end up either saying 'what would you advise, doctor?' or getting the subliminal message that the treatment is one of which the doctor approves.[25]

Expert witnesses

In view of the great importance of expert witnesses in clinical litigation, it may be helpful to summarise their duties. An expert advising either side in litigation now has to sign a declaration acknowledging his duty to the Court. It is not acceptable for an expert to regard himself as 'the Claimant's expert', or 'the Defendant's expert', even when instructed by one side or the other (nowadays, experts are commonly instructed jointly by both sides). An expert is required to put the whole of his opinion into a report, not just that part of it that helps the party that has instructed him. If there is scope for a difference of opinion on an issue, he should say so, and give an idea of the other points of view, even if he disagrees with them.

Once the litigation is under way, and the parties' experts have seen each other's reports, the Court will direct that experts of similar disciplines meet to narrow down the areas of disagreement. It is common for experts to reach almost complete agreement at such meetings, which are held without prejudice to the case. At the end of the meeting, they produce a report setting out those matters that are agreed, and those matters on which they cannot agree, with reasons for their disagreement. The intention is that when the trial takes place, the court's attention is focused on the real issues between the parties.

Cases often end once the experts have met; the gynaecologists, or nephrologists, or urologists, often find it easier to discuss the case among themselves than to answer questions put to them by lawyers.

Conclusion

Clinical considerations should guide clinical decisions. Even the most diehard Claimant's lawyer would not expect doctors to practise with one eye on the Bolam test – and in refining the test over the years the courts have tried to strike a balance between the need to protect patients and the need for the medical profession to have a free hand in taking clinical decisions. Properly interpreted, the law of negligence does not inhibit advances in medicine, nor does it foster conservative treatment for safety's sake.

References

1. Mills DH. Medical Insurance Feasibility Study. West J Med 1978; 128: 360–8.
2. [1985] AC 871 at 897.
3. [1835] 1 C & P 31.
4. [1957] 1 WLR 582 at 587.
5. [1993] MLR 393.
6. [1987] QB 730.
7. [1987] 2 WLR 425 esp. per MUSTILL LJ at 439–40.
8. [1980] 1 All ER 650 at 658.
9. See e.g. *White* v. *Board of Governors of Westminster Hospital* (The Times, 26 October 1961), where the retina was accidentally cut. There is a series of cases following this line: *Kapur* v. *Marshall* (1978) 85 DLR (3d) 567, through to *Ashcroft* v. *Mersey RHA* [1983] 2 All ER 245, which was affirmed on appeal [1985] 2 All ER 96.
10. [1939] 2 KB 14.
11. [1990] 1 MLR 117.
12. [1957] 2 All ER 118, 122.
13. MCNAIR J in Bolam.
14. Jones MA. Professional Negligence.
15. [1954] 2 QB 66.
16. MUSTILL J in *Thompson* v. *Smiths Ship Repairers (North Shields) Ltd* [1984] QB 405 at 422.
17. (1950) 94 SJ 599.
18. *Sidaway* v. *Board of Governors of the Bethlem Royal and Maudsley Hospital* [1985] AC 871.
19. [1955] S.C. 200.
20. (1961) 105 Sol Jo 1008.
21. Supra.
22. Supra.
23. 114 DLR (3d) 1.
24. [1990] 2 MLR 103.
25. See the verb 'to consent', sometimes found in medical records: as in 'the patient was consented'.

42 Informed consent in the management and research of breast cancer

Hazel Thornton

Introduction

The beginning of a new millennium is an appropriate time to take stock and attempt to look ahead to consider how accelerating genetic, pharmacological and technological developments in the field of breast cancer will affect seeking informed consent from women. This will apply to them as citizens when they first consider participating in mammographic screening,[1,2] through to being patients managed by multidisciplinary teams when diagnosed with early breast cancer, and to some as trial participants. It is important for clinicians, researchers, patients, participants and citizens to find ways of improving the negotiation of the consent process for women. It is particularly apt that we consider these issues in an era when the concepts underlying the roles in the doctor–patient relationship are changing, when the culture in which healthcare is practised and delivered in the UK and elsewhere is changing, and when some UK government policies encourage implementation of those changes.

To understand more clearly where we are today, and where we might be heading, it is necessary to examine cultural, political and social influences and interactions. These have shaped the ways in which healthcare is delivered, how research is undertaken, and the change in relationships. Barron Lerner, historian, clinician and scientist, has written an illuminating history of breast cancer in 20th century America that repays close scrutiny.[3] He puts into wider historical and social context how major players, incidents and influences have shaped the history of breast cancer treatment in 20th century America. What will future authors and critics write about the history of breast cancer in the 21st

century, we should wonder, as it is we who will begin to shape it?

In this chapter, I will start by exploring the issues that arise in relation to screening for breast cancer. My key theme is that openness, respectful partnerships and personal accountability, with freedom to contribute constructively, will promote research and treatment that is undertaken with the patient's well-being the main objective of all the stakeholders. Involvement of 'patients' is essential to achieve this.[4,5]

Informed consent for screening

Many people instinctively think of screening programmes as a means of reducing mortality from breast cancer. But screening raises extremely complex and difficult issues. A paper published in 2001,[6] reporting the results of a survey about the public's misconceptions about screening, opened with the statement: 'The current ethos of public health requires that informed consent be given by the users of any health intervention. This obligation is *even stronger* when prospective users do not actively seek help, as often happens with screening.' [my emphasis]. The unrealistic expectations of women concerning the benefits of mammography are exacerbated by the active promotion of screening programmes in order to achieve high population coverage. The conclusion of a paper reporting on a population-based survey of women's perception of the benefits of mammographic screening in four countries (USA, UK, Italy, and Switzerland) was that a high proportion of women overestimated the benefits that can be expected. A majority (68%) believed that screening prevents or reduces the risk of contracting breast cancer, 62% that screening at least halves breast cancer mortality and 75% that 10 years of regular screening will prevent 10 or more deaths per 1000 women. The authors commented:[7] 'This finding raises doubts on informed consent procedures within breast cancer screening programmes.' This is because screening and epidemiological research involving healthy individuals, family groups or communities iatrogenically labels people as 'patients'. It creates a reversal of the usual doctor–patient relationship, requiring particularly sensitive ethical and legal appraisal and consideration. Unfortunately, several problems remain unresolved in relation to screening for breast cancer.

These issues have been difficult to debate because of the often highly emotional arguments that surround screening. The majority of women who accept the invitation to attend for routine mammography will receive 'reassurance' from their results: the voice of the minority who suffer the consequences is drowned by the multitude of the reassured and those who believe their life was saved. The claim for seeking to achieve the greatest good for the greatest number is only sustainable if there is robust evidence that the benefit achieved is greater than the harm occasioned. This continues to be vigorously challenged.[8]

The responsibility of those offering national screening programmes to give healthy members of the population adequate explanation and information to enable them to give informed consent for screening was clearly set out by the General Medical Council (GMC) in November 1998.[9] This advice echoed recommendations that had been in the public arena for some time. However, leaflets issued by the UK NHS Breast Screening Programme (NHSBSP) in October 2001[10] fell far short of these requirements, and also failed to meet established criteria for the production of good-quality patient information leaflets.[11–14] For example, the leaflets do not mention ductal carcinoma in situ (DCIS) as a possible finding following screening, even though one out of five women diagnosed with 'cancer' in the screening programme will have it.[1]

The failure to inform women of the possibility of DCIS results in a range of unwanted consequences. In the clinics, clinicians spend an inordinate amount of time attempting to explain the enigmatic nature of DCIS to the 2000 women per annum sent to them via the NHSBSP who were not advised of this possibility by the screening programme. A woman who is found to have DCIS following participation in the screening programme has the shock of finding she has a borderline 'pseudo-disease'[15] (or, more accurately, one of a range of conditions, which may include lobular carcinoma in situ (LCIS), atypical hyperplasia, low-, intermediate- or high-grade DCIS, microinvasive DCIS and other carcinomas of unknown natural history or significance) where the management is uncertain and the diagnosis can potentially cause the woman subsequent difficult risk-assessment problems. The degree of psychological distress caused by a diagnosis of DCIS has been shown to be the same as that for invasive cancer.[16] The woman experiences an abrupt transition from citizen to patient, and faces uncertainties that may be at least as, if not more, difficult to come to terms with than an invasive diagnosis. These women also acquire the penalties that can be associated with carrying the 'DCIS breast cancer' label. For example, unfair[17] and unfounded[18] intergenerational insurance repercussions have been reported. As I shall describe later, the failure to inform women about DCIS when they consent to screening also raises important problems for those seeking to enrol women into DCIS trials.

The NHSBSP has repeatedly defended its decision not to include DCIS in the invitation leaflets because they claim that their focus group research showed that 'women don't want it' [information about DCIS].[19,20] This is contrary to GMC 1998 guidelines that clearly describe what citizens *ought* to be told,[9] and is clearly a very different situation from the kind of negotiation of preferences for information in doctor–patient relationships that should be available. That 'women don't want it' is still evidently the party line in the NHSBSP, even though they are currently drafting a booklet of supplementary information about DCIS that will be available for women – but only to those who ask for it.

The way in which information and risks are framed influences the decisions that women invited for screening will make.[21,22] There are two distinct aspects to considering 'what women want': the first is content; the second is the amount of information required. To some extent, these overlap. Recent research has confirmed the intuitive assumption concerning heterogeneity of women's desires for information about mammographic screening. There is a wide variety of preference, ranging from wishing to refuse all information through to a need for full and detailed information. The challenge is to cater for all types of preference. This means, as a minimum, that to make an informed decision about whether to be screened, information for DCIS should be made available. Equally, however, it is inappropriate to force unwanted information on those women whose anxiety about attending for screening causes them, at the time, to refuse all information. This is as unsympathetic to women's preferences as is depriving those who want full and detailed information at the moment of invitation.

Decision aids for breast cancer screening have been published, and these appear to offer a way forward.[2,23] These graphic representations would assist women in appreciating firstly their risk of getting breast cancer and secondly their chances of benefiting from or being disadvantaged by mammographic screening.[1] There is already substantial evidence about the effectiveness of these decision aids, particularly on the cognitive and affective outcomes that contribute substantially to informed decision-making. It is felt by many to be approaching a 'class effect' such that evaluation of every innovation may not be necessary. We can act on these findings now to implement supports for consumer decision-making,[24] including appropriate risk-communication tools.[25] These should be incorporated promptly into a new leaflet from the NHSBSP.

As has been discussed, a flexible attitude to responding to the known differences in women's desire for information is to be recommended. What is important is that the 'basic' leaflet be honest, balanced, adequate and complete, and include decision aids and graphics. Links to further sources of information should be provided on the leaflet for those individuals who require full and detailed information. Surely it is a citizen's prerogative to refuse to accept an information leaflet, but it is the provider's responsibility to ensure that good-quality leaflets and other information sources be produced, advertised, available and accessible. The public should not be kept in ignorance concerning the robustness of the evidence, or the need for updating it as fresh evidence becomes available. This will help them to address the uncertainties, controversies and doubts about the benefits and harms of mammographic screening.

'Uncertainty' and 'equipoise'

Once someone has been diagnosed with breast cancer, they will be faced with decisions about treatment, including the possibility of participation in research on breast cancer. Research is necessary to address well-informed uncertainties[26] and to find better ways of caring for people with cancer. Most improvements in treatments, identification of unsatisfactory ones, and detailed profiling of precise benefits and harms are obtained through rigorous evaluation of interventions in good-quality clinical trials. To understand why trials are essential, it is necessary to understand the central concepts of 'uncertainty' and 'equipoise'. These terms are used frequently – and unfortunately sometimes interchangeably – when discussing the ethics of research, but have different meanings. Mann and Djulbegovic[27] have explained why controlled clinical trials are performed to reduce uncertainties about the relative merits of different treatment: '...trials should only be done if physicians and the patients are uncertain which of existing alternatives is better'.[28,29] This requirement is sometimes referred to as 'the uncertainty principle'[30] or 'equipoise'.[31,32]

'Uncertainty' is not a neat concept, as Richard Ashcroft has pointed out (personal communication). There is rational uncertainty, and there is also common-or-garden uncertainty, and we should distinguish between them. The latter might encompass vagueness, dithering, risk aversion or lack of confidence. The former may encompass what Chalmers[26] has termed 'well-informed uncertainties' and the 'residual uncertainty' that can remain after the best possible evidence has been weighed from collective experience, and after taking account of patient preferences. Mann[33] has defined the three levels of uncertainty that are present: the community of 'expert' practitioners (also relevant to research ethics committees who must approve the trial); the patient's doctor (who has to decide whether to participate in the trial and offer enrolment to particular patients); and the patient (who has to decide whether to enrol).

Equipoise, on the other hand, can be more precisely defined. As Lilford[34] states: 'Equipoise is not synonymous with uncertainty. ... Uncertainty is the opposite of certainty and therefore covers a huge range of possibilities, from equipoise all the way to certainty.' Equipose, Lilford and Jackson argue, is:[35]

> 'the point where there is no preference between treatments ... At this point we may be said to be "agnostic" or "resting" on the fulcrum of a decision: we would take odds of 1:1 in a bet. Equipoise is different from simply not "knowing" or being "uncertain", because it implies that we have no (rational) preference whatever. We could have a mild preference for treatment A [over B] and still not "know" which treatment was best: we would be uncertain but not in equipoise.'

Clinical trials therefore turn on the principles of uncertainty and equipoise. Once it has been determined that sufficient uncertainty (equivalent to equipoise) exists about a given clinical question, a trial effectively has a warrant to proceed on scientific grounds. However, I will argue throughout this chapter that a scientific warrant is not sufficient: a trial must also be endorsed by the patients whom it seeks to engage as participants – it must have a patient warrant too.

Public involvement in trials

The reasons why people agree to treatment are obvious, but why should people participate in research? The debate about the moral obligation of patients to join randomised controlled trials rightly occupies many minds. I believe it is important that people do participate in clinical research and that they have responsibilities to do so. The debt to past participants is unfortunately not always recognised or appreciated by patients demanding their rights today. They may not stop to consider that they are beneficiaries of past individuals' efforts, with a responsibility to carry the baton to the next stage in this race without a winning post in sight. The term 'social cost' was coined for this reluctance, used as long ago as 1964 by Edmund Cahn.[36] He said:

> 'To possess the end and yet not be responsible for the means, to grasp the fruit while disavowing the tree, to escape being told the cost until someone else has paid it irrevocably.'

However, while people may have a moral obligation to participate in research, the obligations on trialists are even greater. These include the obligation to undertake high-quality research in true partnership. Chief among the responsibilities that this involves is the need for efforts to move away from viewing trial participants as 'subjects', or as a resource to be used, or as a 'means to an end'. My key argument is that more general public involvement and agreement on the policies and scope of research is the top priority for breast cancer research. Involvement of participants in designing trials, devising recruitment strategies, and providing feedback on their experiences between trials is the key to securing a 'patient' warrant in addition to a scientific warrant. Such an approach would help redress the imbalances between the parties currently funding and conducting research[5,37,38] and would help to address increasing disquiet[39] about conflict of commercial interests with medicine.

Individual and organisational consumer involvement in research

The scope for discussion and debate about clinical trials and consumer involvement in the whole research process has been widened by the emergence of various voluntary, independent organisations in the last decade, enabling the voice of the consumer to be heard in the research process from policy making[40] through to dissemination of research results. Opportunities for consumers to contribute their ideas at conferences, in policy-making fora, on trial steering committees, on data monitoring committees and in leading medical journals[41] have increased, particularly in the last decade and into this new millennium.

My vision of a shared responsibility that I offered when asked to describe 'The patient's role in research' has not dimmed or fundamentally changed since I was given the privilege of presenting my ideas as a layperson to breast cancer health professionals at the first Lancet Conference ('The Challenge of Breast Cancer') in Brugges, in April 1994.[4] Challenged again, later that same year, to translate vision into action, a unique initiative was set up. This took the form of a small facilitative working group of patients and health professionals, with a unique unshakeable ethos – the Consumers' Advisory Group for Clinical Trials (CAG-CT).[42,43] In its short life, this group led the way in turning vision to reality, initially in the world of breast cancer, but subsequently in a broader context.

Dramatic increases in accrual have been made possible through better organisation within the UK cancer research community, and the building of local, regional, and international networks.

In the UK, a significant development has been the establishment in June 2000 of the Consumer Liaison Group (CLG) of the National Cancer Research Institute (NCRI). Patient representatives from the CLG are involved in the work of the Clinical Studies Groups in the National Cancer Research Network (NCRN), each of which covers specific cancer sites. These Groups oversee existing studies, consider new research questions, develop proposals, secure funding and provide advice. Patient representatives help each Group review and develop new trials by providing a patient perspective at all stages of the research process. The NCRN, with Macmillan Cancer Relief, is also developing consumer research panels in each of the 34 UK Cancer Networks.[44]

The most important thing to have changed since my first published patient's viewpoint on breast cancer trials (which generated international debate)[44] is the attitude of many committed health professionals. The patient has to be at the centre of these endeavours, and has an active role to play. The attitude of patients to the profession has also had to change, thus permitting negotiations on respectful and equal terms with other parties engaged in the furtherance of good-quality research. There is no place for either 'doctor-bashing' or excessive subservience! Times are rapidly changing. There is growing realisation that rights may only be claimed upon discharge of responsibilities. Patients have become experts in their own right, whose expertise in guiding and helping to determine the way ahead is as important as that of any other member of a multidisciplinary team. On their shoulders rests the ultimate responsibility of ensuring that various pressures (commercial and professional), baser motivations, and less than honourable ambitions and objectives do not distort the research agenda. Advocates for good-quality research and healthcare have a continuing role to play.

The importance of participants' views

A more patient-led approach to trials would contribute to greater public awareness and involvement in research, both as participants and co-researchers.[46] A trial depends for its speedy success on the cooperation of patients. This cooperation will not occur if research agendas are biased, or there is a mismatch between professional and consumer priorities for research.[47,48] If this mismatch is not addressed then evidence-based medicine will not be representative of consumer needs.[47] The proper management of recruitment needs to be a key area for future research, development and investment.

The first issue that needs to be tackled urgently is general education about the importance of trials. As Iain Chalmers[5] states:

'Engaging the public, patients and the professions in these matters implies the provision of readily accessible information about the rationale for controlled trials; about what is and is not known about the effects of treatments on offer; and about planned and ongoing trials that are addressing important uncertainties. [www.nelh.nhs.uk]'

People should be able, in waiting areas in health service settings, to pick up a very simple leaflet on 'Why do we need clinical trials?'[49] or a booklet such as 'Understanding Cancer Research Trials'.[50] This could encourage a more socially conscious approach, sow the seeds of understanding and lessen the shock of an invitation to join a trial. A further simple leaflet offering expansion of ideas about research can be made available when the patient is on the ward or in the clinic. Research should be promoted as an activity that is conducted by health professional teams in collaboration with patients in order to continuously improve treatment choices and quality of life. Patients also need to be able to identify for themselves clinical trials for which they would be eligible. This kind of promotion of well-regulated research – equating it with hope and progress (but remaining realistic) – in partnership with participants, might go some way to preparing anxious patients by offering them hope, giving them confidence and treating them as partners in the enterprise. This is surely beneficial,

regardless of an individuals' capacity for full intellectual grasp of research concepts or ramifications of specific protocols.

Once people become more engaged in understanding the business of trials, they can become engaged in the business of being partners in those trials. Qualitative research methodologies can play a key role both in informing optimal trial designs and in allowing patients to contribute to trial design and conduct. Such research would ensure that research questions are posed that address issues that are of importance to patients, and would result in trial protocols that are also feasible and acceptable. This would lead to more rapid recruitment. One of the key problems in clinical trials is that too often, too little pretrial qualitative research is undertaken to establish whether the study question is relevant, legitimate and one to which patients ascribe high priority.[51] It is encouraging that the conclusion drawn following a nationwide UK survey was that involvement of consumers in the conduct, design and interpretation of trials was welcomed by most researchers.[52]

The potential for more partnership-based approaches to running trials is especially evident in some areas of trial practice. For example, screening trials (where cluster randomisation might be the most practical, economical and feasible method) can present difficult methodological, social, legal and ethical questions. There are imaginative and practical solutions to some of these questions, including undertaking a citizens' deliberation to secure public legitimacy for undertaking such trials. This provides the added advantage of simultaneously educating and informing wider sections of the public through the publicity afforded by observers who attend.[53]

A citizens' deliberation involves the following:

- A small group of ordinary citizens are selected to represent a cross-section of society by using telephone surveys and criteria such as age, race, gender and education. Jury sizes range from 12 to 24, depending on the scale of the project.
- Deliberations range from 4 to 6 days, facilitated by a trained moderator.
- Jurors are paid a modest daily stipend, which may also be supplemented by compensation for loss of earnings, payments to employers and childcare provision in some countries.
- They are informed about the issues, receive evidence, cross-examine witnesses and engage in full discussion, facilitated by the moderator, who also acts as timekeeper and referee.
- Jurors are sometimes allowed to amend their brief and to call on new sources of information.
- The commissioning body is expected to publicise the jury and its findings, to follow its

recommendations or explain why they have not chosen to do so.

For such a system to be successful, there is a need to ensure that:

- The selection process delivers as representative a sample of the population as possible.
- The initial brief does not unnecessarily limit the jury in their deliberations (framing the question).
- Information is presented in as unbiased a manner as possible.
- There is sufficient time to reach conclusions.
- The jury is not manipulated by either witnesses or moderator.
- The jury's findings are fairly reported and publicised.

Of course, the organisers of a citizens' deliberation have considerable powers: they brief the jury, select the witnesses, organise the presentation of information, moderate the proceedings and report on the findings. They are accountable to the sponsors but not to the wider public. Notwithstanding this caveat, citizens' deliberations are a democratic way of examining important questions, enabling lay people to exercise their citizenship by being involved in the decision-making process, thus sharing the responsibility for initiatives that may be undertaken arising from their conclusions. This is an example of the kind of process that I would like to see informing aspects of trial practice.

However, it is important that the views of people who help to design a trial and its recruitment strategies not be used cynically, as a means of persuading more people to take part: instead, such views must be seen as ensuring that a trial is acceptable to people and reflects their priorities.

I must also emphasise that I do not see the contribution of participants' views as ending when the trial has been designed. The process of actively seeking people's views and experiences must continue throughout the trial, and it is encouraging that trials increasingly include patient-completed quality-of-life assessments that help to reveal issues of concern to patients. For example, a drug may have an unanticipated effect on sexual functioning that would remain hidden if participants were not asked about it, and in particular if there were sole reliance on physicians' assessments. The importance of this is illustrated by evidence showing that patients and doctors evaluated differently the range, severity and importance of known and potential side effects of drugs such as tamoxifen and anastrozole.[54]

Exploration and elicitation of participants' concerns is especially important for informing and directing

marketing strategies. If people's concerns are not known (or ignored), there is a danger that the benefits of a new drug could be eulogised, but the drawbacks muted, thus creating expectations and demands for treatments that may not be appropriate.[55] Merely to qualify with suggestions that it is 'early days yet'[56] may be of unclear significance to a public eager for breakthroughs. Providing information that emerged during the trial is not enough on its own: it is also vital that marketing strategies express caution about the length of time that it can take for evidence about adverse effects to emerge – as was the case with tamoxifen.

Information about research concepts and information about specific trials

There are two distinct needs: firstly, for general education and understanding about the risk limiting practice of undertaking randomised controlled trials and why they are needed; secondly, information about the rationale behind offering a patient a specific clinical trial, what it will involve, and why they are eligible for it.

Involving citizens in the design of trials and ensuring that their views are sought throughout a trial could do much to maintain a focus on patients' priorities. For individuals being asked to join a trial, several specific needs are apparent. Most importantly, they will need information about the rationale behind the offer of a specific clinical trial, what it will involve and why they are eligible for it. Ideally, every opportunity should be taken to educate and inform, so that no patient should feel that they have unmet needs. This is important because patients newly diagnosed with breast cancer tend to feel isolated and have a desperate need for tailored therapies chosen by their physician, and given with the assurance that it is the best for them. New patients should not be surprised to be invited to join a trial: rather, they might be encouraged to ask which trials they might be eligible for.[57] This should be done sensitively and discretely, so that the minority who prefer to cope by 'leaving it to the doctor', or prefer to choose their therapy with their physician, can do so and are not made to feel inadequate because of this.

The main stumbling block for most patients, and indeed for some health professionals, is lack of understanding about randomisation – why it is needed, and what it means in practical terms. This emphasises the urgent need for well-placed, accessible, clearly written general information about clinical trials and the need for them.

It is also important that those patients who choose to inform themselves (e.g. via the internet) be respected and accommodated. Some patients have access to the internet and may come to the clinic forearmed (for better or worse – depending on their sources) with questions and information. Information from various websites will engage those patients who have internet access, and who wish to use it, in positive, constructive ways of helping them to feel in some personal control. These include addresses for reliable sources of information, registers of available trials,[58] brief consumer-orientated summaries and information,[59] and narrative accounts.[60] Providing such information would give a firm signal of respect for the dignity of the patient's desire to enter a more meaningful, mutually beneficial partnership with her physician and team through a better level of understanding, communication and shared decision-making. This can lead to a higher level of satisfaction for both clinician and patient, both within the consultation itself and in the overall outcome.

Trust and altruism: faith and hope

Trust is an essential component of the therapeutic liaison between a patient and the team within a breast unit. A survey has demonstrated that for 21.1% of women it is the main reason for participating in a trial.[61] If a further 23.1% state that their main reason is that 'others will benefit', should this not cause us to question the inflexibility of those who demand that prospective trial participants should have understanding of the 'fullest possible information'? Where is the humanity and beneficence in such imposition? Whose best interests are served by this instruction? As Jenkins and Fallowfield[61] state: 'This finding has remained stable over a decade and forms an important part of the doctor–patient relationship. The provision of faith and hope is seen as a central feature of a "healing" relationship and are powerful agents in their own right.' The same survey showed that those who declined to participate in the trial were somewhat less satisfied with the amount of written information given to them about the trial, but there was no statistical difference between the groups. Astonishingly, 23% of patients in this survey were not provided with written information leaflets, despite the fact that this is a mandatory requirement for ethics approval of any randomised controlled trial. Incentives other than the patient's best interests have been shown to result in 'short-cutting' the consent process – a deplorable and unethical state of affairs that partly explains why all patients may not have been given trial patient information leaflets.[62]

Seeking consent to research participation

Once it has been determined that a woman is eligible for a breast cancer trial and has been invited to participate, she is then faced with the decision about whether to consent. I believe that the aim of seeking consent is to ensure that the patient is, with the help of the whole breast team and the resources at their disposal, able to reach a satisfactory shared decision.[63] People who are candidates for trials should receive 'the right types of information, given in ways optimal for their own level of understanding'[64] and any necessary help to achieve 'substantial understanding',[65] and should be free and able to consider it in the light of their own individual circumstances, values and preferences. Informed consent is a progressive dynamic process – not a single event.[66]

The informed consent process should begin for the citizen or patient with the first encounter with the medical profession, and is an ongoing process throughout that patient's experience of a particular condition. This fact needs to be recognised and accepted by practitioners in healthcare and shared across the barriers dividing department from department, or public health practitioners from practicing clinicians and trialists. It can often appear that these organisations and people work in isolation and have little concept of the need for a common accountability and shared responsibility for ensuring a timely and seamless route for an individual's information needs.[67] Mark Hockhauser,[68] for example, cogently argues that adequate information should be provided at the time of offering screening and prevention, and this should cover possible known consequences of accepting an invitation.

However, while it is important that all relevant information be available and provided in response to patients' requests, it is also desirable that the provision of information be tailored to a patient's individual preferences and requirements. There is a danger that dogmatic insistence by some advocates for full information and consent in all circumstances could interfere with common sense and good practice. Removing flexibility insults the good intentions and integrity of the majority of caring physicians and the common sense of ordinary people who can ask their own questions, or eschew that which is inherently unethical or unacceptable.[69] However, at present, ethical and professional advice on requirements for consent to treatment and consent to research are striking in their divergence. Those entering treatment outside a trial are accorded the respect and kindness of being supplied with a measured quantity of information according to what the patient would like to know.[9] This conforms with the recommendations from the GMC, which suggest that: 'the amount of information you give each patient *will vary*, according to factors such as the nature of the condition, the complexity of the treatment, the risks associated with the treatment or procedure *and the patient's own wishes*.'

Contrast this approach with the principles set out by the same body for consent to research. The 1998 GMC guidelines state that prospective trial participants *must* be given 'the fullest possible information'. This is presumably meant to ensure that patients are not 'used' for experimentation and that they know in advance what will happen to them and why it is being done. Such a ruling deprives doctors of scope for exercising their discretion in situations where they see that the patient's best interests would be served by perhaps euphemistic assurances rather than textbook coverage of all risks, benefits, limitations and consequences of a given course of action.[70] 'Why should randomisation – often to treatments that are "standard" – require especially onerous informed consent? Much more useful would be a flexible approach that recognises that a trusting relationship between doctor and patient is the bedrock of any satisfactory consultation, relationship, dialogue or potential health gain'.[71,72] Perhaps 'given every opportunity of easy access to the fullest possible information' would be a more suitable recommendation.

Early breast cancer patients requiring treatment and care either within or outside trials are presumably equally variable in the amount of information that they desire, their degree of anxiety and fear, their ability to understand it in the time available, and any other attributes that a sensitive clinician will take into account when in dialogue with a patient. Why should the research team be forced to give 'the fullest possible information', with the potential for severely upsetting that category of patient who prefers to 'leave it to the doctor'? Investment in improving the communication skills of health professionals would be a better strategy than rigid insistence on full disclosure.

On balance, there is surely a case for supporting flexibility in seeking patients' consent to take part in randomised controlled trials.

Both the heart and the mind, both belief and reason, are brought to bear in varying proportions by a patient who is considering joining a trial. For many individuals, adequate information is an essential component of the decision-making process, as it is in standard clinical practice, provided at least both verbally and written.[72] One of the most frequent complaints of patients is lack of suitable and adequate information.[73–75] But for others, trust in the experience, knowledge, honesty and integrity of the doctor is the over-riding factor that causes them to go forward to receive treatment within a trial. This is independent of the level of understanding of either the research process or the specifics of the particular trial protocol. Why then should this category, together with the numerous 'partial-understanders', be compelled to have 'the fullest possible information' if it is against their wishes? Is this the penalty that has to be paid to protect the doctor against threat of litigious action by a very small minority of patients? Intimidation of doctors can take many forms.[76]

Surely it is far more important that adequate and good-quality information be readily accessible and that all patients be aware of this? They can then obtain this at their own discretion. The 'bad news' consultation is usually not the moment to overload a frightened patient who will have just received the diagnosis of cancer. What *is* important is for patients to be assured that members of the breast care team are there to help them find out what they need to know. This may relate to their diagnosis and treatment or trial requirements, and research concepts.

Communication – verbal and written

Training in communication skills is particularly important when the issues are complex and demand the kind of flexibility and sensitivity I have alluded to above. Proper balance of power in research endeavours is difficult to achieve,[45] but depends crucially on access to information and the opportunity to share decisions. We would do well to bear in mind Lesley Fallowfield's dictum that desire for information is not the same as a desire to participate in decision-making. The key is flexibility, so that discussions are sensitive to each patient's individual requirements. Providing this flexibility and sensitivity means that doctors' values have to be at the heart of their acquisition of communication skills.

In discussing trials with their patients, ideally doctors should be in equipoise not only about the options being offered within the trial, but also about any other interventions available outside the trial, including the possibility of participation in any other relevant trial. Patients themselves also need to be told about any other options that ought to be considered if they are to make a properly informed decision whether to participate or not. For example, the UK DCIS trial (1989) offered four very different treatment options following complete local excision.[78] These were: (a) no further treatment, (b) tamoxifen 20 mg daily for 5 years, (c) radiotherapy to the breast and (d) tamoxifen 20 mg daily for 5 years plus radiotherapy to the residual ipsilateral breast tissue. If they were to be enabled to achieve equipoise, prospective participants also needed to know that at least two other options were available outside the trial: mastectomy (circa 99% effective) or 'watchful waiting' after diagnosis (this is now termed 'active monitoring'[79]). But this second possibility was no longer an option that was open to potential participants because invitation to be randomised in this trial occurred after complete local excision. Both the imbalance of treatments offered and the failure to include other options resulted in a trial where equipoise (even if adequately informed) was very difficult to achieve. This contributed to the protracted recruitment period for this trial.

Being able to explain uncertainty clearly demands skills and a certain degree of humility on the part of doctors. Much attention has been focused on doctors' intense dislike of having to admit to uncertainty when they are trying to explain to potential trial participants that it is unknown which treatment is best.[80,81] But the public's attitude has changed: arrogant doctors who 'act like God' are given short shrift. We need to focus on training doctors who are not ashamed to admit they are human and that they need the help and participation of patients in research to provide a higher degree of certainty about choices of treatments.

Unfortunately, research on exploring ways of enhancing communication to improve the quality of the doctor–patient relationship[82] and recruitment rates for research,[79,83] has not always been given the priority it deserves. Too often this type of research has been viewed as a soft, optional extra by policy-makers and fundholders, instead of a fundamental necessity.[84] Qualitative research is finally being recognised as having as rigorous a methodology as quantitative research.[85,86] Increasingly, this sort of research must be used to address issues of communication, including how to address cultural variations in the increasingly diverse society in which we practise.[87]

There are encouraging findings from recent developments. A randomised controlled trial seeking evidence for the efficacy of a communication skills training model for oncologists[84] found that the communication problems of senior doctors working in cancer medicine were not resolved by time and clinical experience. The trial showed that training courses significantly improved key communication skills as well as contributing to more rewarding consultations, both personally and professionally. Researchers believe that this can have a significant impact on clinical care and on doctors' and patients' well-being. These findings were corroborated in a randomised trial of professional skill development, informed throughout by patient and consumer engagement.[88] Communication skills are now formally taught as part of the curriculum for medical students,[89–93] and such developments are to be warmly welcomed.

However, there are less cheering signs, particularly relating to written information. Preliminary research undertaken to evaluate the quality of patient information sheets for patients entering cancer trials[94] showed that they were extremely variable in quality. Many failed to meet basic quality criteria when assessed using a prototype evaluation tool. More work is needed to develop and validate such tools in order to facilitate those involved in running clinical trials and the ethics committees who approve trials.

The quality of information provided on websites is also extremely variable, as has been shown in a report of a cross-sectional study that analysed website content concerning presentation of possible benefits and harms of screening.[95] The researchers found that 'consumer sites' were much more balanced and comprehensive than other sites. They found that the information material provided by professional advocacy groups and governmental organisations is information-poor and severely biased in favour of screening. They commented that few websites live up to accepted standards for informed consent such as those stated in the GMC's guidelines.

Thus far, however, there is a lack of systematic research-based guidelines on patients' own priorities for leaflets and summaries.[50] The participant information sheet should be the 'shop window of the trial'.[96] It should accurately reflect the content of the trial, not only for the prospective participants, but also for ethics research committees, and for those seeking information on current ongoing trials. The patient information sheet should set out the trial's aims and objectives so that the patient understands the purpose of her participation – both short-term and long-term. Failure to do this properly can result in unforeseen consequences for patient participants. Involvement of patients in the production of information leaflets enhances their quality, particularly with regard to their use of suitable language, adequacy and 'tone'.

Given the right motivation and attitude, information providers can be assisted to create written materials that will enable citizens to engage in meaning creation, both for their own purposes and satisfaction and so that they might more fruitfully engage in discussion and public debate. The most important driver for change is attitude. In an analysis of published discourses about the use of patient information leaflets by Mary Dixon-Woods,[97] two very differing attitudes towards patient information are identified. The analysis considers two contrasting discourses, each revealing its own motivation for providing information to patients and the resultant mode and framing of that information. As she says: 'the first …. derives its interest in printed information not from an imperative for democratisation, but from a concern with how communication might affect outcomes defined as *biomedically* important. The second discourse shows evidence of engagement with sociology and the social sciences, and much of its motivation for exploring the use of printed information comes from its interest in the role of information materials in "empowering" patients.' The first discourse offers the pervasive view of patients as 'irrational, passive, forgetful and incompetent'. The second discourse depicts 'a view of patients as competent, rational and resourceful, and engaged in continuous processes of meaning creation'. Clearly, it is this second attitude that must underlie our efforts at improving information provision for breast cancer patients.

'Information science' is now a discipline in its own right. Guidance and criteria for health professionals writing for the public or patients are available.[11–14,98,99] Aside from content and language, aspects such as design and layout, navigability, accessibility, suitability and 'tone' are addressed. One of the tenets of good information provision is that patients shall have been involved in its production. A specific tool to encourage easier and better production of patient information leaflets would constitute a big step towards producing trial leaflets that will enable prospective participants to engage in 'meaning creation'.[97]

Information about fulfilment of trial aims

It is very important to convey to potential trial participants that interpretation of trial findings ultimately depends on faithful fulfilment of the trial aims, including attainment of recruitment targets in a reasonable timespan. If a trial is stopped prematurely, inadequate recruitment may compromise the ability to draw satisfactory conclusions from the data, including data on longer-term adverse effects. Early disclosure of data when a trial is discontinued can also prejudice satisfactory completion of similar trials. Editorial comments in the New England Journal of Medicine (NEJM),[100,101] following public release of findings from the first interim analysis of a randomised trial of letrozole therapy in postmenopausal women with breast cancer who had completed 5 years of tamoxifen therapy, are pertinent to the issue of early disclosure. The independent data and safety monitoring committee had recommended termination of the trial and prompt communication of the results to the participants.[102] The model consent form included the statement:

'If new side effects or information about my disease or treatment are discovered during the study, I will be told.'

As the NEJM editorial pointed out, one of the consequences of that decision to unblind is that critical information will be lost so that the primary aim of the study will not be fully achieved. This, and similar instances, should lead us to consider very thoroughly the precise management and implementation of early-stopping rules, and the need for care in wording consent forms. Precipitous decisions made by the data monitoring committee, with no patient input, on the basis of specifics in the protocol, and statements made in the consent form, require challenging. The ethical dimensions are considerable. Moreover, such decisions ignore factors that are known causes for fluctuation of early 'events'; they ultimately fail future potential beneficiaries.

Is this what participants would have wanted had they been fully aware of the implications of signing up to that condition? Given that one of the main motivations that patients have for joining clinical trials is altruism,[60] it is possible that many patients will be disappointed that the trial they participated in has not been allowed to run its full course. In effect, the contract they signed up to has been breached – this is unethical. More reliable data that would have been produced if full recruitment had been achieved will no longer be forthcoming. Because patients on placebo were given the option of active therapy after premature stoppage, we shall never know the true effect on overall survival, or be able to provide patients with an accurate harm–benefit analysis. Inclusion of trained, experienced advocates on the trial steering committee, and on the data monitoring and ethics committee (DMEC) might have contributed to a more balanced consideration of interim data.[103] Decisions to stop a trial prematurely should involve all stakeholders, including users.

It can be useful to set up a trial patient advisory group, comprising trained advocates, at the outset of a trial.[104] Such advocates are able to take a more concerned but detached view of 'participation' and extend their horizons away from self-interested concerns. They would recognise the extended responsibility of trialists and participants to fulfil the trial contract, if at all possible, for the sake of future patient beneficiaries. Study designs, including stopping rules, should favour collection of data about long-term benefits and harms, and should make this aim explicit in the patient information leaflets.

But, as I indicated earlier, perhaps too much emphasis has been placed on achieving complete understanding within the consent-seeking dialogue, and too little on general activity to overhaul the process and ensure that only high-quality research that is relevant to patients' needs is undertaken.[5] Constant critical appraisal of the whole gamut of research activity is occurring. This concerns and involves not just clinical teams, but also dedicated organisations, sponsors, funders, charities, government departments, independent volunteer lay groups, pharmaceutical companies, reviewers, medical editors and publishers.

Prevention trials

Many of the issues that I have already discussed are vividly highlighted in the case of prevention trials, which raise especially important and complex questions. Breast cancer drugs, tested first in advanced disease, then in early breast cancer, are finding their way ever more rapidly into 'prevention' trials that invite participants who sometimes have high-risk borderline pathologies.[105] The draft protocol of a prevention trial can be on the drawing board and nearing finalisation long before any preliminary data from trials evaluating the 'new' treatments in early breast cancer patients are available or published. In turn, trials of adjuvant treatment, such as in the ATAC trial, can start recruiting before the publication of trials from advanced settings.[106] One might question whether such haste is acceptable in terms of safety, particularly as prevention trials involve healthy women, and not patients. Trials of this kind need very large numbers of participants to have sufficient 'events' in as short a time as possible in order to draw reliable conclusions quickly. Comparison of the 'standard' therapy with a newer agent in a prevention trial presents a very different set of trade-offs for healthy (even if high-risk) women than they do for participants in metastatic, advanced disease trials.[107] Even greater care should be taken to make sure that these healthy volunteers are aware that unpleasant side-effects (perhaps only slowly emerging from data in trials of women with invasive breast cancer as quality-of-life data are analysed) may only become apparent later. These data are usually not available until after the main scientific and clinical results of a trial have been published and can give rise to concern about unexpected self-reported side-effects not 'on-protocol'. A woman with invasive disease might be prepared to accept these side-effects in return for likely clinical gain, but in the preventive situation it is particularly important that healthy participants should be made aware of this uncertainty, as the majority will never suffer breast cancer.

These issues appear to have been neglected in the latest breast cancer prevention trial, IBIS II,[108] launched in October 2003 amid much razzamatazz about the latest wonder drug for breast cancer, anastrozole (Arimidex®).[109] This trial is seeking 6000 healthy but high-risk participants, and 4000 participants with DCIS. Clearly, the important issues regarding consent to be screened for DCIS that I described earlier in this chapter are extremely pertinent here. Ethical problems arise if women are to be recruited to a trial of DCIS prevention based on their consent to a screening programme that does not inform them of a DCIS outcome. Women who refuse information, and who are later detected with an abnormality that makes them an eligible candidate for the IBIS II prevention trial, may, with hindsight, regret not having considered the pros and cons of screening at the time of invitation. The IBIS II lead investigator evaded these issues in June 2003 by telling me that clinicians will have already informed the potential DCIS participants about DCIS,[110] or, more recently when responding to concerns that I had raised in The Lancet,[107] that they 'would suggest the BACUP website as a source'.[111] However, it is also acknowledged that 'more information about DCIS should be made available to women involved in screening'.[112] Actions would speak louder than words.[113] It could be argued that recruitment to the DCIS arm of this trial is dependent on the screening programme for recruitment, where potential participants have not been properly informed or consented: a curious symbiotic arrangement.

Ethical governance: research ethics committees (RECs)

It is evident that many of the issues that I have been discussing need to be addressed within a rigorous framework for ethical governance. However, there is extensive support for Iain Chalmers' statement[114] that 'research ethics committees (RECs) could serve the interests of the public more efficiently'. He refers to two particular principles: (i) proposals for new research should be informed by scientifically defensible systematic reviews; (ii) the study will be published in full within a reasonable time. Ethics committees have ethical obligations with regard to the public that they serve: currently, their standards are justifiably subjected to frequent comment and criticism that urgently requires remedial attention. There is understandable concern that they have failed to measure up to the high standards of efficiency and effectiveness required in today's pressurised and complicated research climate.

The governance of medical research ethics committees was reviewed in 2001 in order to provide revised governance arrangements to address the changing role of ethics committees in regulating research applications.[115] The Central Office for Research Ethics Committees (COREC) invited comment in June 2001 on a draft document covering the proposed governance arrangements for NHS RECs. This consultation process[116] provided a democratic opportunity to propose adjustments for consideration. The Research Governance Framework[117] had indicated this need for a review of local research ethics committees (LRECs) and multicentre research ethics committees (MRECs). The consultation document was offered as providing 'a framework for the process of review of the ethics of all proposals for research in the NHS which is efficient, effective and timely, and which will command public confidence'. Regrettably, the objective that the review would command public confidence seems not to have been met. Some of the new NHS governance arrangements will go some way towards ensuring that the full results of approved studies are available for public scrutiny These include, for example, that every research ethics committee should keep a register of all proposals that it reviews and that it should request a final report, to be delivered within 3 months. But there are still many shortcomings in the workings of ethics committees that need to be considered and rectified if the public is to be convinced of the adequacy, transparency and openness of their working arrangements. This is necessary if they are to demonstrate proper fulfilment of the implicit contract between research participants and researchers, in order that the public may see for themselves that they have contributed to the growth of publicly accessible knowledge.

Ethical approval needed for the multiplicity of large and small projects before RECs, some at the cutting edge of science and clinical endeavour, demands skills and expertise that many members of RECs do not have, or cannot be expected to have. The sheer volume of proposals that come before these well-meaning, public-spirited volunteers is daunting. How can they be expected to adequately assess numerous projects, by meeting once monthly, for a few hours outside a normal working day? Various strategies to change systems and processes have resulted in some improvements, but fall short of an ideal and professional system. Furthermore, aside from other inadequacies, unacceptable delays can result from this method of vetting research projects. Do all patient information leaflets, which are so essential for the successful implementation of informed consent and ultimately for the production of reliable trial data, receive the proper scrutiny and assessment against protocol that they should have?

Moreover, a comparison of requirements of RECs in 11 European countries for a non-invasive intervention study showed that there were striking variations in their requirements for approval, with those for the UK being most onerous.[118] This finding will add to the existing body of evidence about variations in the working of RECs. Does this mean that some are too careful or that some are too lax? It identified the risk that inappropriate requirements leading to unnecessary delays and extra costs will not be compensated for by increased protection for participants. A further area of concern is disintegration of research protocols whereby UK partners may be unwelcome in international studies. Further costs include researchers' time, delays, photocopying time and 'paper' costs for documentation demanded. The UK compared unfavourably with other European countries surveyed, and had the most stringent requirements combined with the least flexibility.

Commentators remind us that ethics review is an 'intervention' in the system of healthcare with cost consequences, where the trade-off of benefits and harms must be considered.[119] Surely, the main outcome measure is how this affects the patients' best interests. If unnecessary and/or inappropriate demands are being made that impede or prevent the conduct of research studies to the detriment of patient choice and care then, in order to progress in testing treatments, ethics committee processes and systems should be challenged on ethical, economic and practical grounds, as are other interventions. Excessively onerous requirements imposed by RECs across the board, without distinction between different types of study, result in inhibition of trialists' efforts to the extent that they may not even begin the process. The boundaries between research, audit and practice are becoming less and less clear. The conclusion of Glaziou and Chalmers[119] is that a more concerted effort should now be made to assess the benefits, harms and costs of different approaches to ethics review for different types of evaluation. Commanding public confidence demands a far more acute appreciation by those producing governance frameworks, of public and professional perception of their current suitability and adequacy to be the gatekeepers of research.[120,121]

Guidelines

There is a demonstrable need for flexibility and sensitivity on the part of health professionals in their dealings with patients. It is crucially important that communication and healthcare interventions be tailored to each patient's individual requirements. However, the advent of guidelines for managing breast cancer threatens professionals' ability to deliver on this. History shows us that advances are made not by a regulated grey majority, but rather by the courageous contribution of colourful characters, (from both profession and patients), who speak out and buck the trend.[3] Rose Kushner, Betty Westgate and Vicky Clement Jones were three informed and courageous breast cancer activists of the 20th century who did more for millions of breast cancer patients than a shelf-full of guidelines could ever achieve! In their passion for information and reform, these women were not prepared to be passive recipients of current thinking. Rose Kushner's book, published in 1975,[122] was a rallying call to women 'to have a finger in their own destiny'. Betty Westgate's experience led her to set up in 1972 an information, education and support group that is still active and valuable today as Breast Cancer Care[123] (with branches in London, Scotland and Wales). Following her own experience of cancer, Vicky Clement Jones founded CancerBACUP in 1985, and this now provides a service for almost 50 000 people each year.[111]

The negotiation and content of transactions between a health professional and a patient is now subject to conflicting demands and impositions in the context of delivery within a multidisciplinary team. Antagonisms and differences influence the establishment of various regulatory mechanisms and shape health policies that govern the way medicine is practised. Guidelines, policies and exhortation for changes of culture come from very different parts of the health service that show little evidence of communication, between each other.[124]

How can a patient hope to receive truly 'patient-centred' care, or give informed consent that is founded on information tailored to her specific needs, or engage in meaningful 'shared decision-making'[88] if a consultant is obliged to work to guidelines? How are 'patient preferences' to be accommodated if guidelines are strictly adhered to? If they are accommodated, what is the position of the clinician who has negotiated a treatment plan that does not conform to the guidelines?

Let us consider, for example, those patients where the likelihood of axillary node metastases is quite small. In a Royal Marsden Hospital review of 355 cases, women aged over 55, with breast cancers up to 10 mm in size, with oestrogen receptor-positive and lymphovascular invasion-negative lesions, had an incidence of lymph node metastases of only 2% for grade 1 tumours, and 11% for grade 2 tumours.

In over 90% of cases, only one positive node was found. If the incidence of nodal metastases is between 2% and 11%, then between 5000 and 500 patients will need to receive axillary surgery, and between 98 and 99 patients will need to receive adjuvant chemotherapy, for every 1 or 2 patients who receive a benefit from chemotherapy (see Chapter 37).[125] Is it not imperative to inform patients of this very slim likelihood of benefit before arriving at a decision with them? To do this *and* strictly adhere to guidelines is impossible – a basic incompatibility unless guidelines are used only as a general indication, rather than being enforced.

The British Association of Surgical Oncologists (BASO) guidelines require that 'histopathological node status should be obtained in all invasive tumours to ensure that all necessary data are obtained for making decisions on adjuvant radiotherapy or systemic therapy'. However, the Quality Assurance Guidelines for Surgeons in NHS Breast Cancer Screening state that nodal status should be obtained in over 90% of patients. Not only do these statements conflict, but the former allows no room for consideration of the consequences of undertaking removal of the statutory 10 lymph nodes, in terms of costs both to the patient (physical and psychological) and to the health service (financial). The same criticism applies to blanket statements about the value of chemotherapy to all node-positive patients. Not only will the degree of benefit afforded by adjuvant systemic therapy vary greatly from patient to patient, but the perception of the patient concerning the worth of adjuvant therapy will also vary widely. Some patients will demand that 'everything possible' be done, even though the chance of benefit may be small; others will prefer to decline axillary clearance to avoid possible morbidity and decline an adjuvant treatment to avoid toxicity or short- and long-term side-effects of the treatment. This may be done with or without the patient understanding the degree of benefit. This leaves the doctor with a difficult dilemma.

It is interesting to speculate that breast cancer specialists may be challenged for non-compliance with guidelines. Yet, at the same time, the move away from 'compliance' to 'concordance' with respect to patients' behaviours in medicine-taking is being given increased scrutiny and resources for research. The NHS Service Delivery and Organisation R&D Programme (NHS SDO R&D) is conducting a programme of research on patient- and carer-centred services on Concordance, Adherence and Compliance in Medicine Taking.[126] The lead editorial in the BMJ of 11 October 2003[127] stated: 'Concordance means shared decision making and arriving at an agreement that respects the wishes and beliefs of the patient. What it should not be is a more gift-wrapped version of compliance'. The editorial concluded by stating: 'The biggest challenge for concordance and the most difficult to research will be a change in values'. It is ironic that the move seems to be in the opposite direction from 'concordance' when it comes to controlling health professionals' behaviour through imposition of guidelines.

The production of guidelines involves much discussion amongst many well-intentioned people, with much redrafting and modification. This consumes a huge amount of time and energy – and endless reams of paper. When finally published and ready for the consultant's shelf, it is evident that there is often not complete agreement with similar guidelines produced equally carefully by other experts on the same subject. We have all witnessed, or been involved in, closing 'round table' sessions at prestigious and influential international breast cancer meetings such as St Gallen,[128] where there is difficulty in arriving at a suitable form of wording that will satisfy those present. Cultural differences and antagonisms will be evident, for example with regard to the aggressiveness of treatments that are deemed acceptable, desirable, beneficial or necessary in different countries by different cultures.[129] One must also question what biases are introduced into such guidelines by being decided only by the conscientious delegates who remain to the end of a long conference on a Saturday morning? How representative are they of the breast cancer fraternity? Who, in fact, should decide guidelines, and what disciplines should be involved? Surely it should be required that health economists and statisticians be asked to undertake a cost–benefit analysis of the implementation of specific guidelines to determine their value in terms of mortality and number of relapses, financial cost to providers, and personal costs in terms of morbidity to the patients.

Equity and global considerations

I started this chapter by arguing that research is necessary to find new and better treatments for breast cancer. However, the outcomes of research need to be considered too. Business economics demands that return on outlay is as rapid as possible. Drugs such as tamoxifen currently have an extensive actual and potential market in the prevention and treatment of breast cancer and its price is relatively low in its out-of-licence phase. By contrast, targeted drugs such as trastuzumab (Herceptin; licensed in the UK in 2001, and approved by the National Institute for Clinical Excellence (NICE) in 2002) will only be suitable for a relatively small percentage of patients, thereby limiting demand and dictating price structures.

Market take-up will also vary, depending upon political choice in the use and availability of financial resources and the health systems of individual countries.[130]

Important ethical and social issues arise in relation to equity, concerning the affordability of expensive new drugs. The costs are not easy to calculate – for example, approximately 1000 women will need to be screened to determine the 200 (approximately 20%) who might benefit from trastuzumab. Those who are not going to benefit from the drug therefore incur costs too. Financial cost–benefit analyses are difficult to undertake with any degree of accuracy due to the wide variety of health settings. They must be costed in relation to the national economy of the particular country in which they operate, and even locally within that country. There are other variable factors that affect the calculations and that must be taken into account, such are the huge variations between prescribing in well- or underdeveloped countries, or between systems of private, public or mixed healthcare provision. This difficulty was made very clear in a presentation and discussion comparing costs between anastrozole and tamoxifen in a UK setting,[131] from which it was evident that it is not just a simple matter of comparing drug costs at a particular moment in time.

The advent of pharmacogenetics raises further issues. Full and equitable access to treatment will be increasingly difficult to achieve as increasing numbers of expensive patient-adapted therapies for pathological subclasses become identified and available.[132] Only some individuals will be suitable for these targeted treatments, and only a proportion of those targeted will benefit. Greater openness and debate, not just among health professionals, but also with the wider public, would help explore the legitimacy of these approaches. Both the ethics and economics of blanket prescribing are intertwined and difficult to define or assess. Is it right to knowingly prescribe an inexpensive drug that will be of little or no benefit to the majority,[133,134] in the knowledge that, for some patients, alternative targeted therapies are available? This choice is further complicated by the fact that they are expensive and cannot be infallibly targeted.

These issues are well illustrated in the case of trastuzumab. The sting in the tail of a patient finding that she is eligible for this drug is to find consequently that she has a worse prognosis. Moreover, eligibility is determined by a test that is only 80% accurate. This demands the very highest degree of communication skills for clinicians and research nurses. There is great potential for harm to patients' psychological well-being. Incorrect categorisation will inevitably bring disappointment to some individuals. Risk assessment and weighing harms against benefits will be particularly difficult for both patients and health professionals in these difficult decision-making situations.[135]

Many more of these types of drugs are in the scientific and pharmaceutical pipelines. The balance could be further disturbed by pharmaceutical companies locating themselves where they will be able to obtain greatest return for their efforts. 'Outsourcing' is becoming more prevalent generally. The price of progress will be high. Citizens would do well to consider these checks and balances. The developing and concerned research partnerships in the developed world must work to ensure that benefits are available worldwide to all who have cancer. Participants in underdeveloped countries should equally be assured of the best available standard therapy in the control arms of trials, and be accorded equal care and respect in gaining consent as their more fortunate co-sufferers in well-developed countries. Those more fortunate members of society must shoulder responsibility for this.

Conclusions

The momentum of development and interest in the practical and ethical aspects of informed consent, and the involvement of active patient advocates, has significantly accelerated in the last decade compared with the previous 50 years. Nonetheless, 'informed consent' still remains a limitation to progress, particularly in traumatic conditions such as early breast cancer: obstacles to its satisfactory attainment are manifold and complex. It is now time to centre on trust-based partnerships that will serve to remove barriers and impediments that stand in the way of realising the potential for improved care and hope for cure. Altruistic intent must not be thwarted by the demands of a minority of aggressive patients, bureaucratic protectionism or powerful commercial pressures. Overzealous ethicists are so often overconcerned to protect 'vulnerable' patients rather than encourage proper lay contribution through equal partnerships. There is a danger that such overprotection will slow and prevent progress to the detriment of huge numbers of sufferers. We should heed the warning in the MRC-led Impact assessment:[136] 'The EU Clinical Trials Directive aims to protect trial participants and to simplify and harmonise trials across Europe, but could unnecessarily delay or stop publicly funded clinical trials.'

However, it is also important that 'patient involvement' does not unwittingly become just another tiresome hoop for trialists and commercial organisations to jump through. Even worse, it should not become a way of 'kite-marking' for research that does not genuinely have 'patient-centred' objectives. The more complicated and difficult trials become to understand, the more difficult it will be for citizens to resist relentless commercialism and medicalisation of healthy individuals. Use of consumers' advisory panels, facilitated focus group work, independently facilitated research project planning, and other interactive methodologies employing skilled qualitative researchers and facilitators could all contribute to partnerships with potential for mutual education and improvement. In turn, this would produce protocols of high scientific quality with patient-centred objectives. The James Lind Alliance, a coalition of organisations representing patients and clinicians collaborating to confront important uncertainties about the effects of treatments, offers a constructive way forward.[137]

Acknowledgements

I am indebted to Dr Mary Dixon-Woods of the Department of Health Sciences, University of Leicester for her incisive and sensitive review of this chapter. Her reorganisation of the material, improving the structure and narrative flow, was invaluable. I thank the Royal College of Physicians of Edinburgh for permission to reproduce short extracts from my paper 'The informed patient', which was published in the Journal of the Royal College of Physicians of Edinburgh in May 2004, volume 34, pp. 75–6.

References

1. Thornton H, Edwards E, Baum M. Women need better information about routine mammography. BMJ 2003; 327: 101–3.

2. Marshall T, Adab P. Informed consent for breast screening: What should we tell women? J MedScreen 2003; 10: 22–6.

3. Lerner BH. The Breast Cancer Wars. Fear Hope and the Pursuit of a Cure in Twentieth Century America. New York: Oxford University Press, 2003.

4. Thornton H. The patient's role in research'. Paper presented at The Lancet 'Challenge of Breast Cancer' Conference, Brugge, April 1994. In: Health Committee Third Report. Breast Cancer Services. London: HMSO, 1995: 112–14.

5. Chalmers I. The James Lind Initiative. J R Soc Med 2003; 96: 575–6.

6. Chamot E, Perneger TV. Misconceptions about efficacy of mammography screening: a public health dilemma. J Epidemiol Community Health 2001; 55: 799–803.

7. Domenighetti G, D'Avanzo B, Egger M et al. Women's perception of the benefits of mammography screening:

population-based survey in four countries. Int J Epidemiol 2003; 32: 816–21.

8. Olsen O, Goetszche P. Cochrane Review on screening for breast cancer with mammography. Lancet 2001; 358: 1284–5.

9. General Medical Council. Seeking Patients' Consent: The Ethical Considerations. November 1998. http://www.gmc-uk.org/standards/consent.htm

10. NHS Cancer Screening Programme. Breast Screening – The Facts. http://cancerscreening.org.uk/breastscreen/publication/nhsbsp-the-facts.pdf.

11. Last M. High Quality Matters, Winter 2000, Issue 8. The BMA Patient Information Award. (http://www.library.bma.org.uk/html/patinfox.html#app1)

12. Charnock D. The DISCERN Handbook: Quality Criteria for Consumer Health Information on Treatment Choices (User Guide and Training Resource). Oxford: Radcliffe Medical Press, 1998.

13. Duman M, Farrell C. The Practicalities of Producing Patient Information: The POPPI Guide. London: BMJ Books, 2000.

14. Duman M. Promoting Patient Choice – Some Do's For Producing Quality Evidence Based Patient Choice Information. London: King's Fund, 1998.

15. Welch HG. Should I Be Tested for Cancer? Maybe Not and Here's Why. Berkeley: University of California Press, 2004.

16. Rakovitch E, Franssen E, Kims J et al. A comparison of risk perception and psychological morbidity in women with ductal carcinoma in situ and early breast cancer. Breast Cancer Res Treat 2003; 77: 285–93.

17. Davey C, White V, Ward JE. Insurance repercussions of mammographic screening: What do women think? Med Sci Monitor 2003; 8: LE 44–5.

18. Thornton H. Pairing accountability with responsibility: the consequences of screening 'promotion'. Med Sci Monitor 2001; 7: 531–3.

19. Patnick J. Screens for survival. Chem Ind 2003; 19: 17.

20. Patnick J. Women's needs inform contents of screening literature. BMJ 2003; 327: 868–9.

21. Marshall TP. Framing is important in presenting risk information. BMJ 2003; 327: 868.

22. Gigerenzer, G. Reckoning with Risk: Learning to Live with Uncertainty. London: Penguin, 2002.

23. Burne J. More than you need to know?. The Guardian Weekend, 15 November 2003: 51–3, 75–7.

24. O'Connor AM, Stacey D, Rovner D et al. Decision aids for people facing health treatment or screening decisions. Cochrane Database Syst Rev 2004; (4) CDOO1431.

25. Thornton H, Edwards A, Baum M. Authors' reply: Women need better information on routine mammography. BMJ 2003; 327: 869.

26. Chalmers I. Well-informed uncertainties about the effects of treatments: How should clinicians and patients respond? BMJ 2004; 328: 475–6.

27. Mann H, Djulbegovic B. Biases due to differences in the treatments selected for comparison (comparator bias).

James Lind Library (www.jameslindlibrary.org) (accessed 30 January 2004).

28. Hill AB. Medical ethics and controlled trials. BMJ 1963; i: 1043–9.

29. Djulbegovic B. Acknowledgment about uncertainty: a fundamental means to ensure scientific and ethical validity in research. Curr Oncol Rep 2001; 3: 389–95.

30. Peto R, Baigent C. Trials: the next 50 years. BMJ 1998; 317: 1170–1.

31. Freedman B. Equipoise and the ethics of clinical research. N Engl J Med 1987; 317: 141–5.

32. Edwards SJL, Lilford RJ, Braunholtz DA et al. Ethical issues in the design and conduct of randomized controlled trials. Health Technol Assess 1998; 2: 1–130.

33. Mann H. Thrombolysis for acute ischaemic stroke: trial participants need to be informed of the uncertainty principle. BMJ 2002; 325: 1363.

34. Lilford RJ. Equipoise is not synonymous with uncertainty. BMJ 2001; 323: 574.

35. Lilford RJ, Jackson J. Equipoise and the ethics of randomisation. J R Soc Med 1995; 88: 552–9.

36. Cahn E. Drug experimentation and the public conscience. In: Talalay P, ed. Drugs in our Society. Baltimore: The John Hopkins Press, 1964: 258–61.

37. Sharma R. WHO calls for closer monitoring of commercial interests. BMJ 2002; 324: 6.

38. Harrison T. Getting the Right Medicines. Putting Public Interests at the Heart of Health-Related Research. London: The King's Fund, 2003.

39. Editorial: Just how tainted has medicine become? Lancet 2002; 359: 1167.

40. Sleath B, Rucker DT. Consumer participation in health policy decisions: empowerment or puffery? J Health Care for the Poor and Undeserved. 2001; 12: 35–49.

41. Baum M. Clinical trials – a brave new partnership: a response to Mrs. Thornton. J Med Ethics 1994; 20: 23–5.

42. Consumers' Advisory Group for Clinical Trials (CAG-CT). The British Oncological Association (BOA) Newsletter 1999: 2(1).

43. Consumer's Advisory Group for Clinical Trials: its genesis. NCCA Newsletter (National Centre for Clinical Audit) 1998; Issue 8.

44. Stevens T, Wilde D, Hunt J, Ahmedzai S. Overcoming the challenges to consumer involvement in cancer research. Health Expectations 2003; 6: 81–8.

45. Thornton HM. Breast cancer trials: the patient's viewpoint. Lancet 1992; 339: 44–5.

46. Chalmers I, Rounding C, Lock K. Descriptive survey of non-commercial randomised controlled trials in the United Kingdom 1980–2002. BMJ 2003; 327: 1017–19.

47. Tallon T, Chard J, Dieppe P. Relation between agendas of the research community and the research consumer. Lancet 2000; 355: 2037–40.

48. Grant-Pearce C, Miles I, Hills P. Mismatches in priorities for health research between professionals and consumers. In: Involvement Works. London: NHS Executive, 1999.

49. Thornton H. Why do we need clinical trials? BACUP News 1997; 30: 7.

50. CancerBACUP. Understanding Cancer Research Trials (Clinical Trials). CancerBACUP, 2003. http://www.cancerbacup.org.uk/Trials/Search

51. Thornton H, Dixon-Woods M. Recruitment of women into trials. Lancet 2002; 359: 164–5.

52. Hanley B, Truesdale A, King A et al. Involving consumers in designing, conducting, and interpreting randomised controlled trials: questionnaire survey. BMJ 2001; 322: 519–23.

53. McIver S. Independent Evaluation of Citizens' Juries in Health Authority Settings. London: The King's Fund, 1998.

54. Fellowes D, Fallowfield L, Saunders CM, Houghton J. Tolerability of hormone therapies for breast cancer: how informative are documented symptom profiles in medical notes for 'well-tolerated' treatments? Breast Cancer Res Treat 2001; 66: 73–81.

55. Vass A. Breast cancer drug 'surpasses' tamoxifen. BMJ 2001; 323: 1387.

56. Batten M. A Special Report: Breastlink talks with Dr. Michael Baum. Breastlink 2001; 2.

57. de Takats P, Harrison J. Clinical trials in stroke. Lancet 1999; 353: 150.

58. www.controlled-trials.com.

59. www.cochraneconsumer.com.

60. www.dipex.org.

61. Jenkins V, Fallowfield L. Reasons for accepting or declining to participate in randomised clinical trials for cancer therapy. Br J Cancer 2000; 82: 1783–8.

62. Larkin M. Clinical trials: What price progress? Lancet 1999; 354: 1534.

63. Edwards A, Elwyn G, Atwell C et al. Consumers' views of quality: identifying the consultation outcomes of importance to consumers, and their relevance to 'shared decision-making' approaches. Health Expectations 2001; 4: 151–61.

64. Fallowfield L. Participation of patients in decision about treatment for cancer. BMJ 2001; 323: 114.

65. Mazur DJ. Information disclosure and beyond? How do patients understand and use the information they report they want? Med Decis Making 2000; 20: 132–3.

66. Cox K. Enhancing cancer clinical trial management: recommendations from a qualitative study of trial participants' experiences. Psycho-oncology 2000; 9: 314–22.

67. Editorial: The globalisation of the NHS. Lancet 2002; 359: 1447–8.

68. Hockhauser M. Risk communication: consent delayed is consent denied. http://bmj.bmjjournals.com/cgi/eletters/327/7417/731#38336 (accessed 23 October 2003).

69. Goodare H. Studies that do not have informed consent from participants should not be published. In: Doyal L, Tobias JS, eds. Informed Consent in Medical Research. London: BMJ Books, 2001: 131–3.

70. Brewin T. 'Blanket' consent to trials would be a good idea. In: Len Doyal L, Tobias JS, eds. Informed Consent in Medical Research. London: BMJ Books, 2001: 118.

71. Brewin TB. Consent to randomised treatment. Lancet 1982; ii: 919–22.

72. Tobias JS. BMJ's present policy (sometimes approving research in which patients have not given fully informed consent) is wholly correct. BMJ 1997; 314: 1111–14.

73. Thomas R, Thornton H, Mackay J. Patient information materials in oncology: are they needed and do they work? Clin Oncol 1999; 11: 225–31.

74. Bell S, Brada M, Coombes C, National Cancer Alliance. Patient-Centred Services? What Patients Say. Oxford: National Cancer Alliance, 1996.

75. Audit Commission. What Seems to be the Matter: Communication Between Hospitals and Patients. London: HMSO, 1993.

76. Meredith C, Symonds P, Webster L et al. Information needs of cancer patients in the West of Scotland: cross-sectional survey of patients' views. BMJ 1996; 313: 724–6.

77. Seymour J. Doctors frightened to speak out against trust, says report. BMJ 2001; 323: 650.

78. Protocol of the UK Randomised Trial for the Management of Screen-detected Ductal Carcinoma in Situ (DCIS) of the Breast. UKCCCR, December 1989.

79. Donovan J, Mills N, Brindle L et al. Improving the design and conduct of randomised trials by embedding them in qualitative research: the ProtecT study. BMJ 2002, 325: 766–7.

80. Tobias J, Souhami R. Fully informed consent can be needlessly cruel. BMJ 1993; 307: 119–20.

81. Baum, M. The ethics of randomised controlled trials. Eur J Surg Oncol 1995; 21: 136–7.

82. Edwards A, Elwyn G, Hood K et al. The development of COMRADE – a patient-based outcome measure to evaluate the effectiveness of risk communication and treatment decision making in consultation. Patient Education and Counselling 2003; 50: 311–22.

83. Koops L, Lindley R. Thrombolysis for acute ischaemic stroke: consumer involvement in design of new randomised controlled trials. BMJ 2002; 325: 415–17.

84. Fallowfield L, Jenkins V, Farewell V et al. Efficacy of a Cancer Research UK communication skills training model for oncologists: a randomised controlled trial. Lancet 2002; 359: 650–6.

85. Atwell C, Pill R, Edwards A, Elwyn G. A qualitative analysis of patient accounts of routine consultations with specially trained practitioners. In: Report to 'Health in Partnership' Programme, UK Department of Health. Cardiff: Department of General Practice, University of Wales College of Medicine, 2002 (http://www.healthinpartnership.org/studies/edwards.html).

86. Dixon-Woods M, Agarwal S, Young B et al. Integrative approaches to qualitative and quantitative evidence. Report for NHS Health Development Agency, 2004 (www.had.nhs.uk).

87. Baum M. Philosophy and theology in relation to the understanding and teaching of medical ethics. Surgery 2002; 20: 1–2.

88. Edwards A, Elwyn G, Atwell C et al. Shared decision making and risk communication in general practice – a study incorporating systematic literature reviews, psychometric evaluation of outcome measures, and

quantitative, qualitative and health economic analysis of a cluster randomised trial of professional skill development. In: Report to 'Health in Partnership' programme, UK Department of Health. Cardiff: Department of General Practice, University of Wales College of Medicine, 2002 (http://www.healthinpartnership.org/studies/edwards.html).

89. Kurtz S, Silverman J, Draper J. Teaching and Learning Communication Skills in Medicine. Oxford: Radcliffe Medical Press, 1998.

90. Silverman J, Kurtz S, Draper J. Skills for Communicating with Patients. Oxford: Radcliffe Medical Press, 1998.

91. Kurtz S, Silverman J. Benson J, Draper J. Marrying content and process in clinical method teaching. Enhancing the Calgary–Cambridge Guides. Acad Med 2003; 78: 802–9.

92. General Medical Council. Tomorrow's Doctors: Recommendations on Undergraduate Medical Education. London: General Medical Council, 2002.

93. Wass V, Richards T, Cantillon P. Monitoring the medical education revolution. The impact of new training programmes must be evaluated. BMJ 2003; 327: 1362.

94. Lees N, Dixon-Woods M, Young B et al. CaTLET: Evaluation of information leaflets for patients entering cancer trials. Psycho-Oncology 2001; 10: 266.

95. Jorgensen KT, Goetzsche PG. Presentation on websites of possible benefits and harms from screening for breast cancer: cross sectional survey. BMJ 2004; 328: 148.

96. Duley L, Farrell B, eds. Clinical Trials: Into the New Millennium. London: BMJ Books, 2001: 123.

97. Dixon-Woods M. Writing wrongs. An analysis of published discourses about the use of patient information leaflet. Social Sci Med 2001; 52: 1417–32.

98. Wager E, Tooley PJH, Emanuel BM, Wood SF. Get patients' consent to enter clinical trials. BMJ 1995; 311: 734–7.

99. DISCERN: An Instrument for Judging the Quality of Written Consumer Health Information on Treatment Choices. Oxford: Radcliffe Medical Press, 1997.

100. Bryant J, Wolmark N. Letrozole after tamoxifen for breast cancer – What is the price of success? N Engl J Med 2003; 349: 1855–7.

101. Burstein HJ. Beyond tamoxifen – extending endocrine treatment for early-stage breast cancer. N Engl J Med 2003; 349: 1857–9.

102. Goss PE, Ingle JN, Martino S et al. A randomised trial of letrozole in postmenopausal women after five years of tamoxifen therapy for early-stage breast cancer. N Engl J Med 2003; 340: 1793–802.

103. Protocol for INIS (International Neonatal Immunotherapy Study). Non-specific intravenous immunoglobulin therapy for suspected or proven neonatal sepsis: an international, placebo controlled, multicentre randomised trial. May 2003. ISRCTN 94984750: 17.

104. Dickersin K, Braun L, Mead M et al. Development and Implementation of a science training course for breast cancer activists: Project LEAD (Leadership, Education and Advocacy Development). Health Expectations 2001; 4: 213–20.

105. Thornton H. Anastrozole as a preventive agent in breast cancer. Lancet 2003; 361: 1911–12.

106. Baum M. Current status of aromatase inhibitors in the management of breast cancer and critique of the NCIC MA-17 trial. Cancer Control 2004; 11: 217–21.

107. Thornton, H. Questions about anastrozole for early breast cancer. Lancet 2002; 360: 1890.

108. IBIS Investigators. IBIS-II: an international multicentre study of anastrozole vs placebo in postmenopausal women at increased risk of breast cancer, and of anastrozole vs tamoxifen in postmenopausal women with ER+ve ductal carcinoma in situ (DCIS). Current National Trials. National Cancer Research Institute, 2002.

109. Laurance J. Hailed as the biggest advance in decades, can this drug prevent 70% of breast cancers? Independent, 1 October 2003: 3.

110. Cuzick J. Personal communication. 2003.

111. Renamed 'CancerBACUP' 5 January 1998; see www.cancerbacup.org.uk.

112. Cuzick J, O'Neill C, Howell A, Forbes J. Anastrozole for ductal carcinoma in situ. Lancet 2003; 362: 832.

113. Lock S. Britain prefers talk to action. Which is why it has failed to tackle research misconduct. BMJ 2003; 327: 940–1.

114. Chalmers I. Lessons for research ethics committees. Lancet 2002; 359: 174.

115. Department of Health. Governance arrangements for NHS Research Ethics Committees. July 2001 (www.doh.gov.uk/research/rd1/researchgovernance/corec.htm#ethics).

116. http://www.corec.org.uk/wordDocs/fred.doc.

117. Research Governance Framework (www.nhsetrent.gov.uk/trentrd/resgov/main.htm).

118. Hearnshaw H. Comparison of requirements of research ethics committees in 11 European countries for a non-invasive interventional study. BMJ 2004; 328: 140–1.

119. Glasziou P, Chalmers I. Ethics review roulette: what can we learn? That ethics review has costs and one size does not fit all. BMJ 2004; 328: 121–2.

120. Refractor: Guardianship. Lancet 2001; 357: 1808.

121. Benson J. Guardianship in research. Lancet 2001; 358: 1013.

122. Kushner R. Breast Cancer: A Personal and Investigative Report. New York: Harcourt Brace Jovanovitch, 1975.

123. http://breastcancercare.org.uk.

124. Department of Health. The NHS Plan. London: DoH, 2000 (http://www.nhs.uk/nationalplan/summary/htm) (accessed 26 November 2003).

125. Querci della Rovere G, Benson JR. The case for axillary dissection. Adv Breast Cancer 2004; 1: 3–8.

126. http://www.sdo.lshtm.ac.uk/concordance.htm.

127. Jones G. Prescribing and taking medicines. Concordance is a fine theory but is mostly not being practised. BMJ 2003; 327: 819.

128. Goldhirsch A, Glick JH, Gelber RD et al. Meeting

Highlights: International Consensus Panel on the Treatment of Primary Breast Cancer. J Clin Oncol 2001; 19: 1817–27.

129. Payer L. Medicine and Culture: Notions of Health and Sickness in Britain, the U.S., France and Western Germany. London: Victor Gollancz, 1989.

130. Sen A. Economics and Health. Lancet 2000; 354 (Suppl): siv20.

131. Simons R, Bassi R, Jones D, Barrett-Lee P. Cost analysis of treatment-related adverse events with anastrozole (Arimidex) versus tamoxifen in postmenopausal women with hormone receptor-positive (HR+) advanced breast cancer (ABC): a UK perspective. Paper and discussion, 3rd European Breast Cancer Conference, Barcelona, 19–23 March 2002. EJC Abstract Book 2002; 37 (Suppl 3): S132.

132. Ahr A, Karn T, Solbach C et al. Identification of high risk breast-cancer patients by gene expression profiling. Lancet 2002; 359: 131–2.

133. Smith R. Editor's Choice: The drugs don't work. BMJ 2003; 327.

134. Dyer O. City reacts negatively as GlaxoSmithKline announces plans for new drugs. BMJ 2003; 327: 1366.

135. Communicating risks: illusion or truth? BMJ 2003; 327.

136. http://www.mrc.ac.uk/index/current-research/current-clinical_research/funding.

137. http://www.jameslindlibrary.org/jla.html (accessed 8th September 2004).

Index